Medical Radiology

Diagnostic Imaging

Series Editors

Hans-Ulrich Kauczor
Paul M. Parizel
Wilfred C. G. Peh

For further volumes:
http://www.springer.com/series/4354

Emilio Quaia

Editor

Imaging of the Liver and Intra-hepatic Biliary Tract

Volume 2: Tumoral Pathologies

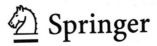 Springer

Editor
Emilio Quaia
Radiology Unit
Department of Medicine - DIMED
University of Padova
Padova
Italy

ISSN 0942-5373   ISSN 2197-4187   (electronic)
Medical Radiology
ISBN 978-3-030-39023-5   ISBN 978-3-030-39021-1   (eBook)
https://doi.org/10.1007/978-3-030-39021-1

This Springer imprint is published by the registered company Springer Nature Switzerland AG
The registered company address is: Gewerbestrasse 11, 6330 Cham, Switzerland

Contents

Part I

Hepatic Tumoral Pathology: Normal Liver

Hepatic Hemangioma, Focal Nodular Hyperplasia, and Hepatocellular Adenoma

Luigi Grazioli, Barbara Frittoli, Roberta Ambrosini, Martina Bertuletti, and Francesca Castagnoli

Contents

Abstract

Benign focal liver lesions can originate from all kind of liver cells: hepatocytes, mesenchymal and cholangiocellular line. Their features at imaging may sometimes pose difficulties in differential diagnosis with malignant primary and secondary lesions. In particular, the use of MDCT and MRI with extracellular and hepatobiliary Contrast Agents may help in correct interpretation and definition of hepatocellular or mesenchymal and inflammatory nature, allowing to choose the best treatment option. The peculiarities of main benign liver lesions at US, CT and MRI are described, with special attention to differential diagnosis and diagnostic clue.

The identification and imaging characterization of benign liver lesions is fundamental for differential diagnosis with malignant primary and secondary lesions. Likewise, differentiating between various benign lesions is of paramount importance because of their distinct management, which can range from no therapeutic treatment, to follow-up or biopsy for definitive confirmation, to surgical resection.

L. Grazioli (✉)
Department of Radiology, ASST-Spedali Civili di Brescia, Brescia, Italy

B. Frittoli · R. Ambrosini
Radiology Service, Imaging Diagnostic Department, ASST-Spedali Civili di Brescia, Brescia, Italy

M. Bertuletti · F. Castagnoli
University of Brescia, ASST "Spedali Civili" University Hospital, Brescia, Italy

© Springer Nature Switzerland AG 2021
E. Quaia (ed.), *Imaging of the Liver and Intra-hepatic Biliary Tract*,
Medical Radiology Diagnostic Imaging, https://doi.org/10.1007/978-3-030-39021-1_1

Incidental focal liver lesions are for the most part benign, even in oncological patients. The most common benign focal liver lesions are hemangiomas which originate from the mesenchymal cellular line, followed by focal nodular hyperplasia (FNH) and hepatocellular adenoma (HCA), both originating from the hepatocellular line.

We can identify and characterize these lesions by using various imaging techniques: US scan can identify liver lesions, but the use of contrast agents is in most cases necessary for correct characterization, whether during US (CEUS), CE-MDCT, or MRI with extracellular or hepatobiliary contrast agents.

The peculiarities of the most common benign liver lesions at US, CT, and MRI are described with particular attention given to differential diagnosis and diagnostic clues. Recent guidelines about post-diagnostic management are also shown below.

1 Hepatocellular Origin

1.1 Hepatocellular Adenoma

Hepatocellular adenoma (HCA) is a rare benign liver lesion with an incidence of 1 case for 1,000,000 people: the incidence increases to 1–3 cases for 100,000 in females who use or have used oral contraceptives (OCPs) for long term (Cogley and Miller 2014). Although the precise pathogenic mechanism leading to hepatic adenomas is still unknown, the use of oral contraceptive and anabolic steroids and some congenital diseases such as glycogen storage diseases and metabolic syndrome are considered risk factors for development and progression of HCA. Men with metabolic syndrome are at a much higher risk (10 times more likely than females) for malignant degeneration of liver adenomas, although this is rare (<5%). Other risk factors for degeneration are androgen use, large tumors (>5 cm), and histological subtype (β-catenin-mutated) (Lee et al. 2014; Neri et al. 2016). More than ten adenomas widespread into liver parenchyma configure "liver adenomatosis."

HCA can be classified at least into four immunohistological subtypes (Lee et al. 2014; Kaltenbach et al. 2016; Katabathina et al. 2011):

1. *Inflammatory type (I-HCA) with serum amyloid A overexpression*: they represent 45–55% of adenomas, initially described as telangiectatic FNH, characterized by inflammatory infiltrates and frequent sinusoidal dilatation, peliotic areas, dystrophic vessels, and ductular dilatations.

2. *Hepatocyte nuclear factor 1α-mutated type (H-HCA)*: they represent 25–45% of adenomas and are characterized by predominant intralesional fat component due to activation of lipogenesis.

3. *β-catenin mutated type with upregulation of glutamine synthetase (β-HCA)*: they represent approximately 5–10% of adenomas, they are considered borderline lesions between HCA and HCC, and they occur more frequently in men and are associated with male hormone administration, glycogen storage disease, and familial adenomatous polyposis.

4. *Unclassified type*: this subtype encompasses HCAs without any genetic abnormalities (<5–10% of cases) (Dhingra and Fiel 2014; Margolskee et al. 2016; Wang et al. 2016).

Small HCAs (<5 cm) are generally asymptomatic; large lesions (6–30 cm) can determine right upper discomfort or pain due to liver capsule strain; acute and dangerous outset is possible if a large peripheral or exophytic HCA breaks and bleeds into abdominal cavity (Lee et al. 2014); other risk factors for rupture and bleeding are lack of capsule, pregnancy, and left lateral lobe location.

Spontaneous hemorrhage is more likely to occur in I-HCA and β-HCA, due to their weak or even absent connective support stroma.

The accurate characterization of HCAs and possibly their subtype is essential because of their different therapeutic options: liver biopsy is the gold standard, but it represents an invasive procedure not devoid of risks such as pain, bleeding, infection, and possible accidental correlated injuries.

Imaging techniques (US, CT, MR) can rightly define different HCAs in a high percentage of cases because they show different characteristics at "basal" acquisitions and different patterns of enhancement after contrast media administration, thus reflecting their histological subtype.

I-HCA is the most common type of HCA: it appears as well-delineated, often hyperechoic, and heterogeneous nodules on ultrasound. Doppler signals are commonly seen and may mimic central arteries (Cogley and Miller 2014; Gangahdar et al. 2014). On unenhanced CT, HCAs may appear hypo-heterogeneously attenuating with spontaneously hyperattenuating areas related to recent intralesional bleeding (Katabathina et al. 2011; Gangahdar et al. 2014). At real-time CEUS (contrast-enhanced US), they show rapid centripetal filling in the arterial phase and persistent peripheral rim enhancement with central washout during portal and late phases. On CECT, their characteristic pattern is the strong arterial enhancement and a persistent enhancement in delayed phases (Kaltenbach et al. 2016; Katabathina et al. 2011; Gangahdar et al. 2014).

On MR, I-HCAs show discrete hyperintense signal on T2-weighted images and iso- to hyperintense signal on T1-weighted sequences with and without fat suppression. Some lesions may contain a small amount of fat, visible as a signal dropout in opposed-phase T1-weighted sequences (Kaltenbach et al. 2016; Katabathina et al. 2011; Darai et al. 2015). Hyperintensity on T1 images can be seen if glycogen component, or less commonly hemorrhage, is present (Kaltenbach et al. 2016; Katabathina et al. 2011; Darai et al. 2015). Most I-HCAs show diffusion restriction on diffusion-weighted imaging (DWI) (Grazioli et al. 2013). After Gd chelate administration, the pattern of enhancement is similar to CECT, with arterial enhancement which persists on delayed phases; it seems that the persistent enhancement on delayed phases is less frequently observed after ethoxybenzyl diethylenetriamine pentaacetic acid (EOB-DTPA), due to its rapid intake from hepatocytes (pseudo-washout). After hepatocyte liver-specific agent administration, such as EOB-DTPA or gadobenate dimeglumine (Gd-BOPTA), I-HCA may show generally poor uptake in the hepatobiliary phase, and in the majority of cases, it appears hypointense. In about 20–25% of cases, peripheral hyperintensity (atoll sign) reflects the abnormal

ductal reaction with altered biliary excretion in the peripheral portion of the lesion (Kaltenbach et al. 2016; Katabathina et al. 2011; Hartleb and Gutkowski 2011). This particular condition may also determine a hyperintense lesion rim on T2w sequences.

Marked T2 hyperintensity associated with persistent delayed enhancement has a sensitivity of 85–88% and a specificity of 87–100% for the diagnosis of inflammatory HCA (Jharap et al. 2015). In a small percentage of cases, inflammatory HCAs may appear isointense on T2w and T1w images with discrete enhancement in the arterial phase and a quite rapid washout (Lee et al. 2014; Kaltenbach et al. 2016; Katabathina et al. 2011; Darai et al. 2015) (Fig. 1).

H-HCAs is the second most frequent type of HCA: on ultrasound examination, they typically appear as very homogeneous hyperechoic lesions because of marked and diffuse fat within the lesions; rare and poor flow signal can be detected at color Doppler examination (Kaltenbach et al. 2016).

On non-enhanced CT, H-HCAs are generally hypoattenuating in relation to the percentage of fat content.

MR plays a decisive role in characterizing H-HCA, demonstrating the presence of intralesional fat unequivocally: it shows, in fact, homogeneous and intense signal dropout on in- and opposed-phase T1-weighted sequences (Katabathina et al. 2011; Gangahdar et al. 2014). On T2w images, H-HCAs generally appear iso- or hypointense without significant restriction on DWI (Grazioli et al. 2013).

At real-time CEUS and on CECT and CE-MRI, the presence of abundant intralesional fat influences the degree of enhancement of H-HCAs. It shows a variable grade of contrast enhancement during the arterial phase (in most cases not very intense) and rapid washout during portal and late dynamic phases. On MR hepatobiliary phase images, after administration of Gd chelates with hepatocyte affinity, they appear homogeneously hypointense in almost 100% of cases (Gangahdar et al. 2014; Grazioli et al. 2013) (Figs. 2 and 3).

β-catenin-mutated type adenoma (β-HCA) and *unclassified HCAs* are rarer, and they have

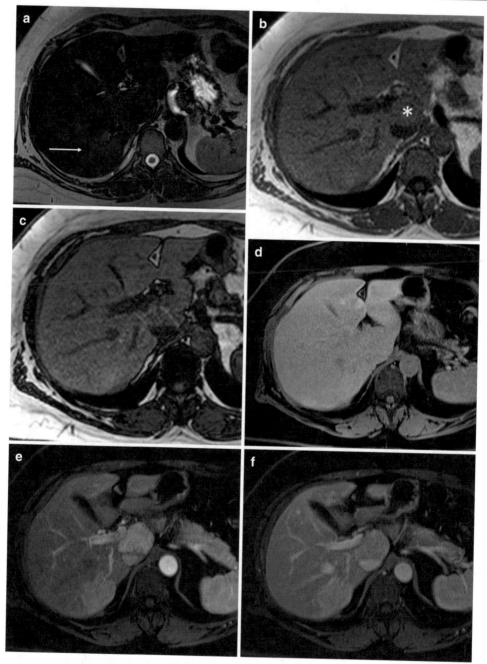

Fig. 1 41 years old, female, chronic slight pain in right hypochondrium. A large nodule in segment VII is homogeneously hyperintense on T2w images (arrow in **a**) and appears iso-slightly hyperintense in T1w in/opposed (opp) phase (**b**, **c**) and in T1w with fat saturation (FS) acquisition (**d**). During dynamic acquisition after injection of Gd-BOPTA, the mass shows intense enhancement in arterial phase (**e**), without washout in portal and delayed phases (**f**, **g**). After 10′ (* in **h**), the lesion is isointense to the surrounding parenchyma. After 2 h (HBP), it appears markedly hypointense with thin hyperintense peripheral rim named "atoll sign" (arrow in **i**): inflammatory hepatic adenoma at biopsy. In caudate lobe, another lesion is isointense on T1w (*) and T2w images (**a–d**); it shows intense and homogeneous enhancement in arterial phase (**e**) and becomes isointense during the next phases of dynamic study (**f**, **g**), till 5 min (**h**); the lesion appears hyperintense on HBP (**i**): typical FNH without central scar

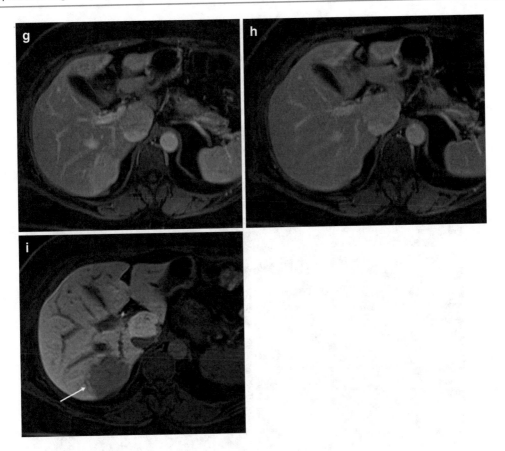

Fig. 1 (continued)

less specific characteristics on imaging, more similar to HCC pattern. They can appear hypoechoic on ultrasound examination and spontaneously iso- to hypoattenuating on unenhanced CT (Katabathina et al. 2011; Gangahdar et al. 2014). At CEUS and CECT, they show arterial enhancement and portal or delayed washout (Vijay et al. 2015; Wang et al. 2016). They may have heterogeneous content. On MR imaging, β-catenin-mutated HCA appears as a nodule with homogeneous or heterogeneous hyperintense signal intensity on T1- and T2-weighted images, depending on the presence of hemorrhage and/or necrosis. After Gd chelate contrast media administration, they commonly appear as homogeneous or, more often, heterogeneous hypervascular masses with persistent or non-persistent enhancement during the delayed dynamic phase images. Hypointensity at the hepatobiliary phase is the prevalent pattern (90–92%) (Lee et al. 2014; Kaltenbach et al. 2016; Katabathina et al. 2011; Darai et al. 2015). Malignant transformation simulates HCC on imaging (Figs. 4 and 5).

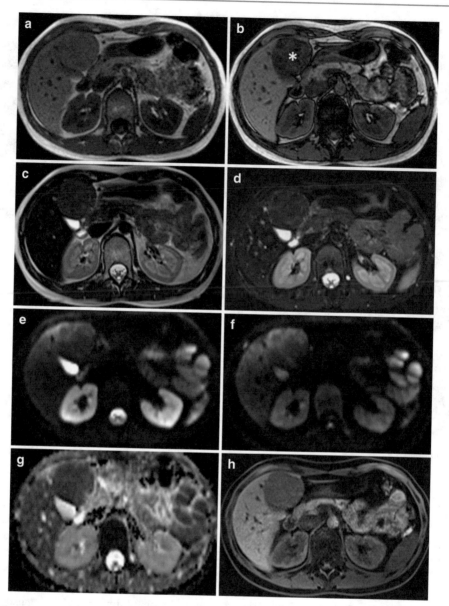

Fig. 2 32 years old, female, asymptomatic; previous Ewing sarcoma. A large nodule in segment V appears isointense on T1 in-phase acquisition (**a**) and shows intense signal dropout on T1 opp-phase acquisition (* in **b**); it's slightly hyperintense on T2w images (**c**), and it shows signal dropout on T2w images with fat saturation (**d**) because of intralesional fat. No signs of restriction of the signal at DWI study (b0–b1000, ADC map: **e–g**). The lesion appears hypointense on T1w with fat satura- tion (FS) (**h**) and shows heterogeneous slight enhance- ment after injection of gadoxetate disodium during arterial phase (**i**). The nodule has rapid washout and appears hypointense in portal and delayed phases (**j, k**). On hepa- tobiliary phase (HPB), 15 min after contrast medium injection (**l**), the lesion is markedly hypointense: hepato- cyte nuclear factor 1α-mutated adenoma ("steatotic" ade- noma) at biopsy

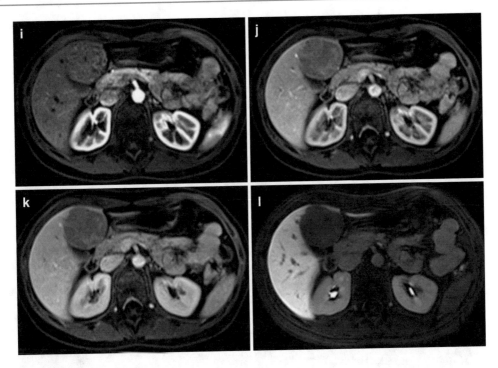

Fig. 2 (continued)

Other lesions in the same clinical setting, such as FNH (especially in the presence of atypical findings like the absence of central scar, fat infiltration, or regressive changes within the nodule), can mimic HCAs, but iso- or slightly hyperintensity on T1w and T2w sequences, lack of washout in the dynamic evaluation, and hyperintensity on hepatobiliary phase are peculiar for FNH (Kaltenbach et al. 2016). Furthermore, in rare cases, I-HCAs and β-catenin HCAs may mimic FNH, showing iso-hyperintensity in the hepatobiliary phase (Fig. 6). This could happen, using contrast media with hepatocyte affinity, when there is an overexpression of the organic anionic transport protein (OATP1B1 and OATP1B3), which mediates the uptake of gadoxetic acid or Gd-BOPTA into the hepatocyte. Clinical information, such as obesity, alcohol consumption, and use of oral contraceptives, may help to distinguish them in these cases correctly, but a biopsy is mandatory for the definitive diagnosis (Agarwal et al. 2014).

Another situation that may determine the difficulty in terms of differential diagnosis is the presence of fat and abundant vascular structures within the lesion (PEComas) (Fig. 7).

Given that the introduction of liver-specific contrast agents has improved diagnostic accuracy for benign hepatocellular lesion, according to the recently published EASL clinical practice guidelines, there is not a preferred MRI contrast agent, nor are there data indicating diagnostic superiority of one agent over another. However, some studies suggest that Gd-EOB-DTPA is more accurate than Gd-BOPTA when it comes to differentiating between HCAs and FNHs, especially if the lesion is intrinsically hyperintense on precontrast T1-weighted images, due to glycogen content or hemorrhage within the lesion (Vanhooymissen et al. 2019).

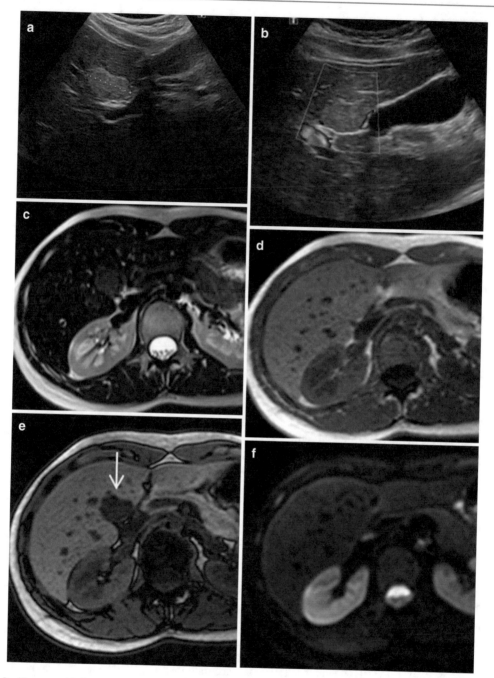

Fig. 3 45 years old, female, asymptomatic; incidental finding on US examination. Large hyperechoic mass at US (**a**), not significantly vascularized at color Doppler evaluation (**b**). At MR examination, the lesion in S4b is slightly hyperintense on T2w images (**c**); it appears isointense on T1 in-phase acquisition (**d**) and shows intense signal drop on T1 opp-phase acquisition (arrow in **e**) because of intralesional steatosis. No signs of restriction of the signal at DWI study with b values 50 (**f**) and 800 (**g**) and ADC map (**h**). The lesion appears hypointense on T1w with fat saturation (**j**) and shows mild enhancement after injection of gadoxetate disodium during arterial phase (**l**). The nodule has rapid washout and appears hypointense in portal and delayed phases (**k**, **l**). On HPB, 15 min after contrast medium injection (**m**), the lesion is markedly hypointense. The nodule shows 18FDG avidity at PET-CT (**n**). Hepatocyte nuclear factor 1α-mutated adenoma ("steatotic" adenoma) at biopsy

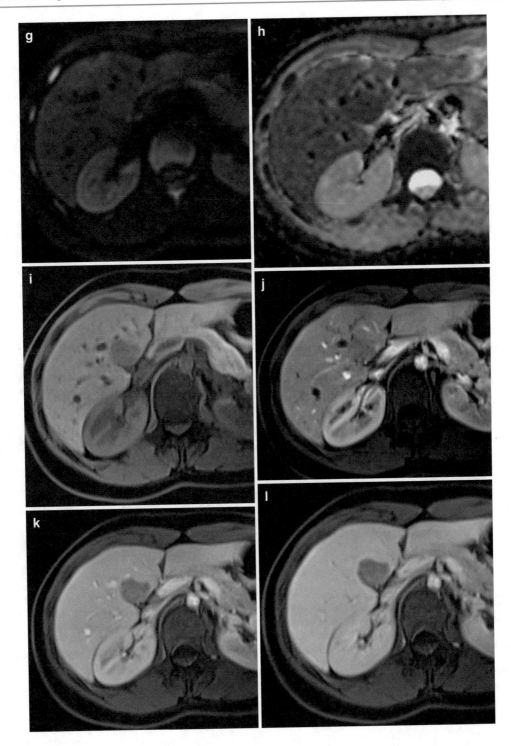

Fig. 3 (continued)

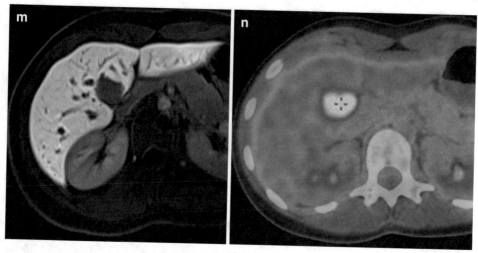

Fig. 3 (continued)

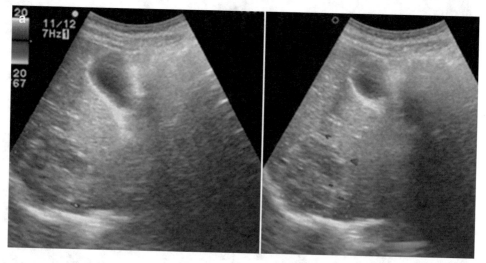

Fig. 4 38 years old, male, acute pain in right hypochondrium. On US examination (**a**), a large heterogeneous lesion in VIIIs, without evident intralesional vascularization at color Doppler evaluation, suspected for atypical cavernous hemangioma. At MR examination, on T2w images (**b**), it appears almost homogeneously isointense in the right posterior part (*) and hyperintense, with some hypointense irregular components in its left anterior part (arrow). The central portion of the lesion appears hyperintense in unenhanced T1w images (**c**), as for intraparenchymal bleeding. After Gd-BOPTA injection, the lesion shows intense enhancement in its central portion during arterial phase (**d**) with rapid washout in the next dynamic acquisitions, while the left anterior part remains hypointense (**e–g**). At MRI evaluation after pre-surgical embolization, the lesion shows cystic degeneration (arrow in **h**) on T2w images and heterogeneous hyperintense signal on T1w (**i**): β-catenin-mutated adenomas with foci of HCC at histologic examination after surgery

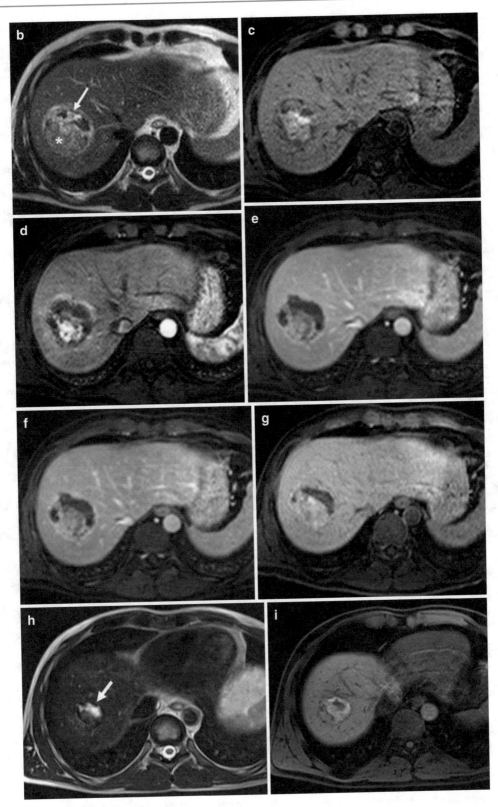

Fig. 4 (continued)

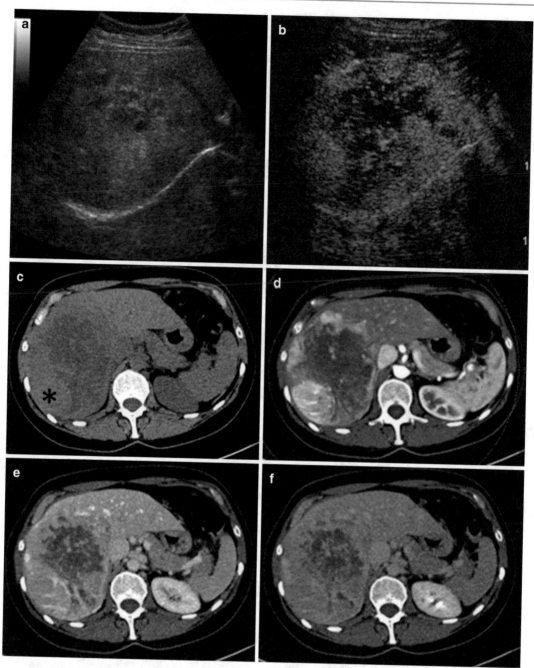

Fig. 5 54 years old, female, acute pain in right hypochondrium. On US examination (**a**), huge heterogeneous mass in right hepatic lobe that shows intense enhancement with central hypovascular area at CEUS (**b**) is found. At unenhanced CT (**c**), the lesion appears hypointense with iso-/slightly hyper-posterior area (*). During arterial phase of CECT (**d**), it shows heterogeneous peripheral enhancement, stronger and more homogeneous in the posterior area; on portal venous phase (PVP) (**e**) and delayed phases (**f**), the solid posterior area doesn't show significant washout, and the central zone presents slow pooling. At MR examination, two different components are confirmed: on T2w images (**g**), it appears not homogeneously hyperintense in the central portion and iso/slightly hyper in its posterior part (*). Any lipid component is evident on T1 in-/opp-phase acquisitions (**h**, **i**). No evident signs of restriction of the signal at DWI study (**j**, **k**) and ADC map (**l**). The mass is iso-/hypointense on T1w image with fat saturation (**m**). After gadoxetic acid, the lesion shows intense enhancement in its solid component during arterial phase with rapid washout in the next dynamic acquisitions (**n**–**p**). On HPB (**q**), the lesion is hypointense with some pooling in the central necrotic area; multiple other hypointense nodules are evident (arrows in **q**) in the left lobe: β-catenin-mutated adenomas with foci of HCC at biopsy

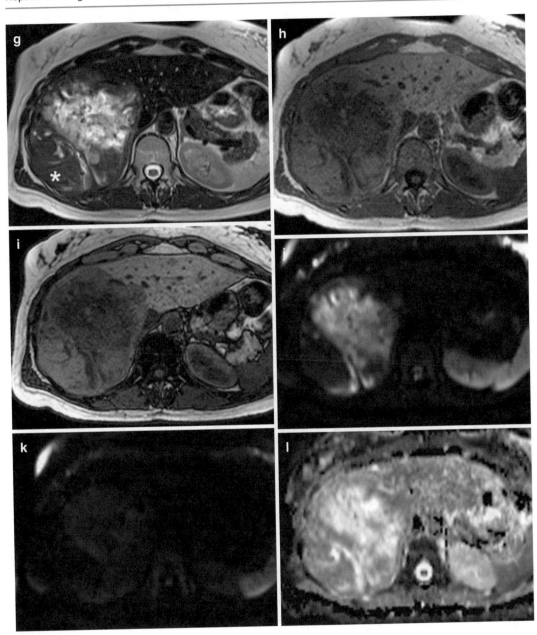

Fig. 5 (continued)

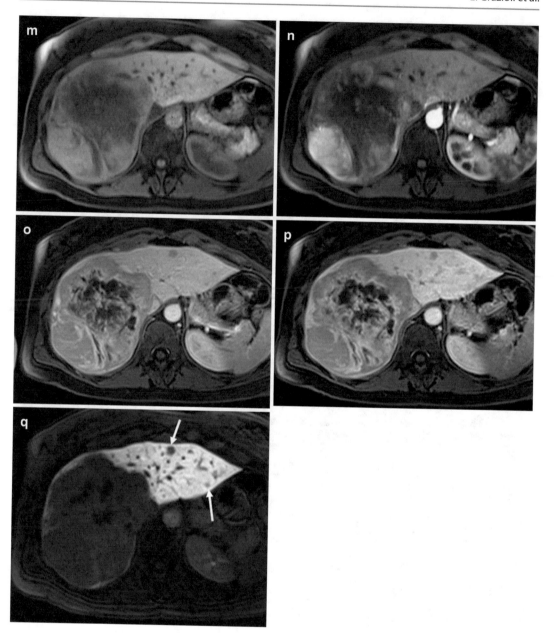

Fig. 5 (continued)

HCC in non-cirrhotic liver and fibrolamellar HCC, because they affect the same population (young patients, with no history of hepatopatic diseases), may mimic HCAs: they show heterogeneously hyperintense signal on T2-weighted images and hypointense on T1-weighted sequences; they may show intense and heterogeneous enhancement during the arterial phase of dynamic study, subsequent washout, and hypointensity at hepatobiliary phase. A fat intralesional component can be present in HCC. Since the precise risk of malignant transformation is little known (5–9%) and the differential diagnosis between a very well-differentiated HCC and borderline HCA (subtypes inflammatory and β-catenin) with the current pathological criteria is

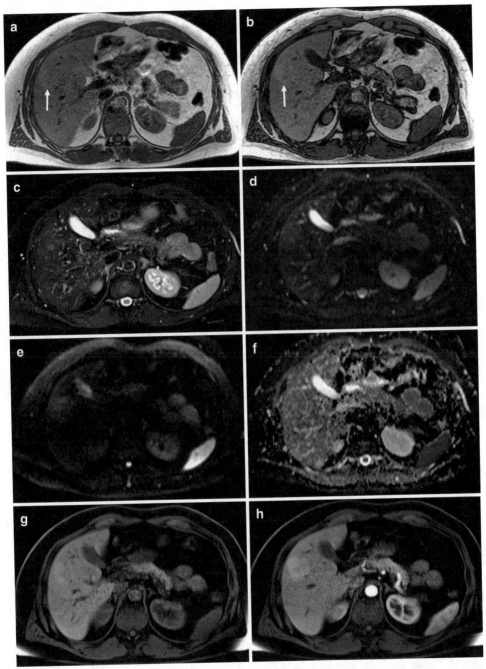

Fig. 6 44 years old, male, incidental finding. An iso-/slightly hyperintense lesion can be seen on T1 in-/opp-phase acquisition (arrows in **a**, **b**) and appears isointense on T2w FS imaging (**c**); the nodule doesn't show restriction at DWI acquisition (b0–b800, ADC map, **d**–**f**). On T1w image with fat saturation before Gd-EOB i.v. injection (**g**), the nodule is slightly iso-/hyperintense. During arterial phase (**h**), it shows discrete homogeneous enhancement, without any washout during portal venous (**i**); during transitional phase, the lesion is iso-/slightly hyperintense (**j**). On HBP after 20′ (**k**), the lesion is isointense with tiny hypointense eccentric scar (arrow in coronal view); not typical FNH was suspected at MRI; at histology (**l**): I-HCA—the iso-/hyperintense signal on HBP was the manifestation of OATP1 B3 overexpression

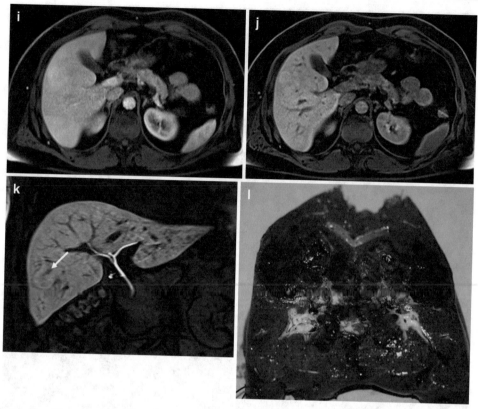

Fig. 6 (continued)

indeed challenging (Cogley and Miller 2014; Lee et al. 2014; Katabathina et al. 2011; Darai et al. 2015), these cases should be characterized with immunohistochemistry (E-cadherin and metalloproteinases; Tretiakova et al. 2009).

American and European guidelines slightly differ from one another when it comes to HCA management: according to the former, the decision tree is based first and foremost on the size of the lesion, whereas the latter provides for a different treatment based first on patient sex and lifestyle changes.

However, both approaches state that withdrawal from exogenous hormone therapy consumption should be mandatory for all adenoma patients (surgical and nonsurgical candidates).

Management options for HCA include surgery for all adenomas >5 cm, adenomas with dysplastic foci, and β-catenin-activated HCA, increasing size or imaging features of malignant transformation and increase in alpha-fetoprotein (AFP), male sex, and presence of glycogen storage diseases (GSD).

Adenomas that are <5 cm and present in anatomically challenging locations and those that undergo regression on steroid withdrawal can be managed conservatively with follow-up imaging (CT/MRI) at 6- to 12-month intervals for the first 2 years. Following this, annual imaging may be modulated based on lesion stability and growth patterns (EASL Clinical Practice Guidelines on the management of benign liver tumours 2016; Vijay et al. 2015) (Fig. 8).

Pregnancy is no longer considered a contraindication in HCA <5 cm; in these cases, it is recommended conservative management, with

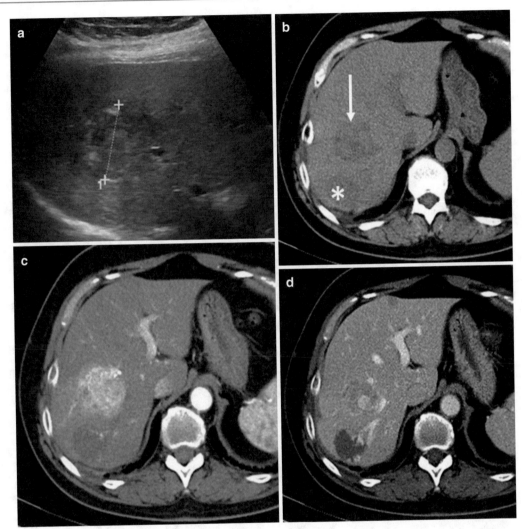

Fig. 7 A 53-year-old female patient, with multiple sclerosis and overactive bladder. At US, incidental finding of a heterogeneously hypoechoic lesion with hyperechoic spots in VIIIS (a). At CT the lesion in segment VIII (white arrow) is iso-/slightly hypoattenuating at baseline (b), with intense but heterogeneous arterial enhancement (c), followed by progressive washout during portal and late phase (d, e), and therefore was deemed as a possible inflammatory HA. In segment VII, another lesion (* in b) shows globular enhancement during dynamic acquisition (c–e), typical for cavernous hemangioma. At MRI the lesion in segment VIII appears hypointense on T1w in-/opp-phase images (f, g), without detectable fat content; it's heterogeneously hyperintense on T2w (h) and doesn't show diffusion restriction at DWI (b0–b800) (i) or on ADC map (j). At the dynamic study (k–n) after gadoxetic acid injection, the lesion shows early and homogeneous arterial enhancement (l), with progressive washout during portal venous and transitional phases (m, n), without contrast uptake at hepatobiliary phase T1w images (o), and was categorized as possible inflammatory HA. At histopathologic examination, the lesion was proven to be an epithelioid angiomyolipoma/PEComa

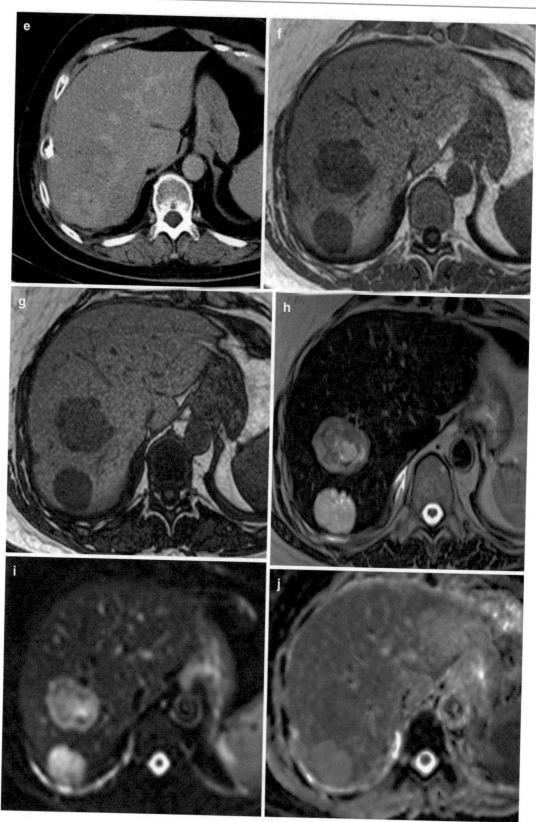

Fig. 7 (continued)

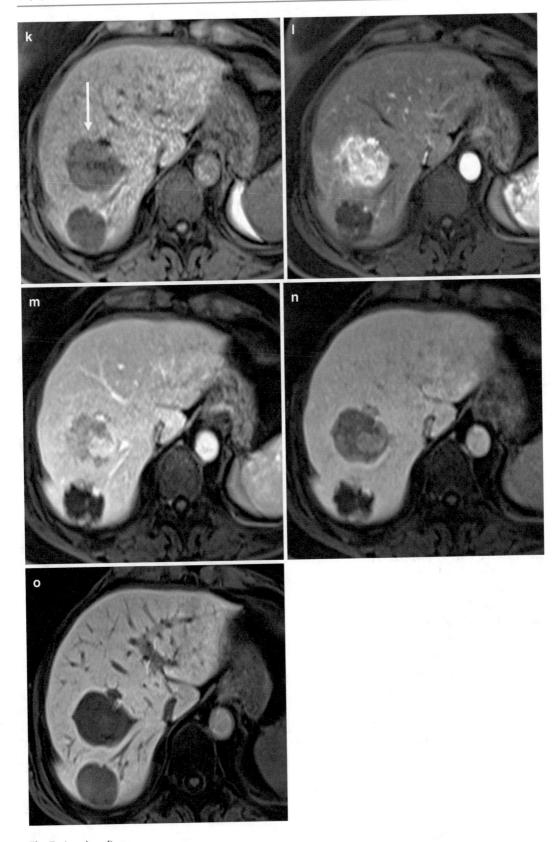

Fig. 7 (continued)

Fig. 8 Flowchart for the management of FNH (from EASL guidelines 2016). Imaging modalities may include US, CEUS, and CE-MRI. For large (>3 cm), MRI sensitivity is very good. Different imaging modalities can be complementary, and for lesions <3 cm, where sensitivity and certainty may be less, a second imaging modalities, such as CEUS, is advised. If doubt remains after two imaging modalities, the patients should be referred to a specialist center, where percutaneous or resection biopsy may be considered

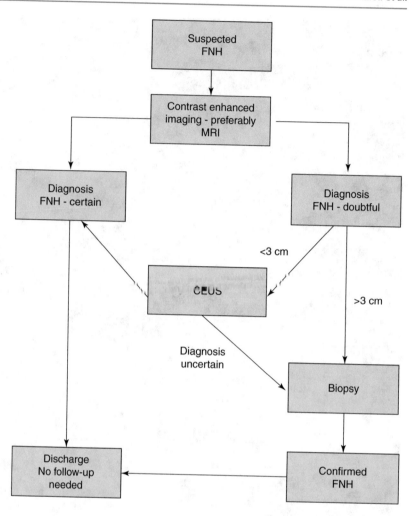

ultrasound monitoring every 6 weeks. Given that the increased level of endogenous hormones during pregnancy has been postulated toward the increase in size of adenomas and that hyperdynamic circulation combined with increased liver vascularity may further increase the risk of adenoma rupture during the third trimester, HCA > 5 cm or those who experienced adenoma-related complications in previous pregnancies should undergo resection prior to pregnancy. If an HCA is detected incidentally during pregnancy, an individualized approach is to be taken into consideration (radiofrequency ablation [RFA], transarterial embolisation [TAE], or surgical resection).

The diagnosis at imaging of HCAs can be challenging, as both benign and malignant lesions may simulate them; furthermore, if H-HCAs and I-HCAs are often typical and relatively easy to characterize on MR, the same is not valid for B-catenin HCAs and unclassified HCAs.

The differential diagnosis can depend on clinical/epidemiological features and imaging findings (especially signal intensity and enhancement patterns at MR) (Kaltenbach et al. 2016).

2 Focal Nodular Hyperplasia (FNH)

Focal nodular hyperplasia (FNH) is the second most common benign hepatic tumor (8–9% of all primary hepatic tumors). Its origin is probably due to the presence of a vascular abnormality that under hormonal stimulation determines a hyperplastic response with ensuing disorganized growth of hepatocytes and bile ducts representing a hamartomatous malformation.

In a normal liver, the artery within the portal tract supplies the peribiliary vascular plexus, the portal vein wall, and the portal tract interstitium. FNH results from portal tract injury, leading to arterioportal or hepatic venous shunts, arterialized sinusoids with hepatocellular hyperplasia, and, often, cholestasis. Portal tract remodeling leads to ductular reaction and portal-periportal fibrosis. Arterial hyperperfusion (and resultant hyperoxemia) leads to increased expression of vascular endothelial and somatic growth factors and activation of hepatic stellate cells, which are thought to be responsible for the formation of the characteristic central scar (Roncalli et al. 2016). FNH is more frequent in females (8:1) and in the third–fifth decades, in most cases with a history of oral contraceptive consumption (Cogley and Miller 2014; Neri et al. 2016). Frequently FNH nodules are incidental findings, generally asymptomatic, or can determine vague abdominal pain (10–15%) if very large (>5 cm) or pedunculated. FNH typically presents as a single lesion in 70% of patients and with two to four lesions in the remaining 30%. In 10–20% of cases, it is associated with the presence of one or more hemangiomas (Cogley and Miller 2014; Katabathina et al. 2011; Jharap et al. 2015).

Histologically it appears as a homogeneous mass formed by aggregation of nodules of organized connective tissue and liver parenchyma, with well-definite margins and fibrous septa; rarely it may contain fat, triglycerides, and glycogen. Lesions more than 5 cm frequently show a central scar which consists of fibrous connective tissue, inflammatory cell infiltration, cholangiocellular proliferation, and malformed vessels (arteries, capillaries, and veins) (Katabathina et al. 2011).

At US, FNH is usually lobulated isoechoic or slightly hypoechoic (especially in the steatotic liver); hypoechoic halo can be observed. In 20% of the cases, a central, slightly hyperechoic scar can be visualized. At color Doppler examination, a central feeding artery with a stellate or spoke-wheel appearance can be identified (Cogley and Miller 2014).

On unenhanced CT, FNH is seen generally as a solitary lesion with central focal low attenuation scar (30%) surrounded by well-defined homogeneously iso-/slightly hypoattenuating tissue. Calcifications may rarely be present in the scar (1–2%) (Kaltenbach et al. 2016; Katabathina et al. 2011).

At MR examinations, FNHs generally appear homogeneously iso- or mildly hypointense on T1- and T2-weighted sequences (Figs. 9 and 10).

Rarely (but more often in steatotic livers), FNH may contain fat (with a dropout of signal intensity on T1-weighted out-phase acquisition), and in this case, it can mimic hepatocyte nuclear factor 1- alpha mutated type (H-HCA) (Jharap et al. 2015; Vijay et al. 2015). Usually the diagnosis of steatotic FNH can be reached on imaging with very high specificity, as long as all common imaging findings are observed in the lesion, and in particular the homogeneous or heterogeneous iso-hyperintensity on hepatobiliary phase images (Ronot and Vilgrain 2014) (Fig. 11).

In the literature, the sensitivity of contrast-enhanced ultrasound for the diagnosis of FNH varies depending on the studies between 80 and 100%, with a specificity value between 85 and 95%. Early, centrifugal, spoke-wheel arterial contrast uptake is the typical pattern of enhancement at CEUS; nodule appears hyperechoic at the end of the arterial phase, and it is iso- or dis-

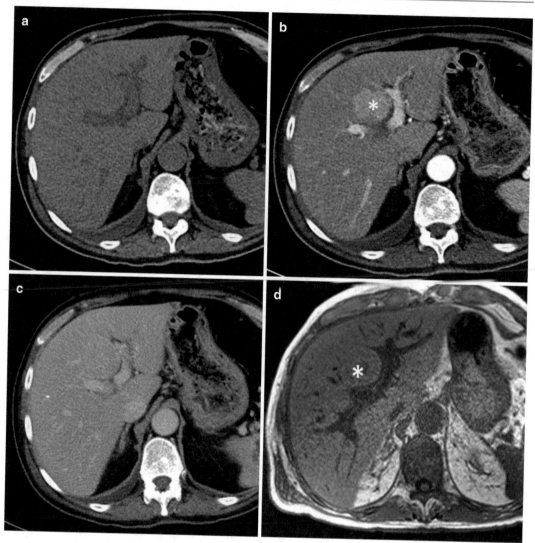

Fig. 9 74 years old, male, chronic diarrhea after returning from a trip to Thailand. Incidental finding at CT. In IVs an isodense lesion at unenhanced CT (**a**) shows intense and homogeneous enhancement during arterial phase (* in **b**) and appears isodense on PVP (**c**). On MR examination, the lesion is iso-slightly hypointense on T1 in-phase acquisition (* in **d**) and appears more hypointense on T1 opposed-phase sequence (**e**) for likely small intralesional steatosis; on T2w images (**f**), it appears fairly hyperintense. On DWI images (**h**), the mass shows signs of restriction, and it appears hypointense on ADC map (**g**). On T1w image with fat saturation before contrast medium injection (**i**), the nodule is fairly hypointense. After Gd-EOB, the lesion shows very rapid and intense enhancement during arterial phase (**j**); during PVP (**k**) and delayed (**l**) phases, it appears hyperintense. On HBP (**m**), the lesion is markedly hyperintense: FNH without any scar

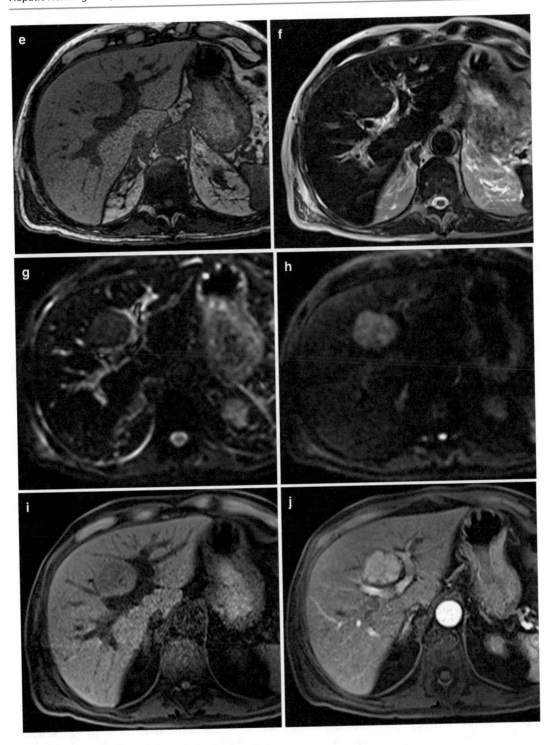

Fig. 9 (continued)

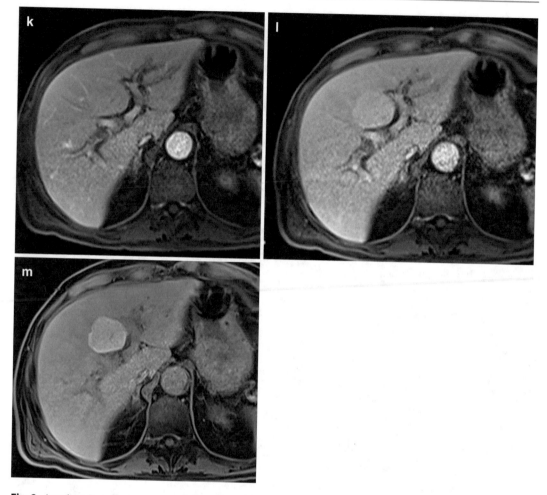

Fig. 9 (continued)

cretely hyperechoic in the portal and late phases (Dioguardi Burgio et al. 2016).

Both on CT and MR, after contrast media administration, during the arterial phase, FNH is homogeneously and strongly enhanced (96%) except for the central scar. During portal phase, it becomes isodense/isointense to the liver parenchyma, and the central scar remains relatively hypodense/hypointense. In MRI using a Gd chelate contrast medium with long interstitial phase, the central scar shows enhancement in the delayed phase (presence of abundant myxomatous stroma); differently, using Gd-EOB–DTPA, the scar often remains hypointense also in the delayed phase. With hepatobiliary MR contrast agents, the sensitivity for diagnosing FNH has increased up to 90%. Iso-hyperintensity on the hepatobiliary phase has high sensitivity and specificity to differentiate FNH from HCA with Gd-BOPTA or gadoxetic acid MRI (92%–96.9% and 91%–100%, respectively). On the hepatobiliary phase, FNH appears more frequently iso-hyperintense with respect to the surrounding liver, without or with hypointense central scar (Katabathina et al. 2011; Darai et al. 2015; Grazioli et al. 2013; Hartleb and Gutkowski 2011).

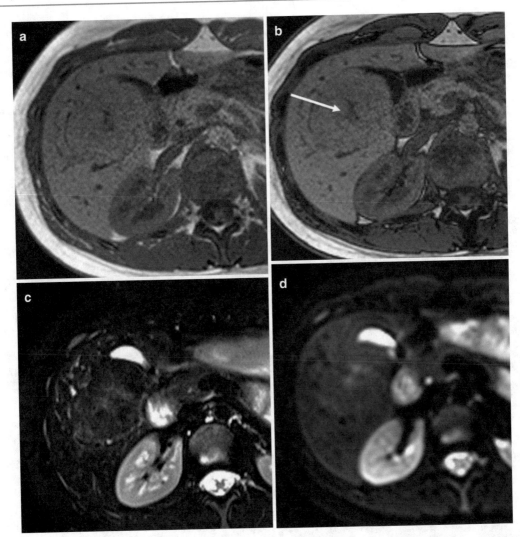

Fig. 10 24 years old, female, hyperechoic mass in VS, incidental finding during US for right hypochondrium discomfort. At MR examination, the lesion located in VS, with partial exophytic development, appears iso-slightly hypointense on T1 in/opp phases (**a**, **b**), with tiny hypointense central scar (arrow in **b**); on T2w images (**c**), it's isointense, and the scar appears slightly hyperintense. The mass doesn't show restriction on DW imaging (B800, ADC map: **d**, **e**). During dynamic study before and after Gd-EOB injection (**f–i**), the mass shows very intense enhancement during arterial phase (**g**) and becomes progressively isointense in PVP (**h**) and slightly hyperintense on delayed phase (**i**); because of Gd-EOB short interstitial distribution and rapid hepatocellular uptake, central scar doesn't show significant enhancement in any phase of this dynamic study, and the lesion appears brightly hyperintense after only 15 min (coronal view: **j**): typical FNH with central starred scar

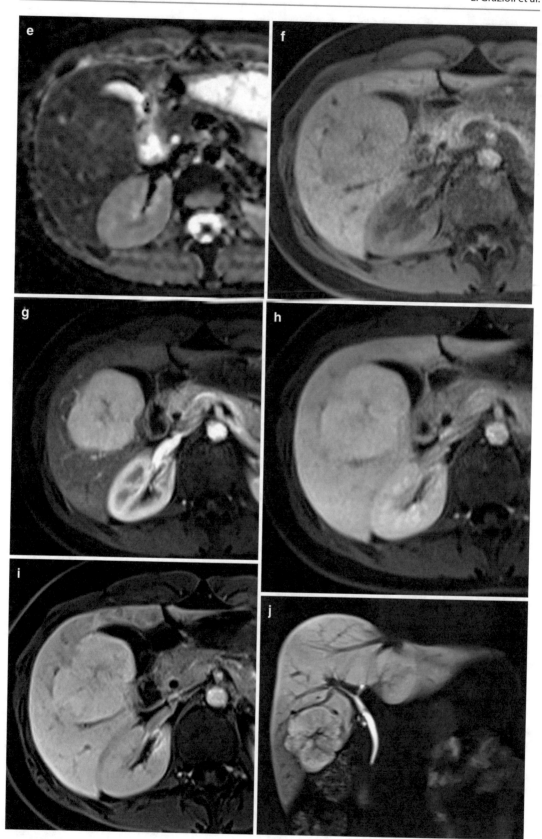

Fig. 10 (continued)

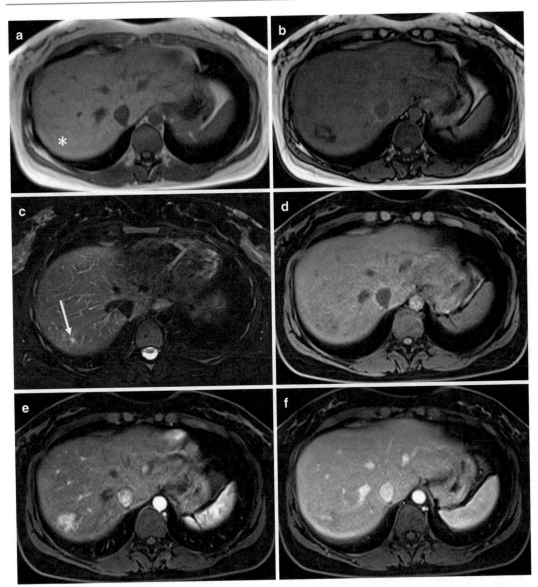

Fig. 11 38 years old, female, incidental findings on US examination. From T1 in-phase (**a**) to T1 opp-phase acquisitions (**b**), the signal intensity of liver drops because of diffuse steatosis. In liver segment VII a lesion is isointense on in-phase (* in **a**) and appears heterogeneously hypointense on T1 opp-phase sequence (**b**) because of intralesional fat; on T2w images with fat saturation, only a tiny portion of the nodule appears fairly hyperintense (arrow in **c**). On T1w image with fat saturation before contrast medium injection (**d**), the nodule is fairly hypointense. After Gd-EOB administration, the lesion shows very rapid but heterogeneous enhancement (**e**); during PVP (**f**) and delayed (**g**) phases, it appears iso-/slightly hyperintense. On HBP, after 10′ (**h**) and 20′ (**i**), the lesion is isointense, with thin hypointense rim (arrow) and eccentric slightly hypointense area/scar (* in **i**); at biopsy, FNH with intralesional fat

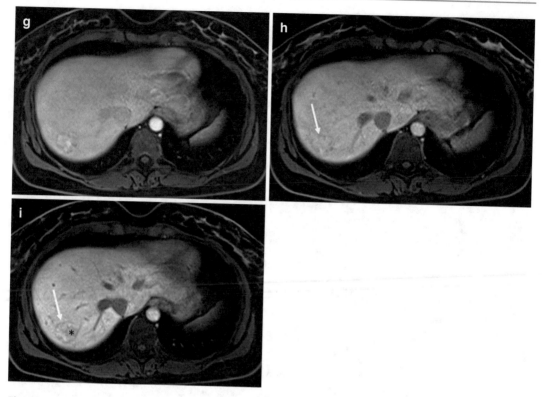

Fig. 11 (continued)

In some cases, it can have a heterogeneous appearance with a so-called "salt-and-pepper" aspect or with hyperintense ring (Vijay et al. 2015). Other atypical findings include nodules with a dominant central scar with strong hyperintensity on T2-weighted imaging (Fig. 12), pseudocapsule that can mimic true capsule, and washout during dynamic acquisition. In atypical cases on imaging, liver biopsy is indicated.

Peculiar features suggesting surgical management have to be reported: pedunculated/exo- phytic lesions, rapid growth, and compression on biliary or vascular branches with functional parenchymal alterations (EASL 2016).

When the diagnosis is confident without any patient's symptoms, follow-up imaging is not required. There is no indication for discontinuing OCPs, and follow-up during pregnancy is not necessary. Annual follow-up using US for 2–3 years is prudent in women diagnosed with FNH who wish to continue OCP use (EASL 2016; Marrero et al. 2014) (Fig. 13).

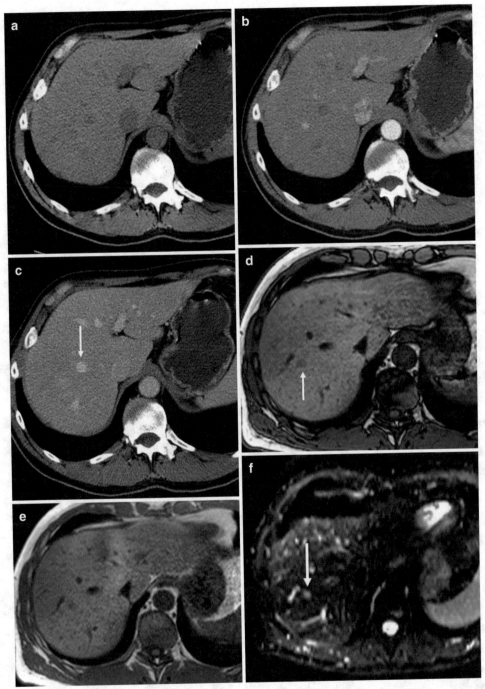

Fig. 12 54 years old, male, during US follow-up for previous colon cancer. At dynamic contrast-enhanced CT (**a–c**), the lesion shows enhancement during portal venous phase (arrow), which was deemed as a possible hemangioma. At MR examination, the lesion (arrow) appears hypointense on T1 in-/opp-phase acquisition (**d, e**). The nodule appears fairly hyperintense on DW images with different b values (arrows in 50–800; **f, g**); it has high values (2000 cm/s⁻¹) on ADC map (**h**). Before contrast medium injection (**i**), the nodule is hypointense. After Gd-EOB injection during arterial phase (**j**), the lesion shows strong enhancement, without washout at portal phase (**k**). On HBP (**l**), the lesion presents markedly hyperintense peripheral rim (cellular component) and large central heterogeneously hypointense round scar (mesenchymal component). At biopsy, FNH with large scar

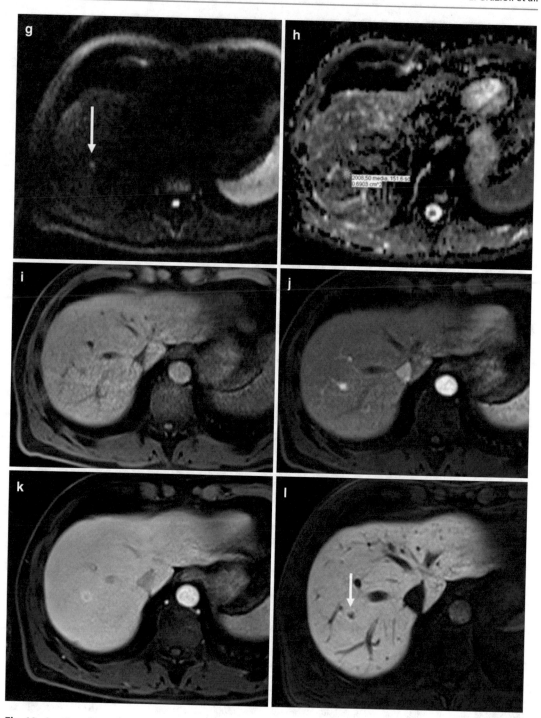

Fig. 12 (continued)

Fig. 13 Flowchart for the management of presumed HCA (from EASL guidelines 2016). Baseline MRI is necessary to help to confirm a diagnosis of HCA and characterize it. In men, resection is the treatment of choice. In women, a period of 6 month's observation, after lifestyle change, is appropriate. Resection is indicated in lesions persistently greater than 5 cm or increasing in size. In smaller lesions, a conservative approach with interval imaging can be adopted. In specialist centers practicing MRI subtyping, longer intervals between scans may be preferred for H-HCA

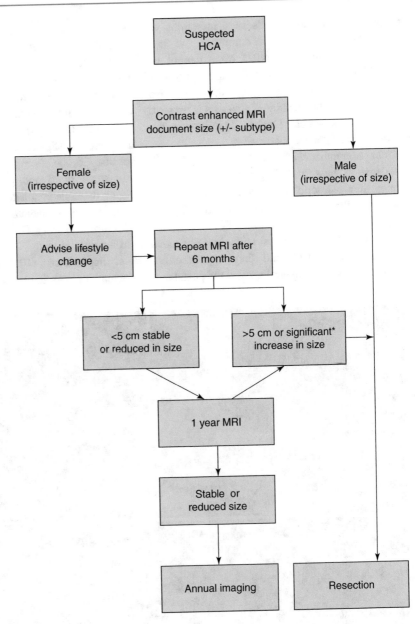

3 Nodular Regenerative Hyperplasia (NRH)

Nodular regenerative hyperplasia (NRH) is a rare liver condition characterized by a diffuse micronodular transformation of the hepatic parenchyma with associated portal hypertension.

There are several hypotheses behind the pathogenesis of NRH: the "vascular hypothesis" considers the chronic parenchymal ischemia related to a reduction of portal blood flow (due to obstruction or thrombosis of main and/or peripheral vessels) as the stimulus to regenerative proliferation. A second theory states that NRH is a primitive proliferative disorder of the liver and that it is bound to become the cause of portal hypertension because of portal vessel compression by regenerative nodules (Maillette et al. 2010).

The alteration of portal perfusion can be triggered by several causes, being autoimmune, neoplastic, or hematological diseases, infections, or drug-related causes the most common.

At US examination, NRH often cannot be appreciable because nodules are generally isoechoic to liver parenchyma; they can also appear slightly hypoechoic if steatosis is present. In these cases, at color Doppler examination, the nodules can show vascularity.

On non-enhanced CT, NRH is generally isodense to the surrounding parenchyma; sometimes, if a siderotic intralesional component is present, the nodules can appear slightly hyperdense.

At CECT, the nodules have homogeneous arterial enhancement, and they appear either isodense or slightly hyperdense on the portal and delayed phases (Kaltenbach et al. 2016; Dioguardi Burgio et al. 2016).

On unenhanced T1w MR images, NRH is generally isointense or slightly hyperintense compared to the surrounding liver parenchyma, without intralesional fat.

On T2w images, the nodules can appear iso- or, if siderotic, slightly hypointense. After liver-specific Gd chelate injection, the nodules generally show rapid and progressive enhancement during dynamic acquisition, and they appear iso-/hyperintense on hepatobiliary phase (the same with a central scar). Differential diagnosis can be challenging: indeed, NRH often shows an FNH-like appearance (Kaltenbach et al. 2016; Katabathina et al. 2011; Dahl et al. 2015) (Fig. 14).

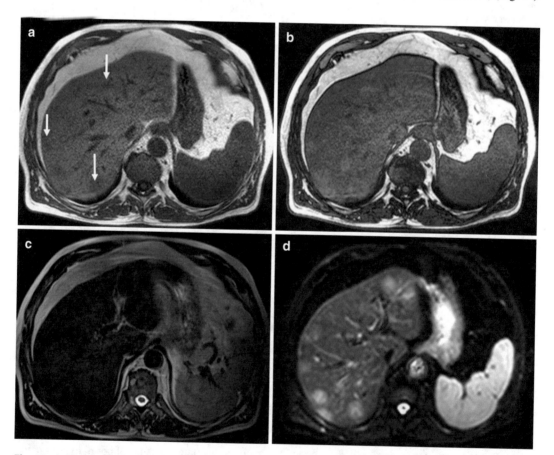

Fig. 14 A 60-year-old man, chronic steroidal therapy for lumbar discal hernia; US follow-up for liver steatosis: multiple hypoechoic nodules suspected for metastases. On T1w in-phase acquisition, multiple lesions can be observed in all hepatic segments, iso-/slightly hypointense (arrows in **a**); they appears slightly hyperintense on T1w opp phase (**b**) because of parenchymal diffuse steatosis. At T2w imaging, the nodules are isointense (**c**), and they don't show any restriction at DWI (**d**, **e**) or ADC map (**f**). On T1 FS acquisition, the lesions are isointense (**g**); after injection of Gd-BOPTA, they show intense enhancement during arterial phase (**h**), and they appear slightly hyperintense on portal venous (**i**) and delayed phases after 3 min (**j**) and 10 min (**k**). The particular of the bigger lesion in VII S during HBP (**l**): a thin scar can be noted. At biopsy: regenerative nodular hyperplasia

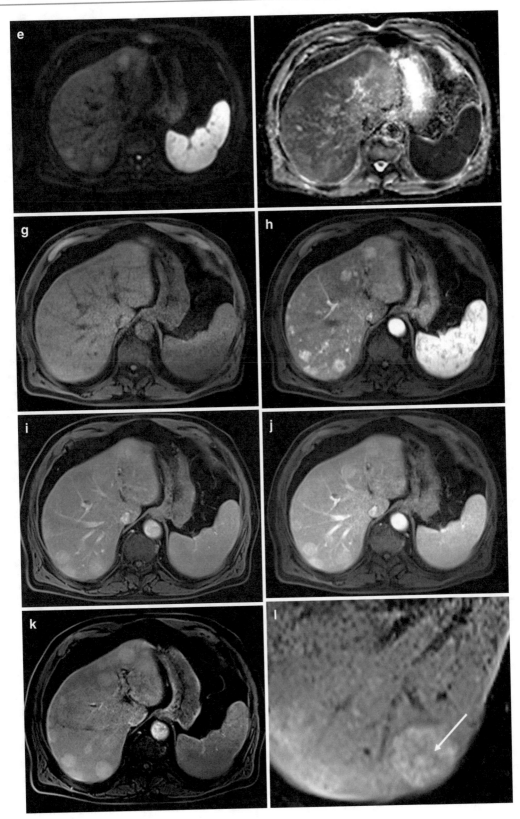

Fig. 1.14 (continued)

4 Mesenchymal Origin

4.1 Hepatic Hemangioma

Hepatic hemangiomas (HHs) are the most common benign liver lesions with an incidence that may reach 20% of the general population (Caseiro-Alves et al. 2007). The lesion is often found incidentally in asymptomatic patients during routine radiologic examinations, but its high prevalence may sometimes be a diagnostic clue in oncologic patients or when the lesion does not show a typical structure, enhancement on imaging techniques, or atypical T2 signal intensity at imaging MR, especially when the background liver parenchyma is altered. The lesion consists of blood-filled vascular cavities of different sizes, lined by a single layer of flat endothelial cells supported by connective tissue (Ishak et al. 2000). HH is typically fed by the hepatic artery circulation, with very slow blood flow within the lesional vessels, being asymptomatic in the majority of patients. Recent retrospective cohort studies (Hasan et al. 2014) have shown that nearly 40% of HH may exhibit lesional grow, usually with a slow rate (2 mm/year in linear dimension and 17.4%/year per volume). HH has been histologically categorized into three different subtypes, with a possible continuity in evolution among them: capillary, cavernous, and sclerosed. The pathologic structure of the lesion conditions its echogenicity, attenuation, signal intensity, and enhancement pattern at contrast-enhanced radiologic examinations. Moreover, the alterations of the background liver parenchyma may cause differences in lesion detection and characterization, and for its superior contrast resolution capacities, MRI is considered the best imaging modality for detection and characterization of HHs, with high sensitivity and specificity (100% and 95%, respectively) (Rodríguez de Lope et al. 2012).

Cavernous hemangioma is the most common type, usually less than 3 cm in size and with few internal connective components, for the prevalence of large vascular spaces. At ultrasonography (US), cavernous hemangioma typically appears as a hyperechogenic, homogeneous lesion with sharp outlines, frequently with poste-

rior acoustic enhancement. This pattern is related to histology and hemodynamic behavior (Yu et al. 1998). In fact, it can be related to the many and extensive interfaces between the vascular spaces and the fibrous stroma as well as to the slow blood flow in these large vascular spaces. Color and power Doppler evaluation usually does not show any vascular signal within the lesion, due to the very slow blood flow that characterizes it. Contrast-enhanced US (CEUS) more easily allows the characterization of the vascular nature of the lesion (Quaia et al. 2006). At unenhanced CT on a background of normal liver parenchyma, HH (<3 cm) is typically isoattenuating to vessels and adjacent parenchyma. The typical pattern of cavernous HH at contrast-enhanced examinations, on CEUS, CT, or MRI (with extracellular contrast agents), is the presence of peripheral nodular enhancement in the arterial phase, with a centripetal progression and fill-in in the extended portal venous phase and late phases (Brannigan et al. 2004). In particular, the correlation between internal HH architecture and dynamic CT findings in cavernous hemangiomas, showing that the diameters of the vascular spaces are smaller in the early peripheral zones of enhancement compared with the central zone of progressive centripetal filling, has been analyzed in the literature (Yamashita et al. 1997) (Fig. 15).

Sometimes, especially in giant HH (>5 cm), a residual central hypodense/hypointense portion resembling a scar may be observed, but also in this pattern, the enhanced components are characterized by density/intensity values similar to blood vessels on all phases of dynamic imaging. At MRI examination, the high water content of HH correlates to homogeneous and high signal intensity on T2w images and maintains hyperintensity on longer echo times (TE > 120 ms), with low signal intensity on T1w sequences (Klotz et al. 2013; Chan et al. 2002). In the case of "giant" HH, a central T2w hypointense portion may be observed, corresponding to hyalinized or thrombosed areas, sometimes with calcifications, with incomplete contrast filling (Fig. 16).

Diffusion-weighted (DW) MRI is considered a useful technique for the detection and characterization of focal liver lesions. Using this

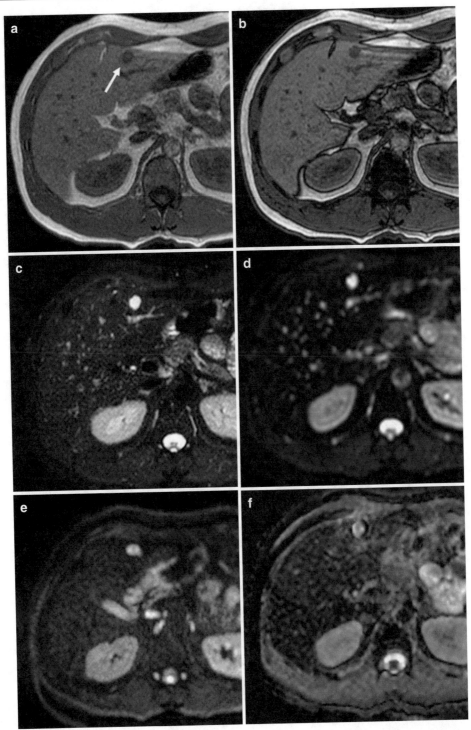

Fig. 15 A 52-year-old male, chronic abdominal pain. US finding of nodular hyperechoic lesion in IIS. On T1w in/opp imaging (**a**, **b**), the lesion appears hypointense (arrow in **a**); it's brightly hyperintense on T2w acquisition with fat saturation (**c**). At DWI imaging (b0–b800), the signal intensity of the lesion is high due to shine-through effect (**d**, **e**), but the lesion doesn't show restriction in the ADC map (**f**). During dynamic acquisition before and after i.v. administration of gadoxetic acid (**g–j**) with a slow flow injection rate (1 mL/s), the lesion shows globular enhancement (arrow in **h**) and almost complete fulfilling during PVP. The lesion appears slightly hypointense after 3 min during transitional phase (**j**), and it's markedly hypointense after 10 min (HBP in **k**): cavernous hemangioma

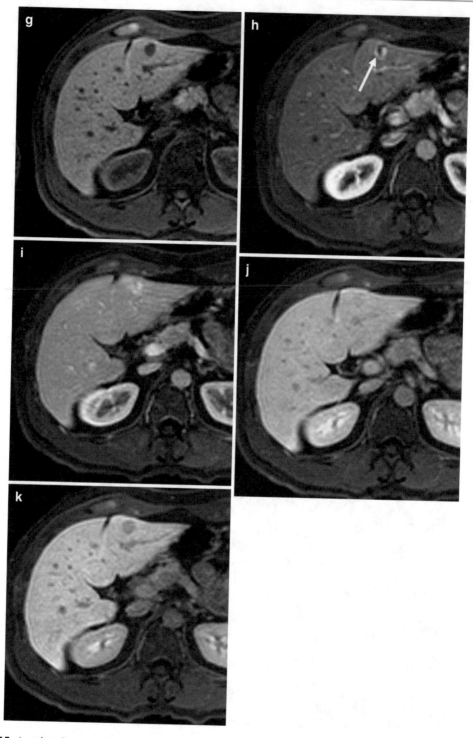

Fig. 1.15 (continued)

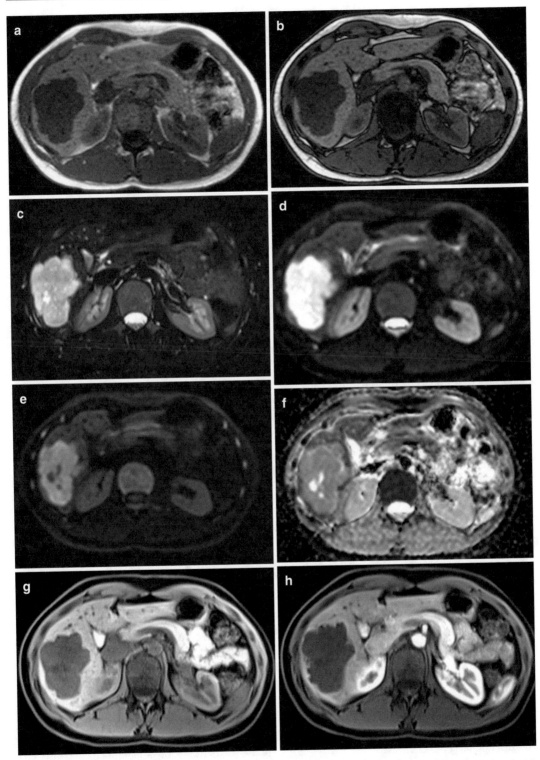

Fig. 16 A 48-year-old, female, abdominal discomfort. US finding of heterogeneously hyperechoic mass in S5–S6. At MR examination the lesion is hypointense on T1 in/opp-phase acquisitions (**a**, **b**) and brightly hyperintense T2-w image (**c**); the lesion does not show restriction on b50 (**d**), b800 (**e**) and ADC map (**f**); at T1w images with fat saturation (**g**) the lesion is hypointense. After Gd-BOPTA administration (**h–j**) the lesion shows typical globular enhancement, incomplete after 5′ (**j**): giant cavernous hemangioma

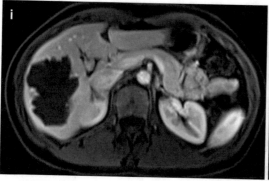 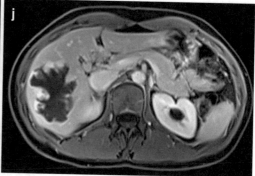

Fig. 16 (continued)

approach, benign lesions (mostly cyst and hemangioma) can be correctly categorized if they show high signal intensity on both T2w and b0 s/mm², with a progressive and significant signal intensity decrease at high b values 500/750 s/mm² and an apparent diffusion coefficient (ADC) signal that is subjectively higher than the adjacent liver (Parikh et al. 2008). Some HHs may demonstrate residual high signal intensity on high b value images (500–750 s/mm²) and are more difficult to characterize at the qualitative assessment of DW MR images. This phenomenon, known as "T2w shine-through effect," is explained by the influence of T2w properties to the DW images (being the other two factors involved in DW signal intensity the ADC and the spin density of the examined tissue). Moreover, the absence of restricted diffusion on a qualitative evaluation is supported by the quantitative assessment on the ADC map, with values that are always higher than hepatic parenchyma $(2.17 \pm 0.36 \times 10 - 3 \text{ mm}^2/\text{s})$ (Duran et al. 2014).

The same peculiar aspect can be observed after bolus administration of EOB-DTPA due to its rapid hepatocyte intake. Indeed EOB vascular profile, in terms of globular and progressive fill-in, could not be typically evaluated, and, in late phases of dynamic evaluation, hemangiomas tend to appear iso- or hypointense, differently from what is seen when using vascular interstitial contrast agents (Fig. 17).

Capillary hemangioma may be observed in almost 16% of all HH, 42% less than 1 cm in size. It consists of small vascular spaces, with more abundant connective components, that may be the explanation for the different hemodynamic and contrast enhancement behavior (Klotz et al. 2013; Vilgrain et al. 2000). It may appear more frequently iso-hypoechogenic at US, due to tight vascular spaces and faster blood flow, with less reverberation of acoustic echoes and possible demonstration of intralesional flow at color Doppler evaluation. In steatotic liver, small capillary HH may demonstrate a perilesional hypoechogenicity at US, corresponding to the hyperattenuating rim at baseline CT and hyperintensity on T1w "chemical shift" images due to peritumoral sparing of fatty infiltration. At CT examination, the lesion may appear slightly hypodense or isodense before contrast medium injection, with early, homogeneous, and rapid and intense contrast enhancement, that follows the aortic enhancement in each phase, without any washing (Caseiro-Alves et al. 2007; Youssef et al. 2015). Furthermore, especially in small lesions (<1 cm), a transient perilesional parenchymal enhancement may be observed, due to the presence of arterioportal shunting (Kim et al. 2001, 2006). A similar "flash-filling" kinetic of contrast enhancement may be observed using CEUS and CE-MRI with extracellular gadolinium contrast agents. In the differential diagnosis from hypervascular metastases, it is essential to observe delayed-phase CT/MR lesion appearance, because HH remains hyperattenuating/hyperintense, whereas hypervascular metastases do not (Vilgrain et al. 2000) (Figs. 18 and 19).

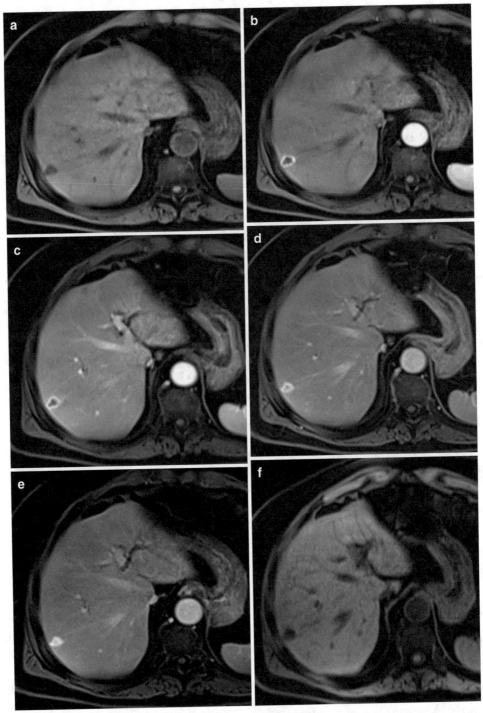

Fig. 17 A 62-year-old male, hospitalization for cerebral stroke. At thoracic unenhanced CT, hypodense lesion in the liver (segment VI). At MRI dynamic study with Gd-BOPTA (**a–e**), the lesion shows globular progressive enhancement, and the enhancement is complete only after 10 min (**e**). At MRI dynamic study with gadoxetic acid (**f–l**), the enhancement of the lesion is recognizable in arterial (**g**), PVP (**h**), and transitional phase (3′ after contrast media injection, **i**); after 10′ (**j**), the lesion appears hypointense because of rapid gadoxetic acid uptake by liver cells and consequent intense liver enhancement on T1w acquisition. Sclerotic hemangioma

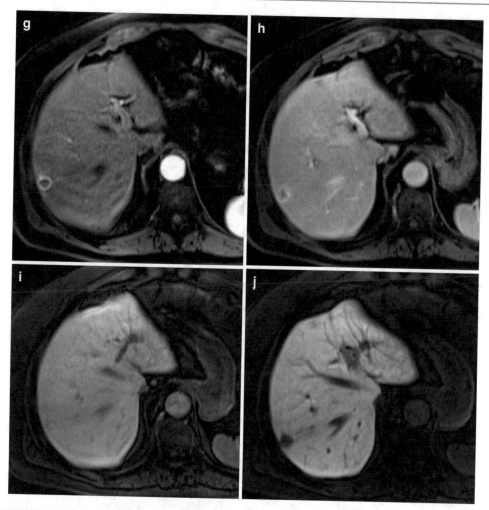

Fig. 17 (continued)

Sclerosed/hyalinized hemangioma occurs when HH degenerates and develops extensive fibrosis, which usually begins at the center of the lesion, causing obliteration of the vascular spaces and changes in US echogenicity, attenuation, and signal intensity at MRI. The preoperative diagnosis of sclerosed HH is very challenging, both for its rarity and for its radiological features that resemble those of hepatic malignancies (cholangiocarcinoma or metastatic lesions). The lesional heterogeneity is conditioned by different grades of fibrotic or hemorrhagic and cystic degeneration which determine the absence of typical early enhancement, sometimes showing a slow and inhomogeneous contrast progression both at CEUS, CT, and MRI, with a late or absent centripetal filling within the central scar. Moreover, if typical HH is characterized by marked high signal intensity on T2w MR images, sclerosed HH shows only slight T2w hyperintensity, more often at the periphery of the lesion (Vilgrain et al. 2000; Miyamoto et al. 2015; Ridge et al. 2014). These atypical radiological structural and enhancement features may cautiously suggest the diagnosis, which most often remains histological.

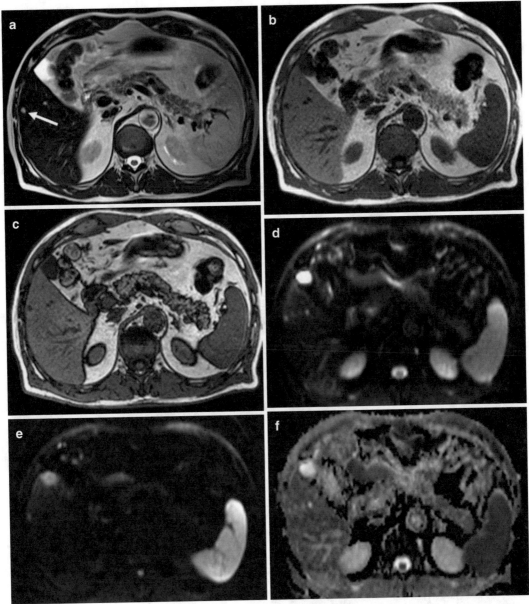

Fig. 18 A 67-year-old male, suspected geographic fatty liver at US. On T2w imaging, a tiny bright hyperintense lesion (arrow in **a**) can be noted in VS. It appears homogeneously hypointense on T1 in-/opp-phase acquisition (**b**, **c**). No restriction of diffusivity can be observed at DWI (b0–b800, ADC map) (**d–f**). During dynamic study after gadoxetic acid injection (**g–k**), the tiny lesion shows rapid and homogeneous enhancement (**h**, **i**); it's slightly hypointense at transitional phase after 3′ (**j**) and hypointense after 10′ (**k**): capillary hemangioma

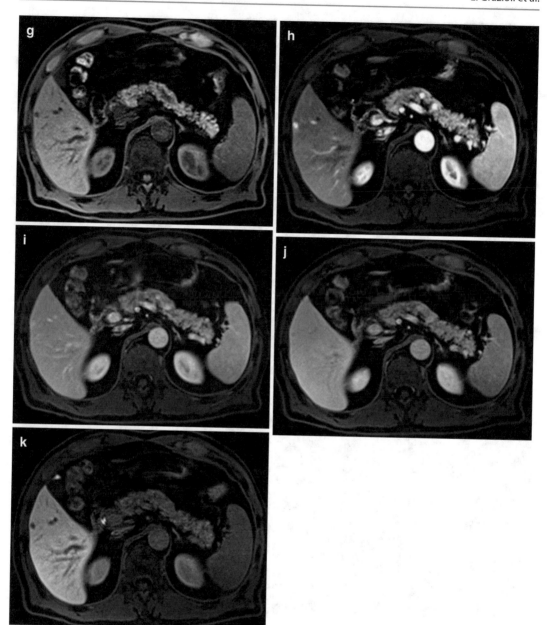

Fig. 1.18 (continued)

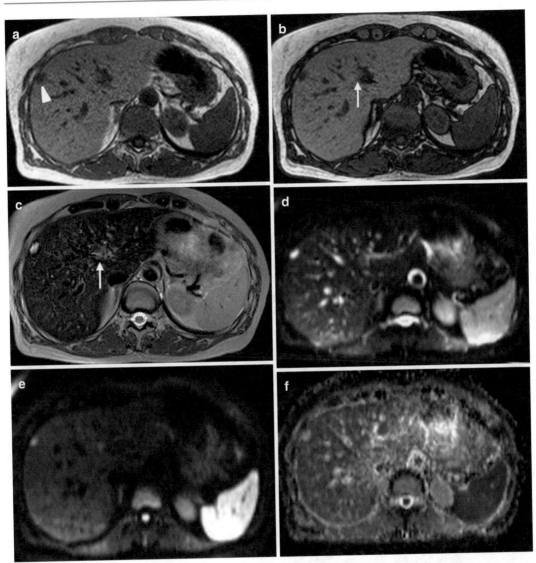

Fig. 19 A 55-year-old, female, US finding during staging for breast cancer. Hyperechoic lesion in S8 and iso-/hypoechoic lesion in S4. At MR examination, the lesion in S8 is hypointense on T1 in-/opp-phase acquisition (point of arrow in **a**) and shows homogeneous hyperintense signal on T2w imaging (**c**); the nodule doesn't show restriction at DWI acquisition (**d**–**f**); on T1w image with fat saturation before contrast medium injection (**g**), the nodule is hypointense. After Gd-EOB administration, the lesion shows very rapid but not homogeneous enhancement during arterial phase (**h**): a polygonal-shaped area of transient enhancement surrounds it; during PVP (**i**), the lesion is homogeneously hyperintense; during transitional phase, after 3 min (**j**), it appears slightly hypointense. On HBP after 10′ (**m**), the lesion is hypointense: high-flow hemangioma. The lesion in S4 is isointense on T1w (**a**–**g**, arrow in **b**), T2w (**c**), and DWI (**d**–**f**) acquisitions; during dynamic acquisition, it shows intense and homogeneous enhancement on arterial phase (**h**); it appears isointense on PVP (**i**) and slightly hyperintense on transitional phase (**j**); on HPB, the lesion shows typical hyperintense peripheral rim (arrow in **k**) and central rounded hypointense scar: typical FNH

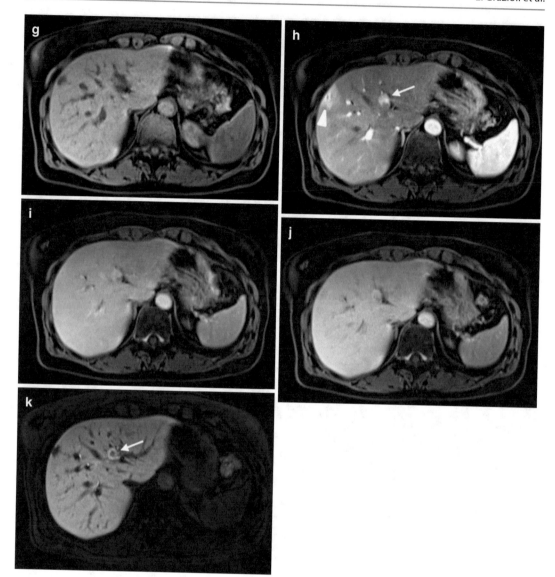

Fig. 1.19 (continued)

References

Agarwal S, Fuentes Orrego JM et al (2014) Inflammatory hepatocellular adenomas can mimic focal nodular hyperplasia on gadoxetic acid-enhanced MRI. AJR Am J Roentgenol 203(4):W408–W414. https://doi.org/10.2214/AJR.13.12251

Brannigan M, Burns PN, Wilson SR (2004) Blood flow patterns in focal liver lesions at microbubble-enhanced US. Radiographics 24(4):921–935

Caseiro-Alves F, Brito J, EirasAraujo A, Belo-Soares P, Rodrigues H, Cipriano A, Sousa D, Mathieu D (2007) Liver haemangioma: common and uncommon findings and how to improve the differential diagnosis. Eur Radiol 17:1544–1554

Chan YL, Lee SF, Yu SC, Lai P, Ching AS (2002) Hepatic malignant tumour versus cavernous hemangioma: differentiation on multiple breath-hold turbo spin-echo MRI sequences with different T2 weighting and T2w-relaxation time measurements on a single slice multi-echo sequence. Clin Radiol 57(4):250–257

Cogley JR, Miller FH (2014) MR imaging of benign focal liver lesions. Radiol Clin North Am 52(4):657–682

Darai N, Shu R et al (2015) Atypical CT and MRI features of focal nodular hyperplasia of liver: a study with radiologic-pathologic correlation. Open J Radiol 5:131–141

Dhingra S, Fiel MI (2014) Update on the new classification of hepatic adenomas. Clinical, molecular, and pathologic characteristics. Arch Pathol Lab Med 138(8):1090–1097

Dioguardi Burgio M, Ronot M, Salvaggio G, Vilgrain V, Brancatelli G (2016) Imaging of hepatic focal nodular hyperplasia: pictorial review and diagnostic strategy. Semin Ultrasound CT MRI 37(6):511–524

Duran F, Ronot M, Kerbaol A, Van Beers B, Vilgrain V (2014) Hepatic hemangiomas: factors associated with T2 shine-through effect on diffusion-weighted MR sequences. Eur J Radiol 83(3):468–478

EASL Clinical Practice Guidelines on the management of benign liver tumours (2016) J Hepatol 65(2):386–398

Gangahdar K, Santhosh D et al (2014) MRI Evaluation of masses in the noncirrhotic liver. Appl Radiol 2014:20–28

Grazioli L et al (2013) MR imaging of hepatocellular adenomas and differential diagnosis dilemma. Int J Hepatol 374170, 20 p

Hartleb M, Gutkowski K (2011) Nodular regenerative hyperplasia: evolving concepts on underdiagnosed cause of portal hypertension. World J Gastroenterol 17(11):1400–1409

Hasan HY, Hinshaw L, Borman EJ, Gegios A, Leverson G, Winslow E (2014) Assessing normal growth of hepatic hemangiomas during long-term follow-up. JAMA Surg 149(12):12661271

Ishak KG, Anthony PP, Niederau C, Nakanuma Y. Mesenchymal tumours of the liver(2000) In: Hamilton SR, Aaltonen LA (eds) World Health Organization classification of tumours. Pathology and genetics of tumours of the digestive system. IARC, Lyon, pp 191–198

Jharap B, van Asseldonk DP et al (2015) Diagnosing nodular regenerative hyperplasia of the liver is thwarted by low Interobserver agreement. PLoS One 10(6):e0120299

Kaltenbach T, Engler P et al (2016) Prevalence of benign focal liver lesions: ultrasound investigation of 45,319 hospital patients. Abdom Radiol (NY) 41:25–32

Katabathina VS, Menias CO et al (2011) Genetics and imaging of hepatocellular adenomas. Radiographics 31(6):1529–1543. https://doi.org/10.1148/rg.316115527

Kim KW, Kim TK, Han JK, Kim AY, Lee HJ, Choi BI (2001) Hepatic hemangiomas with arterioportal shunt: findings at two-phase CT. Radiology 219(3):707–711

Kim KW, Kim TK, Han JK et al (2006 Oct) Hepatic hemangiomas with arterioportal shunt: sonographic appearances with CT and MRI correlation. AJR Am J Roentgenol 187(4):W406–W414

Klotz T, Montoriola P-F, Da Ines D, Petitcolin V, Joubert-Zakeyh J, Garcier J-M (2013) Hepatic hemangioma: common and uncommon imaging features. Diagn Interv Imaging 94:849–859 34

Lee NK, Kim S, Kim DU, Seo HII, Kim HS, Jo HJ et al (2014) Diffusion-weighted magnetic resonance imaging for non-neoplastic conditions in the hepatobiliary and pancreatic regions: pearls and potential pitfalls in imaging interpretation. Abdom Imaging 40(3):643–662

Maillette L et al (2010) Focal nodular hyperplasia and hepatic adenoma: epidemiology and pathology. Dig Surg 27:24–31

Margolskee E, Bao F et al (2016) Hepatocellular adenoma classification: a comparative evaluation of immunohistochemistry and targeted mutational analysis. Diagn Pathol 11:27

Marrero JA, Ahn J, Rajender Reddy K, ACG Clinical Guideline (2014) The diagnosis and management of focal liver lesions. Am J Gastroenterol 109(9):1328–1347

Miyamoto S, Oshita A, Daimaru Y, Sasaki M, Ohdan H, Nakamitsu A (2015) Hepatic sclerosed hemangioma: a case report and review of the literature. BMC Surg 15:45

Neri E, Bali MA, Ba-Ssalamah A et al (2016) ESGAR consensus statement on liver MR imaging and clinical use of liver-specific contrast agents. Eur Radiol 26:921–931

Parikh T, Drew SJ, Lee VS, Wong S, Hecht EM, Babb JS, Taouli B (2008) Focal liver lesions detection and characterization with diffusion-weighted MR imaging-comparison with standard breath-hold T2-weighted imaging. Radiology 246:812–822

Quaia E, Bartolotta TV, Midiri M ct al (2006) Analysis of different contrast enhancement patterns after microbubble-based contrast agent injection in liver hemangiomas with atypical appearance on baseline scan. Abdom Imaging 31:59–64

Ridge CA, Shia J, Gerst SR, Do RK (2014 Apr) Sclerosed hemangioma of the liver: concordance of MRI features with histologic characteristics. J Magn Reson Imaging 39(4):812–818

Rodríguez de Lope C, Reig ME, Darnell A, Forner A (2012) Approach of the patient with a liver mass. Frontline Gastroenterol 3(4):252–262. https://doi.org/10.1136/flgastro-2012-100146

Roncalli M, Sciarra A, Di Tommaso L (2016) Benign hepatocellular nodules of healthy liver: focal nodular hyperplasia and hepatocellular adenoma. Clin Mol Hepatol 22(2):199–211

Ronot M, Vilgrain V (2014) Imaging of benign hepatocellular lesions: current concepts and recent updates. Clin Res Hepatol Gastroenterol 38(6):681–688

Tretiakova M, Hart J et al (2009) Distinction of hepatocellular adenoma from hepatocellular carcinoma with and without cirrhosis using E-cadherin and matrix metalloproteinase. Mod Pathol 22(8):1113–1120

Vanhooymissen I, Maarten GT et al (2019) Intrapatient comparison of the hepatobiliary phase of Gd-BOPTA and Gd-EOB-DTPA in the differentiation of hepatocellular adenoma from focal nodular hyperplasia. J Magn Reson Imaging 49(3):700–710

Vijay A, Elaffandi A, Khalaf H (2015) Hepatocellular adenoma: An update. World J Hepatol 7(25):2603–2609

Vilgrain V, Boulos L, Vullierme MP, Denys A, Terris B, Menu Y (2000) Imaging of atypical hemangiomas of the liver with pathologic correlation. Radiographics 20(2):379–397

Wang W, Liu JY et al (2016) Hepatocellular adenoma: comparison between real-time contrast-enhanced ultrasound and dynamic computed tomography. Springerplus 5:951

Yamashita Y, Ogata I, Urata J, Takahashi M (1997) Cavernous hemangioma of the liver: pathologic correlation with dynamic CT findings. Radiology 203(1):121–125

Youssef E, Baron RL, Elsayes KM (2015) Diagnostic approach of focal and diffuse hepatic diseases, Chapter 2. In: Elsayes KM (ed) Cross-sectional imaging of the abdomen and pelvis: a practical algorithmic approach. Springer, New York, pp 11–76

Yu JS, Kim MJ, Kim KW, Chang JC, Jo BJ, Kim TH et al (1998) Hepatic cavernous hemangioma: sonographic patterns and speed of contrast enhancement on multiphase dynamic MR imaging. AJR Am J Roentgenol 171(4):1021–1025

Inflammatory Liver Lesions

Anna Sara Fraia, Silvia Brocco, and Emilio Quaia

Contents

Abstract

Inflammatory lesions, such as pyogenic abscess and inflammatory pseudotumor, represent an important subgroup of focal liver lesions. As they could mimic primary or metastatic tumor, the knowledge of radiological features of these inflammatory diseases in a multimodality approach allows to differentiate them between other entities, early establishing diagnosis and management of the patient.

A. S. Fraia · S. Brocco · E. Quaia (✉)
Radiology Unit, Department of Medicine - DIMED,
University of Padova, Padova, Italy
e-mail: emilio.quaia@unipd.it

1 Pyogenic Abscess

1.1 Definition and Epidemiology

Hepatic abscess can be defined as a localized or multifocal collection of suppurate material in the liver associated with destruction of liver parenchyma and stroma (Oto et al. 1999), caused by invasion and multiplication of bacterial, parasitic, or, more rarely, fungal pathogens (Lardière-Deguelte et al. 2015). Frequently the etiology could be mixed (pyogenic superinfection of parasitic abscess).

Among the several liver diseases caused by bacterial infections, such as granulomatous disease and acute hepatitis, pyogenic abscess (PA) is a relatively uncommon entity characterized by a varying epidemiology according to geographical regions but still burdened by significant morbidity and mortality worldwide (Kaplan et al. 2004).

E. Quaia (ed.), *Imaging of the Liver and Intra-hepatic Biliary Tract*,
Medical Radiology Diagnostic Imaging, https://doi.org/10.1007/978-3-030-39021-1_2

In the early 1900s, mortality was as high as 75–80% (Huang et al. 1996). Recently, the improvements in antibiotic therapy and interventional procedures for the treatment of PA markedly decreased mortality, ranging from 10 to 40% (Law and Li 2012); however, it still remains high, making early diagnosis of PA important to improve clinical outcome (Mavilia et al. 2016).

Prevalence of PA is higher in East Asian countries, and it is endemic in some areas, such as Taiwan, where the estimated incidence increased from 10.8 to 15.4 cases per 100,000 per year between 2000 and 2011 (Chen et al. 2016).

In contrast, the incidence of bacterial abscesses is lower in Europe and Canada, ranging from 1.1 to 2.3 cases per 100,000 per year (Kaplan et al. 2004; Jepsen et al. 2005), but it represents about 80% of the total hepatic abscesses that occur in Western countries (Lardière-Deguelte et al. 2015).

American studies suggest a male PA predominance describing that incidence is 3.92 cases per 100,000 per year for male compared to 1.87 cases per 100,000 per year for female; furthermore, it was reported a correlation with increasing age because older individuals are more susceptible to bacterial infection and thus abscess formation (Sharma et al. 2018).

As shown by several recent population-based studies from different countries, these data will likely change in the nearby future: the rising frequency of hepatobiliary interventions (e.g., ERCP, RFA, and TACE), the higher prevalence of liver transplantation, the frequency of organisms with multidrug resistance, and the predisposing medical conditions are already modifying the PA global incidence, which will increase especially in Western world (Sharma et al. 2018; Meddings et al. 2010).

Particularly, risk factors predisposing patients to develop PA are male gender, advanced age, diabetes mellitus (Lee et al. 2001), liver cirrhosis (Mølle et al. 2001), general immunocompromised state (Eltawansy et al. 2015), and use of proton pump inhibitor (PPI) medications (Wang et al. 2015).

Other factors contributing to higher mortality rates include malignancy, multiorgan failure, respiratory distress, hypotension, PA rupture, large abscess size (<5 cm), jaundice, and extrahepatic involvement (Chen et al. 2014).

1.2 Etiology

PA etiopathogenesis is multifactorial and depends on the variability in geographical region, the predisposing factors, and the source of initial infection. Based on the underlying conditions, PA can be divided into three main subgroups that can overlap: infectious, malignant, and iatrogenic (Mavilia et al. 2016).

1.2.1 Infectious

Bacteria can gain access to the liver from biliary tract diseases, hematogenous dissemination of a gastrointestinal infection via the portal vein, systemic bacteremia via the hepatic artery, direct extension from a contiguous septic focus, or trauma (Huang et al. 1996). Around 20% of PAs are still cryptogenic, with unknown etiology.

The most frequent causes are the biliary diseases, which represent approximately 40–50% of cases (Meddings et al. 2010). Biliary duct obstruction, especially if partial, due to gallstone disease, malignancy (cholangiocarcinoma), strictures (sclerosing cholangitis), or congenital disease (e.g., Caroli disease), causes proliferation of bacteria in the biliary tract, ascending cholangitis, and invasion of liver parenchyma.

Portal pyaemia may be leaded by intra-abdominal infections with gastrointestinal or pelvic source, such as appendicitis (Kumar et al. 2015), empyema of the gallbladder, diverticulitis (Murarka 120 et al. 2011), regional enteritis, perforated gastric or colonic ulcers, pancreatitis (Ammann et al. 1992), infected hemorrhoids, and leaking gastrointestinal anastomoses.

Formation of liver PAs can be associated with non-metastatic colon-rectal cancer, because of tumor erosion of the mucosa, bacterial invasion of portal vessels, and thus liver infection (Jeong et al. 2012).

Traumatic and penetrating accidents may cause direct inoculation and bacterial liver seeding.

Systemic bacteremia usually causes multiple abscesses, while solitary abscess originates from spreading of contiguous tissue infection. Direct invasion of pathogens can follow cholecystitis and subphrenic or perinephric abscess.

1.2.2 Malignant

Malignant liver abscess can follow secondary infection of primary or metastatic tumor and a superinfection of spontaneous necrosis (Mavilia et al. 2016).

Pyogenic abscess may be the initial manifestation of HCC due to the infection of central necrosis or secondary to the ascending cholangitis leading to tumor biliary obstruction. More rarely, PA could complicate hepatic localization of metastatic melanoma, colon-rectal cancer, esophageal carcinoma, and pancreatic cancer.

1.2.3 Iatrogenic

Patients affected by inoperable HCC or hepatic metastases may undergo local treatment of liver lesions by transarterial chemoembolization (TACE) or radiofrequency ablation (RFA) (Shin et al. 2014). PA may develop following these procedures: TACE and RFA induce necrosis of the tumor and the contiguous hepatic parenchyma and produce directly and indirectly immunosuppressive effects (Huang et al. 2003; Sun et al. 2011). In literature, the incidence of PA after TACE and RFA has been reported to range from 0 to 1.4% (Shin et al. 2014) and 0.1–0.7% (Iida et al. 2014), respectively.

High risk of iatrogenic PA is related to several surgical, endoscopic, or radiological procedures, despite the use of prophylactic antibiotic therapy. More frequently, the placement of biliary stenting, enterobiliary anastomosis, and sphincterotomy may lead to develop abscesses (Montvuagnard et al. 2012).

Hepatic arterial injury during surgery (e.g., cholecystectomy or arterial embolization of abdominal trauma) can induce ischemic necrosis and subsequent development of PA.

Hepatic arterial thrombosis complicating liver transplant may be also associated with development of pyogenic abscesses. Also, the immunosuppressive drugs in transplant recipients, systemic chemotherapies, inherited immunodeficiency syndromes, and acquired immunodeficiency states (HIV/AIDS) could be considered in etiology of PA (Lardière-Deguelte et al. 2015).

Depending on the source of initial infection, several bacteria, aerobes and anaerobes, can be involved in PA formation. If the bacteria derive from the gut, such as in PA associated with biliary disease and intra-abdominal sepsis, the prevalent causative agents are *Escherichia coli*, *Klebsiella pneumoniae*, *Streptococcus faecalis*, and *Proteus vulgaris*.

Prior to 1980, *Escherichia coli* was the most common pathogen that caused PA (Keller et al. 2013), and most abscesses were polymicrobial, ranging from 11 to 65% (Johannsen et al. 2000), but during the past two decades, this trend has changed. Highly virulent strains of *K. pneumoniae*, particularly serotypes K1 and K2, have emerged as the predominant isolate in patients particularly from Asia (Li et al. 2010), United States (Rahimian et al. 2004), and Europe (Moore et al. 2013), and this trend tends to spread globally (Turton et al. 2007). This may be related to rising incidence of diabetes mellitus and more susceptibility of diabetic patient to *K. pneumoniae* infections. Furthermore, *K. pneumoniae* distant infections, including endophthalmitis, meningitis, septic pulmonary emboli, and empyema, appear to be associated with developing of occult liver PA (Webb et al. 2014). Other causative pathogens include *Staphylococcus* and *Streptococcus* species associated with direct trauma and percutaneous procedures or embolization or *Yersinia enterocolitica* in patient with hemochromatosis (Johannsen et al. 2000). Resistant *Enterobacter* or *Pseudomonas* species can cause liver abscesses, also as a complication following biliary stenting and endoprosthesis. Rare cases include *Brucella* species, *Nocardia* species, *Clostridium perfringens*, and *Mycobacterium* species (Meddings et al. 2010).

1.3 Clinical Aspects, Management, and Prognosis

PA diagnosis may be quite difficult based on the clinical manifestations, because signs and symptoms are highly variable and non-specific. The most common clinical features are fever, severe right-sided abdominal pain with hepatomegaly, hypotension, nausea, and vomiting, but the onset may be more insidious in clinically occult ("cold") abscesses, which cause only weight loss and vague abdominal tenderness. Multiple abscesses are more often acute, associated with a timely diagnosis. Occasionally, patients may present with peritonitis and sepsis as a sign of the rupture of the abscess. If the abscess causes a diaphragmatic irritation, the patient may refer right shoulder pain, cough, and pleural rubbing. Jaundice is usually a late manifestation, unless there is an underlying biliary disease (Mohsen et al. 2002; Singh et al. 2013).

Approximately 80% of abscesses involves the right liver lobe and less commonly the left liver lobe (15%) or both (5%) liver lobes (Singh et al. 2013).

Laboratory findings are non-specific and include hypoalbuminemia and elevated levels of blood cell count, C-reactive protein, aspartate aminotransferase, alanine aminotransferase, alkaline phosphatase, gamma-glutamyl transpeptidase, and total bilirubin.

Laboratory testing and clinical manifestations alone are not diagnostic, as they need correlation with imaging features.

Management of PAs depends on the pathogen and the source of infection and patient's clinical underlying conditions.

In general, both early and proper antibiotic therapy and imaging-guided or surgical drainage are the mainstay of treatment. Early diagnosis and CT-/US-guided percutaneous drainage reduced the mortality rates, from 65 to 2–12% (Mohsen et al. 2002; Huang et al. 1996) and the need for open surgery. Small liver abscesses (<5 cm in diameter) are successfully treated by antibiotic therapy, without any need of drainage (Lardière-Deguelte et al. 2015).

1.4 Multimodality Imaging

Early diagnostic definition and treatment require correlation between clinical, laboratory, and imaging features. Imaging is essential for diagnosis and for specific antimicrobial therapy. CT- or US-guided percutaneous needle aspiration of pus, eventually associated with placement of drainage, allows to isolate pathogen.

Diagnosis of PA is made by imaging in 90% of cases (Lardière-Deguelte et al. 2015). The primary methods of diagnostic imaging are conventional ultrasound (US) and computed tomography (CT), respectively, with 85% (Lin et al. 2009) and 97% (Halvorsen et al. 1984) of sensitivities.

The radiological features of PA depend on size and pathologic stage of the abscess formation. In the early phase, the abscess frequently appears as microabscesses (<2 cm) with a scattered distribution into hepatic parenchyma or as a cluster of multiple small lesions focally coalescing into a single larger cavity (Jeffrey et al. 1988). The diffuse miliary pattern typically occurs in sepsis caused by staphylococcal infection, while the cluster pattern is associated with enteric origin of infection, especially by coliform bacteria. During evolution, the abscess cavity may appear as unilocular or multilocular cystic lesion filled by purulent material and lined by a fibrous cuff.

1.4.1 US and CEUS

The sonographic pattern of PA is correlated with its evolution. In the initial phase, it may appear as an ill-defined hypoechoic area with a surrounding hypervascular liver parenchyma, demonstrated at the color Doppler ultrasound (CDUS). The colliquative phase is characterized by an anechoic area with hyperechoic spots in suspension, increased posterior acoustic transmission, and lateral acoustic shadows (Figs. 1 and 2). During the resolution phase, the lesion tends to reduce in size according to the progressive reduction of the liquid component (Ralls et al. 1987).

Microabscesses appear as hypo-anechoic nodules or ill-defined areas of distorted liver parenchyma, while larger abscess may appear as

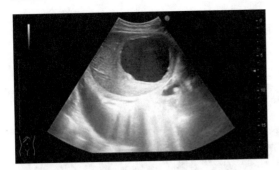

Fig. 1 Ultrasound (US) demonstrates a large, well-defined abscess in colliquative phase, as an anechoic lesion with fine internal echoes in suspension localized in right hepatic lobe

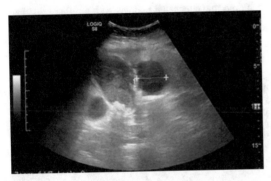

Fig. 2 Ultrasound shows synchronous pyogenic liver abscess and acute cholecystitis. The abscess (calipers) appears as an anechoic lesion with small internal echoes in suspension

hypoechoic lesions or hyperechoic areas, according to the varying presence of internal thickened septa and debris (Mortelé et al. 2004). In this case, the PA may simulate a solid mass, especially in *K. pneumoniae* monomicrobial hepatic abscess (Hui et al. 2007).

At unenhanced US, factors as acoustic through-transmission and absence of internal signal at Doppler US may help to differentiate PA from solid neoplasm, but if the necrosis is predominant within the lesion, diagnosis may be challenging. In this case, CT, MR, and also contrast-enhanced ultrasound (CEUS) may allow to characterize the lesion and to make diagnosis.

On CEUS, the characteristic features of PA after microbubble injection are the rim enhance-ment in arterial phase, the progressive washout of the lesion during the late phase, and the enhancement of septa with a honeycomb appearance in loculated abscesses. Based on these three findings, Popescu et al. suggested that CEUS may be more accurate than conventional US in detecting abscesses. They evaluated 41 patients with confirmed diagnosis of liver abscess and concluded that the method provides a definitive diagnosis in 93% of cases (Popescu et al. 2015). In contrast, according to Liu et al., these findings are not specific: they examined patients with various focal liver lesions and demonstrated that other entities such as infected granulomas and inflammatory pseudotumors may show peripheral or septal enhancement and late phase washout (Liu et al. 2008). Therefore, it may be difficult to make a conclusive diagnosis by CEUS as suggested by Popescu et al., although CEUS may better detect the presence of septations within the abscess and the consistency of the central area, guiding a better treatment approach.

1.4.2 CT

CE-CT represents an important method to detect abscess, to define the underlying clinical condition of the patient, and to reveal vascular, biliary, or systemic complications.

Particularly, among the complications of hepatic abscess, the most frequent are septic shock, empyema, thoracoabdominal fistula, right pleural effusion, portal thrombosis, inferior vena cava thrombosis, gastric perforation, pancreatitis, peripancreatic abscess, intra-abdominal collections, and peritonitis (Reyna-Sepúlveda et al. 2017).

A variety of CT aspects can be recognized, depending on the number and size of the lesions, the source of infections, and the underlying clinical patient's conditions. In case of single abscess, the radiological manifestations range from non-loculated fluid collection to multiloculated cystic mass and solid (phlegmonous) process (Halvorsen et al. 1984; Alsaif et al. 2011). Multiple abscesses may present a miliary or a cluster pattern distribution, with evidence of multiple low attenuation lesions scattered into liver parenchyma (miliary distribution) (Fig. 3a–c) or evidence of aggregation in a localized area and coalescence into a larger abscess (Fig. 4a–d) ("cluster sign") (Jeffrey et al. 1988).

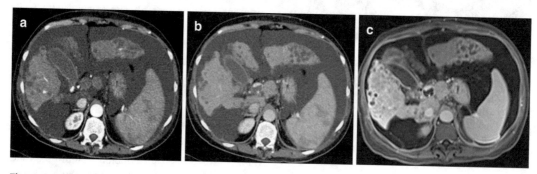

Fig. 3 Multiple small nodules representing pyogenic microabscesses scattered throughout a cirrhotic liver. Large ascites volume and portal vein thrombosis coexist. (*). (**a, b**) Axial arterial and portal venous phase CT show multiple low-attenuated nodules with a miliary distribution within the liver. (**c**) Axial MR image shows the signal void due to the portal vein thrombosis (*)

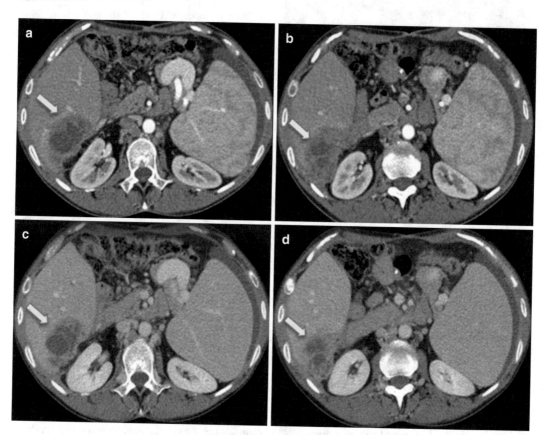

Fig. 4 Contrast-enhanced computed tomography (CT) of coalescent pyogenic abscesses in a 50-year-old woman who underwent liver transplantation for congenital biliary atresia. Splenomegaly and ascites coexist (**a, b**) Axial arterial phase CT shows peripheral enhancement of abscesses that aggregate in a single large cavity (cluster sign). (**c, d**) Axial portal venous phase CT shows the late enhancement of the outer layer, corresponding to perilesional edema

The most common findings at CE-CT of PA are a well-defined round mass, with a central low attenuation fluid-filled area, and an enhancing peripheral rim, surrounded by a low attenuation outer ring (Fig. 5a, b). The inner layer represents the pyogenic capsule that shows an early contrast enhancement persisting in delayed phases. The outer hypodense ring is a localized perilesional edema of surrounding liver parenchyma that enhances only in delayed phases. This appearance reflects the "double target sign," a characteristic imaging features of PA seen on CE-CT images (Mathieu et al. 1985).

A transient segmental wedge-shaped hepatic enhancement has been associated with hepatic PAs. This transient hepatic attenuation is visible in the early phase of dynamic CT and equilibrates in late phases, resulting in a reduction of portal venous flow surrounding the abscess, due to the compression of small portal venules by inflammatory cell infiltration, and a compensatory increase in arterial inflow. Typically, the segmental enhancement associated with liver abscesses has a wedge shape and decreases in size on follow-up dynamic CT: these findings may help to differentiate hepatic abscess from hepatic tumor with segmental enhancement caused by portal or hepatic vein stenosis or occlusion and other nontumorous arterioportal shunts (Gabata et al. 2001).

1.4.3 MR

At MR imaging, abscess cavity may show homogeneous or heterogeneous signal intensity, depending on the protein content. Small lesions may enhance homogeneously similar to small hemangiomas (Basilico et al. 2002), but in general, PA appears as an area of low intensity on T1-weighted images and of high intensity on T2-weighted images (Fig. 6a).

On T2-weighted MR image, it may be visible the "double target sign" of the abscess wall, with hyperintense content of the abscess surrounded by an iso- to hypointense inner layer and a moderately hyperintense outer layer (Fig. 6e).

Similar to dynamic CE-CT, in T1-weighted MR images after gadolinium administration, the inner layer shows an early enhancement in arterial phase that persists in delayed phase (Fig. 6b–d). Internal septations also show an enhancement pattern comparable to the abscess wall. The internal area of necrosis does not show enhancement, but on the delayed hepatobiliary phase images, a central pooling due to diffusion of the contrast agent may be seen.

A peripheral edema can be identified in 35% of hepatic abscesses, and it is characterized by a delayed enhancement in T1-weighted MR images after contrast medium administration and a high signal intensity on T2-weighted images (Balci et al. 1999; Mendez et al. 1994). The presence of peripheral edema can be used to differentiate a

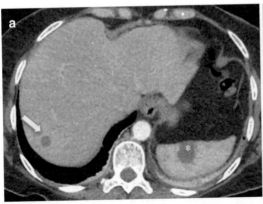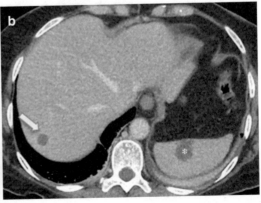

Fig. 5 Hepatic and splenic pyogenic abscesses. (**a, b**) Axial arterial and portal venous contrast-enhanced CT images show a small abscess localized in VII hepatic segment (arrow), with a persisting enhanced peripheral rim corresponding to the enhancing pyogenic capsule. A second abscess is localized in the spleen (*)

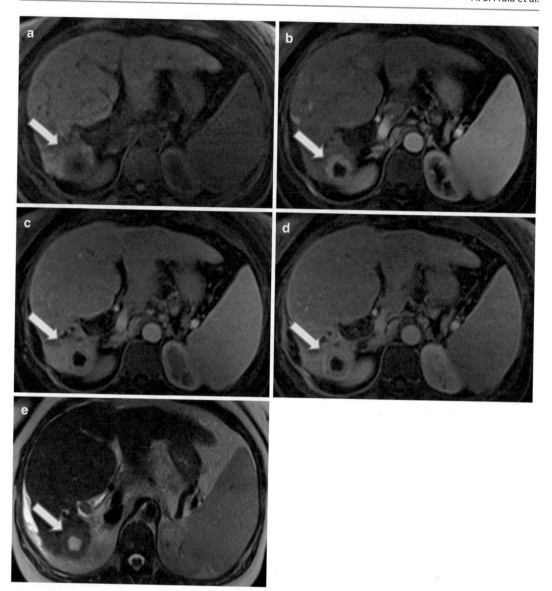

Fig. 6 Magnetic resonance (MR) of pyogenic abscess (arrow) in a 59-year-old woman with recurrent pyogenic cholangitis and chronic hepatopathy. (**a**) Axial non-enhanced fat-suppressed T1-weighted MR image shows an iso-hypointense nodule with a necrotic core localized in VI hepatic segment. (**b**) Axial contrast-enhanced arterial phase fat-suppressed T1-weighted MR image shows early enhancement of the inner layer of abscess wall. (**c**,

d) Axial contrast-enhanced portal venous and delayed phase fat-suppressed T1-weighted MR images show late enhancement of the outer layers, due to perilesional edema. The necrotic area does not show enhancement during dynamic phases. (**e**) T2-weighted image shows an iso-hypointense inner layer and a moderately hyperintense outer layer surrounding the high signal intensity content of the abscess

hepatic abscess from a benign cystic lesion, while primary or secondary hepatic malignancy may also be surrounded by a localized perilesional edema. A variety of malignant hepatic tumors, including intrahepatic cholangiocarcinoma, scirrhous hepatocellular carcinoma, epithelioid hemangioendothelioma, hepatic metastasis, and necrotic or cystic tumor, may show arterial rim enhancement, and they can mimic PA in clinical practice. The overlap of radiological features can make challenging the differentiation between liver PA and its malignant mimickers on conventional MR imaging. According to Chan et al., the diffusion-weighted images (DWI) and apparent diffusion coefficient (ADC) may allow to characterize PA lesions from cystic or necrotic tumor. In their study, they demonstrated that cystic or necrotic tumors show a greater degree of signal drop on high b-value DWI and a higher ADC value, while high viscosity pus in abscesses reveals a high signal intensity on high b-value DWI and iso-hypointensity on ADC map (Fig. 7a–d) (Chan et al. 2001).

Gas bubbles or air-fluid level is described in up to 20% of PAs, suggesting septic origin of the lesion (Fig. 8a–c). Nevertheless, it is possible to detect nonseptic gas in necrotic liver after tumor ablation or other similar procedures, and it represents a potential pitfall. At US, gas shows posterior acoustic reverberations and shadowing, while at MR imaging, it appears as a signal voids within the abscess, better detected on T1-weighted GE MRI images with a long TE . In *K. pneumoniae* infection is common to see gas within the abscess that appears as an air-fluid level or numerous thin arborizing internal bands that resemble the turquoise mineral ("turquoise sign").

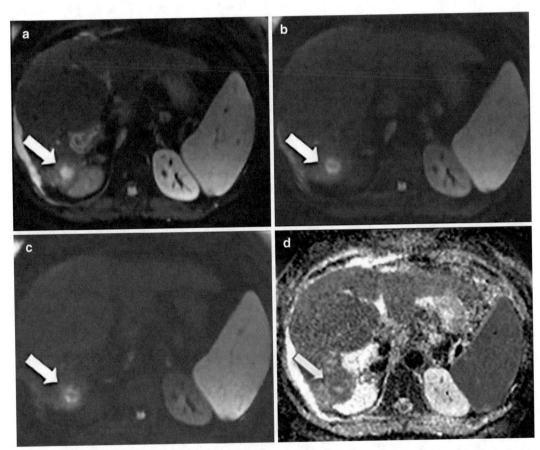

Fig. 7 (**a–c**) Axial diffusion-weighted MR image shows internal high signal intensity of the abscess (arrow) persisting even on high b-value, due to restricted water diffusion. (**d**) Corresponding ADC map demonstrates decreased water diffusivity as iso-hypointensity of the abscess; the inter necrotic liquid content of the abscess persists with high ADC value

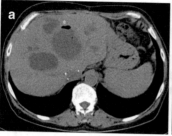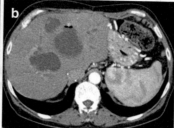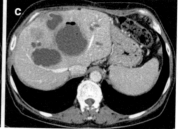

Fig. 8 Axial unenhanced (**a**) and contrast-enhanced hepati arterial (**b**) and portal venous phase (**c**) on CT of multiple abscesses localized in the right hepatic lobe. Gas (*) within the major abscess cavity is present

2 Inflammatory Pseudotumor of the Liver

2.1 Definition and General Features

Inflammatory pseudotumors (IPT), or inflammatory myofibroblastic liver tumors, are rare conditions characterized by exaggerated inflammatory response of unknown origin (Faraj et al. 2011).

IPT is believed to be, from some authors (Hedlund et al. 1999; Dehner 2000), a low-grade fibrosarcoma with inflammatory lymphomatous cells because it can be locally aggressive and multifocal and can progress occasionally to a true malignant tumor.

In some cases, IPT is thought to result from inflammation linked to trauma and surgery and other malignancies (Sanders et al. 2001; Maves et al. 1989), to immune-autoimmune mechanism (Stark et al. 1995), or to infection (Dehner 2000).

IPT presents feature of acute and chronic inflammation with accumulation of lymphocytes, plasma cells, myofibroblastic spindle cells, and collagen as fibrous reaction. Histiocytic cells seem to predominate in IPT linked to infections, whereas myofibroblastic cells characterize the lesions to be considered true neoplasms (Dehner 2000).

The lesions commonly relapses locally and rarely metastasize to distant sites; there are several studies of histologic predictors of aggressive behavior of IPT (presence of ganglion-like cells, p53 expression, aneuploidy, absence of ALK expression) (Hussong et al. 1999; Jiang et al.

2009; Coffin et al. 2007; Mariño-Enríquez et al. 2011); but there are case reports of spontaneous regression of IPT reflecting its inflammatory nature (Sugiyama and Nakajima 2008).

It was first observed in the lung by Brunn in 1939, while the term IPT was first mentioned in 1954 because the lesion can mimic a malignant tumor (Umiker and Iverson 1954).

IPT has been described most commonly in the lung (Patnana et al. 2012) but can be found also in the heart, head and neck, abdomen, pelvis, gastrointestinal tract, mesentery, omentum, retroperitoneum, hepatobiliary system, genitourinary tract, and soft tissues of trunk and extremities (Coffin et al. 1995).

IPT was first described in the liver in 1953 (Pack and Baker 1953).

It is more frequent in children and young adults, affects males more than females with a ratio of 8:1, (Horiuchi et al. 1990), and has a higher incidence in Asia.

Frequent symptoms are fever and abdominal pain with eventually portal hypertension and liver failure; sometimes signs of biliary obstruction as jaundice are present if porta hepatis or bile ducts are involved (Tang et al. 2010). Other symptoms include abdominal pain and weight loss.

Laboratory tests may be normal or present abnormalities like leukocytosis, elevated erythrocyte sedimentation rate, C-reactive protein, liver enzyme, and lactate dehydrogenase values (Horiuchi et al. 1990).

In some cases, liver IPT was associated with sclerosing cholangitis, phlebitis, retroperitoneal fibrosis (Torzilli et al. 2001), and immunosuppressive therapy after transplantation; Epstein-Barr virus has also been implicated (Pollock et al. 1995).

Spontaneous regression of hepatic IPT has been reported (Levy et al. 2001).

The knowledge of such entity is fundamental because it can affect treatment. In case of peripheral hepatic mass with recognized features of IPT and exclusion of malignancies, the patients can be treated with observation and nonsteroidal anti-inflammatory drugs. Sometimes the diagnosis is not clear and surgical resection may be required (Tang et al. 2010).

2.1.1 Multimodality Imaging

The imaging findings are heterogeneous, variable, and non-specific. IPT can present as a single or multifocal mass; most hepatic cases are solitary solid tumors, mainly arising from the right hepatic lobe. The most common differential diagnosis based on imaging is HCC (Figs. 9 and 10).

2.1.2 US

On ultrasound images, hepatic IPTs appear as hypo- or hyperechoic masses with well-defined or ill-defined margins (Horiuchi et al. 1990; Milias et al. 2009). They can have solid or cystic pattern with heterogeneous internal echotexture mimicking liver abscess or cystic lesions (Horiuchi et al. 1990; Milias et al. 2009; Celik et al. 2005). They can present multiple internal thin septae with posterior acoustic enhancement (Nam et al. 1996).

2.1.3 CT

On non-enhanced CT, IPTs present a low attenuation relative to the surrounding liver. They can show calcifications and present indistinct and irregular margins (Nam et al. 1996; Levy et al. 2001).

With contrast-enhanced CT imaging, they usually present a variable degree of portal venous enhancement that can show various patterns: heterogeneous enhancement, homogeneous enhancement, enhancement of septa, peripheral enhancement with delayed central filling; segments with no enhancement can be also present. Usually they can exhibit a degree of delayed peripheral enhancement probably related to the fibrous component of the lesion (Nam et al. 1996).

Central necrosis may occur in particular in larger lesions (Nam et al. 1996, Levy et al. 2001). Mass effect with dilatation of intrahepatic biliary tree may be present (Horiuchi et al. 1990, Milias et al. 2009).

2.1.4 MR

On MR images, these masses show variable pattern. They are usually hypointense in T1-weighted images and hyperintense in T2-weighted images. Heterogeneous enhancement after administration of gadolinium has been described with cases of delayed enhancement (Yan et al. 2001; Torzilli et al. 2001; Horiuchi et al. 1990).

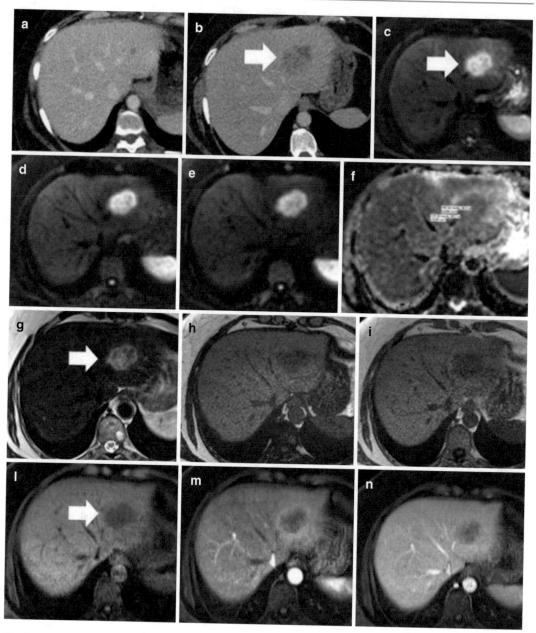

Fig. 9 Female 53 years old with previous resection of sigmoid carcinoma. (**a**, **b**) Contrast-enhanced CT, portal venous (**a**) and late phase (**b**). Evidence of hypodense lesion (arrow) on late phase (**c–r**) MR imaging. (**c–f**) Diffusion-weighted MR imaging with b = 0 (**c**), b = 400 (**d**), b = 800 (**e**), and ADC map (**f**). Evidence of signal restriction (arrow) on diffusion-weighted imaging. Lesion hyperintensity on T2-w images (**g**) and hypointensity on in-phase (**h**) and out-of-phase (**i**) T1-w MRI images (arrow). (**l**) Unenhanced and (**m–r**) contrast-enhanced MRI. Evidence of rim-like peripheral enhancement on arterial phase after gadoxetic acid injection (**m**). Evidence of lesion hypointensity on portal venous (**n**), transitional phase (**o–q**), and hepatobiliary phase (**r**). Surgical specimen analysis revealed granulomatous fibro-inflammatory lesion with lymphocyte infiltration (courtesy of Prof. Luigi Grazioli and Dr. Barbara Frittoli)

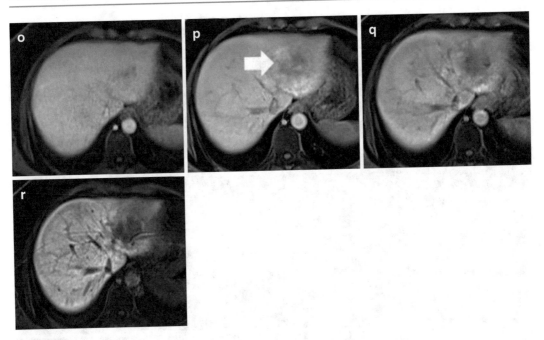

Fig. 9 (continued)

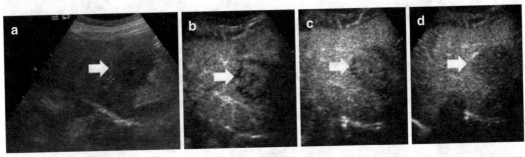

Fig. 10 (a–r) Male 30 years old with persistent epigastric pain and weight loss. (**a**) Unenhanced US. Single hypoechoic lesion (arrow) 5 cm in diameter. (**b–d**) Contrast-enhanced US. On arterial phase (**b**), there is clear enhancement (arrow) with evidence of contrast washout on portal venous (**c**) and late phase (**d**). Unenhanced (**e**) and contrast-enhanced CT (**f–h**). Enhancement pattern is not typical with evidence of lesion mild enhancement on arterial phase (**f**) and mild contrast washout on portal venous (**g**) and late phase (**h**) and evidence of peripheral hypodense rim. (**i–k**) MR imaging. Lesion hypointensity on in-phase (**i**) and out-of-phase (**j**) T1-w MRI (arrow) and lesion mild hyperintensity with central core hyperintensity on T2-w MRI (**k**). Unenhanced (**l**) and contrast-enhanced MRI (**m–p**). Evidence of mild enhancement on arterial phase after gadoxetic acid injection (**m**) with evidence of peripheral hypointense rim. Evidence of mild lesion hypointensity on portal venous (**n**), transitional phase (**o**), and hepatobiliary phase (**p**). Surgical specimen analysis revealed myofibroblastic inflammatory lesion with lymphocyte infiltration. After 6 months of antibiotic treatment, the lesion disappeared (courtesy of Prof. Luigi Grazioli and Dr. Barbara Frittoli)

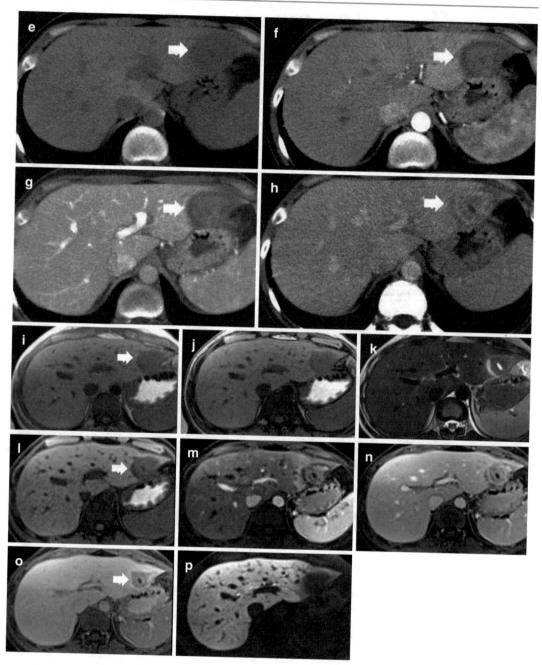

Fig. 10 (continued)

References

Alsaif HS, Venkatesh SK, Chan DS et al (2011) CT appearance of pyogenic liver abscesses caused by Klebsiella pneumoniae. Radiology 260:129–138

Ammann R, Münch R, Largiadèr F et al (1992) Pancreatic and hepatic abscesses: a late complication in 10 patients with chronic pancreatitis. Gastroenterology 103:560–565

Balci NC, Semelka RC, Noone TC et al (1999) Pyogenic hepatic abscesses: MRI findings on T1- and T2-weighted and serial gadolinium-enhanced gradient-echo images. J Magn Reson Imaging 9:285–290

Basilico R, Blomley MJ, Harvey CJ et al (2002) Which continuous US scanning mode is optimal for the detection of vascularity in liver lesions when enhanced with a second generation contrast agent? Eur J Radiol 41:184–191

Celik H, Ozdemir H, Yücel C et al (2005) Characterization of hyperechoic focal liver lesions: quantitative evaluation with pulse inversion harmonic imaging in the late phase of Levovist. J Ultrasound Med 24:39–47

Chan JH, Tsui EY, Luk SH et al (2001) Diffusion-weighted MR imaging of the liver: distinguishing hepatic abscess from cystic or necrotic tumor. Abdom Imaging 26:161–165

Chen CH, Wu SS, Chang HC et al (2014) Initial presentations and final outcomes of primary pyogenic liver abscess: a cross-sectional study. BMC Gastroenterol 14:133

Chen YC, Lin CH, Chang SN et al (2016) Epidemiology and clinical outcome of pyogenic liver abscess: an analysis from the National Health Insurance Research Database of Taiwan, 2000-2011. J Microbiol Immunol Infect 49:646–653

Coffin CM, Watterson J, Priest JR et al (1995) Extrapulmonary inflammatory myofibroblastic tumor (inflammatory pseudotumor): a clinicopathologic and immunohistochemical study of 84 cases. Am J Surg Pathol 19:859–872

Coffin CM, Hornick JL, Fletcher CD (2007) Inflammatory myofibroblastic tumor: comparison of clinicopathologic, histologic, and immunohistochemical features including ALK expression in atypical and aggressive cases. Am J Surg Pathol 31:509–520

Dehner LP (2000) The enigmatic inflammatory pseudotumors: the current state of understanding, or misunderstanding (editorial). J Pathol 192:277–279

Eltawansy SA, Merchant C, Atluri P et al (2015) Multi-organ failure secondary to a Clostridium perfringens liver abscess following a self-limited episode of acute gastroenteritis. Am J Case Rep 16:182–186

Faraj W, Ajouz H, Mukherji D et al (2011) Inflammatory pseudo-tumor of the liver: a rare pathological entity. World J Surg Oncol 9:5

Gabata T, Kadoya M, Matsui O et al (2001) Dynamic CT of hepatic abscesses: significance of transient segmental enhancement. AJR Am J Roentgenol 176:675–679

Halvorsen RA, Korobkin M, Foster WL et al (1984) The variable CT appearance of hepatic abscesses. AJR Am J Roentgenol 142:941–946

Hedlund GL, Navoi JF, Galliani GA et al (1999) Aggressive manifestation of inflammatory pulmonary pseudotumor in children. Pediatr Radiol 29:112–116

Horiuchi R, Uchida T, Kojima T et al (1990) Inflammatory pseudotumor of the liver. Clinicopathologic study and review of the literature. Cancer 65:1583–1590

Huang CJ, Pitt HA, Lipsett PA et al (1996) Pyogenic hepatic abscess. Changing trends over 42 years. Ann Surg 223:600–607

Huang SF, Ko CW, Chang CS et al (2003) Liver abscess formation after transarterial chemoembolization for malignant hepatic tumor. Hepatogastroenterology 50:1115–1118

Hui JY, Yang MK, Cho DH et al (2007) Pyogenic liver abscesses caused by Klebsiella pneumoniae: US appearance and aspiration findings. Radiology 242:769–776

Hussong JW, Brown M, Perkins SL et al (1999) Comparison of DNA ploidy, histologic, and immunohistochemical findings with clinical outcome in inflammatory myofibroblastic tumors. Mod Pathol 12:279–286

Iida H, Aihara T, Ikuta S et al (2014) Risk of abscess formation after liver tumor radiofrequency ablation: a review of 8 cases with a history of enterobiliary anastomosis. Hepatogastroenterology 61:1867–1870

Jeffrey RB Jr, Tolentino CS, Chang FC et al (1988) CT of pyogenic hepatic microabscesses: the cluster sign. AJR Am J Roentgenol 151:487–489

Jeong SW, Jang JY, Lee TH et al (2012) Cryptogenic pyogenic liver abscess as the herald of colon cancer. J Gastroenterol Hepatol 27:248–255

Jepsen P, Vilstrup H, Schønheyder HC et al (2005) A nationwide study of the incidence and 30-day mortality rate of pyogenic liver abscess in Denmark, 1977-2002. Aliment Pharmacol Ther 21:1185–1188

Jiang YH, Cheng B, Ge MH et al (2009) Comparison of the clinical and immunohistochemical features, including anaplastic lymphoma kinase (ALK) and p53, in inflammatory myofibroblastic tumours, J Int Med Res 37:867–877

Johannsen EC, Sifri CD, Madoff LC (2000) Pyogenic liver abscesses. Infect Dis Clin N Am 14:547–563

Kaplan GG, Gregson DB, Laupland KB (2004) Population-based study of the epidemiology of and the risk factors for pyogenic liver abscess. Clin Gastroenterol Hepatol 2:1032–1038

Keller JJ, Tsai MC, Lin CC et al (2013) Risk of infections subsequent to pyogenic liver abscess: a nationwide population-based study. Clin Microbiol Infect 19:717–722

Kumar D, Ramanathan S, Al Faki A et al (2015) Faecolith migrating from the appendix to produce liver abscess after subhepatic laparoscopic appendectomy. Trop Dr 45:241–244

Lardière-Deguelte S, Ragot E, Armoun K et al (2015) Hepatic abscess: diagnosis and management. J Visc Surg 152:231–243

Law ST, Li KK (2012) Is hepatic neoplasm-related pyogenic liver abscess a distinct clinical entity? World J Gastroenterol 18:1110–1116

Lee KT, Wong SR, Sheen PC (2001) Pyogenic liver abscess: an audit of 10 years' experience and analysis of risk factors. Dig Surg 18:459–465

Levy S, Sauvanet A, Diebold M et al (2001) Spontaneous regression of an inflammatory pseudotumor of the liver presenting as an obstructing malignant biliary tumor. Gastrointest Endosc 53:371–374

Li J, Fu Y, Wang JY et al (2010) Early diagnosis and therapeutic choice of Klebsiella pneumoniae liver abscess. Front Med China 4:308–316

Lin AC, Yeh DY, Hsu YH et al (2009) Diagnosis of pyogenic liver abscess by abdominal ultrasonography in the emergency department. Emerg Med J 26: 273–275

Liu GJ, Lu MD, Xie XY et al (2008) Real-time contrast-enhanced ultrasound imaging of infected focal liver lesions. J Ultrasound Med 27:657–666

Mariño-Enríquez A, Wang WL, Roy A et al (2011) Epithelioid inflammatory myofibroblastic sarcoma: an aggressive intra-abdominal variant of inflammatory myofibroblastic tumor with nuclear membrane or perinuclear ALK. Am J Surg Pathol 35:135–144

Mathieu D, Vasile N, Fagniez PL et al (1985) Dynamic CT features of hepatic abscesses. Radiology 154: 749–752

Maves CK, Johnson JF, Bove K et al (1989) Gastric inflammatory pseudotumor in children. Radiology 173:381–383

Mavilia MG, Molina M, Wu GY (2016) The evolving nature of hepatic abscess: a review. J Clin Transl Hepatol 4:158–168

Meddings L, Myers RP, Hubbard J et al (2010) A population-based study of pyogenic liver abscesses in the United States: incidence, mortality, and temporal trends. Am J Gastroenterol 105:117–124

Mendez RJ, Schiebler ML, Outwater EK et al (1994) Hepatic abscesses: MR imaging findings. Radiology 190:431–436

Milias K, Madhavan K, Bellamy C et al (2009) Inflammatory pseudotumors of the liver: experience of a specialist surgical unit. J Gastroenterol Hepatol 24:1562–1566

Mohsen AH, Green ST, Read RC et al (2002) Liver abscess in adults: ten years experience in a UK centre. QJM 95:797–802

Mølle I, Thulstrup AM, Vilstrup H et al (2001) Increased risk and case fatality rate of pyogenic liver abscess in patients with liver cirrhosis: a nationwide study in Denmark. Gut 48:260–263

Montvuagnard T, Thomson V, Durieux M et al (2012) A superinfection of focal liver lesions after bile duct procedures. Diagn Interv Imaging 93:e191–e195

Moore R, Shea DO, Geoghegan T et al (2013) Community-acquired Klebsiella pneumoniae liver abscess: an emerging infection in Ireland and Europe. Infection 41:681–686

Mortelé KJ, Segatto E, Ros PR (2004) The infected liver: radiologic-pathologic correlation. Radiographics 24:937–955

Murarka S, Pranav F, Dandavate V (2011) Pyogenic liver abscess secondary to disseminated Streptococcus anginosus from sigmoid diverticulitis. J Glob Infect Dis 3:79–81

Nam KJ, Kang HK, Lim JH (1996) Inflammatory pseudotumor of the liver: CT and sonographic findings. AJR Am J Roentgenol 167:485–487

Oto A, Akhan O, Ozmen M (1999) Focal inflammatory diseases of the liver. Eur J Radiol 32:61–75

Pack GT, Baker HW (1953) Total right hepatic lobectomy: report of a case. Ann Surg 138:253–258

Patnana M, Sevrukov AB, Elsayes KM (2012) Inflammatory pseudotumor: the great mimicker. AJR Am J Roentgenol 198:W217–W227

Pollock AN, Newman B, Putnam PE et al (1995) Imaging of post-transplant spindle cell tumors. Pediatr Radiol 25:S118–S121

Popescu A, Sporea I, Sirli R et al (2015) Does contrast enhanced ultrasound improve the management of liver abscesses? A single Centre experience. Med Ultrason 17:451–455

Rahimian J, Wilson T, Oram V et al (2004) Pyogenic liver abscess: recent trends in etiology and mortality. Clin Infect Dis 39:1654–1659

Ralls PW, Barnes PF, Radin DR et al (1987) Sonographic features of amebic and pyogenic abscesses: a blinded comparison. AJR Am J Roentgenol 149: 499–501

Reyna-Sepúlveda F, Hernández-Guedea MA, García-Hernández S et al (2017) Epidemiology and prognostic factors of liver abscess complications in northeastern Mexico. Medicina Universitaria 19:178–183

Sanders BM, West KW, Gingalewski C et al (2001) Inflammatory pseudotumor of the alimentary tract: clinical and surgical experience. J Pediatr Surg 36:169–173

Sharma A, Mukewar S, Mara KC et al (2018) Epidemiologic factors, clinical presentation, causes, and outcomes of liver abscess: a 35-year Olmsted County study. Mayo Clin Proc Innov Qual Outcomes 2:16–25

Shin JU, Kim KM, Shin SW et al (2014) A prediction model for liver abscess developing after transarterial chemoembolization in patients with hepatocellular carcinoma. Dig Liver Dis 46:813–817

Singh S, Chaudhary P, Saxena N et al (2013) Treatment of liver abscess: prospective randomized comparison of catheter drainage and needle aspiration. Ann Gastroenterol 26:332–339

Stark P, Sandbank JC, Rudnicki C et al (1995) Inflammatory pseudotumor of the heart with vasculitis and venous thrombosis. Chest 102:1884–1885

Sugiyama K, Nakajima Y (2008) Inflammatory myofibroblastic tumor in the mediastinum mimicking a malignant tumor. Diagn Interv Radiol 14:197–199

Sun Z, Li G, Ai X et al (2011) Hepatic and biliary damage after transarterial chemoembolization for malignant hepatic tumors: incidence, diagnosis, treatment, outcome and mechanism. Crit Rev Oncol Hematol 79:164–174

Tang L, Lai EC, Cong WM et al (2010) Inflammatory myofibroblastic tumor of the liver: a cohort study. World J Surg 34:309–313

Torzilli G, Inoue K, Midorikawa Y et al (2001) Inflammatory pseudotumors of the liver: prevalence and clinical impact in surgical patients. 48: 1118–1123

Turton JF, Englender H, Gabriel SN et al (2007) Genetically similar isolates of Klebsiella pneumoniae serotype K1 causing liver abscesses in three continents. J Med Microbiol 56:593–597

Umiker WO, Iverson LC (1954) Post inflammatory tumor of the lung: report of four cases simulating xanthoma, fibroma or plasma cell granuloma. J Thorac Surg 28:55–62

Wang YP, Liu CJ, Chen TJ et al (2015) Proton pump inhibitor use significantly increases the risk of cryptogenic liver abscess: a population-based study. Aliment Pharmacol Ther 41:1175–1181

Webb GJ, Chapman TP, Cadman PJ et al (2014) Pyogenic liver abscess. Frontline Gastroenterol 5:60–607

Yan FH, Zhou KR, Jiang YP et al (2001) Inflammatory pseudotumor of the liver: 13 cases of MRI findings. World J Gastroenterol 7:422–424

Infectious Liver Diseases and Parasitic Lesions

Ali Devrim Karaosmanoglu, Aycan Uysal,
and Musturay Karcaaltincaba

Contents

A. D. Karaosmanoglu · A. Uysal
M. Karcaaltincaba (✉)
Liver Imaging Team, Department of Radiology,
Hacettepe University School of Medicine,
Ankara, Turkey

Abstract

Infectious diseases of the liver include pyogenic and amebic abscesses and viral, fungal, parasitic and granulomatous infections. Imaging plays a fundamental role in diagnosis and follow-up of infectious liver diseases. All imaging modalities including ultrasonography, computed tomography, and magnetic resonance imaging may be helpful for detection and characterization of most hepatic infections. In certain patients, imaging may provide very specific signs to characterize the pathogen and confidently exclude other non-infectious clinical entities with similar imaging features.

1 Introduction

Hepatic infections are among the diseases in which prompt diagnosis and treatment are crucial for preventing potentially devastating outcomes. Pyogenic and amebic abscesses are the most common forms of liver infections; however, infections due to fungal and parasitic agents are not uncommon. The infectious organisms may gain access into the liver by several ways. Hematogenous seeding, ascending infection from the biliary tract, or direct external inoculation during trauma should be mentioned among the common routes.

As for the source organisms, the demographics of the liver infections are also diverse. Although *Entamoeba histolytica* is globally the most common causative organism for liver abscesses, pyogenic infections are the most common form of liver abscesses in the developed world. Adding more to the confusion, some parasites that are highly uncommon in the other parts of the world are endemic in certain countries, which are located in Asia, Africa, and South America.

Prompt diagnosis and early intervention, whether it is surgical, medical, or percutaneous, are the most crucial factors for a favorable clinical outcome in the victims. This situation is even more important in patients with pyogenic abscesses or fungal infections, as these diseases are almost uniformly fatal if left untreated.

Cross-sectional imaging revolutionized the diagnosis of the liver infections. With the support of the suggestive patient history and demographic findings, the diagnosis can be made promptly and efficiently.

2 Pyogenic Liver Abscess

2.1 Clinical Findings

The most common routes of pyogenic liver abscesses in the western hemisphere are the ascending biliary infections and hematogenous dissemination from other infectious sources, like the diverticulitis and appendicitis. Historically, pyogenic liver abscesses were regarded as a fatal disease; however, with the advance of the diagnostic tools and antibiotic treatments, the mortality rates have now significantly improved. In an early review of 470 patients with pyogenic liver abscesses, diagnosed between 1954 and 1979, the mortality rate was as high as 57% (McDonald and Howard 1980), while more recent studies demonstrated mortality rates around 15% for single liver abscesses and 41% for multifocal liver abscesses (Ralls 1998). Lower mortality rates have also been described around 2% (1/54 patients) in newer studies (Stain et al. 1991). The highest mortality rates were reported among the elderly patients with underlying malignancies who develop multiple liver abscesses from septicemia (Land et al. 1985). Pyogenic liver abscesses may present as solitary or multifocal lesions, while solitary pyogenic liver abscesses are generally cryptogenic with no identifiable underlying source. In patients with multiple abscesses, hematogenous dissemination from the gastrointestinal tract, generalized septicemia, or ascending biliary infections should be considered (Mortele et al. 2004). While appendicitis is the leading underlying abnormality in the pre-antibiotic era, biliary tract diseases, underlying malignancy, trauma, or surgery should be counted among the common reasons in today's medicine (Ralls 1998).

The diagnosis may sometimes be problematic, and a delay in the diagnosis is the main contributing factor to increased patient morbidity and mortality. Clinical findings may be deceptive and indolent, without any signs or symptoms. Fever is not universal and may be seen in less than half of the patients (Halvorsen et al. 1984). Patients may present with non-specific and vague symptoms like weight loss, malaise, vomiting, anorexia, or fatigue (Benedetti et al. 2008). Common causative agents are *Escherichia coli* and *Klebsiella pneumoniae*; however, polymicrobial infections are common and detected in more than half of the cases (Benedetti et al. 2008). The blood cultures are negative in a significant portion of the patients, and the biochemical studies generally don't point any specific agent.

2.2 Imaging Findings

Advance of the new, fast, and reliable cross-sectional imaging modalities had revolutionized the diagnosis of pyogenic liver abscesses. With the accumulation of the experience and the widespread availability, pyogenic liver abscess is today a generally straightforward diagnosis, especially in the setting of suggestive clinical history.

2.2.1 Computed Tomography

Computed tomography (CT) is the single most common and successful method for diagnosing liver abscesses with a remarkable sensitivity as high as 97% (Ros et al. 2015). Several CT features of the pyogenic liver abscesses had been described in the literature (Kim et al. 2007a, b). CT is the preferred imaging modality in patients with open abdominal wounds and multiple surgical drains. The classical imaging finding on CT is a low attenuation round mass with well-defined borders. The lesions can be single, multiple, loculated, or non-loculated. The so-called cluster sign is the most characteristic finding (Fig. 1). This sign basically refers to coalescence of several neighboring infectious foci into a single, larger cavity (Jeffrey et al. 1984). In the wall of some abscesses, a high attenuation inner ring and a low attenuation outer zone, due to perilesional parenchymal edema, surrounding the abscess cavity may be detected, known as the "double target" sign (Halvorsen et al. 1984). The presence of gas within the cavity is another sign, which is highly suggestive of an abscess. Gas may be seen

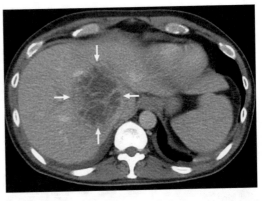

Fig. 1 A 34-year-old man hospitalized for perforated appendicitis. Abdominal US revealed a heterogenous, partly ill-defined mass within right liver parenchyma. Axial postcontrast abdominal CT image showed multi-loculated, heterogenously enhancing, hypodense lesion (arrows) consistent with a liver abscess. Percutaneous drainage revealed pus and the patient placed on IV antibiotic treatment

as an air-fluid level or scattered bubbles, but is seen to be present in only 20% of the patients (Halvorsen et al. 1984). The presence of gas had generally been regarded as suggestive of *Klebsiella pneumoniae* abscesses (Chou et al. 1995; Yang et al. 1993); however, this notion has been challenged in a different study (Kim et al. 2007a). The presence of gas within the abscess cavities tends to be more common in patients with diabetes (Fig. 2). There are also other helpful imaging clues for *Klebsiella pneumoniae* abscesses that were reported in the imaging literature. "Septal breakage" sign refers to arborizing patterns of septa within the abscess cavity, and the "turquoise" sign refers to numerous septal breakages. The "hair ball sign" defines a tangled pattern of blurring amorphous hairlike content within the abscess cavity (Kim et al. 2007a). The abscesses may also be named based on their sizes, where lesions smaller than 2 cm are called as microabscesses and larger lesions are named as macroabscesses (Fig. 3) (Mortele et al. 2004).

Amebic abscess, fungal and parasitic abscesses, hematoma, cystadenoma/cystadenocarcinoma, necrotic metastases, and liver infarct

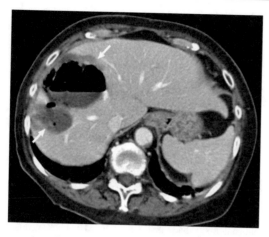

Fig. 2 A 59-year-old woman with uncontrolled type 2 diabetes presented with right upper quadrant pain and fever. Abdominal US study shows thick-walled cystic lesion with fluid content. Postcontrast abdominal CT image demonstrated a large, bilobulated lesion with air-fluid level within right hepatic lobe consistent with a liver abscess (arrows). Also note peripheral hypodense area representing parenchymal edema. Percutaneous drainage revealed pus, and cultures grew *Klebsiella pneumoniae*

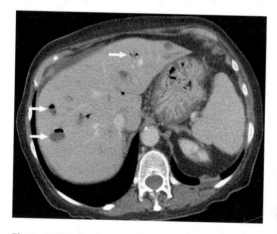

Fig. 3 A 68-year-old woman who has undergone Whipple surgery due to pancreatic cancer now presenting with abdominal pain, fever, and septicemia. Axial postcontrast abdominal CT image shows multiple, small-sized, hypodense lesions (arrows) containing air-fluid levels. Findings were consistent with parenchymal microabscesses

2.2.2 Ultrasound

Ultrasound (US) is another commonly utilized modality. It is a robust and highly efficient modality; however, its use may be difficult in patients who have large body mass. In early post-surgical period, it may be difficult to scan the patients with US due to multiple bandages and surgical drains. The bowel distension, which is not uncommon in the setting of an intraabdominal infection, may also further decrease the sensitivity of the study. The pyogenic abscesses are generally detected as focal hypoechoic lesions in the liver parenchyma; however, the appearance of an abscess may be highly variable in different patients. It is not uncommon to detect the collection as a complex multiseptated mass with minimal fluid content (Fig. 4). Color Doppler sonography may be helpful by outlining the hyperemic ring in the periphery of the abscess with absence of vascularity inside the collection. Intense echogenicity due to gas accumulation within the lesion may also be problematic and sometimes even may end up completely overlooking the lesion, especially in abscesses from *Klebsiella pneumoniae* and *Clostridium* (Hui et al. 2007). Special attention must be paid in the setting of a gangrenous cholecystitis, as abscesses

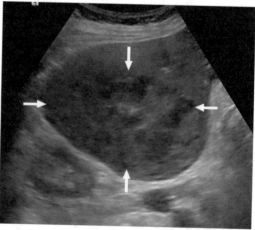

Fig. 4 A 46-year-old woman who was operated for perforated appendicitis a week ago now presenting with right upper quadrant pain and fever. Abdominal US image shows a large, complex, heterogenous, predominantly hypoechoic lesion (arrows) within the right liver lobe suggestive for a liver abscess. Subsequent abdominal CT scan confirmed this putative diagnosis. Image-guided percutaneous drainage revealed pus

in transplanted kidneys may all mimic pyogenic liver abscesses. Accurate diagnosis may be extremely difficult in certain situations, especially in patients with vague clinical symptoms. Percutaneous aspiration may be used for diagnosis in these cases.

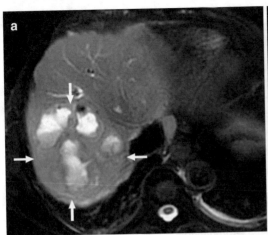

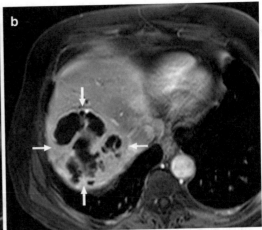

Fig. 5 A 66-year-old man who has been hospitalized recently for acute diverticulitis started to complain with right upper quadrant pain and resistant fever. (**a**) Axial T2W MR image demonstrates multiloculated, thick-walled hyperintense lesion (arrows). (**b**) Axial postcon- trast T1W MR image of the same patient demonstrates intense peripheral enhancement with internal fluid content (arrows). Image-guided percutaneous drainage revealed pus

may easily be missed due to sound wave attenuation from the gas (Benedetti et al. 2008).

2.2.3 Magnetic Resonance Imaging

The imaging findings of pyogenic abscesses are variable in the magnetic resonance imaging (MRI) studies. Although, MRI is generally not the first imaging method employed in the evaluation of these patients, its increasing popularity and application in abdominal imaging mandates the radiologists to make themselves familiarize with the findings of liver abscesses. These lesions are generally of low intensity in T1- and high on T2-weighted (T2W) images (Mendez et al. 1994; Schmiedl et al. 1988). The cluster sign is the most specific finding for a pyogenic liver abscess, as in CT (Fig. 5). Diffuse enhancement of the cavity wall may be suggestive for an abscess (Doyle et al. 2006). The presence of air may be detected as signal-void areas on T1-weighted (T1W) images, which become more prominent on in-phase images compared to out-of-phase T1W images due to magnetic susceptibility. Perilesional T2 hyperintense edema has been detected in 50% of the patients, but this finding may be unreliable, as this can also be detected in only 20–30% of the primary and secondary liver malignancies (Fig. 6) (Pastakia et al. 1988).

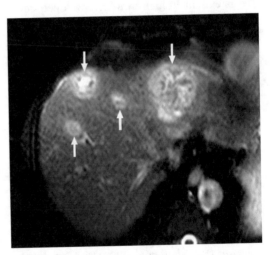

Fig. 6 A 63-year-old man with a history of bladder cancer and known choledocholitiasis now presenting with right upper quadrant pain, fever, and elevated liver function tests. T2W abdominal MR image demonstrated multiple, centrally hyperintense lesions (arrows) consistent with an inner cystic or a necrotic content. Also note perilesional hyperintensity consistent with parenchymal edema. Percutaneous aspiration and drainage revealed pus

3 Amebic Liver Abscess

3.1 Clinical Findings

Amebic liver abscess is caused by the protozoan *Entamoeba histolytica* and is a very common pathogen, especially in India, Africa, Far East, and Central and South Americas. It has been assumed that 10% of the world population is infected with this agent (Ralls 1998). Although in most of the patients it is clinically silent, it may be highly symptomatic and fatal in certain individuals. An estimated 40,000–100,000 people die yearly from amebiasis, making it the second most common leading cause of death among parasitic diseases (Walsh 1988). Although the disease symptoms have been known since the ancient times, the pathogen could be isolated only in 1875 by a physician from St. Petersburg, Fedor Aleksandrovich Losch, in the stool and the colonic ulcerations of a fatal dysentery case (Lösch 1875).

Unlike many other protozoans, *E. histolytica* has a simple life cycle, and humans seem to be their natural hosts. The prevalence of the infection is extremely high in underdeveloped countries, where the barriers between the human feces and food and water are inadequate (Stanley 2003). Although amebiasis most commonly results in asymptomatic colonization of the gastrointestinal tract, it can also cause hepatic disease by the ascension into the portal venous system. Liver involvement is the second most common location of the parasites after the intestines. Fever, right upper quadrant pain, and diarrhea are the most common symptoms. Another distinguishing feature of amebic liver abscess is its tendency to cause solitary abscess in most of the patients, in contrast to pyogenic liver abscesses, which tend to be multifocal in 50% of the cases (Benedetti et al. 2008). Enzyme immunoassays are very useful in the diagnosis with sensitivities up to 99% and specificities of greater than 90% (Hughes and Petri 2000).

3.2 Imaging Findings

US and CT are the most commonly employed modalities for the diagnosis and are quite sensitive for correct identification of the disease. Imaging features, alone, may not be sensitive, and it may be hard to reliably differentiate them from the pyogenic liver abscesses. Needle aspiration may be helpful in some patients, especially who are negative serologically in the early phases of the disease (first 7–10 days).

3.2.1 Ultrasonography

In general, sonography is the first imaging choice in patients with a clinical suspicion of liver abscesses. This point may be even more valid in cases of amebic liver abscesses. There are well-defined sonographic diagnostic criteria for amebic liver abscesses (Ralls et al. 1982):

1. Absence of significant wall echoes
2. Oval or rounded shape
3. Homogenous abscess content with low-level internal echoes
4. Location near or touching the liver capsule
5. Enhanced through transmission of the sound waves deep to the lesion

However, only 30% of proved amebic abscesses demonstrate all these five features (Fig. 7a). Target pattern may also be detected with a dense echogenic center and a hypoechoic periphery (Ralls et al. 1982). During the first 2 weeks of treatment, the imaging findings may even look worse with enlargement of the index lesion (Landay et al. 1980). Successfully treated lesions may be anechoic or calcified (Landay et al. 1980; Ralls et al. 1983).

3.2.2 Computed Tomography and MRI

Classical CT appearance is round to oval hypodense lesion with well-defined borders. The lesion is almost always of fluid attenuation. A very helpful imaging finding, although not specific, is the detection of the enhancing wall (3–15 mm) and a peripheral zone of edema (Fig. 7b) (Mortele et al. 2004). The appearance of the collection is highly variable with septations, fluid-debris levels, and, rarely, gas or hemorrhage (Radin et al. 1988).

MR imaging findings are similar to CT findings. Classically, the lesion is detected as a well-circumscribed lesion with wall enhancement on dynamic imaging.

Pyogenic infections, necrotic metastases, cystadenoma, cystadenocarcinoma, hematoma,

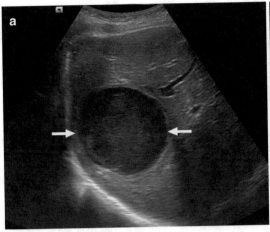
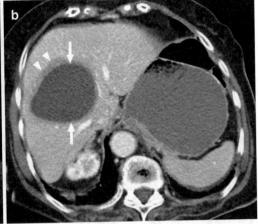

Fig. 7 A 70-year-old woman with a recent history of travel to North Africa presented with malaise, right upper quadrant pain, and subclinical fever. (**a**) Abdominal US shows a well-defined, round-shaped, peripherally located, cystic mass (arrows) with internal echoes. (**b**) Axial post-contrast CT image demonstrates the same lesion as well-defined hypodense cystic mass (arrows) with peripheral hypodense rim (arrowheads) suggestive of neighboring parenchymal edema. Image-guided percutaneous drainage confirmed hepatic amebic abscess

and infarction may all be confused with amebic abscesses. Epidemiologic and clinical information are the key sources of information for accurate diagnosis. Associated thickening of the cecum (although concomitant involvement with the liver is rare) and elevation of the right hemidiaphragm are important clues for the diagnosis. Individuals may present with amebic liver abscess after months to years of their travel to endemic areas; therefore, careful history with special attention, even to the minute details, is of fundamental importance. Atelectasis and transudative pleural effusion, especially on the right side, are common findings. The presence of treatment-resistant cough, pleuritic chest pain, and respiratory distress are among the signs of pleuropulmonary amebiasis, which typically appears after abscess rupture into the chest cavity through the diaphragm (which occurs in 7–20% of the patients) (Stanley 2003). Rupture of the liver abscess into the peritoneum is another serious clinical situation which occurs in 2–7% of the patients with liver involvement. Sudden onset of peritonitis and shock are typical clinical findings in peritoneal rupture (Stanley 2003). Pericardial rupture and subsequent cardiac tamponade are rare and most commonly detected in left-sided amebic liver abscesses. This is a very serious clinical condition with a mortality rate of 30% (Adams and Macleod 1977).

Urogenital and central nervous system involvements are rare and have been reported as anecdotal case reports (Stanley 2003).

4 Acute Cholangitis

Acute bacterial cholangitis (ABC) is the bacterial inflammation of the biliary system. Fever, pain, and jaundice, also called as Charcot's triad, are characteristic clinical symptoms. If not treated properly, the symptoms may quickly progress to diffuse septicemia and metabolic shock. Biliary system obstruction due to calculi is the most common underlying cause, which is detected in around 80% of the cases (Csendes et al. 1992). Instrumentation of the biliary system, obstructing malignant disease, and sclerosing cholangitis may be mentioned among the other causes (Catalano et al. 2009).

Imaging is critical for detecting the underlying abnormality and suggestive biliary and parenchymal features. Biliary obstruction is typical in obstructive cases of ABC. Associated wall thickening, that is typically smooth and symmetric, is present in 85% of the cases (Bader et al. 2001).

Postcontrast enhancement of the intrahepatic bile duct walls is another characteristic imaging finding (Fig. 8) and has been reported in 92% of the cases in patients who are evaluated with MR imaging (Fig. 9), most prominent in delayed-phase fat-suppressed sequences after contrast injection (Catalano et al. 2009).

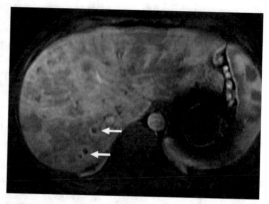

Fig. 10 A 52-year-old man with known pancreatic adenocarcinoma now presenting with right upper quadrant pain, chills, and fever. Abdominal US revealed mild dilatation of the intrahepatic bile ducts and several small-sized hypoechoic lesions within liver parenchyma. Axial postcontrast T1W MR image demonstrates heterogenous enhancement of the liver parenchyma and small peripherally enhancing lesions (arrows) within the right liver lobe which were later confirmed to be microabscesses on post IV antibiotic treatment scan

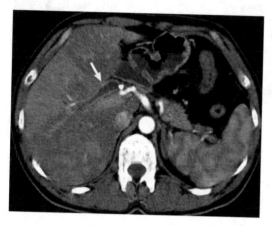

Fig. 8 A 44-year-old man with a history of recently implanted plastic biliary stent for pancreatic adenocarcinoma now presenting with right upper quadrant pain and fever. Blood count showed leukocytosis. Axial postcontrast arterial phase image demonstrates dilatation, wall thickening, and enhancement of the main bile duct (arrow). Also note heterogenous enhancement of the liver parenchyma in arterial phase

Parenchymal changes are also common in patients with ABC, and this association is most likely related to the extension of the inflammatory reaction into the periportal areas. Dilation of the peribiliary plexus and increased arterial blood flow have also been implicated in the etiology (Bader et al. 2001; Arai et al. 2003). MRI is more sensitive to detect these changes, and increased signal intensity on T2W images (mostly wedge-shaped or around the peribiliary areas) is typical. On postcontrast imaging, parenchymal changes appear to be most prominent on arterial phase (Fig. 10). Liver abscesses and portal vein thrombosis may be detected in a subgroup of patients with ABC (Bader et al. 2001). Magnetic resonance cholangiopancreatography (MRCP) is the preferred test to detect choledochal stones and is superior to CT in this regard.

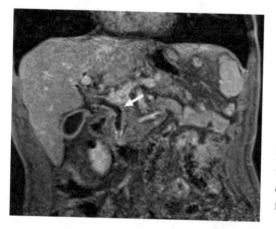

Fig. 9 A 75-year-old man with a remote history of gastrectomy for gastric lymphoma and cholelithiasis now presenting with jaundice, rigors, and fever. Blood tests revealed leukocytosis and elevated liver function tests. Coronal reformatted postcontrast T1W image demonstrates pronounced mural enhancement of the main bile duct (arrow)

5 Acute Viral Hepatitis

Acute viral hepatitis is most commonly caused by hepatitis A, B, C, or E viruses. Clinical manifestations may be highly variable from no symptoms to fever, abdominal discomfort, and jaundice (Ryder and Beckingham 2001). The diagnosis is mostly based on clinical symptomatology, serologic studies, or histopathology, and imaging does not play a major role in the diagnosis. Despite this seemingly secondary role of imaging, cross-sectional studies are commonly used to rule out other clinical conditions that may present with similar symptomatology such as cirrhosis, biliary obstruction, and metastatic liver disease (Bächler et al. 2016).

US findings are mostly non-specific but include hepatomegaly and diffuse decrease in parenchymal echogenicity, which results in relatively increased echogenicity of the portal triads (a situation also called as the "starry sky" pattern) (Bächler et al. 2016; Kurtz et al. 1980). Periportal edema, heterogenous parenchymal enhancement, and gallbladder wall edema and thickening are other commonly detected imaging findings on CT and MRI studies (Mortele et al. 2004).

6 Fungal Infection

6.1 Clinical Findings

Hepatic fungal infections are opportunistic infections and most commonly occur after prolonged neutropenia in leukemic patients under chemotherapy. Several fungal organisms may be counted among the causative organisms, where *Candida* is the most common followed by *Aspergillus*, *Cryptococcus*, *Histoplasma*, and *Mucor*. Infections with *Aspergillus* have also been reported sporadically (Eckburg and Montoya 2001). The fungus likely enters the bloodstream via the breakdown of the gastrointestinal mucosa (Benedetti et al. 2008). The initial manifestation is of neutropenic fever that does not clinically respond to conventional antibiotics. At this stage, the laboratory and imaging findings may be normal due to the inability of the patient to mount an inflammatory reaction. Once the neutrophil counts begin to recover, imaging findings may appear in the liver and/or the spleen.

6.1.1 Ultrasonography

US is almost always the first utilized imaging modality. It can be performed at the bedside, without putting the already infection-prone patient to additional risks of microbial exposure during the travel to CT or MR unit. The diagnostic accuracy of US may be high, especially in experienced hands. Four patterns of hepatic fungal infection were described on US (Pastakia et al. 1988):

1. Uniform hypoechoic nodule (Fig. 11a)
2. Echogenic nidus (inflammation) with hypoechoic rim (fibrosis) ("bull's eye")
3. Diffusely echogenic lesion
4. Central echogenic nidus (necrotic fungal debris), inner hyperechoic ring (inflammatory cells), and peripheral hypoechoic ring (fibrosis) ("wheel-within-a-wheel" appearance).

The first pattern is the least specific one, which may also be seen in lymphomatous or leukemic liver involvement and other solid organ metastases. In general, wheel-within-a-wheel pattern and bull's eye pattern are detected in the active phase of infection, and relatively normal white blood cell counts are common. The other two patterns are seen in the late phases of the disease and may also represent resolution (Ralls 1998; Pastakia et al. 1988).

6.1.2 Computed Tomography

Contrast-enhanced CT is a very sensitive examination for diagnosing the fungal microabscesses. On CT, they are seen as low attenuation lesions with discrete margins. They are rarely larger than 20 mm in some patients, and target appearance may be seen with a central focus of high attenuation (Pastakia et al. 1988). Peripheral enhancing rim may be detected in some patients and likely represent compressed adjacent liver parenchyma. CT is also useful in the follow-up of the patients by demonstrating the resolution of the lesions. Chemotherapy may be resumed after documentation of the disappearance of the microabscesses by CT. Persistence of splenic abscesses, despite anti-fungal therapy, is associated with a mortality rate of 60% (Berlow et al. 1984).

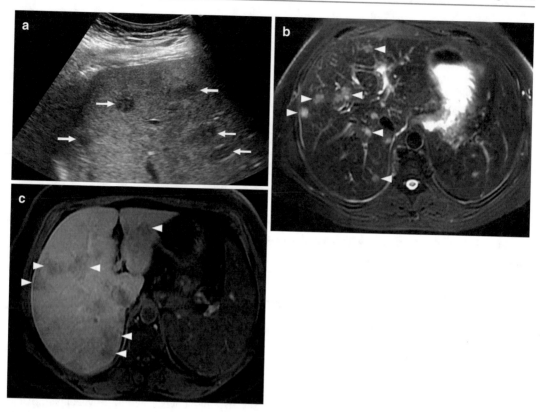

Fig. 11 A 43-year-old woman with leukemia who is currently undergoing inpatient chemotherapy treatment now presenting with high fever, malaise, and elevated liver function tests. (**a**) Abdominal US showed multiple well-defined hypoechoic lesions (arrows). (**b**) Axial T2W MR image of the same patient demonstrates multiple, brightly hyperintense lesions with well-defined borders (arrowheads). (**c**) Axial postcontrast T1W image shows multiple hypointense lesions (arrowheads). Percutaneous biopsy revealed active inflammation, and microbiologic evaluation of the specimen was consistent with *Candida* infection

6.1.3 MR Imaging

The MR imaging appearances are not specific. The lesions tend to be minimally hypointense on T1- and brightly hyperintense on T2W sequences (Fig. 11b, c) (Mortele et al. 2004). Completely treated lesions are minimally hypointense on T1- and isointense to mildly hyperintense on T2W images (Semelka et al. 1992). They may demonstrate gadolinium enhancement on delayed phases (Fig. 12). Addition of short tau inversion recovery sequence has been reported to increase the sensitivity in the detection of the focal abscesses (Antilla et al. 1996).

Definitive diagnosis of the fungal infections may be difficult. The blood culture is positive in only 20% of the patients (Masood and Sallah 2005). In some patients, liver biopsy may be necessary to confirm the diagnosis. The nidus

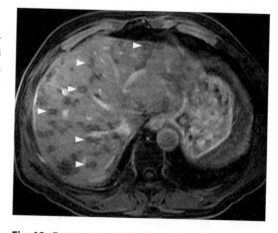

Fig. 12 Posttreatment follow-up study of a 45-year-old male patient with a history of leukemia and hepatic candidiasis. Axial postcontrast T1W image shows multiple, small-sized hypointense nodules demonstrating central enhancement suggestive of resolution phase of the disease (arrowheads)

of the infection should be sampled in biopsy for correct diagnosis (Masood and Sallah 2005).

7 Granulomatous Infections

By definition, granulomatous diseases of the liver are defined as inflammatory processes of the liver associated with granuloma formation in the liver parenchyma. The definitive diagnosis is almost always made with tissue analysis. Histologically, they appear as sharply defined nodular infiltrates consisting of aggregates of epithelioid cells or macrophages. In tuberculosis, the granulomas may undergo central liquefaction necrosis (Balci et al. 2001). Tuberculosis and histoplasmosis are the most common granulomatous infections of the liver.

7.1 Tuberculosis

Tuberculosis (TB) is among the most common and fatal infectious diseases of the world, especially in the developing countries. The liver may be involved in tuberculosis in different ways: (1) disseminated miliary TB, (2) primary nodular TB only involving the liver, and (3) primary TB abscess or granulomas of the liver (Jain et al. 1999; Hickey et al. 1999). Miliary form is the most commonly detected form of the disease and is reported to occur in 50–80% of the patients with terminal pulmonary tuberculosis (Mortele et al. 2004). Micronodular liver involvement may be seen as hyperechoic on US, or the liver may be seen as overall hyperechoic and enlarged (Hulnick et al. 1985). CT findings are not specific, and the liver may be enlarged or normal in size with/without micronodules (Fig. 13). When nodules are present, they are frequently very small, measuring between 0.5 and 2 mm, and difficult to detect with CT (Doyle et al. 2006). Diffuse calcification occurs in 50% of the cases with healing (Alvarez 1998). In cases where imaging findings are absent or non-specific, liver

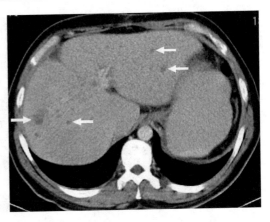

Fig. 13 A 45-year-old man with a history of pulmonary miliary tuberculosis now presents with mild fever, fatigue, and elevated liver function tests. Axial postcontrast abdominal CT image demonstrates multiple, small, hypodense lesions (arrows) within the liver parenchyma which were later confirmed to represent hepatic TB nodules on percutaneous biopsy

biopsy may be used for diagnosis in selected cases (Mortele et al. 2004). On MR imaging, tuberculomas may appear as hypointense on T1- and hypo-isointense on T2W images (Fig. 14) (Hickey et al. 1999).

Abscess formation in tuberculosis is rare (Fig. 15). Abdominal pain, fever, weight loss, anorexia, night sweats, and jaundice have all been reported among the clinical manifestations of the patients (Oliva et al. 1990). It is also a well-known fact that the liver TB abscesses may form even after the start of therapy for the treatment of extrahepatic tuberculosis (Gracey 1965).

7.2 Histoplasmosis

Histoplasmosis of the liver is rare, and almost all of the patients (99%) exposed to histoplasmosis develop subclinical infection (Mortele et al. 2004). In acute setting, hepatomegaly may be detected with accompanying hypoattenuated lymph nodes. Liver involvement is not uncommon in disseminated histoplasmosis. Small punctate calcifications may be detected in the liver of healed patients.

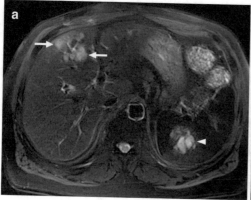

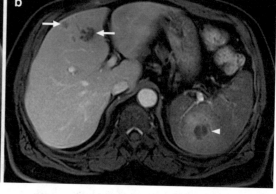

Fig. 14 A 70-year-old man with a remote history of lung tuberculosis now presents with right upper quadrant pain, fever, and night sweats. Abdominal US showed a hypoechoic lesion within the right liver parenchyma. (**a**) Axial T2W MR image shows clustering, hyperintense lesions (arrows). (**b**) Axial postcontrast T1W MR image shows peripheral enhancement within these lesions (arrows). Also note the lesion in the splenic parenchyma with the same imaging features. Percutaneous biopsy of the liver lesion confirmed hepatic TB granuloma

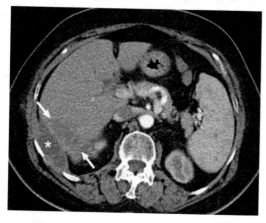

Fig. 15 A 62-year-old woman with no significant past medical history now presents with recently gradually increasing right upper quadrant pain, fever, and night sweats. Axial postcontrast abdominal CT image demonstrates peripherally located, ill-defined, hypoechoic liver lesion (arrows) and an adjacent perihepatic fluid collection (asterisk). Percutaneous drainage of the fluid collection confirmed active TB infection

8 Parasitic Infections

8.1 Ecchinococcal Infection

Hydatid disease is a worldwide zoonosis due to the larval form of the *Echinococcus* tapeworm (Pedrosa et al. 2000). After ingestion of the contaminated food or water, the eggs start to hatch in the duodenum, and the parasites penetrate the intestinal mucosa. After this penetration the pathogen gains access into the portal circulation and subsequently spread throughout the body. The liver is the most commonly affected organ; however, virtually every organ system has been reported to be involved, especially with *Echinococcus granulosus*. *Echinococcus granulosus* is the most common cause of the infection followed by *Echinococcus multilocularis* and *Echinococcus vogeli* which has been reported in Central and South America. The cyst rupture is the most important potential complication of the disease, which may end up with anaphylaxis and dissemination of the disease (Czermak et al. 2008).

8.1.1 *E. granulosus* Infection

E. granulosus infection is endemic in the Mediterranean Basin. Humans are infected by ingesting the food contaminated by the parasite or from contact with the dogs. Sheep are the intermediate hosts, while dogs and foxes are the definitive hosts. Humans may become the intermediate hosts by ingesting the eggs infested with larvae, also called as the oncospheres. The ingested embryos proceed to the liver by the portal venous system. Although most of these embryos are filtered and eliminated by the liver, some surviving embryos may cause the infection. Infected patients may be asymptomatic for many years when these cysts are small in size. With the gradual expansion of these cysts, patients may begin to experience abdominal pain, right upper quadrant mass, or obstructive jaundice when the cysts get large enough to compress or open into the biliary system.

In the liver, the cyst consists of (a) outer pericyst, which corresponds to the compressed and fibrosed liver tissue; (b) endocyst, an inner germinal layer; and (c) ectocyst, the thin, translucent interleaved membrane located in between the endocyst and pericyst (Mortele et al. 2004). Brood capsules (germinating cyst) and daughter cysts develop from the inner surface of the endocyst. The cysts expand slowly over years and when the brood capsules rupture the viable protoscoleces form (which are seen as white sediments floating within the cyst fluid, also called as hydatid sand) (Eckert and Deplazes 2004).

8.1.1.1 Ultrasound

E. granulosus cysts may have a laminar appearance of the thick cyst wall, which is visualized as "double-line" sign (Czermak et al. 2008). Freefloating protoscoleces (hydatid sand) in the cysts may be observed as "snowflake" on sonography ("snowflake" becomes even more prominent when the patient is repositioned) (Fig. 16).

Daughter cysts are observed in 75% of patients and may be observed as "wheel-like," "rosette-like," or "honeycomb-like" structures (Czermak et al. 2008). Daughter cysts are the most sensitive sonographic finding, and sonography is the most sensitive modality for the detection of membranes, septa, and hydatid sand (Fig. 17) (Oto et al. 1999). When the viability of the parasite is lost, intracystic pressure decreases, and the endocytic membrane detaches from the wall and float freely within the cyst fluid. The observation of floating membranes in the cyst gives rise to "water lily" appearance (Fig. 18). These cysts represent a transitional form in which the integrity of the cyst has been compromised (Czermak et al. 2008). Degenerated cysts consist of heterogenous, solid-looking pseudotumor that may look like a "ball of wool" as the cyst gradually shrinks and degenerates (Fig. 19). Finally, inactive dead cysts demonstrate heavy wall calcifications. Wall calcifications with intense posterior shadowing due to acoustic attenuation are detected in 50% of the cases (Mortele et al. 2004; Doyle et al. 2006).

The World Health Organization Informal Working Group on Echinococcus has published classification of echinococcosis, which is based on sonographic findings relating to the viability of the hydatid cyst (WHO Informal Working Group 2003).

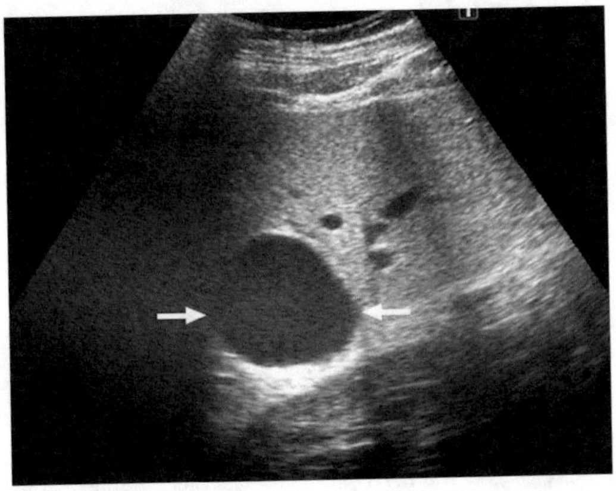

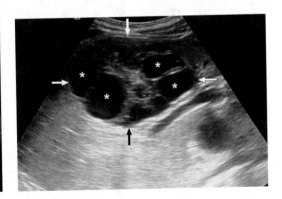

Fig. 16 A 29-year-old man with no known medical history underwent an abdominal US for right flank pain. Abdominal US study demonstrates a well-defined purely cystic mass (arrows) within the liver parenchyma. Serologic tests and percutaneous drainage confirmed hydatid cyst

Fig. 17 A 24-year-old man with no known medical history presented with right upper quadrant pain. Abdominal US shows well-defined complex mass (arrows) with peripherally located cysts which were found to be consistent with daughter vesicles. The lesion was then treated with percutaneous approach

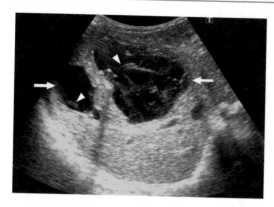

Fig. 18 A 9-year-old girl with no medical history has underwent an abdominal ultrasound for screening hydatid cyst because her mother has been diagnosed with active disease. Abdominal US demonstrates two cystic lesions (arrows) with internal linear echogenic structures which showed mobility in real-time US exam (imaging findings were found to be suggestive for hydatid cyst with detached membrane (arrowhead)). The patient subsequently underwent percutaneous treatment

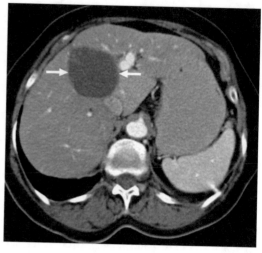

Fig. 20 A 70-year-old woman with a remote history of colon cancer (in clinical and imaging remission) underwent a follow-up CT. Axial postcontrast abdominal CT image demonstrates well-defined, thin-walled, round-shaped purely cystic-appearing mass (arrows) within the liver parenchyma. Percutaneous drainage confirmed hydatid cyst

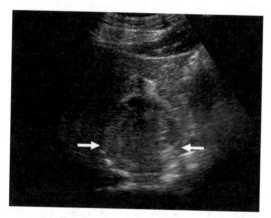

Fig. 19 A 26-year-old man who is on follow-up for percutaneously treated liver hydatid cyst. Abdominal US shows well-defined, solid lesion with heterogenous content, consistent with degenerated, inactive hydatid cyst (arrows)

8.1.1.2 Computed Tomography and Magnetic Resonance Imaging

E. granulosus cysts are almost always seen as hypoattenuating lesions in the liver parenchyma on CT studies (Fig. 20). Daughter cysts have even lower attenuation than the cyst fluid (Fig. 21). Daughter cysts are observed in the majority of the cases, and "water lily" sign may also be appreciated (Fig. 23). Dense or curvilinear calcification within the cyst wall is almost always a sign of a biologically inactive cyst (Fig. 23).

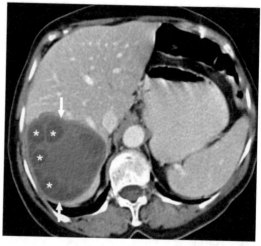

Fig. 21 A 66-year-old woman with no significant past medical history now presents with right upper quadrant pain. Axial postcontrast abdominal CT image demonstrates well-defined, complex-looking mass with peripherally located hypodense daughter vesicles (asterisks) which is a typical finding for hydatid cyst (arrows). Note daughter vesicles are more hypodense than the central matrix of the mother cyst. Percutaneous drainage confirmed the diagnosis

Hypointense wall of 4–5 mm in thickness is hypointense in both T1- and T2-weighted images and represents the pericyst (Fig. 24) (Czermak

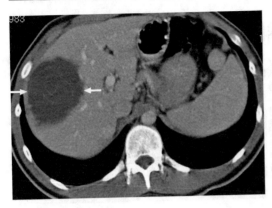

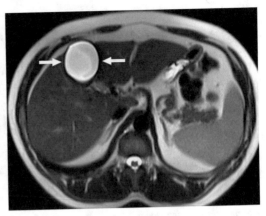

Fig. 22 A 20-year-old man with no significant medical history underwent a CT exam for acute right lower quadrant pain. Axial postcontrast abdominal CT image incidentally detected a large cystic lesion (arrows) with internal hyperintense linear structures which were thought to be consistent with detached hydatid cyst membranes. Percutaneous aspiration and treatment confirmed the diagnosis

Fig. 24 A 36-year-old man with no significant past medical history underwent MRI for a cystic liver mass that was incidentally detected on US exam. Axial T2W MR image demonstrates well-defined, round-shaped hyperintense cystic mass (arrows) with a hypointense wall which was suggestive for pericyst. Percutaneous drainage confirmed hydatid cyst

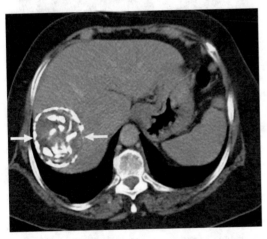

Fig. 23 A 40-year-old man with a history of percutaneously treated hydatid cyst 5 years ago underwent a follow-up CT. Axial postcontrast abdominal CT image demonstrates a round well-defined mass (arrows) with scattered internal and peripheral calcifications. The constellation of imaging findings is typical for inactive hydatid cyst

et al. 2008). The hydatid matrix or hydatid sand represents the free-floating scolices and appears hypointense on T1W and brightly hyperintense on T2W images (Fig. 25). Daughter cysts are typically hypointense on T1W images than the matrix of the mother cyst (Fig. 26) (Mortele et al.

2004). They typically appear as hyperintense on T2W images (Fig. 27).

The differential diagnosis includes biliary cystadenoma-cystadenocarcinoma, pyogenic abscess, cystic metastases from the pancreas or the ovaries, and hemorrhagic or infected liver cyst (Mortele and Ros 2001). Curvilinear calcification within the daughter cysts is the most characteristic imaging finding.

8.1.2 *Echinococcus multilocularis* Infection

Echinococcus multilocularis can affect any organ or tissue, but the liver is the most commonly affected site. The characteristic feature of this parasite is its capability of multilocular alveolar cyst formation (1–10 mm in diameter) that resembles the lung alveoli. Another important feature of this agent is its highly invasive biological manner. As a reaction of the liver parenchyma to the invasion of the germinal layer, severe fibrosis is induced that further increases the detrimental effect of the parasite. The disease's biological behavior is reminiscent of a malignant neoplasm.

8.1.2.1 Imaging Findings

Typical imaging finding is an infiltrative hepatic lesion with ill-defined borders. The lesion may

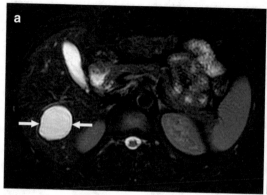

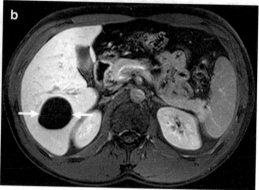

Fig. 25 (a) Axial T2W MR image of the same patient in "Fig. 16" demonstrates brightly hyperintense cystic lesion (arrows). (b) Axial postcontrast T1W image demonstrates the same lesion (arrows) as uniformly hypointense without any mural or internal contrast enhancement. Percutaneous drainage confirmed hydatid cyst

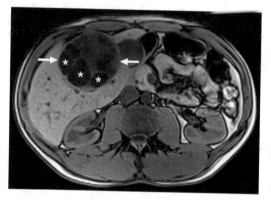

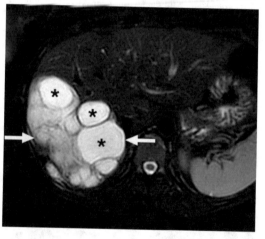

Fig. 26 Axial postcontrast T1W image of the same patient in "Fig. 17" demonstrates the same lesion as non-enhancing, well-defined mass (arrows) with internal daughter cysts (asterisks) and hypointense central matrix. Note daughter cysts are typically more hypointense than the matrix

Fig. 27 A 39-year-old woman with no significant medical history now presents with right upper quadrant pain. Axial T2W MR image demonstrates a complex, well-defined mass (arrows) with multiple internal thin-walled, round hyperintense daughter vesicles (asterisks). These are typical for hydatid cyst

contain cystic and solid parts. The solid parts include coagulation necrosis, granuloma, and calcifications, whereas the cystic components comprise of metacestodal vesicles and liquefactive necrosis (Czermak et al. 2008). As the small-sized lesions generally consist of small clustered cysts (metacestodal vesicles), invasively enlarging *E. multilocularis* infections tend to form central liquefactive necrosis. This necrosis is induced by the ischemia associated with vascular invasion. The contrast enhancement is either completely absent or very faint. Enlarged lymph nodes are generally not seen which may be a useful sign in differentiating *E. alveolaris* infection

from true malignant processes (Akin and Isiklar 1999).

On US, the lesions appear as hypo-/hyperechoic mass with indistinct margins; however, cystic or vesicular appearance is not unusual (Fig. 27a). Color Doppler flow shows the absence of vascularity in the lesion and may help the diagnosis (Coskun et al. 2004).

On CT and MRI, lesions display irregular, ill-defined margins invading the liver tissue. The lesions are hypodense on CT (Fig. 28b) and

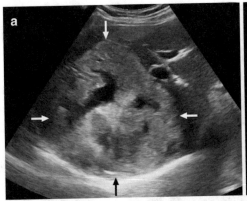

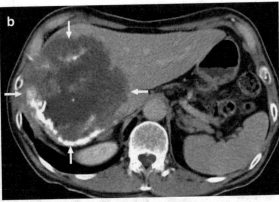

Fig. 28 A 65-year-old man recently presented with right upper quadrant pain and elevated liver function tests. (**a**) Abdominal ultrasound demonstrates lobulated, predominantly hyperechoic mass (arrows) with centrally located, hypoechoic cystic component. (**b**) Axial postcontrast CT image of the same patient demonstrates a large, hypoattenuating, centrally cystic/necrotic liver mass (arrows) with peripheral calcifications. Percutaneous biopsy confirmed alveolar hydatid cyst

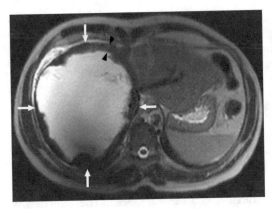

Fig. 29 A 45-year-old woman with no known significant past medical history now presents with right upper quadrant pain and a palpable mass at the same location. Axial T2W MR image demonstrates a large, almost completely cystic mass (arrows) with irregularly thickened wall (arrowheads). Percutaneous biopsy of the lesion wall confirmed alveolar hydatid cyst

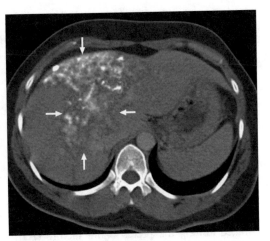

Fig. 30 A 30-year-old woman with no significant past medical history now presents with weight loss, right upper quadrant pain, and elevated liver function tests. Axial postcontrast abdominal CT image demonstrates an infiltrative, hypodense lesion (arrows) within the liver parenchyma. Also note the scattered calcifications within the same lesion. Percutaneous biopsy confirmed alveolar hydatid cyst

hypointense on T1W images. On T2W images, the lesions may be hypo-, hyper-, or isointense. On MR, solid and cystic parts of the lesions may be better delineated compared to CT (Fig. 29). Multiple round cysts with solid components or solid structures encircling the large and/or irregular cysts can be characteristic for *E. multilocularis* infection (Kodama et al. 2003). Calcifications are common (found in 90% of the subjects), and poor contrast enhancement is almost always present (Fig. 30) (Czermak et al. 2008). Hilar infiltration is frequent which may result in mechanical biliary obstruction and invasion/occlusion of the portal vein (Fig. 31). Hepatic veins may also be involved during the process. Lobar atrophy is also another characteristic feature of the disease (Rozanes et al. 1992).

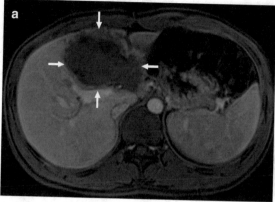 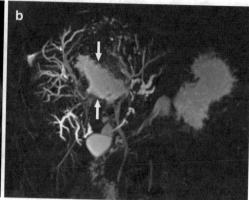

Fig. 31 A 27-year-old man with no known past medical history now presents with right upper quadrant pain and abnormal liver function tests. US exam showed a hypoechoic mass in the left liver lobe (not shown). (**a**) Axial postcontrast T1W MR image demonstrates a well-defined, centrally cystic/necrotic liver mass (arrows) extending into the hepatic hilum. (**b**) MRCP image better demonstrates the cystic character of the lesion (arrows). Also note the markedly dilated intrahepatic bile ducts

The pancreas, right kidney, right adrenal gland, peritoneum, or vascular structures may all be involved as a result of direct spread of the infection (Czermak et al. 2008).

8.2   Actinomycosis of the Liver

Actinomycosis is a rare cause of liver infection. The bacteria typically gain access to the liver via the hematogenous route. Prior to abdominal surgery, loss of integrity in the gastrointestinal system mucosa and immunosuppression may be counted among the predisposing factors (Avila et al. 2015). Despite these several predisposing factors, around 80% of the hepatic actinomycosis cases are cryptogenic (Lall et al. 2010; Christodoulou et al. 2004).

Imaging diagnosis may be difficult as most of the cases present with non-specific features on cross-sectional imaging. In 66% of the cases, a solitary lesion is typical, but multifocal hepatic lesions are also not rare. Right lobe is the most commonly affected part of the liver, and imaging characteristics of these lesions may be easily confused with neoplastic liver disease (Avila et al. 2015). The lesions mostly appear as hypodense on CT studies. On MRI exams, they are typically seen as hypointense on T1W images and hyperintense on T2W images (Fig. 32) (Kim et al. 2007b). As the imaging findings may closely mimic parenchymal neoplastic processes, histopathologic diagnosis is almost always necessary for diagnosis and treatment planning.

8.3   Schistosomiasis of the Liver

Schistosomiasis is endemic in the tropical and subtropical areas of the Africa, Asia, South America, and the Caribbean. The infection is transmitted via the freshwater snails. An estimated 200 million people are infected with this parasite. Schistosomiasis of the liver is caused by trematodes *Schistosoma mansoni* and *Schistosoma japonicum*. Both of these parasites live inside the lumens of the mesenteric veins, and the final end result is liver fibrosis. They penetrate the human skin and subsequently migrate to their residence in the mesenteric veins. The eggs are carried by the portal vein to the liver where they lodge within the venules, causing granuloma formation, periportal fibrosis, and, finally, portal hypertension. Infections with *S. japonicum* are more virulent than those with *S. mansoni*, because each adult worm pair of *S. japonicum* produces 10 times as many eggs as of their *S. mansoni* counterparts (Manzella et al. 2008).

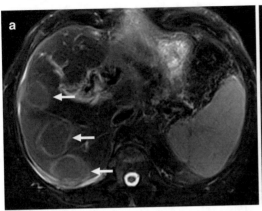

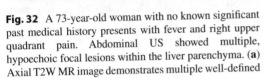

Fig. 32 A 73-year-old woman with no known significant past medical history presents with fever and right upper quadrant pain. Abdominal US showed multiple, hypoechoic focal lesions within the liver parenchyma. (**a**) Axial T2W MR image demonstrates multiple well-defined mildly hyperintense lesions (arrows). (**b**) Axial postcontrast T1W MR image demonstrates the same lesions (arrows) as hypointense compared to the neighboring liver parenchyma. Percutaneous biopsy confirmed active inflammation and *Actinomyces* colonies

8.3.1 Imaging Findings

Periportal fibrosis is the hallmark abnormality of both parasites which is caused by deposition of their eggs. As *S. japonicum* eggs are smaller than the *S. mansoni* eggs, they tend to lodge in the peripheral veins, whereas the eggs of *S. mansoni* tend to lodge in the central veins (Manzella et al. 2008). Therefore, the distribution of periportal fibrosis may be helpful in the differential diagnosis. Periportal fibrosis is detected as thickening alongside the peripheral branches of the portal vein with increased echogenicity. Bands of periportal fibrosis give rise to Symmers' pipe stem fibrosis with hyperechoic septae in a polygonal arrangement mimicking a "fish scale" appearance and so-called "turtle back" appearance (Manzella et al. 2008). The hyperechoic bands seen on US in peripheral locations in *S. japonicum* infections are detected as curvilinear calcifications at the same locations on CT. *S. japonicum* eggs tend to calcify as they die which is in contrast with the eggs of *S mansoni*, which is an useful clue in the differential diagnosis.

Computed tomography findings of *S. mansoni* infection are primarily hypodense low attenuation bands or rings around the central portal vein branches with marked enhancement of these areas after contrast injection. Calcification is not observed in CT in contrast to *S. japonicum* infection. Extensive widening of the hepatic fissures in the hilum and along the portal vein branches with diffuse atrophy is typical of schistosomiasis. MR imaging findings are similar to the morphological findings described above in US and CT. Fibrous tissues around the portal vein are typically hypointense on both T1- and T2-weighted images.

8.4 Toxocariasis

Toxocariasis is caused by the larvae of the dog ascarid, *Toxocara canis*, or less commonly by the cat ascarid, *Toxocara cati*. Ingestion of the egg or encapsulated larvae excreted in the feces of the dogs is the typical mode of infection. The larvae are liberated in the human intestine and reach the liver via the portal circulation. Infections of the lung, eye, brain, and heart have all been reported (Lim 2008). When larvae reach the liver, they move to different places in the liver tissue (larva migrans) (Beaver 1969). During its migration in the liver, it prompts the formation of eosinophilic liver abscesses, eosinophilic infiltration, and granuloma formation within the liver parenchyma. The granulomas or abscesses are small measuring between 1 and 1.5 cm in diameter (Lim 2008).

8.4.1 Imaging Features

The lesions in the liver appear as small, multiple, hypoechoic lesions in the liver parenchyma on

US (Chang et al. 2006). The margins of the lesions are not well-defined, and the lesions are not perfectly round. On CT, the lesions appear as multiple hypodense lesions scattered through the liver parenchyma. The lesions are generally ill-defined, oval or irregularly shaped, typically low-attenuating nodules. The lesions are small with a diameter between 1 and 1.5 cm (Chang et al. 2006). On MR, lesions are detected as multiple lesions scattered throughout the liver parenchyma that are mildly hypointense on T1W images, while on T2W images, they are mildly hyperintense. On postcontrast imaging, they are again best detected on portal venous phase and isointense or nearly isointense in arterial and equilibrium phase images (Lim 2008).

8.5   Fascioliasis

Fascioliasis is caused by a liver trematode named as *Fasciola hepatica*. The pathogen particularly affects the sheep and the cows, and humans are accidentally infected by ingesting contaminated watercress. The ingested larvae encyst in the stomach, penetrate the duodenal wall, escape into the peritoneal cavity, and then penetrate the liver capsule. In the liver, the flukes make small holes and cavities during its migration. This migration ends when the fluke reaches the larger bile duct and penetrates into its lumen, which is the permanent residence of the fluke (Lim et al. 2008).

8.5.1   Imaging Findings

During its migration in the liver, which may last for months, the mature flukes digest the liver parenchyma and "dig tunnels and caves." During its migration within the liver parenchyma, the parasite leaves multiple small necrotic cavities and abscesses (Han et al. 1999). The abscesses of hepatic fascioliasis do not coalesce, a feature which is in contrast to pyogenic abscesses (Fig. 33). The underlying reason is most likely that they are caused by the necrosis of the liver parenchyma rather than the inflammation (Llorente et al, 2002). The entire path of migration may be detected on cross-sectional imaging as a "tunnel-like tract" from the entry site at the liver capsule into the depths of the liver parenchyma (Fig. 34) (Lim et al. 2008). Subcapsular abscesses have been reported in a patient with hepatic fascioliasis (Llorente et al. 2002). The "tunnels and caves" sign was reported to be a useful sign in the differentiation from the cholangiocellular carcinoma, which may sometimes mimic fasciolar infection (Lim et al. 2008). Although MR and US have also been reported to be useful, CT seems to be the most beneficial modality (Lim et al. 2008).

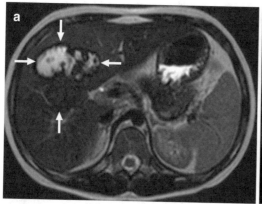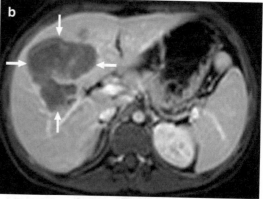

Fig. 33 A 10-year-old girl with no significant past medical history now presents with right upper quadrant pain and fever. Abdominal US showed hypointense heterogeneous ill-defined mass within liver parenchyma (not shown). (**a**) T2W MR image demonstrates a complex-appearing mass with cystic and solid components (arrows). (**b**) Axial postcontrast T1W MR image of the same patient demonstrates the hypovascular nature of this mass (arrows). Percutaneous biopsy confirmed hepatic fasciolar disease

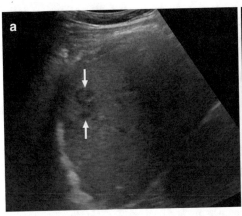

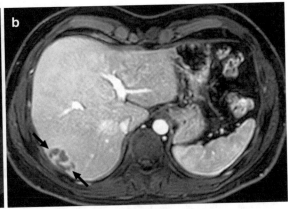

Fig. 34 A 39-year-old man with a remote history of surgically treated testicular germ cell tumor. (**a**) Follow-up US study showed intraparenchymal tubular-shaped, hypoechoic structure (arrows) close to the liver capsule.

(**b**) Axial postcontrast T1W MR image of the same patient in "Fig. 33" demonstrates the same lesion (arrows) just beneath the liver capsule. Percutaneous biopsy confirmed fasciolar disease

When the adult flukes are in the biliary system, they grow and enlarge in size and may reside in the biliary system for years. They can be detected in both the intra- and extrahepatic compartments of the biliary system, as well as within the lumen of the gallbladder (Lim et al. 2008; Ooms et al. 1995). Chronic inflammation may cause the thickening in the walls of the affected parts of the biliary system and the gallbladder; however, cholangiocarcinoma development due to chronic presence of the parasites has not been reported before (Kabaalioglu et al. 2007).

9 Conclusion

Hepatic infections are relatively common infections, and prompt diagnosis and relevant treatment are of paramount importance for preventing the potential, sometimes deadly, complications. All imaging modalities may be used for diagnosis, but imaging findings can sometimes be rather non-specific for a definitive diagnosis. In these patients, percutaneous biopsy may also be used for the diagnosis.

References

Adams EB, MacLeod IN (1977) Invasive amebiasis: amebic liver abscess and its complications. Medicine (Baltimore) 56:325–334

Akin O, Isiklar I (1999) Hepatic alveolar echinococcosis. Acta Radiol 40:326–328

Alvarez SZ (1998) Hepatobiliary tuberculosis. J Gastroenterol Hepatol 13:833–839

Antilla VJ, Lamminen AE, Bondestam S et al (1996) Magnetic resonance imaging is superior to computed tomography and ultrasonography in imaging infectious liver foci in acute leukaemia. Eur J Haematol 56:82–87

Arai K, Kawai K, Kohda W et al (2003) Dynamic CT of acute cholangitis: early inhomogeneous enhancement of the liver. AJR Am J Roentgenol 181: 115–118

Avila F, Santos V, Massinha P et al (2015) Hepatic actinomycosis. GE Port J Gastroenterol 22:19–23

Bächler P, Baladron MJ, Menias C et al (2016) Multimodality imaging of liver infections. Radiographics 36:1001–1023

Bader TR, Braga L, Beavers KL, Semelka RC (2001) MR imaging findings of infectious cholangitis. Magn Reson Imaging 19:781–788

Balci NC, Tunaci A, Akinci A et al (2001) Granulomatous hepatitis: MRI findings. Magn Reson Imaging 19:1107–1111

Beaver PC (1969) The nature of visceral larva migrans. J Parasitol 55:3–12

Benedetti NJ, Desser TS, Jeffrey RB (2008) Imaging of hepatic infections. Ultrasound Q 24:267–278

Berlow ME, Spirit BA, Weil L (1984) CT follow-up of hepatic and splenic fungal microabscesses. J Comput Assist Tomogr 8:42–45

Catalano OA, Sahani DV, Forcione DG et al (2009) Biliary infections: spectrum of imaging findings and management. Radiographics 29:2059–2080

Chang S, Lim JH, Choi D et al (2006) Hepatic visceral larva migrans of Toxocara canis: CT and sonographic findings. Am J Roentgenol 187:622–629

Chou FF, Sheen-Chen SM, Chen YS et al (1995) The comparison of clinical course and results of treatment between gas-forming and non-gas-forming pyogenic liver abscess. Arch Surg 130:401–405

Christodoulou N, Papadokis I, Velegrakis M (2004) Actinomycotic liver abscesses. Case report and review of the literature. Chir Ital 56:141–146

Coskun A, Ozturk M, Karahan OI et al (2004) Alveolar echinococcosis of the liver: correlative color Doppler US, CT, and MRI study. Acta Radiol 45:492–498

Csendes A, Diaz JC, Burdiles P et al (1992) Risk factors and classification of acute suppurative cholangitis. Br J Surg 79:655–658

Czermak BV, Akhan O, Hiemetzberger R et al (2008) Echinococcosis of the liver. Abdom Imaging 33:133–143

Doyle DJ, Hanbidge AE, O'Malley ME (2006) Imaging of hepatic infections. Clin Radiol 61:737–748

Eckburg PB, Montoya JG (2001) Hepatobiliary infections. In: Wilson WR, Sande MA (eds) Diagnosis and treatment in infectious diseases. McGraw-Hill, New York, pp 269–286

Eckert J, Deplazes P (2004) Biological, epidemiological, and clinical aspects of echinococcosis, a zoonosis of increasing concern. Clin Microbiol Rev 17:107–135

Gracey L (1965) Tuberculous abscess of the liver. Br J Surg 55:442–443

Halvorsen RA, Korobkin M, Wl F et al (1984) The variable CT appearance of hepatic abscesses. Am J Roentgenol 142:941–946

Han JK, Jang HJ, Choi BI et al (1999) Experimental hepatobiliary fascioliasis in rabbits: a radiology-pathology correlation. Investig Radiol 34:99–108

Hickey N, McNulty JG, Osborne H, Finucane J (1999) Acute hepatobiliary tuberculosis: a report of two cases and a review of the literature. Eur Radiol 9:886–889

Hughes MA, Petri WA Jr (2000) Amebic liver abscess. Infect Dis Clin N Am 14:565–582

Hui JY, Yang MK, Cho DH et al (2007) Pyogenic liver abscesses caused by Klebsiella pneumoniae: US appearance and aspiration findings. Radiology 242:769–779

Hulnick DH, Megibow AJ, Naidich DP et al (1985) Abdominal tuberculosis: CT evaluation. Radiology 157:199–204

Jain R, Sawhney S, Gupta RG et al (1999) Sonographic appearances and percutaneous management of primary tuberculous liver abscess. J Clin Ultrasound 27:159–163

Jeffrey RB Jr, Tolentino CS, Chang FC et al (1984) CT of small pyogenic hepatic abscesses. Am J Roentgenol 142:941–946

Kabaalioglu A, Ceken K, Alimoglu E et al (2007) Hepatobiliary fascioliasis: sonographic and CT findings in 87 patients during the initial phase and long-term follow-up. Am J Roentgenol 189: 824–828

Kim HS, Park NH, Park KA, Kang SB (2007b) A case of pelvic actinomycosis with hepatic actinomycotic pseudotumour. Gynecol Obstet Investig 64:95–99

Kim SB, Je BK, Lee KY et al (2007a) Computed tomographic differences of pyogenic liver abscesses caused by Klebsiella pneumoniae and non-Klebsiella pneumoniae. J Comput Assist Tomogr 31:59–65

Kodama Y, Fujita N, Shimizu T et al (2003) Alveolar echinococcosis: MR findings in the liver. Radiology 228:172–177

Kurtz AB, Rubin CS, Cooper HS et al (1980) Ultrasound findings in hepatitis. Radiology 136:717–723

Lall T, Shehab TM, Valenstein P (2010) Isolated hepatic actinomycosis: a case report. J Med Case Rep 4:45

Land MA, Moinuden M, Biano AL (1985) Pyogenic liver abscess: changing epidemiology and prognosis. South Med J 78:1426–1430

Landay MJ, Setiawan H, Hirsch G et al (1980) Hepatic and thoracic amebiasis. Am J Roentgenol 135:449–454

Lim JH (2008) Toxocariasis of the liver: visceral larva migrans. Abdom Imaging 33:151–156

Lim JH, Mairiang E, Ahn GH (2008) Biliary parasitic diseases including clonorchiasis, opisthorchiasis and fascioliasis. Abdom Imaging 33:157–165

Llorente JG, Domingo AH, Gonzalez PC et al (2002) Subcapsular abscess: an unusual CT finding in hepatic fascioliasis. Am J Roentgenol 178:514–515

Lösch F (1875) Massenhafte Entwickelung von Amöben in Dickdarm. Arch F Path Anat 65:196–211

Manzella A, Ohtomo K, Monzawa S et al (2008) Schistosomiasis of the liver. Abdom Imaging 33:144–150

Masood A, Sallah S (2005) Chronic disseminated candidiasis in patients with acute leukemia: emphasis on diagnostic definition and treatment. Leuk Res 29:493–501

McDonald AP, Howard RJ (1980) Pyogenic liver abscess. World J Surg 4:369–380

Mendez RJ, Schiebler ML, Outwater EK et al (1994) Hepatic abscesses: MR imaging findings. Radiology 190:431–436

Mortele KJ, Ros PR (2001) Cystic focal liver lesions in the adult: differential CT and MR imaging features. Radiographics 30:1112–1116

Mortele KJ, Segatto E, Pos PR (2004) The infected liver: radiologic-pathologic correlation. Radiographics 24:937–955

Oliva A, Duarte B, Jonasson O et al (1990) The nodular form of local hepatic tuberculosis—a review. J Clin Gastroenterol 12:166–173

Ooms HWA, Puylaert JBCM, Van der Werf SDJ (1995) Biliary fascioliasis: US and endoscopic retrograde cholangiopancreatography findings. Eur Radiol 5:196–199

Oto A, Akhan O, Ozmen M (1999) Focal inflammatory diseases of the liver. Eur J Radiol 32:61–75

Pastakia B, Shawker TH, Thaler M et al (1988) Hepatosplenic candidiasis: wheels within wheels. Radiology 166:417–421

Pedrosa I, Saiz A, Arrazola J et al (2000) Hydatid disease: radiologic and pathologic features and complications. Radiographics 20:795–817

Radin DR, Ralls PW, Colletti PM et al (1988) CT of amebic liver abscess. Am J Roentgenol 150:1297–1301

Ralls PW (1998) Inflammatory disease of the liver. Radiol Clin N Am 36:377–389

Ralls PW, Colletti PM, Quinn MF et al (1982) Sonographic findings in hepatic amebic abscess. Radiology 145:123–126

Ralls PW, Quinn MF, Boswell WD et al (1983) Patterns of resolution in successfully treated hepatic amebic abscess: sonographic evaluation. Radiology 149:541–543

Ros PR et al (2015) Focal hepatic infections. In: Richard MG, Marc SL (eds) Textbook of gastrointestinal radiology, 2nd edn. Saunders, Philadelphia, pp 1569–1572

Rozanes I, Acunas B, Celik L et al (1992) CT in lobar atrophy of the liver caused by alveolar echinococcosis. J Comput Assist Tomogr 16:216–218

Ryder SD, Beckingham IJ (2001) ABC of diseases of liver, pancreas, and biliary system: acute hepatitis. BMJ 322:151–153

Schmiedl U, Paajanen H, Arakawa M et al (1988) MR imaging of liver abscesses: application of Gd-DTPA. Magn Reson Imaging 6:9–16

Semelka RC, Shoenut JP, Greenberg HM et al (1992) Detection of the acute and treated lesions of hepatosplenic candidiasis: comparison of dynamic contrast-enhanced CT and MR imaging. J Magn Reson Imaging 2:341–345

Stain SC, Yellin AE, Donovan AJ et al (1991) Pyogenic liver abscess. Modern treatment. Surgery 126:991–996

Stanley SL (2003) Amoebiasis. Lancet 361:1025–1034

Walsh J (1988) Prevalence of Entamoeba histolytica infection. In: Ravdin JI (ed) Amebiasis: human infection by Entamoeba histolytica. Wiley, New York, pp 93–105

WHO Informal Working Group (2003) International classification of ultrasound images in cystic echinococcosis for application in clinical and field epidemiological settings. Acta Trop 85:253–261

Yang CC, Chen CY, Lin XZ et al (1993) Pyogenic liver abscess in Taiwan: emphasis of gas forming liver abscess in diabetics. Am J Gastroenterol 88:1911–1915

Imaging of Hepatic Cystic Tumors

Vishal Kukkar and Venkata S. Katabathina

Contents

Abstract

Cystic tumors of the liver are a heterogeneous group of neoplasms with characteristic histogenesis, clinico-biological features, and pathologic findings. They include both epithelial and mesenchymal liver tumors and commonly originate from the biliary epithelium. Mucinous cystic neoplasm (MCN) and intraductal papillary neoplasm of the bile duct (IPNB) are the most common cystic neoplasms of the liver. Cystic changes can develop in hepatocellular carcinoma (HCC) and hepatic metastases due to cystic degeneration and necrosis. Rarely, mass-forming intrahepatic cholangiocarcinoma and giant cavernous hemangioma may also show cystic appearance with necrotic areas. Rare hepatic tumors such as mesenchymal hamartoma, undifferentiated embryonal carcinoma, lymphangioma, and inflammatory myofibroblastic tumors are also cystic in nature. Select cystic hepatic tumors show characteristic cross-sectional imaging findings that permit an accurate diagnosis. Imaging is also pivotal in the follow-up and long-term surveillance of cystic hepatic tumors.

V. Kukkar · V. S. Katabathina (✉)
Department of Radiology,
University of Texas Health Science Center at San Antonio, San Antonio, TX, USA
e-mail: katabathina@uthscsa.edu

© Springer Nature Switzerland AG 2021
E. Quaia (ed.), *Imaging of the Liver and Intra-hepatic Biliary Tract*,
Medical Radiology Diagnostic Imaging, https://doi.org/10.1007/978-3-030-39021-1_4

1   Introduction

Cystic liver tumors are a rare, diverse group of neoplasms that include both benign and malignant entities as well as primary and secondary tumors. Cystic nature in hepatic cystic tumors either represents an innate architectural characteristic of the tumor or significant biliary dilation or may be related to extensive tumor necrosis. According to the 2010 World Health Organization (WHO) classification schemata of the tumors of the digestive system, primary epithelial cystic liver tumors include mucinous cystic neoplasm (MCN) and intraductal papillary neoplasm of the bile duct (IPNB) (Bosman et al. 2010). Primary cystic mesenchymal liver tumors include mesenchymal hamartoma, undifferentiated embryonal sarcoma, lymphangioma, inflammatory myofibroblastic tumor, and epithelioid hemangioendothelioma (Bosman et al. 2010). Also, extensive necrosis and cystic degeneration in hepatocellular carcinoma (HCC), metastases, intrahepatic cholangiocarcinoma, and giant cavernous hemangioma may result in cystic change and mimic cystic hepatic tumors (Table 1) (Qian et al. 2013). Cystic liver tumors demonstrate characteristic ontogeny, clinico-biological features, pathologic findings, and cross-sectional imaging features that permit better characterization. Cystic liver tumors should be differentiated from the wide spectrum of benign cystic focal lesions of the liver, including congenital, developmental, post-traumatic, infectious/inflammatory, and miscellaneous entities (Mortele and Ros 2001; Qian et al. 2013; Vachha et al. 2011). Accurate preoperative characterization of cystic liver tumors and their differentiation from the other benign entities is pivotal in management and prognostification.

A wide array of imaging techniques are helpful in the diagnosis, management, and follow-up of hepatic cystic tumors. They include ultrasonography (US), computed tomography (CT), and magnetic resonance imaging (MRI) with magnetic resonance cholangiopancreatography (MRCP). US is generally the initial imaging modality used to investigate the focal liver lesions as it is widely available, cost-effective, and without risk of radiation. US helps to differentiate cystic liver lesions from solid liver masses and can demonstrate internal septations and solid components within the cystic liver lesions (Borhani et al. 2014; Mortele and Peters 2009; Mortele and Ros 2001; Qian et al. 2013). CT is helpful to further characterize cystic liver lesions by identifying the enhancing wall, internal septations, and mural nodularity. CT is also useful in the morphological classification of cystic liver lesions, such as MCN and IPNB (Qian et al. 2013). MRI with MRCP is the primary imaging modality for evaluating the hepatic cystic masses due to high soft tissue contrast, development of hepatobiliary-specific contrast agents, and multiplanar capability. MRCP is very useful to identify the communication of the cystic lesion with biliary ducts better than any other imaging modality, provide excellent delineation of associated ductal obstruction, and can also identify internal septations and hence aid in differentiating lesions such as MCN and IPNB (Billington et al. 2012; Lewin et al. 2006). Also, endoscopy-guided procedures such as endoscopic retrograde cholangiopancreatography (ERCP) and endoscopic US (EUS) are useful in the direct visualization of the biliary tract and obtaining tissue biopsy to confirm the diagnosis (Natov et al. 2017; Tsuchida et al. 2010). In this chapter, we will present the cross-sectional imaging spectrum of the common and relatively rare cystic tumors of the liver.

Table 1 Common and uncommon cystic hepatic tumors

Biliary epithelial cystic tumors	Non-biliary cystic tumors	Rare cystic tumors
Mucinous cystic neoplasm of liver (MCN) Intraductal papillary neoplasm of the bile duct (IPNB)	Cystic hepatocellular carcinoma Cystic metastases	Intrahepatic cholangiocarcinoma Giant cavernous hemangioma Mesenchymal hamartoma Undifferentiated embryonal sarcoma Inflammatory myofibroblastic tumor

1.1 Mucinous Cystic Neoplasm of the Liver

Previously known as biliary cystadenoma/cystadenocarcinoma, the 2010 WHO classification defines mucinous cystic neoplasms of the liver (MCN) as biliary epithelial cystic tumors usually showing no communication with the bile ducts, composed of cuboidal to columnar, variably mucin-producing epithelium, and associated with ovarian-type subepithelial stroma (Bosman et al. 2010). MCNs are further classified into three types based on the severity of epithelial dysplasia and invasiveness: (1) MCN with low- or intermediate-grade intraepithelial neoplasia, (2) MCN with high-grade intraepithelial neoplasia, and (3) MCN with an associated invasive carcinoma (Bosman et al. 2010). MCN is a distinct entity that differs clinicopathologically and radiologically from cystic IPNB and carries different natural histories and prognosis (Soares et al. 2014; Zen et al. 2011). MCNs likely represent about 5% of all symptomatic liver cysts referred for surgical treatment with a strong female preponderance and usually occurs in middle-aged women with earlier age of presentation in benign/noninvasive tumors (Zen et al. 2011).

The cell of origin of hepatic MCNs is controversial given the presence of ovarian-like stroma in almost all cases, and the hypothesis should explain this unusual feature as well as structural similarity with pancreatic MCNs. One theory suggests the possibility of MCN development from immature endodermal stroma or primary yolk cells or ectopic ovarian tissue implanted in the liver during embryogenesis, whereas others suggest that hepatic MCNs develop from the intrahepatic peribiliary glands as a biliary counterpart of pancreatic MCN (Fragulidis et al. 2017; Nakanuma et al. 2014; Zen et al. 2011). While the high prevalence of hepatic MCN in segment 4 of the liver supports "the implant theory" as hamartomatous lesions commonly develop in segment 4, the pathologic and immunohistochemical similarities between the pancreatic and hepatic MCNs favor the origin from peribiliary glands (Erdogan et al. 2010; Nakanuma et al. 2014; Zen et al. 2011). The fusion of both theories could explain the origin of MCN in a better way: the cell of origin is in the peribiliary glands that eventually receive stimulation by ectopic ovarian stroma resulting in the tumor formation (Nakanuma et al. 2014; Zen et al. 2011). On gross pathology, MCNs appear as a multilocular cystic mass containing clear fluid or thick mucus or hemorrhagic fluid with multiple papillary areas/mural nodules along the wall, surrounded by a thick fibrous capsule and without definite, identifiable communication with adjacent larger bile ducts (Bosman et al. 2010; Simo et al. 2012; Zen et al. 2011). At histology, cuboidal or low columnar type, the mucin-producing epithelium lining the wall with cellular spindle cell mesenchymal stroma that resembles ovarian stroma and tumor cells are positive for CK7, MUC2, MUC5AC, estrogen receptor, and progesterone receptor on immunohistochemistry (Bosman et al. 2010; Zen et al. 2011).

Hepatic MCNs are slow-growing tumors with the majority being asymptomatic, but some may present with abdominal pain/discomfort or a palpable mass (Del Poggio and Buonocore 2008). Rarely, hepatic MCNs may distend liver capsule resulting in rupture and spontaneous bleeding or cause bile duct invasion and obstruction with obstructive jaundice (Soares et al. 2014). Imaging plays an important role to identify MCN and preoperative planning and differentiate this from other benign/malignant cystic lesions of the liver (Pitchaimuthu and Duxbury 2017; Qian et al. 2013). MCN is typically a moderate to large cystic mass on cross-sectional imaging and has multiple internal septations. At US, MCN appears as a large, complex cystic mass with multiple internal septations, low-level internal echoes, and peripheral nodularity (Fig. 1) (Mortele and Peters 2009; Qian et al. 2013; Soares et al. 2014). US is very helpful in demonstrating internal septations better than any other imaging modality. On color Doppler interrogation, septations and mural nodularity may show increased vascularity. On CT, MCN appears commonly as a multilocular cystic lesion with the enhancing wall, a well-defined fibrotic capsule, internal septations, and solid

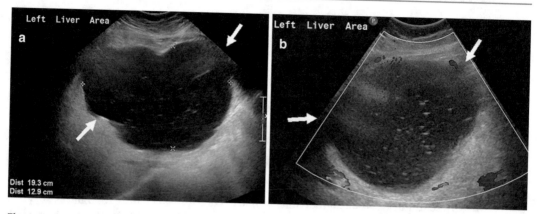

Fig. 1 (**a**, **b**) A 79-year-old woman with mucinous cystic neoplasm (MCN) of the liver. Transverse grayscale (**a**) and color Doppler (**b**) US images of the right upper quadrant demonstrate a well-defined, lobulated cystic lesion in the liver with multiple thin internal septations and without any increased vascularity on Doppler interrogation (arrows). This cystic mass was proven to be hepatic MCN on pathology

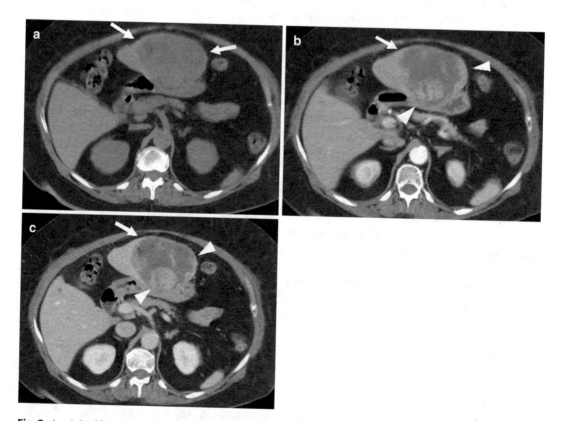

Fig. 2 (**a–c**) An 82-year-old woman with mucinous cystic neoplasm (MCN) of the liver. Axial contrast-enhanced CT images of the upper abdomen obtained during the noncontrast (**a**), arterial (**b**), and portal venous (**c**) phases demonstrate a well-defined cystic lesion in the left lobe of the liver (arrows) with irregularly thickened wall and containing enhancing septations and solid components (arrowheads). This complex cystic mass was proven to be hepatic MCN on surgical resection

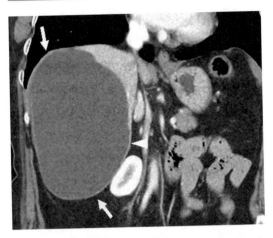

Fig. 3 A 78-year-old woman with mucinous cystic neoplasm (MCN) of the liver. Coronal contrast-enhanced CT image of the abdomen demonstrates a unilocular, well-defined cystic lesion in the right lobe of the liver (arrows) with minimally thickened wall (arrowhead). This cystic liver lesion was proven to be hepatic MCN on pathology

nodules and may also contain discontinuous peripheral calcifications (Fig. 2) (Borhani et al. 2014; Mortele and Peters 2009). MCN may also appear as a large unilocular cystic liver lesion with peripheral lobulations and without any identifiable septations or mural nodules (Fig. 3) (Mortele and Ros 2001; Qian et al. 2013; Soares et al. 2014). Hepatic MCNs show variable internal signal intensities on MRI, depending upon the amount of mucinous material, hemorrhage, proteinaceous debris, internal septations, or solid components; on MRI, the cyst content is variable in signal intensity on T1-weighted and usually hyperintense on T2-weighted images (Fig. 4) (Borhani et al. 2014; Pitchaimuthu and Duxbury 2017). MCN shows a thick, T2 hypointense wall that may demonstrate delayed enhancement; and, the

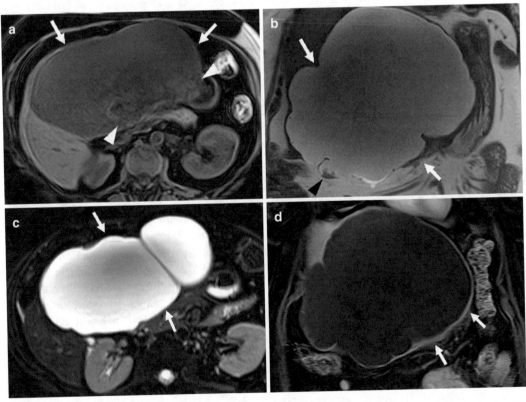

Fig. 4 (a–d) Mucinous cystic neoplasm (MCN) of the liver in a 79-year-old woman with abdominal distension. Axial T1-weighted (**a**), coronal T2-weighted (**b**), axial fat-saturated T2-weighted (**c**), and gadolinium-enhanced coronal T1-weighted (**d**) MR images of the abdomen demonstrate a large, multilobulated, septated cystic mass in the left lobe of the liver, extending into the right hepatic lobe (white arrows). The contents of this cystic mass are heterogeneously hyperintense on T1-weighted image (white arrowheads in **a**) and T2 hypointense peripheral nodules (black arrowheads in **b**). Irregularly thickened wall is seen that demonstrates heterogeneous enhancement after gadolinium administration. This mass was proven to be MCN of the liver on surgical resection

internal septations and solid nodules may show variable enhancement after gadolinium administration (Fig. 4). Typically, MCN demonstrates no adjacent bile ductal dilation or definite communication with the adjacent bile ductal system on MRI or MRCP (Vachha et al. 2011). The presence of a large, solitary cystic liver lesion in a middle-aged or older women without adjacent biliary duct dilatation or communication should raise the suspicion of MCN (Kim et al. 2010).

Risk of malignant transformation to invasive cholangiocarcinoma in hepatic MCNs can be as higher as 20% (Fragulidis et al. 2017). Benign tumors have thinner septa and less papillary projections and less likely to be hypervascular or show contrast enhancement when compared to their malignant counterparts. Although the presence of enhancing mural nodules and septations suggest the possibility of malignant MCN, it is sometimes not possible to diagnose malignancy preoperatively, and surgical resection is recommended in all cases of MCNs (Del Poggio and Buonocore 2008; Pitchaimuthu and Duxbury 2017). Aim of the treatment is the complete excision of MCN because of the high incidence of local recurrence in the liver after partial resection or marsupialization and a slow progression toward malignant transformation with a reasonable frequency (Pitchaimuthu and Duxbury 2017). However, considering the low biologic potential of hepatic MCNs wide resection margin is not mandatory. Management of the peripherally located MCNs is complete surgical resection, and the MCNs located centrally and close to biliary and vascular structures can be managed by enucleation of the tumor (Pitchaimuthu and Duxbury 2017). The presence of invasion, metastatic disease, and completeness of resection dictates the prognosis in hepatic MCNs. The prognosis of completely resected, noninvasive MCN is excellent and prolonged survival even in patients with invasive cholangiocarcinoma if treated appropriately; however, if MCNs are incompletely excised, drained, or marsupialized the prognosis is less favorable (Pitchaimuthu and Duxbury 2017; Zen et al. 2011).

1.2 Intraductal Papillary Neoplasm of the Bile Duct

Intraductal papillary neoplasm of the bile duct (IPNB) is recognized as a distinct clinicopathologic entity in the 2010 WHO classification and defined as a biliary epithelial cystic neoplasm with dilated intrahepatic bile ducts filled with papillary or villous biliary tumors covering delicate fibrovascular stalks, with and without mucin secretions, and absence of ovarian-like stoma (Bosman et al. 2010; Zen et al. 2006a). Previously described biliary tumors such as biliary papilloma or papillomatosis, intraductal type of cholangiocarcinoma, papillary type of bile duct carcinoma, and mucin-producing bile duct tumor are currently considered as IPNBs (Wan et al. 2013). IPNB is regarded as the biliary counterpart of the intraductal papillary mucinous neoplasm of the pancreas (IPMN) (Nakanuma et al. 2014). IPNBs are further classified into three types based on the severity of epithelial dysplasia and invasiveness: (1) IPNB with low- or intermediate-grade intraepithelial neoplasia, (2) IPNB with high-grade intraepithelial neoplasia, and (3) IPNB with an associated invasive carcinoma (Bosman et al. 2010). Along with MCN and biliary intraepithelial neoplasia, IPNB is regarded as a precursor lesion of cholangiocarcinoma (Park et al. 2018). The classification of IPNBs has been evolving as new information is identified regarding tumor origin and growth patterns; however, based on morphology, IPNB can be classified into three major groups that include duct-ectatic type, cystic type, and an intermediate type. Duct-ectatic type is characterized by multiple papillary tumors within a diffusely dilated duct, and cystic type shows a predominantly cystic lesion with communication with the adjacent intrahepatic bile duct. Intermediate type is characterized by a cystic lesion containing a solid component that communicates with the dilated mucin-filled bile ducts (Kim et al. 2011a).

IPNB is relatively rare biliary tumor comprising 9–38% of all bile duct carcinomas (Barton et al. 2009). IPNBs are typically found in patients from the Far East due to the high prevalence of hepatolithiasis and clonorchiasis (Park et al.

2018). IPNBs are slightly more common in older men rather than women and occur between the ages of 50–70 years. The most common symptoms are intermittent abdominal pain, infection, and jaundice (Kim et al. 2012; Yang et al. 2012). Abdominal pain is probably related to the presence of biliary stones, cholangitis, or mucin secretion, causing high pressure in the biliary tract. Recurrent cholangitis is probably due to a large amount of mucin in the bile ducts intermittently impeding bile flow, leading to repeated episodes of cholangitis (Rocha et al. 2012). Intrahepatic bile duct is the most common site of origin for IPNB (69%) followed by extrahepatic bile duct (22%) and hilar location (9%); also, for unclear reasons, left side biliary system is predominantly involved, although the primary site of tumor origin does not affect the progress or prognosis of the disease (Kim et al. 2012; Wan et al. 2013; Wang et al. 2015).

IPNBs develop from stem cells in the bile ductules, bile duct epithelium, or peribiliary glands; the interplay between the two factors, epithelial proliferation and mucus production, decides the morphologic subtype of IPNB (Kim et al. 2011a; Lim et al. 2011). Recent developments indicate the development of the cystic IPNB from the peribiliary glands located within the wall of bile ducts or scattered in the surrounding connective tissue. These are the IPNBs which correspond to pancreatic IPMN of the branch duct type (Lim et al. 2011; Nakanishi et al. 2011, 2009; Nakanuma and Sato 2012; Sato et al. 2014). Some other authors have proposed that aberrations in the biliary stem/progenitor cells located in the peribiliary glands predispose to the development of IPNB and mucin-producing cholangiocarcinoma (Cardinale et al. 2012). On gross pathology, IPNBs demonstrate papillary growth/mass within the lumen of the bile ducts with a superficial spreading pattern of growth and demonstrate mucin production in about one-third of cases. Sometimes, they also manifest as multilocular cystic mass (Wan et al. 2013). Microscopically, IPNB is characterized as papillary proliferation with a fibrovascular core; sometimes, tubulopapillary architecture can be seen in IPNB without mucin hypersecretion.

There are four epithelial subtypes of IPNB, namely: (1) pancreaticobiliary, which is most common, (2) intestinal, (3) gastric, and (4) oncocytic type (Zen et al. 2006b). Cystic type of IPNB has morphological features similar to MCN, but ovarian-like stoma is never seen in IPNB, which is one of the defining characteristics of the MCN (Zen et al. 2006a, 2011). IPNBs may share many genetic aberrations associated with biliary intraepithelial neoplasia (BilIN), a precursor associated with the development of nonpapillary invasive cholangiocarcinoma (Kim et al. 2011a; Lim et al. 2011; Wan et al. 2013).

Imaging plays an important role in the diagnosis and management of patients with IPNB. Most common imaging findings of IPNB on CT/MRI are dilated intrahepatic bile ducts with or without associated intraductal masses, and gross cystic dilatations are originating from the biliary tract (Fig. 5) (Park et al. 2018; Wang et al. 2015). Multiple intraductal masses may show heterogeneous enhancement and associated bile ductal wall thickening (Lim et al. 2011; Park et al. 2018). IPNBs appear as iso- to hypointense masses on T1-weighted and hyperintense masses on T2-weighted images (Fig. 5) (Yoon et al. 2013). Cholangioscopy including PTCS (percutaneous transhepatic cholangioscopy) and POCS (peroral cholangioscopy) can be performed to assess tumor location and extension, including superficial spreading along the biliary epithelium (Sakai et al. 2010; Tsou et al. 2008).

IPNBs can be categorized into different subtypes depending on the size and morphology of the intraductal mass, degree of mucin secretion, tumor location, and biliary duct dilatation. Many authors have described different radiological/morphological classification systems, which, for the most part, are similar, although with slight variations (Park et al. 2018; Ying et al. 2018). Park et al. (2018) classified IPNBs into four subtypes: (1) masses with proximal ductal dilatation, (2) disproportionate dilatation without masses, (3) mass with proximal and distal ductal dilatation, and (4) cystic lesions. Out of these four varieties, "mass with proximal and distal ductal dilatation" subtype is the most common. Ying et al. (Ying et al. 2018) recently described seven

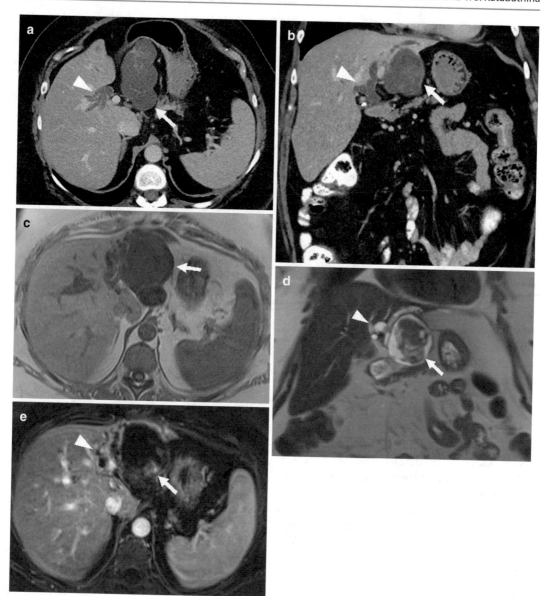

Fig. 5 (a–e) Intraductal papillary neoplasm of the bile duct (IPNB) in a 58-year-old woman with abdominal pain and jaundice. Axial (**a**) and coronal (**b**) contrast-enhanced CT images and axial T1-weighted (**c**), coronal T2-weighted (**d**), and gadolinium-enhanced T1-weighted (**e**) MR images of the liver demonstrate a multiloculated cystic lesion in the left hepatic lobe with enhancing septa-tions and solid components (arrows) with associated dilation of the intrahepatic bile ducts in the left lobe as well as dilation of the common bile duct (arrowheads). These imaging findings are highly concerning for mixed type of IPNB, which was subsequently proved on pathologic examination after surgical resection

radiological/morphological subtypes of IPNB: (1) upstream-ductectatic type, (2) typical, (3) superficial spreading, (4) no mass-forming type; (5) intrahepatic-cystic type; (6) extrahepatic-cystic type, and (7) infiltrating type. This classifi-cation system is most appropriate, with contrast-enhanced CT, and MRI can display dif-ferent types of IPNB (Ying et al. 2018). Morphological classification of IPNB facilitates the management of the disease.

Type I (upstream-ductectatic type): This type demonstrates intraductal mass with proximal upstream biliary dilatation. Due to the absence of mucin production, only upstream biliary ducts are dilated owing to ductal obstruction by the tumor. Contrast-enhanced CT or MRI demonstrates tumoral enhancement similar to the hepatic parenchyma on arterial phase; also notable is the absence of intense delayed contrast enhancement demonstrated by the conventional cholangiocarcinoma, which can be attributed to the lack of substantial fibrosis in IPNB (Wan et al. 2013). T2-weighted MRI demonstrates papillary filling defect with a high signal of the background bile. Type II (typical type): This is the most common type with intraductal tumors and dilation of both proximal and distal bile ducts secondary to mucin. Dilatation in bile ducts containing tumors may be the most prominent feature (Aoki et al. 2005; Zen et al. 2006b). Type III (superficial spreading type): Tumors spread along the inner walls of dilated bile ducts without obvious intraluminal projection or mass. Mucin production is usually present. Type IV (no mass-forming type): Bile ducts are dilated due to excessive mucin production without any obvious visible mass or tumor. Mucin, which is often not visible radiologically by either CT or MRI, can sometimes be detected on MRCP as linear and curved hypointense stripes in dilated ducts (Hong et al. 2016). The tumor is most often present in the disproportionately dilated portion of the biliary tree (Lim et al. 2008, 2004) with associated lobar atrophy. This subtype can be confused with choledochal cyst and recurrent pyogenic cholangitis. Type V (intrahepatic-cystic type) demonstrates spherical dilatation of the intrahepatic bile duct with the visible intraluminal tumor. Type VI (extrahepatic-cystic type) demonstrates spherical dilatation of the bile duct protruding outside of the liver contour with a visible intraluminal tumor. Type VII (infiltrating type) is where tumors not only grow within the bile duct but also invade the liver parenchyma outside of the bile duct with associated bile duct dilatation.

Risk of malignant transformation to invasive cholangiocarcinoma in IPNBs can be as higher as 80% and all IPNBs should be treated as malignant lesions (Park et al. 2018; Wan et al. 2013; Ying et al. 2018). MRI and MRCP are helpful to differentiate IPNB with an invasive carcinoma from IPNB with intraepithelial neoplasia preoperatively. The presence of visible intraductal mass, tumor size greater than 2.5 cm, the multiplicity of the tumor, bile duct wall thickening, and adjacent organ invasion suggest the possibility of invasive carcinoma in IPNB (Lee et al. 2019). MRI findings of invasive IPNB have a negative impact on recurrent-free survival; additionally, tumor multiplicity on MRI is an independent risk factor for tumor recurrence of IPNB after surgical resection (Lee et al. 2019). Cystic type of IPNB has to be differentiated from MCN as the management and prognosis vary significantly, and imaging plays an important role in this task (Park et al. 2018). While the presence of multiple intracystic septations with minimal intramural nodularity, absence of significant solid components, and absence of definite communication or dilation of adjacent intrahepatic bile ducts suggest the diagnosis of MCN, multilocular cystic lesion with multiple solid enhancing areas, adjacent bile ductal dilation, and communication raise the suspicion of cystic IPNB (Kim et al. 2011a; Lim et al. 2011; Park et al. 2018; Ying et al. 2018). However, there are rare case reports of MCN with bile ductal dilation and communication, and it is important to assess overall morphology and growth pattern in these cases for definite preoperative characterization (Kunovsky et al. 2018).

Surgical resection is the mainstay of treatment in IPNBs, and it has been shown that IPNBs carry a favorable prognosis when compared to nonpapillary cholangiocarcinomas. Treatment depends upon the location of the tumor. If the tumor is located only in the intrahepatic bile ducts, hepatectomy is commonly performed, and if extrahepatic bile ducts are involved, pancreaticoduodenectomy and bile duct resection is performed. It should be noted that extensive resection is advisable even in benign varieties, as the preoperative biopsy cannot always reflect the architectural atypia (Wan et al. 2013). The intraoperative frozen section at the stumps of the bile duct is essential to confirm the cancer-free surgical margin (Wang et al. 2015; Yeh et al. 2006). Liver transplantation is an option if extensive multifocal or diffuse involvement of the biliary tract is found preoperatively. In addition, invasive cholangiocarcinomas may develop after initial surgical resection of primary tumor; thus long-term imaging surveillance with MRI and MRCP is very important in patients with IPNB (Fig. 6). Development of invasive adenocarcinoma, particularly those with mucinous carcinomas, has more favorable prognoses than cholangiocarcinoma (Park et al. 2018).

1.3 Cystic Hepatocellular Carcinoma

Cystic hepatocellular carcinoma (HCC) is rare malignancy and could present as a multilocular cystic mass with enhancing septations and solid components mimicking a hepatic MCN on imaging (Vachha et al. 2011). Cystic changes in HCC are likely secondary to either spontaneous internal necrosis/hemorrhage or cystic degeneration in the rapidly growing tumor or due to liquefactive necrosis after locoregional therapies such as radiofrequency ablation (RFA), microwave ablation (MWA), and trans-arterial chemoembolization (TACE) (Mortele and Ros 2001). While the cystic component of the tumor denotes either

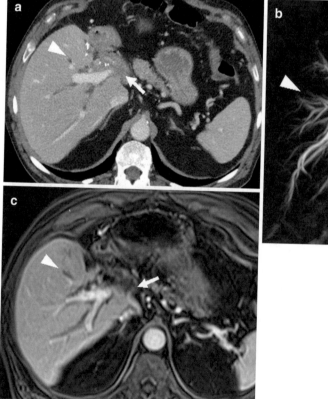
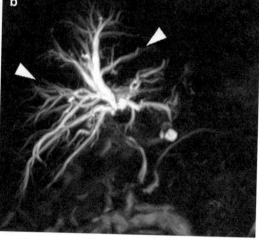

Fig. 6 (a–c) Invasive cholangiocarcinoma development after surgical resection of intraductal papillary neoplasm of the bile duct (IPNB) involving the left hepatic lobe in a 73-year-old man. Axial contrast-enhanced CT image (a), and 3D MRCP (b), and gadolinium-enhanced T1-weighted (c) MR images of the liver demonstrate an ill-defined, het-

erogeneously enhancing soft tissue mass at the porta hepatis abutting the right portal vein (arrows) resulting in moderate intrahepatic biliary ductal dilation involving the right hepatic lobe (arrowheads). This mass was proven to be invasive cholangiocarcinoma on pathology spontaneous necrosis or hemorrhage, solid nodular components or septa denote the viable malignant portions of the tumor (Alobaidi and Shirkhoda 2004). Patients with cystic HCC may present with clinical signs of inflammation such as fever and elevated white count and imaging findings suggesting a hepatic abscess; however, if there are signs or complications of underlying cirrhosis, cystic HCC should be considered in the differential diagnosis (Powers et al. 1994; Vachha et al. 2011).

On US, cystic HCC appears either as a multilocular cystic mass with solid nodular components and septations or a solid mass with extensive central necrosis/cystic areas (Fig. 7) (Qian et al. 2013). At CT/MR imaging, cystic HCC may have

a varied imaging appearances; it can either appear as an atypical multilocular cystic mass with internal necrotic or hemorrhagic areas or a large, cystic mass with peripheral enhancement (Fig. 7) (Mortele and Ros 2001; Qian et al. 2013; Vachha et al. 2011). Multiple cystic areas with internal septations and solid components may also develop in the infiltrating HCC (Fig. 8) (Alobaidi and Shirkhoda 2004). The solid components of the cystic HCC, including nodules or septations, demonstrate imaging features of HCC, including arterial phase hyperenhancement with portal venous and delayed phase washout and delayed capsular enhancement (Fig. 8). "Abnormal internal vessels and variegated pattern" in the mural nodules is an interesting feature that

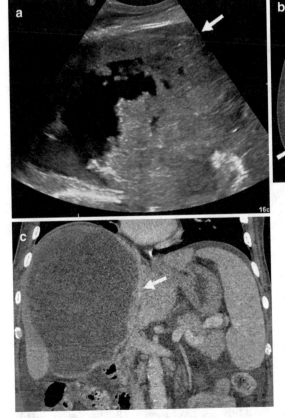

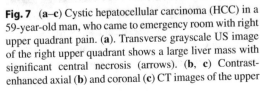

Fig. 7 (a–c) Cystic hepatocellular carcinoma (HCC) in a 59-year-old man, who came to emergency room with right upper quadrant pain. (**a**). Transverse grayscale US image of the right upper quadrant shows a large liver mass with significant central necrosis (arrows). (**b, c**) Contrast-enhanced axial (**b**) and coronal (**c**) CT images of the upper abdomen demonstrate a large, necrotic liver mass (arrows) with peripheral rim enhancement and scattered foci of intralesional air (arrowheads) mimicking an abscess. This mass was proven to be cystic HCC with extensive necrosis on pathology

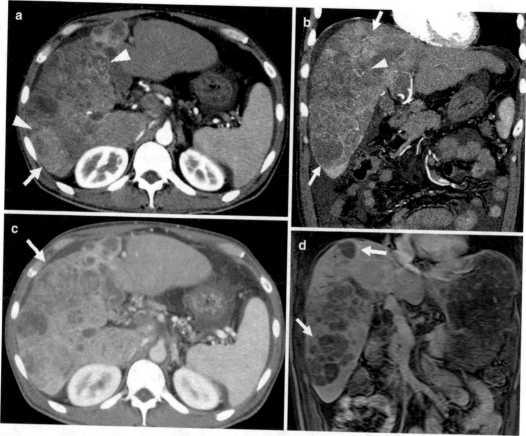

Fig. 8 (**a–d**) Infiltrating hepatocellular carcinoma (HCC) in a 50-year-old man with multifocal cystic areas secondary to extensive necrosis. Axial and coronal contrast-enhanced CT images of the liver obtained during the arterial phase (**a, b**) and axial CT image obtained during the portal venous phase (**c**) demonstrate infiltrating HCC in the right hepatic lobe with multiple cystic areas (arrows) and abnormal internal vessels and variegated pattern in the mural nodules during arterial phase (arrowheads). (**d**). Coronal gadolinium-enhanced T1-weighted image shows multiple cystic foci with the infiltrating HCC (arrows)

strongly suggests the possibility of HCC (Fig. 8) (Qian et al. 2013). These findings are described by Nino-Murcia et al. as either visible internal vessels with an irregular distorted contour or randomly distributed hyperattenuating and hypoattenuating regions in the hepatic mass (Nino-Murcia et al. 2000). Compared to spontaneous necrosis, the coagulative necrosis in the ablative zone appears as an oval or round area with heterogeneously high signal intensity on T1-weighted and low signal intensity on T2-weighted MR images (Fig. 9) (Kim et al. 2011b). At CT, TACE-induced hemorrhagic coagulative necrosis is characterized by hyperattenuating iodized oil retention within the tumor.

Also, adjacent hepatic capsular retraction is common in patients who have undergone prior ablation or TACE (Blachar et al. 2002).

1.4 Cystic Liver Metastases

Metastases are the most common malignant neoplasms of the liver and are far more common than primary liver tumors (Borhani et al. 2014; Sica et al. 2000). Most of the liver metastases arise from the gastrointestinal tract with colorectal cancer being the most common primary tumor; adenocarcinomas are the most frequent primary tumors that metastasize to the liver, fol-

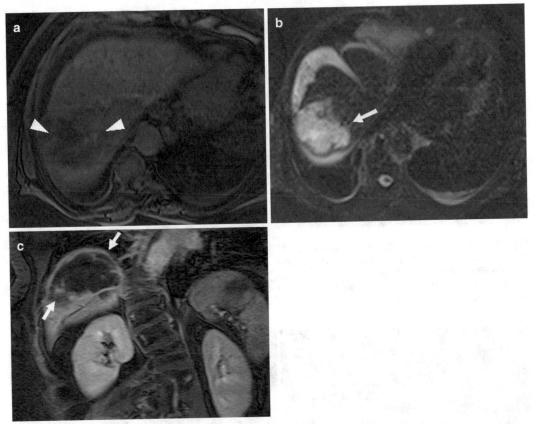

Fig. 9 (a–c) Cystic appearance of hepatocellular carcinoma (HCC) after treatment with microwave ablation in a 65-year-old woman. Axial T1-weighted (**a**), axial T2-weighted (**b**), and gadolinium-enhanced coronal T1-weighted (**c**) MR images of the liver demonstrate treated HCC in the hepatic dome with heterogeneously hyperintense foci on T1-weighted image (arrowheads) suggestive of coagulative necrosis. The treated HCC is diffusely hyperintense on T2-weighted image and shows peripheral rim enhancement after gadolinium administration (arrows)

lowed by squamous cell cancers (Borhani et al. 2014; Qian et al. 2013). While the majority of liver metastases spread by hematogenous route, ovarian carcinoma metastases spread by peritoneal seeding that result in serosal implants on both the visceral peritoneal surface of the liver and the parietal peritoneum of the diaphragm (Mortele and Ros 2001). Majority of the hepatic metastases present as multiple solid lesions that are hypoattenuating to the adjacent liver parenchyma on CT with irregular peripheral rim enhancement. However, select hepatic metastases are partially or entirely cystic in nature. Cystic hepatic metastases are comparatively less common and they are commonly seen secondary to the rapid growth and insufficient vascular supply to the lesion, leading to cystic degeneration and necrosis (Mortele and Ros 2001), which is frequently seen in metastases from a neuroendocrine tumor, pancreatic adenocarcinoma, renal cell carcinoma, lung adenocarcinoma, choriocarcinoma, sarcoma, melanoma, or gastrointestinal stromal tumor (GIST) (Figs. 10 and 11) (Qian et al. 2013). Cystic change can also develop due to abundant mucin production from mucinous adenocarcinomas, such as colorectal or ovarian carcinoma or secondary to systemic or locoregional treatment (Fig. 12) (Kanematsu et al. 2006; Sandrasegaran et al. 2005; Warakaulle and Gleeson 2006).

On CT, cystic hepatic metastases appear as multiple cystic lesions with thick, irregularly

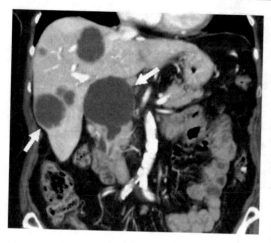

Fig. 10 Cystic metastases to the liver in an 85-year-old woman with pancreatic ductal adenocarcinoma. Coronal contrast-enhanced CT image of the abdomen shows multiple focal cystic lesions in the liver that were proven to be metastatic disease on pathology

enhancing wall, nodular septations, mural nodularity, and internal debris (Figs. 10 and 11). Given the presence of mucin, hemorrhage, and necrosis, attenuation of the cystic component is higher than simple fluid (Qian et al. 2013). Also, mucinous metastases from colorectal or ovarian primary may demonstrate scattered calcifications (Fig. 12). On MR, cystic metastases demonstrate moderately low signal on T1-weighted and moderately high signal on T2-weighted images with a hyperintense center (liquefactive necrosis) surrounded by a less intense rim of viable tumor (Fig. 11). Given the hypervascular nature, hepatic metastases from choriocarcinoma demonstrate peripheral nodular enhancing foci that likely represent pseudoaneurysms (Fig. 13). Differential diagnosis

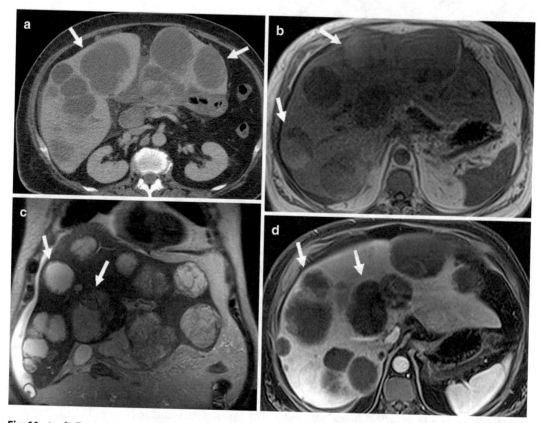

Fig. 11 (a–d) Cystic and necrotic hepatic metastases in a 52-year-old man with pancreatic neuroendocrine tumor. Axial contrast-enhanced CT image of the liver (**a**) and axial T1-weighted (**b**), coronal T2-weighted (**c**), and axial gadolinium-enhanced T1-weighted (**d**) MR images of the liver demonstrate multiple cystic lesions of varying sizes that demonstrate iso- to hyperintense signal on T1-weighted image suggestive of hemorrhagic/proteinaceous contents (arrows). They appear hyperintense on T2-weighted image and heterogeneous enhancement after gadolinium administration with central necrosis and cystic change

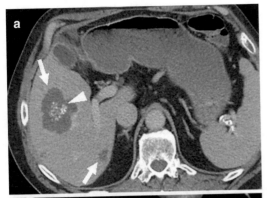

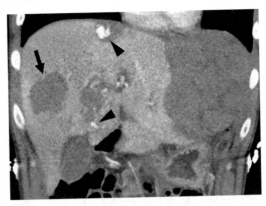

Fig. 13 Cystic metastases from gestational choriocarcinoma in a 33-year-old woman. Coronal contrast-enhanced CT image of the liver demonstrates multiple hypodense, cystic lesions in the liver (arrows) with peripheral enhancing foci (arrowheads) suggestive of pseudoaneurysms. These lesions were proven to be metastatic disease from gestational choriocarcinoma on pathology

2 Rare Cystic Tumors of the Liver

2.1 Intrahepatic Cholangiocarcinoma

Intrahepatic cholangiocarcinoma is usually differentiated into three morphologic subtypes: (1) mass forming, (2) periductal infiltrating, and (3) intraductal growth (Fabrega-Foster et al. 2017; Seo et al. 2017). Mass-forming cholangiocarcinoma (M-CCA) is the most common subtype that demonstrates incomplete peripheral enhancement in the arterial phase that may become iso- or hypodense in the portal venous phase (Ringe and Wacker 2015). The central fibrous stroma enhances most prominently in the delayed phase unless there is abundant central mucin or necrosis (Valls et al. 2000). With necrotic or mucin-producing M-CCAs, the central portion does not enhance in the late phase and remains hypodense throughout all three phases, when it can be confused with other peripherally enhancing multilocular cystic liver lesions (Fig. 14) (Alobaidi and Shirkhoda 2004; Ringe and Wacker 2015). Ancillary features of M-CCA on CT/MR include

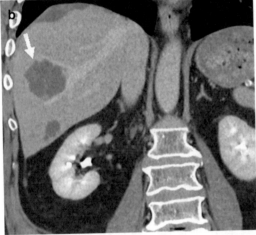

Fig. 12 (**a, b**) Cystic metastases from colonic adenocarcinoma in a 68-year-old woman. Axial (**a**) and coronal (**b**) contrast-enhanced CT images of the liver demonstrate multiple cystic lesions in the liver (arrows) with central calcifications (arrowhead). These lesions were proven to be metastatic disease from mucinous adenocarcinoma of the colon

includes polycystic liver disease and multiple hepatic abscesses. Polycystic liver disease cysts have mostly smooth walls, and they displace adjacent vessels, whereas cystic metastases are heterogeneous with ragged, irregular borders. Multiple liver abscesses are easily distinguished from the cystic metastases by the clinical findings, presence of intralesional air, and the presence of a late faint enhancing peripheral rim on CT/MR when compared to the early arterial enhancing ring observed in the case of metastases (Mortele et al. 2004).

capsular retraction, biliary obstruction, satellite nodules, vascular encasement, lobar atrophy, and lymphadenopathy and these features help to differentiate cholangiocarcinoma from other malignant cystic tumors (Ringe and Wacker 2015).

2.2 Giant Cavernous Hemangioma

Cavernous hemangioma is the second most common cause of focal liver lesions after metastases. Most lesions are solid, are less than 5 cm in size, and are asymptomatic. However, select tumors

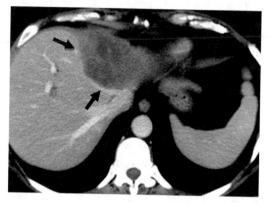

Fig. 14 Cystic cholangiocarcinoma in a 57-year-old woman. Axial contrast-enhanced CT image of the liver shows a centrally necrotic tumor with peripheral heterogeneous enhancement (arrows). This was proven to be a mass-forming intrahepatic cholangiocarcinoma on pathology

can become very large and outgrow their blood supply leading to cystic degeneration. These can cause symptoms such as compression of adjacent structures, rupture, or acute thrombosis (Vachha et al. 2011). On US, a giant cavernous hemangioma may demonstrate similar features as of cavernous hemangiomas, such as a well-circumscribed echogenic periphery with a hypoechoic center (Vachha et al. 2011). On CT/MR, the central cystic component remains non-enhancing in all phases of the post-contrast study. The peripheral portion of the lesion demonstrates discontinuous nodular enhancement in the arterial phase with progressive fill-in in the portal venous and delayed phases similar to the conventional cavernous hemangiomas (Fig. 15) (Vachha et al. 2011).

2.3 Mesenchymal Hamartoma

Mesenchymal hamartoma is an uncommon tumor that usually occurs in children less than 2 years of age (Qian et al. 2013). This tumor is considered as a developmental lesion containing bile ducts, immature mesenchymal cells, and hepatocytes. Imaging appearance of mesenchymal hamartoma is largely dependent on the proportion of the cystic and solid components. Cystic portions are avascular, and stromal portions are relatively hypovascular (Ros et al. 1986). At US, mesenchymal hamartoma appears as a cystic mass with

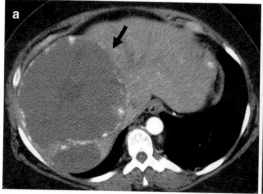

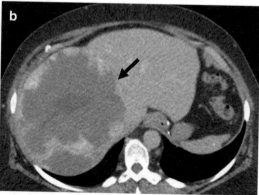

Fig. 15 (**a**, **b**) Cystic appearing giant cavernous hemangioma of the liver in a 25-year-old woman. Axial contrast-enhanced CT images of the liver obtained during the arterial (**a**) and portal venous (**b**) phases demonstrate a large cavernous hemangioma in the liver (arrows) with central necrosis appearing as a cystic mass

thin or thick internal septations (Gow et al. 2009). On CT, these tumors appear as a complex cystic mass with a relatively hypodense stromal component, when compared to the surrounding liver parenchyma. Solid stromal component and septations show post-contrast enhancement. On MR, solid stromal component demonstrates low signal on both T1- and T2-weighted images secondary to fibrosis. Cystic component demonstrates a high T2 signal with the variable signal on T1-weighted images depending upon the protein content of the cyst material (Mortele and Ros 2002; Qian et al. 2013).

2.4 Undifferentiated Embryonal Sarcoma

Undifferentiated embryonal sarcoma (UES) is a rare, malignant hepatic tumor affecting older children and presents as a cystic mass with enhancing septations and solid areas (Lauwers et al. 1997). Hemorrhage and necrosis are frequently seen within the tumor. On CT, UES appears as a well-defined complex but predominantly cystic mass with enhancing solid septations and a pseudo-capsule separating it from adjacent normal liver parenchyma (Mortele and Ros 2001). It appears cystic on CT/MRI and solid on ultrasound due to high myxoid content of the cystic component (Alobaidi and Shirkhoda 2004; Mortele and Ros 2001). On MR, UES demonstrates low T1 and high T2 signal with scattered areas of hemorrhage (Qian et al. 2013). Solid areas demonstrate delayed post-contrast enhancement, and pseudo-capsule demonstrates early arterial enhancement (Buetow et al. 1997; Yoon et al. 1997).

2.5 Inflammatory Myofibroblastic Tumor

An inflammatory myofibroblastic tumor (IMT), also known as "inflammatory pseudotumor," is an uncommon cause of focal hepatic cystic lesions and is presumed to be occurring as a hepatic regenerative response to inflammation (Faraj et al. 2011; Yoon et al. 1999). Symptoms are nonspecific and include right upper quadrant pain, jaundice, and sometimes obliterative phlebitis. Although cross-sectional imaging features are nonspecific, IMT commonly appears as a multilocular, predominantly cystic mass with a remarkable delayed enhancement of internal septa, which is presumably due to delayed washout of contrast medium accumulating in the extravascular space (Anderson et al. 2009; Fukuya et al. 1994; Venkataraman et al. 2003).

3 Conclusion

The increasing availability of cross-sectional imaging has led to a significant increase in the incidental detection of asymptomatic cystic liver lesions, and it is essential to differentiate cystic liver neoplasms from benign entities. Cystic liver tumors demonstrate characteristic pathologic findings, imaging features, natural history, and prognoses. Cross-sectional imaging plays a pivotal role in the initial diagnosis, treatment follow-up, and surveillance of these tumors. Awareness of various cystic liver tumors and familiarity with their cross-sectional imaging findings permit appropriate diagnosis and patient management.

References

Alobaidi M, Shirkhoda A (2004) Malignant cystic and necrotic liver lesions: a pattern approach to discrimination. Curr Probl Diagn Radiol 33(6):254–268. https://doi.org/10.1067/j.cpradiol.2004.08.002

Anderson SW, Kruskal JB, Kane RA (2009) Benign hepatic tumors and iatrogenic pseudotumors. Radiographics 29(1):211–229. https://doi.org/10.1148/rg.291085099

Aoki S, Okayama Y, Kitajima Y, Hayashi K, Imai H, Okamoto T, Akita S, Gotoh K, Ohara H, Nomura T, Joh T, Yokoyama Y, Itoh M (2005) Intrahepatic biliary papilloma morphologically similar to biliary cystadenoma. J Gastroenterol Hepatol 20(2):321–324. https://doi.org/10.1111/j.1440-1746.2005.03242.x

Barton JG, Barrett DA, Maricevich MA, Schnelldorfer T, Wood CM, Smyrk TC, Baron TH, Sarr MG, Donohue JH, Farnell MB, Kendrick ML, Nagorney DM, Reid Lombardo KM, Que FG (2009) Intraductal papillary mucinous neoplasm of the biliary tract: a real disease? HPB (Oxford) 11(8):684–691. https://doi.org/10.1111/j.1477-2574.2009.00122.x

Billington PD, Prescott RJ, Lapsia S (2012) Diagnosis of a biliary cystadenoma demonstrating communication with the biliary system by MRI using a hepatocyte-specific contrast agent. Br J Radiol 85(1010):e35–e36. https://doi.org/10.1259/bjr/52850720

Blachar A, Federle MP, Brancatelli G (2002) Hepatic capsular retraction: spectrum of benign and malignant etiologies. Abdom Imaging 27(6):690–699. https://doi.org/10.1007/s00261-001-0094-8

Borhani AA, Wiant A, Heller MT (2014) Cystic hepatic lesions: a review and an algorithmic approach. AJR Am J Roentgenol 203(6):1192–1204. https://doi.org/10.2214/AJR.13.12386

Bosman FT, Carneiro F, Hruban RH (2010) Theise ND WHO classification of tumours of the digestive system, 4th edn. International Agency for Research on Cancer, Lyon

Buetow PC, Buck JL, Pantongrag-Brown L, Marshall WH, Ros PR, Levine MS, Goodman ZD (1997) Undifferentiated (embryonal) sarcoma of the liver: pathologic basis of imaging findings in 28 cases. Radiology 203(3):779–783. https://doi.org/10.1148/radiology.203.3.9169704

Cardinale V, Wang Y, Carpino G, Reid LM, Gaudio E, Alvaro D (2012) Mucin-producing cholangiocarcinoma might derive from biliary tree stem/progenitor cells located in peribiliary glands. Hepatology 55(6):2041–2042. https://doi.org/10.1002/hep.25587

Del Poggio P, Buonocore M (2008) Cystic tumors of the liver: a practical approach. World J Gastroenterol 14(23):3616–3620

Erdogan D, Kloek J, Lamers WH, Offerhaus GJ, Busch OR, Gouma DJ, van Gulik TM (2010) Mucinous cystadenomas in liver: management and origin. Dig Surg 27(1):19–23. https://doi.org/10.1159/000268110

Fabrega-Foster K, Ghasabeh MA, Pawlik TM, Kamel IR (2017) Multimodality imaging of intrahepatic cholangiocarcinoma. Hepatobiliary Surg Nutr 6(2):67–78. https://doi.org/10.21037/hbsn.2016.12.10

Faraj W, Ajouz H, Mukherji D, Kealy G, Shamseddine A, Khalife M (2011) Inflammatory pseudo-tumor of the liver: a rare pathological entity. World J Surg Oncol 9:5. https://doi.org/10.1186/1477-7819-9-5

Fragulidis GP, Pantiora EV, Kontis EA, Primetis E, Polydorou A, Karvouni E, Polymeneas G (2017) Biliary mucinous cystic neoplasm of the liver with ovarian Stroma and elevated serum and cystic fluid cancer antigen 19-9 levels. Cureus 9(11):e1863. https://doi.org/10.7759/cureus.1863

Fukuya T, Honda H, Matsumata T, Kawanami T, Shimoda Y, Muranaka T, Hayashi T, Maeda T, Sakai H, Masuda K (1994) Diagnosis of inflammatory pseudotumor of the liver: value of CT. AJR Am J Roentgenol 163(5):1087–1091. https://doi.org/10.2214/ajr.163.5.7976880

Gow KW, Lee L, Pruthi S, Patterson K, Healey PJ (2009) Mesenchymal hamartoma of the liver. J Pediatr Surg 44(2):468–470. https://doi.org/10.1016/j.jpedsurg.2008.09.029

Hong GS, Byun JH, Kim JH, Kim HJ, Lee SS, Hong SM, Lee MG (2016) Thread sign in biliary intraductal papillary mucinous neoplasm: a novel specific finding for MRI. Eur Radiol 26(9):3112–3120. https://doi.org/10.1007/s00330-015-4158-5

Kanematsu M, Kondo H, Goshima S, Kato H, Tsuge U, Hirose Y, Kim MJ, Moriyama N (2006) Imaging liver metastases: review and update. Eur J Radiol 58(2):217–228. https://doi.org/10.1016/j.ejrad.2005.11.041

Kim JY, Kim SH, Eun HW, Lee MW, Lee JY, Han JK, Choi BI (2010) Differentiation between biliary cystic neoplasms and simple cysts of the liver: accuracy of CT. AJR Am J Roentgenol 195(5):1142–1148. https://doi.org/10.2214/AJR.09.4026

Kim H, Lim JH, Jang KT, Kim MJ, Lee J, Lee JY, Choi D, Lim HK, Choi DW, Lee JK, Baron R (2011a) Morphology of intraductal papillary neoplasm of the bile ducts: radiologic-pathologic correlation. Abdom Imaging 36(4):438–446. https://doi.org/10.1007/s00261-010-9636-2

Kim YS, Rhim H, Lim HK, Choi D, Lee MW, Park MJ (2011b) Coagulation necrosis induced by radio-frequency ablation in the liver: histopathologic and radiologic review of usual to extremely rare changes. Radiographics 31(2):377–390. https://doi.org/10.1148/rg.312105056

Kim KM, Lee JK, Shin JU, Lee KH, Lee KT, Sung JY, Jang KT, Heo JS, Choi SH, Choi DW, Lim JH (2012) Clinicopathologic features of intraductal papillary neoplasm of the bile duct according to histologic subtype. Am J Gastroenterol 107(1):118–125. https://doi.org/10.1038/ajg.2011.316

Kunovsky L, Kala Z, Svaton R, Moravcik P, Mazanec J, Husty J, Prochazka V (2018) Mucinous cystic neoplasm of the liver or Intraductal papillary mucinous neoplasm of the bile duct? A case report and a review of literature. Ann Hepatol 17(3):519–524. https://doi.org/10.5604/01.3001.0011.7397

Lauwers GY, Grant LD, Donnelly WH, Meloni AM, Foss RM, Sanberg AA, Langham MR Jr (1997) Hepatic undifferentiated (embryonal) sarcoma arising in a mesenchymal hamartoma. Am J Surg Pathol 21(10):1248–1254

Lee S, Kim MJ, Kim S, Choi D, Jang KT, Park YN (2019) Intraductal papillary neoplasm of the bile duct: assessment of invasive carcinoma and long-term outcomes using MRI. J Hepatol 70(4):692–699. https://doi.org/10.1016/j.jhep.2018.12.005

Lewin M, Mourra N, Honigman I, Flejou JF, Parc R, Arrive L, Tubiana JM (2006) Assessment of MRI and MRCP in diagnosis of biliary cystadenoma and cystadenocarcinoma. Eur Radiol 16(2):407–413. https://doi.org/10.1007/s00330-005-2822-x

Lim JH, Yoon KH, Kim SH, Kim HY, Lim HK, Song SY, Nam KJ (2004) Intraductal papillary mucinous tumor of the bile ducts. Radiographics 24(1):53–66. (Discussion 66–57). https://doi.org/10.1148/rg.241035002

Lim JH, Jang KT, Choi D (2008) Biliary intraductal papillary-mucinous neoplasm manifesting only as dilatation of the hepatic lobar or segmental bile ducts: imaging features in six patients. AJR Am J Roentgenol 191(3):778–782. https://doi.org/10.2214/AJR.07.2091

Lim JH, Zen Y, Jang KT, Kim YK, Nakanuma Y (2011) Cyst-forming intraductal papillary neoplasm of the bile ducts: description of imaging and pathologic aspects. AJR Am J Roentgenol 197(5):1111–1120. https://doi.org/10.2214/AJR.10.6363

Mortele KJ, Peters HE (2009) Multimodality imaging of common and uncommon cystic focal liver lesions. Semin Ultrasound CT MR 30(5):368–386

Mortele KJ, Ros PR (2001) Cystic focal liver lesions in the adult: differential CT and MR imaging features. Radiographics 21(4):895–910. https://doi.org/10.1148/radiographics.21.4.g01jl16895

Mortele KJ, Ros PR (2002) Benign liver neoplasms. Clin Liver Dis 6(1):119–145

Mortele KJ, Segatto E, Ros PR (2004) The infected liver: radiologic-pathologic correlation. Radiographics 24(4):937–955. https://doi.org/10.1148/rg.244035719

Nakanishi Y, Zen Y, Hirano S, Tanaka E, Takahashi O, Yonemori A, Doumen H, Kawakami H, Itoh T, Nakanuma Y, Kondo S (2009) Intraductal oncocytic papillary neoplasm of the bile duct: the first case of peribiliary gland origin. J Hepato-Biliary-Pancreat Surg 16(6):869–873. https://doi.org/10.1007/s00534-009-0070-1

Nakanishi Y, Nakanuma Y, Ohara M, Iwao T, Kimura N, Ishidate T, Kijima H (2011) Intraductal papillary neoplasm arising from peribiliary glands connecting with the inferior branch of the bile duct of the anterior segment of the liver. Pathol Int 61(12):773–777. https://doi.org/10.1111/j.1440-1827.2011.02738.x

Nakanuma Y, Sato Y (2012) Cystic and papillary neoplasm involving peribiliary glands: a biliary counterpart of branch-type intraductal papillary mucinous [corrected] neoplasm? Hepatology 55(6):2040–2041. https://doi.org/10.1002/hep.25590

Nakanuma Y, Harada K, Sasaki M, Sato Y (2014) Proposal of a new disease concept "biliary diseases with pancreatic counterparts". Anatomical and pathological bases. Histol Histopathol 29(1):1–10. https://doi.org/10.14670/HH-29.1

Natov NS, Horton LC, Hegde SR (2017) Successful endoscopic treatment of an intraductal papillary neoplasm of the bile duct. World J Gastrointest Endosc 9(5):238–242. https://doi.org/10.4253/wjge.v9.i5.238

Nino-Murcia M, Olcott EW, Jeffrey RB Jr, Lamm RL, Beaulieu CF, Jain KA (2000) Focal liver lesions: pattern-based classification scheme for enhancement at arterial phase CT. Radiology 215(3):746–751. https://doi.org/10.1148/radiology.215.3.r00jn03746

Park HJ, Kim SY, Kim HJ, Lee SS, Hong GS, Byun JH, Hong SM, Lee MG (2018) Intraductal papillary neoplasm of the bile duct: clinical, imaging, and pathologic features. AJR Am J Roentgenol 211(1):67–75. https://doi.org/10.2214/AJR.17.19261

Pitchaimuthu M, Duxbury M (2017) Cystic lesions of the liver-a review. Curr Probl Surg 54(10):514–542. https://doi.org/10.1067/j.cpsurg.2017.09.001

Powers C, Ros PR, Stoupis C, Johnson WK, Segel KH (1994) Primary liver neoplasms: MR imaging with pathologic correlation. Radiographics 14(3):459–482. https://doi.org/10.1148/radiographics.14.3.8066263

Qian LJ, Zhu J, Zhuang ZG, Xia Q, Liu Q, Xu JR (2013) Spectrum of multilocular cystic hepatic lesions: CT and MR imaging findings with pathologic correlation. Radiographics 33(5):1419–1433. https://doi.org/10.1148/rg.335125063

Ringe KI, Wacker F (2015) Radiological diagnosis in cholangiocarcinoma: application of computed tomography, magnetic resonance imaging, and positron emission tomography. Best Pract Res Clin Gastroenterol 29(2):253–265. https://doi.org/10.1016/j.bpg.2015.02.004

Rocha FG, Lee H, Katabi N, DeMatteo RP, Fong Y, D'Angelica MI, Allen PJ, Klimstra DS, Jarnagin WR (2012) Intraductal papillary neoplasm of the bile duct: a biliary equivalent to intraductal papillary mucinous neoplasm of the pancreas? Hepatology 56(4):1352–1360. https://doi.org/10.1002/hep.25786

Ros PR, Goodman ZD, Ishak KG, Dachman AH, Olmsted WW, Hartman DS, Lichtenstein JE (1986) Mesenchymal hamartoma of the liver: radiologic-pathologic correlation. Radiology 158(3):619–624. https://doi.org/10.1148/radiology.158.3.3511498

Sakai Y, Tsuyuguchi T, Ishihara T, Sugiyama H, Miyakawa K, Yasui S, Eto R, Fujimoto T, Ohtsuka M, Miyazaki M, Yokosuka O (2010) Usefulness of peroral cholangioscopy in preoperative diagnosis of intraductal papillary neoplasm of the bile duct. Hepato-Gastroenterology 57(101): 691–693

Sandrasegaran K, Rajesh A, Rydberg J, Rushing DA, Akisik FM, Henley JD (2005) Gastrointestinal stromal tumors: clinical, radiologic, and pathologic features. AJR Am J Roentgenol 184(3):803–811. https://doi.org/10.2214/ajr.184.3.01840803

Sato Y, Harada K, Sasaki M, Nakanuma Y (2014) Cystic and micropapillary epithelial changes of peribiliary glands might represent a precursor lesion of biliary epithelial neoplasms. Virchows Arch 464(2):157–163. https://doi.org/10.1007/s00428-014-1537-2

Seo N, Kim DY, Choi JY (2017) Cross-sectional imaging of intrahepatic cholangiocarcinoma: development, growth, spread, and prognosis. AJR Am J Roentgenol 209(2):W64–W75. https://doi.org/10.2214/AJR.16.16923

Sica GT, Ji H, Ros PR (2000) CT and MR imaging of hepatic metastases. AJR Am J Roentgenol 174(3):691–698. https://doi.org/10.2214/ajr.174.3.1740691

Simo KA, McKillop IH, Ahrens WA, Martinie JB, Iannitti DA, Sindram D (2012) Invasive biliary mucinous cystic neoplasm: a review. HPB (Oxford) 14(11):725–740. https://doi.org/10.1111/j.1477-2574.2012.00532.x

Soares KC, Arnaoutakis DJ, Kamel I, Anders R, Adams RB, Bauer TW, Pawlik TM (2014) Cystic neoplasms of the liver: biliary cystadenoma and cystadenocarcinoma. J Am Coll Surg 218(1):119–128. https://doi.org/10.1016/j.jamcollsurg.2013.08.014

Tsou YK, Liu NJ, Wu RC, Lee CS, Tang JH, Hung CF, Jan YY (2008) Endoscopic retrograde cholangiography in the diagnosis and treatment of mucobilia. Scand J Gastroenterol 43(9):1137–1144. https://doi.org/10.1080/00365520802029856

Tsuchida K, Yamagata M, Saifuku Y, Ichikawa D, Kanke K, Murohisa T, Tamano M, Iijima M, Nemoto Y, Shimoda W, Komori T, Fukui H, Ichikawa K, Sugaya H, Miyachi K, Fujimori T, Hiraishi H (2010) Successful endoscopic procedures for intraductal papillary neoplasm of the bile duct: a case report. World J Gastroenterol 16(7):909–913. https://doi.org/10.3748/wjg.v16.i7.909

Vachha B, Sun MR, Siewert B, Eisenberg RL (2011) Cystic lesions of the liver. AJR Am J Roentgenol 196(4):W355–W366.   https://doi.org/10.2214/AJR.10.5292

Valls C, Guma A, Puig I, Sanchez A, Andia E, Serrano T, Figueras J (2000) Intrahepatic peripheral cholangiocarcinoma: CT evaluation. Abdom Imaging 25(5):490–496

Venkataraman S, Semelka RC, Braga L, Danet IM, Woosley JT (2003) Inflammatory myofibroblastic tumor of the hepatobiliary system: report of MR imaging appearance in four patients. Radiology 227(3):758–763. https://doi.org/10.1148/radiol.2273020572

Wan XS, Xu YY, Qian JY, Yang XB, Wang AQ, He L, Zhao HT, Sang XT (2013) Intraductal papillary neoplasm of the bile duct. World J Gastroenterol 19(46):8595–8604. https://doi.org/10.3748/wjg.v19.i46.8595

Wang X, Cai YQ, Chen YH, Liu XB (2015) Biliary tract intraductal papillary mucinous neoplasm: report of 19 cases. World J Gastroenterol 21(14):4261–4267. https://doi.org/10.3748/wjg.v21.i14.4261

Warakaulle DR, Gleeson F (2006) MDCT appearance of gastrointestinal stromal tumors after therapy with imatinib mesylate. AJR Am J Roentgenol 186(2):510–515. https://doi.org/10.2214/AJR.04.1516

Yang J, Wang W, Yan L (2012) The clinicopathological features of intraductal papillary neoplasms of the bile duct in a Chinese population. Dig Liver Dis 44(3):251–256. https://doi.org/10.1016/j.dld.2011.08.014

Yeh TS, Tseng JH, Chiu CT, Liu NJ, Chen TC, Jan YY, Chen MF (2006) Cholangiographic spectrum of intra-

ductal papillary mucinous neoplasm of the bile ducts. Ann Surg 244(2):248–253. https://doi.org/10.1097/01.sla.0000217636.40050.54

Ying S, Ying M, Liang W, Wang Z, Wang Q, Chen F, Xiao W (2018) Morphological classification of intraductal papillary neoplasm of the bile duct. Eur Radiol 28(4):1568–1578. https://doi.org/10.1007/s00330-017-5123-2

Yoon W, Kim JK, Kang HK (1997) Hepatic undifferentiated embryonal sarcoma: MR findings. J Comput Assist Tomogr 21(1):100–102

Yoon KH, Ha HK, Lee JS, Suh JH, Kim MH, Kim PN, Lee MG, Yun KJ, Choi SC, Nah YH, Kim CG, Won JJ, Auh YH (1999) Inflammatory pseudotumor of the liver in patients with recurrent pyogenic cholangitis: CT-histopathologic correlation. Radiology 211(2):373–379. https://doi.org/10.1148/radiology.211.2.r99ma36373

Yoon HJ, Kim YK, Jang KT, Lee KT, Lee JK, Choi DW, Lim JH (2013) Intraductal papillary neoplasm of the bile duct: description of MRI and added value of diffusion-weighted MRI. Abdom Imaging 38(5):1082–1090. https://doi.org/10.1007/s00261-013-9989-4

Zen Y, Fujii T, Itatsu K, Nakamura K, Konishi F, Masuda S, Mitsui T, Asada Y, Miura S, Miyayama S, Uehara T, Katsuyama T, Ohta T, Minato H, Nakanuma Y (2006a) Biliary cystic tumors with bile duct communication: a cystic variant of intraductal papillary neoplasm of the bile duct. Mod Pathol 19(9):1243–1254. https://doi.org/10.1038/modpathol.3800643

Zen Y, Fujii T, Itatsu K, Nakamura K, Minato H, Kasashima S, Kurumaya H, Katayanagi K, Kawashima A, Masuda S, Niwa H, Mitsui T, Asada Y, Miura S, Ohta T, Nakanuma Y (2006b) Biliary papillary tumors share pathological features with intraductal papillary mucinous neoplasm of the pancreas. Hepatology 44(5):1333–1343. https://doi.org/10.1002/hep.21387

Zen Y, Pedica F, Patcha VR, Capelli P, Zamboni G, Casaril A, Quaglia A, Nakanuma Y, Heaton N, Portmann B (2011) Mucinous cystic neoplasms of the liver: a clinicopathological study and comparison with intraductal papillary neoplasms of the bile duct. Mod Pathol 24(8):1079–1089. https://doi.org/10.1038/modpathol.2011.71

Uncommon Liver Tumors

Ersan Altun and Katrina Anne Mcginty

Contents

Abstract

Uncommon liver tumors do not have specific imaging features, but MRI is still the best imaging modality for the detection and characterization of these uncommon tumors compared to other imaging modalities including CT and US. Due to nonspecific MRI features of these tumors in a significant number of patients, histopathologic diagnosis is usually required for definitive diagnosis. However, some distinctive imaging features could still be detected on MRI in this group of uncommon liver tumors. MRI features of uncommon liver tumors will be reviewed in this chapter, particularly emphasizing distinctive features.

E. Altun (✉) · K. A. Mcginty
Department of Radiology, University of North Carolina at Chapel Hill, Chapel Hill, NC, USA
e-mail: ersan_altun@med.unc.edu

1 Uncommon Liver Tumors

Magnetic resonance imaging (MRI) is the best imaging modality for the detection and characterization of focal liver lesions compared to other imaging modalities including computed tomography (CT) and ultrasound (US) (Matos et al. 2015; Braga et al. 2015). Common primary hepatic benign and malignant lesions including cysts, biliary hamartomas, focal nodular

© Springer Nature Switzerland AG 2021
E. Quaia (ed.), *Imaging of the Liver and Intra-hepatic Biliary Tract*,
Medical Radiology Diagnostic Imaging, https://doi.org/10.1007/978-3-030-39021-1_5

hyperplasia, adenoma, hepatocellular carcinoma (HCC), and cholangiocarcinoma (CCA) can be characterized on MRI with high accuracy due to their specific imaging features (Matos et al. 2015; Braga et al. 2015). However, rare primary hepatic tumors do not have specific MRI features, and therefore histopathologic diagnosis is usually required for definitive diagnosis due to relatively lower accuracy of MRI for characterization of these tumors (Semelka et al. 2018). Although MRI features are not specific, some distinctive MRI features could be helpful in the diagnosis of each entity in this group of tumors (Semelka et al. 2018). CT and US are generally not used for the characterization of uncommon hepatic lesions in the great majority of patients, and therefore in this chapter, MRI features of angiomyolipoma, extramedullary hematopoiesis, mixed HCC-CCA, fibrolamellar HCC, epithelioid hemangioendothelioma, sarcomas, and lymphoma will be reviewed.

1.1 Extramedullary Hematopoiesis

Extramedullary hematopoiesis (EMH) is defined as the production of blood elements outside of the bone marrow (Georgiades et al. 2002). It is a compensatory mechanism that occurs in ineffective erythropoiesis which could be secondary to infiltrative bone marrow processes or secondary to dysfunctional erythrocyte production.

Extramedullary hematopoiesis can occur by direct expansion, when normal hematopoietic tissue expands through the cortex through small erosions. This is the more typical pattern of EMH, manifesting as paraspinal masses with areas of soft tissue and fat attenuation (Georgiades et al. 2002; Orphanidou-Vlachou et al. 2014; Jelali et al. 2006; Roberts et al. 2016).

The other form of EMH occurs through reactivation of previously dormant hematopoietic tissue, which is a site of hematopoietic production during fetal and early life, most commonly the liver, spleen, and lymph nodes (Georgiades et al. 2002; Orphanidou-Vlachou et al. 2014; Jelali et al. 2006; Roberts et al. 2016). However, other

visceral sites, such as the kidneys, adrenal glands, lung, pleura, skin, breasts, dura mater, ovary, thymus, gastrointestinal tract, and CNS, may also be involved (Georgiades et al. 2002; Orphanidou-Vlachou et al. 2014; Jelali et al. 2006; Roberts et al. 2016).

Although EMH frequently involves the liver, it is rarely found only within the liver. More commonly, it presents intraabdominally with nonspecific features of hepatosplenomegaly and adenopathy secondary to diffuse infiltration (Georgiades et al. 2002; Orphanidou-Vlachou et al. 2014; Jelali et al. 2006; Roberts et al. 2016) and could be accompanied by iron deposition (Fig. 1).

Rarely, EMH can manifest as mass-like lesions. MR imaging characteristics will vary, depending on the fat content and hematopoietic elements, and are usually nonspecific (Georgiades et al. 2002; Orphanidou-Vlachou et al. 2014; Jelali et al. 2006; Roberts et al. 2016). These lesions are usually mildly T1 hypointense and T2 hyperintense and show minimal enhancement (Georgiades et al. 2002; Orphanidou-Vlachou et al. 2014; Jelali et al. 2006; Roberts et al. 2016). Rarely, EMH can manifest as a predominantly fatty lesion (Georgiades et al. 2002; Orphanidou-Vlachou et al. 2014; Jelali et al. 2006; Roberts et al. 2016). However, because the imaging findings are nonspecific, EMH should be included in the differential diagnosis of hepatic lesions in patient with myeloproliferative disorders.

1.2 Angiomyolipoma

Angiomyolipomas (AMLs) are commonly found in the kidneys, but they are rare hepatic tumors and often present a diagnostic dilemma (Prasad et al. 2005; Kamimura et al. 2012). Hepatic AMLs could be sporadic or associated with tuberous sclerosis (TS) (Prasad et al. 2005; Kamimura et al. 2012). The patients with AMLs do not have history of chronic liver disease and do not demonstrate symptoms.

Hepatic AMLs are much less common than renal AMLs in patients with TS (Fig. 2). AMLs in patients with TS tend to be smaller and multiple

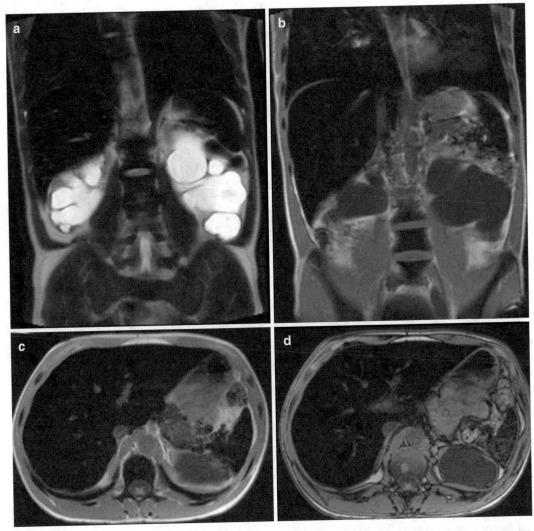

Fig. 1 Extramedullary hematopoiesis. Coronal T2-weighted single-shot echo train spin echo (**a**), coronal T1-weighted two-dimensional gradient echo (**b**), and transverse T1-weighted two-dimensional gradient echo in-phase (**c**) and out-of-phase (**d**) images demonstrate diffuse iron deposition in the liver, spleen, and bone marrow, and this is a common finding of extramedullary hematopoiesis. Please note bilateral severe hydronephrosis

and are most often lipomatous subtype, making them easier to recognize due to their mature fat content. In contrast to AMLs associated with TS, sporadic AMLs are much rarer and are usually solitary.

There are four subtypes of AMLs, classified by the predominant cell subtype: mixed, lipomatous, myomatous, and angiomyomatous (Kamimura et al. 2012). The mixed and lipomatous subtypes are the most easily identified due to mature fatty component, with lipomatous subtype being composed of more than 70% fat.

Angiomyomatous subtype is also easier to recognize, identified by large, malformed vascular components. Because of the large vessels, angiomyomatous subtype may be mistaken for intrahepatic arterial venous malformations. The myomatous subtype is the most difficult to diagnose on imaging due to its low fat content (<10% fat) and overlap in appearance with other hypervascular lesions (Kamimura et al. 2012).

MRI can demonstrate both mature fatty elements with fat-suppressed imaging and microscopic amount of fat on opposed-phase imaging

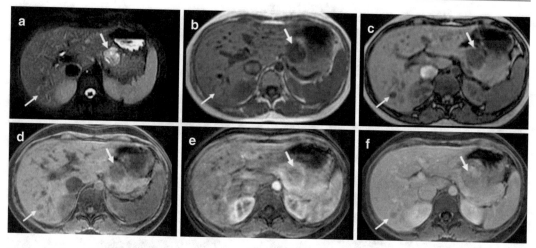

Fig. 2 Angiomyolipoma. Transverse T2-weighted fat-suppressed single-shot echo train spin echo (**a**), transverse T1-weighted two-dimensional gradient echo in-phase (**b**) and out-of-phase (**c**), transverse T1-weighted three-dimensional fat-suppressed precontrast (**d**), and postgadolinium late arterial phase (**e**) and hepatic venous phase (**f**) images demonstrate an angiomyolipoma in the right lobe of the liver (thin arrow, **a–c**, **d**, **f**) and pancreatic neuroendocrine tumor (thick arrows, **a–f**) in a patient with tuberous sclerosis (TS). The angiomyolipoma appears relatively isointense on T2-weighted image but shows signal drop on T1-weighted out-of-phase image (**c**) compared to in phase image (**b**) and on fat-suppressed precontrast which is consistent with fat content. The angiomyolipoma appears hypoenhancing compared to the background liver on postgadolinium images (**e**, **f**). The pancreatic neuroendocrine tumor shows high T2 signal (**a**) and low T1 signal on T1-weighted in-phase (**b**) and out-of-phase (**c**) images and heterogeneous enhancement on postgadolinium images (**e**, **f**)

(Fig. 2). While the presence of mature fatty elements suggests the diagnosis of AML, it is not a specific feature. Other lesions in the liver may contain macroscopic fat, most notably and commonly hepatocellular carcinoma and adenomas. Lipomas, liposarcomas, and teratomas may contain macroscopic fat, but these lesions are extremely rare (Prasad et al. 2005; Kamimura et al. 2012).

AMLs show avid arterial enhancement of their angiomyomatous components which become either isoenhancing or hypoenhancing on portal venous and interstitial phase imaging on postgadolinium T1-weighted sequences. The lipomatous elements may not demonstrate significant enhancement on all phases (Fig. 2). The appearance of central enhancing vessels suggests the diagnosis of AML as well as the presence of a large draining vein extending from the tumor to the IVC or hepatic/portal veins, called early venous return, which is specific to AML. AMLs do not retain contrast with hepatobiliary contrast agents since they lack hepatocytes. Mildly restricted diffusion and hemorrhage could be detected in these lesions (Prasad et al. 2005; Kamimura et al. 2012).

Since hepatocellular carcinomas also show avid arterial enhancement and may contain both mature and microscopic fatty elements, distinguishing between these two entities may be difficult. The presence of intralesional central vessels in arterial phase imaging and early venous return are more specific to AMLs and suggest this diagnosis instead of HCC. Clinical factors are also useful for distinguishing AML from HCC, as AMLs are not associated with tumor markers, cirrhosis, or hepatitis (Lee et al. 2016).

1.3 Mixed Hepatocellular Carcinoma and Cholangiocarcinoma (Mixed HCC-CCA)

These comprise a minority of primary hepatic malignancies, accounting for 0.4–14.5%, and also referred to as biphenotypic tumors (Fowler et al. 2013). In general, the risk factors and patient demographics of mixed HCC-CCA are similar to HCC and CCA including chronic liver disease, male sex, and advanced age. Serum tumor markers including alpha-fetoprotein and CA 19-9 could be helpful in the diagnosis of this tumor. Prognosis has been reported to be worse compared to HCC and CCA (Fowler et al. 2013).

Mixed HCC-CCA can mimic MR imaging features of HCC or CCA or both (Fowler et al. 2013; de Campos et al. 2012; Potretzke et al. 2016). This tumor usually shows mildly high T2 signal and mildly to moderately low T1 signal and could be associated with diffusion restriction, capsular retraction, and biliary ductal dilation. If the tumor contains separate components of HCC and CCA, combined imaging features of HCC and CCA could be distinctive for mixed HCC-CCA. Therefore, while part of the tumor may demonstrate later arterial phase enhancement associated with later washout (Fig. 3) ± capsule on the hepatic venous or interstitial phase, suggestive of HCC, the other part of the tumor

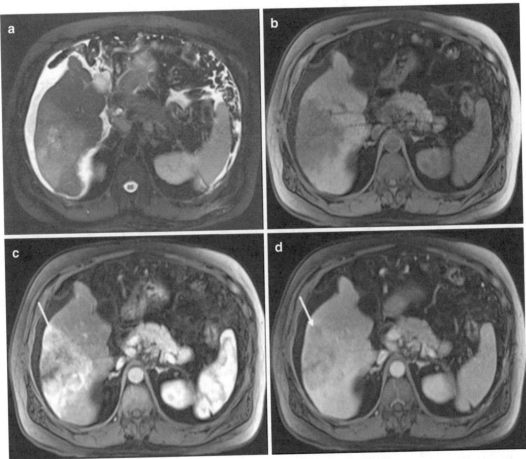

Fig. 3 Mixed hepatocellular carcinoma and cholangiocarcinoma. Transverse T2-weighted fat-suppressed single-shot echo train spin echo (**a**), transverse T1-weighted fat-suppressed precontrast three-dimensional gradient echo (**b**), and postgadolinium late hepatic arterial phase (**c**) and interstitial phase (**d**) images demonstrate mixed hepatocellular carcinoma and cholangiocarcinoma in a cirrhotic liver. The lesion shows mildly high T2 signal (**a**) with central necrosis and moderately low T1 signal (**b**) on precontrast image. Heterogeneous prominent enhancement on the late arterial phase (**c**) is noted with associated areas of washout and areas of persistent predominantly peripheral enhancement on the interstitial phase (**d**). Specifically note that an area of early enhancement on the late arterial phase shows relative washout on the interstitial phase (arrows, **c**, **d**). Ascites and prominent/enlarged portacaval and retroperitoneal lymph nodes are also present

may demonstrate progressive enhancement toward the center which increases particularly on the interstitial phase, suggestive of CCA (Fig. 3). However, the tumor can also show peripheral rim enhancement on the late arterial phase with mild central progressive enhancement on the later phases, and associated peripheral washout may also be detected on the later phases (Fowler et al. 2013; de Campos et al. 2012; Potretzke et al. 2016).

1.4 Fibrolamellar Hepatocellular Carcinoma

Fibrolamellar HCC comprises less than 1% of HCC in the United States and usually exhibits slow growth and more favorable prognosis compared to HCC (Ganeshan et al. 2014). Characteristically 95% of fibrolamellar HCC is seen in patients who do not have underlying chronic liver disease or cirrhosis, and it typically occurs in young adults and more frequently in females (Ganeshan et al. 2014; Smith et al. 2008).

MR imaging features include variable heterogeneous precontrast T1 and T2 signal, but fibrolamellar HCC usually shows mild to moderate high signal on T2-weighted sequences and moderate to markedly low signal on T1-weighted sequences (Ganeshan et al. 2014; Smith et al. 2008). Central scar is a typical imaging feature which is usually large and heterogeneous and demonstrates low T2 signal (Fig. 4) (Ganeshan et al. 2014; Smith et al. 2008). The tumor shows heterogeneous increased enhancement on the late arterial phase with associated persistent or progressive heterogeneous enhancement on the later phases (Fig. 4); however, relative mild fading (Fig. 4) or washout could also be seen on the later phases. The central scar typically does not demonstrate enhancement on the late arterial phase and later phases (Fig. 4) (Ganeshan et al. 2014; Smith et al. 2008).

The differentiation of fibrolamellar HCC from conventional HCC and focal nodular hyperplasia (FNH) is critical. The distinctive feature of fibrolamellar HCC compared to FNH is the large heterogeneous central scar showing T2 dark signal and no or minimal enhancement on the late arterial phase and later phases (Semelka et al. 2018). The central scar of FNH, which is again a typical imaging feature for FNH, is usually small and homogeneous with associated high T2 signal and enhancement on the later phases (Semelka et al. 2018). HCCs may also have central scar or necrosis mimicking central scar, which usually shows high T2 signal. Therefore, the signal intensity of central scar is a helpful feature for the differentiation of HCC from fibrolamellar HCC (Semelka et al. 2018).

1.5 Epithelioid Hemangioendothelioma

Epithelioid hemangioendothelioma (EHE) is a rare malignant slow-growing vascular tumor, usually occurring in middle-aged patients with female predilection (Semelka et al. 2018, Giardino et al. 2016; Paolantonio et al. 2014). These tumors usually have low-grade malignancy and contain fibrotic component (Semelka et al. 2018).

EHE can be nodular or diffuse in form (Semelka et al. 2018, Giardino et al. 2016; Paolantonio et al. 2014). Single or multiple nodules could be present with nodular form (Fig. 5). Diffuse form is characterized by infiltrative masses which usually forms secondary to coalescence of nodules and is usually located at the periphery of the liver (Semelka et al. 2018, Giardino et al. 2016; Paolantonio et al. 2014).

MR imaging features are not specific with variable precontrast T1 and T2 signal intensity although the lesions usually demonstrate mildly to moderately high T2 signal and mildly to moderately low T1 signal (Semelka et al. 2018, Giardino et al. 2016; Paolantonio et al. 2014). Postcontrast imaging findings could also be variable, but the most common finding is peripheral ring enhancement on the late arterial phase (Fig. 5) which may be associated with targetoid appearance on the later phases (Semelka et al. 2018, Giardino et al. 2016; Paolantonio et al. 2014). The targetoid appearance could

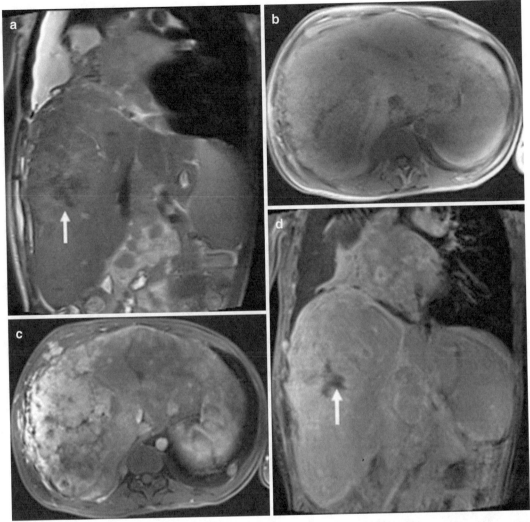

Fig. 4 Fibrolamellar hepatocellular carcinoma. Coronal T2-weighted single-shot echo train spin echo (**a**), transverse T1-weighted two-dimensional gradient echo (**b**), transverse T1-weighted fat-suppressed postgadolinium late hepatic arterial phase (**c**), and coronal T1-weighted fat-suppressed postgadolinium interstitial phase (**d**) images show metastatic fibrolamellar hepatocellular carcinoma. The mass shows mildly high T2 signal and central scar with low T2 signal (arrow, **a**). Heterogeneous intense early enhancement is seen on the late arterial phase with associated persistent heterogeneous enhancement on the interstitial phase. Please note that the central scar shows hypoenhancement (arrow, **d**). Metastatic lesions are seen in the liver, right lateral abdominal wall, porta hepatis, mediastinum and right sided lung

demonstrate peripheral rim enhancement with associated outer hypointense band and central enhancing core and delayed progressive enhancement toward the center (Semelka et al. 2018; Giardino et al. 2016; Paolantonio et al. 2014). However, targetoid appearance is uncommon in lesions smaller than 2 cm (Semelka et al. 2018).

1.6 Undifferentiated Embryonal Sarcomas

Undifferentiated embryonal sarcoma (UES) is a rare mesenchymal tumor occurring most frequently in pediatric patients and accounts for 13% of pediatric hepatic malignancies (Iqbal

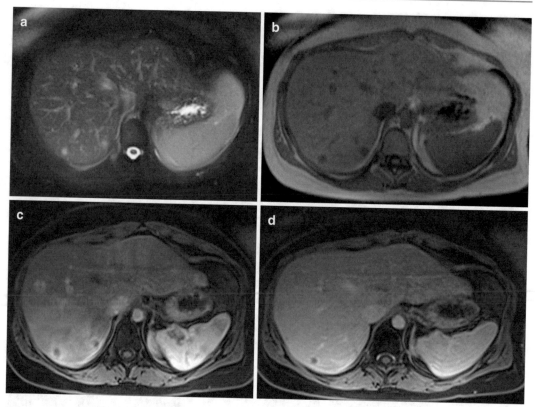

Fig. 5 Epithelioid hemangioendothelioma. Transverse T2-weighted fat-suppressed single-shot echo train spin echo (**a**), transverse T1-weighted two-dimensional gradient echo (**b**), transverse T1-weighted fat-suppressed post-gadolinium late hepatic arterial phase (**c**), and transverse T1-weighted fat-suppressed postgadolinium interstitial phase (**d**) images demonstrate multiple scattered foci of epithelioid hemangioendothelioma. The lesions show mildly to moderately high T2 signal (**a**) and moderately low T1 signal (**b**). Thick peripheral rim enhancement on the late arterial phase (**c**) with later fading of the rim enhancement (**d**) is also noted in the lesions

et al. 2008). A few cases have been reported in adults. The prognosis of UES has been reported to be poor.

These lesions usually present as complex mass lesions with cystic and/or necrotic components or centers (Iqbal et al. 2008; Tsukada et al. 2010). Therefore, these lesions demonstrate moderately to markedly high T2 signal and moderately to markedly low T1 signal (Iqbal et al. 2008; Tsukada et al. 2010). These lesions may also demonstrate areas of hemorrhage showing high T1 signal and low T2 signal. Peripheral rim enhancement is seen on the late arterial phase with associated progressive enhancement of the solid components on the later phases. Cystic and necrotic components and areas of hemorrhage do not demonstrate evidence of enhancement (Iqbal et al. 2008; Tsukada et al. 2010).

1.7 Angiosarcoma

Primary hepatic angiosarcoma is a rare and aggressive malignancy of mesenchymal origin and accounts for less than 2% of all primary liver neoplasms (Thapar et al. 2014). Angiosarcoma most commonly affects men in the fifth–sixth decades and has been reported to be associated with exposure to several environmental carcinogens including thorotrast, arsenic, and vinyl chloride (Thapar et al. 2014; Koyama et al. 2002).

Angiosarcomas demonstrate heterogeneous variable but mostly moderate to markedly high T2 and variable but mostly prominently low T1 signal (Thapar et al. 2014; Koyama et al. 2002). These lesions could demonstrate evidence of

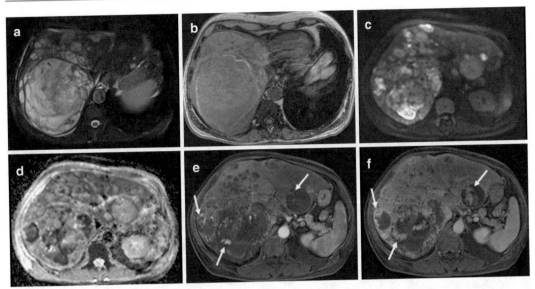

Fig. 6 Angiosarcoma. Transverse T2-weighted fat-suppressed single-shot echo train spin echo (**a**), transverse T1-weighted out-of-phase two-dimensional gradient echo (**b**), and transverse diffusion-weighted echo planar image (**c**) with associated apparent diffusion coefficient map (**d**) and transverse T1-weighted fat-suppressed postgadolinium three-dimensional gradient echo late arterial phase (**e**) and hepatic venous phase (**f**) images show multiple foci of angiosarcoma in the liver. The lesions show heteroge-neous high T2 signal and low T1 signal on precontrast images with associated high signal intensity rim on T1-weighted image and low signal rim on T2-weighted image, suggestive of blood products in the dominant mass Areas of prominent diffusion restriction are noted in these lesions. Predominantly peripheral nodular enhance-ment (arrows, **e**) with progressive central filling (arrows, **f**) is noted in multiple lesions

internal hemorrhage (Fig. 6), which has been reported in 50% of the patients according to some studies (Semelka et al. 2018). These tumors could show variable enhancement patterns; however, nodular enhancement on the late arterial phase with progressive enhancement (Fig. 6) to the center has been reported in 50% of the patients according to some studies (Semelka et al. 2018).

One of the distinctive features of angiosarcoma compared to hemangioma could be the presence of hemorrhage and heterogeneous appearance, which is extremely rare in hemangiomas (Semelka et al. 2018). Another distinctive feature of angiosarcoma could be the presence of oval or round contours compared to lobulated contours of hemangiomas, which is commonly seen in hemangiomas larger than 18 mm (Semelka et al. 2018). The other distinctive feature of angiosarcoma could also be early relatively large peripheral nodular enhancement with progressive central filling, which is different from discontinuous nodular enhancement on the late arterial phase with coalescence of nodules on the later phases with central progressive filling (Semelka et al. 2018).

1.8 Other Sarcomas

Other types of sarcomas can also be seen in the liver including but not limited to leiomyosarcoma or malignant fibrous histiocytoma (Yu et al. 2008). These tumors usually show mildly to moderately high T2 and moderately to marked low T1 signal and are usually associated with the presence of central necrosis (Fig. 7) (Semelka et al. 2018; Yu et al. 2008). Hemorrhagic changes may also be seen in sarcomas (Semelka et al. 2018). Peripheral heterogeneous enhancement on the late arterial phase with progressive enhancement toward the center is the most common enhancement pattern seen on dynamic imaging (Fig. 7) (Semelka et al. 2018; Yu et al. 2008).

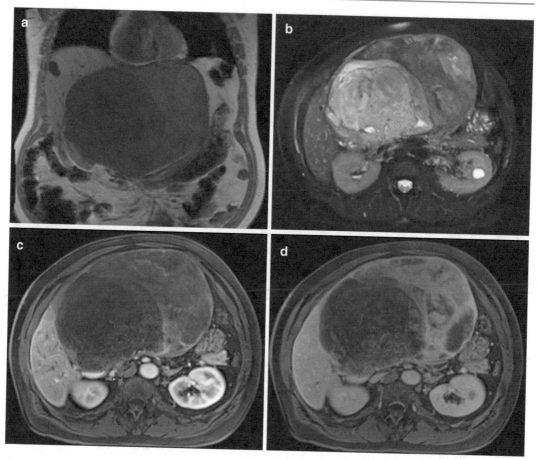

Fig. 7 Sarcoma. Coronal T1-weighted two-dimensional gradient echo (**a**), transverse T2-weighted fat-suppressed single-shot echo train spin echo (**b**), and transverse T1-weighted fat-suppressed postgadolinium late arterial phase (**c**) and interstitial phase (**d**) three-dimensional gra- dient echo images show a large leiomyosarcoma with very heterogeneous T1 and T2 signal. Small areas of central necrosis are seen in the large tumor showing heteroge- neous progressive enhancement with peripheral dominant enhancement and central filling (**c, d**)

1.9 Primary Hepatic Lymphoma

Primary hepatic lymphoma accounts for less than 1% of all non-Hodgkin's lymphoma. Additionally, it is more common in patients with immunosuppression, human immunodeficiency virus (HIV), Epstein-Barr virus, and hepatitis B and C virus.

Primary hepatic lymphoma can present as mass-forming lesions or infiltrative lesions (Semelka et al. 2018; Steller et al. 2012; Maher et al. 2001). These lesions demonstrate variable precontrast T1 and T2 signal although most com- monly these lesions demonstrate mildly to mod- erately high T2 signal and mildly to moderately low T1 signal (Fig. 8) (Semelka et al. 2018; Steller et al. 2012; Maher et al. 2001). These tumors show variable enhancement (Fig. 8) although minimal or mild to moderate progres- sive enhancement on dynamic postgadolinium series is most commonly seen (Semelka et al. 2018; Steller et al. 2012; Maher et al. 2001). Necrosis is not commonly seen in these tumors (Semelka et al. 2018). Although MR imaging findings of mass-forming primary lymphoma are not specific, infiltrative type primary lymphoma encases the vessels without significant compres- sion or deviation, and this feature is a distinctive feature for the identification of primary lymphoma (Semelka et al. 2018).

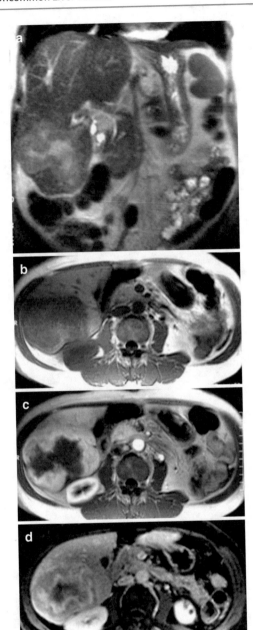

Fig. 8 Primary lymphoma. Coronal T2-weighted single-shot echo train spin echo (**a**), transverse T1-weighted two-dimensional gradient echo (**b**), transverse two-dimensional gradient echo postgadolinium late arterial phase (**c**), and transverse two-dimensional fat-suppressed gradient echo hepatic venous phase (**d**) images show primary lymphoma of the right lobe of the liver. The lesion shows heterogeneous mildly high T2 signal with central necrosis and lobulated contours. The lesion shows heterogeneous early enhancement on the late arterial phase and peripheral washout on the interstitial phase

References

Braga L, Altun E, Armao D, Semelka RC (2015) Liver. In: Semelka RC, Brown M, Altun E (eds) Abdominal-pelvic MRI, vol 2, 4th edn. Wiley-Blackwell, Hooken, pp 39–393

de Campos RO, Semelka RC, Azevedo RM et al (2012) Combined hepatocellular carcinoma-cholangiocarcinoma: report of MR appearance in eleven patients. J Magn Reson Imaging 36:1139–1147

Fowler KJ, Sheybani A, Parker RA et al (2013) Combined hepatocellular and cholangiocarcinoma (biphenotypic) tumors: imaging features and diagnostic accuracy of contrast-enhanced CT and MRI. Am J Roentgenol 201:332–339

Ganeshan D, Szklaruk J, Kundra V, Rashid AK, Elsayesl KM (2014) Imaging features of fibrolamellar hepatocellular carcinoma. AJR Am J Roentgenol 202:544–552

Georgiades CS, Neyman EG, Francis IR, Sneider MB, Fishman EK (2002) Typical and atypical presentations of extramedullary hemopoiesis. AJR Am J Roentgenol 179:1239–1243

Giardino A, Miller FH, Kalb B et al (2016) Hepatic epithelioid hemangioendothelioma: a report from three university centers. Radiol Bras 49:288–294

Iqbal K, Xian ZM, Yuan C (2008) Undifferentiated liver sarcoma—rare entity: a case report and review of the literature. J Med Case Rep 2:20

Jelali MA, Luciani A, Kobeiter H et al (2006) MRI features of intrahepatic extramedullary haematopoiesis in sickle cell anaemia. Cancer Imaging 6:182–185

Kamimura K, Nomoto M, Aoyagi Y (2012) Hepatic angiomyolipoma: diagnostic findings and management. Int J Hepatol 2012:410781

Koyama T, Fletcher JG, Johnson CD et al (2002) Primary hepatic angiosarcoma: findings at CT and MR imaging. Radiology 222:667–673

Lee SJ, Kim SY, Kim KW et al (2016) Hepatic angiomyolipoma versus hepatocellular carcinoma in the noncirrhotic liver on Gadoxetic acid-enhanced MRI: a diagnostic challenge. AJR Am J Roentgenol 207:562–570

Maher MM, Mcdermott SR, Fenlon HM et al (2001) Imaging of primary non-hodgkin's lymphoma of the liver. Clin Radiol 56:295–301

Matos AP, Velloni F, Ramalho M, AlObaidy M, Rajapaksha A, Semelka RC (2015) Focal liver lesions: practical magnetic resonance imaging approach. World J Hepatol 7:1987–2008

Orphanidou-Vlachou E, Tziakouri-Shiakalli C, Georgiades CS (2014) Extramedullary hemopoiesis. Semin Ultrasound CT MR 35:255–262

Paolantonio P, Laghi A, Vanzulli A et al (2014) MRI of hepatic epithelioid Hemangioendothelioma (HEH). J Magn Reson Imaging 40:552–558

Potretzke TA, Tan BR, Doyle MB, Brunt EM, Heiken JP, Fowler KJ (2016) Imaging features of biphenotypic primary liver carcinoma (hepatocholangiocarcinoma) and the potential to mimic hepatocellular carcinoma: LIRADS analysis of CT and MRI features in 61 cases. AJR Am J Roentgenol 207:25–31

Prasad SR, Wang H, Rosas H et al (2005) Fat-containing lesions of the liver: radiologic-pathologic correlation. Radiographics 25:321–331

Roberts AS, Shetty AS, Mellnick VM, Pickhardt PJ, Bhalla S, Menias CO (2016) Extramedullary haematopoiesis: radiological imaging features. Clin Radiol 71:807–814

Semelka RC, Nimojan N, Chandana S et al (2018) MRI features of primary malignancies of the liver: a report from university centres. Eur Radiol 28:1529–1539

Smith MT, Blatt ER, Paul Jedlicka P, Strain JD, Fenton LZ (2008) Fibrolamellar hepatocellular carcinoma. Radiographics 28:609–613

Steller EJA, Leeuwen MSV, Hillegersberg RV et al (2012) Primary lymphoma of the liver: a complex diagnosis. World J Radiol 4:53–57

Thapar S, Rastogi A, Ahuja A, Sarin S (2014) Angiosarcoma of the liver: imaging of a rare salient entity. J Radiol Case Rep 8:24–32

Tsukada A, Ishizaki Y, Nobukawa B, Kawasaki S (2010) Embryonal sarcoma of the liver in an adult mimicking complicated hepatic cyst: MRI findings. J Magn Reson Imaging 31:1477–1480

Yu R-S, Chen Y, Jiang B, Wang L-H, Xu X-F (2008) Primary hepatic sarcomas: CT findings. Eur Radiol 18:2196–2205

Intrahepatic Cholangiocarcinoma and Mixed Tumors

Jelena Kovač

Contents

Abstract

Intrahepatic cholangiocarcinoma (ICC) represents the second most common primary liver tumor after hepatocellular carcinoma. These tumors arise from the bile ducts epithelium, peripheral to the secondary bifurcation of the left or right hepatic duct. Although most cholangiocarcinomas occur sporadically, the disease incidence is higher, and it develops earlier in the patients with primary sclerosing cholangitis (PSC), choledochal cyst, Caroli disease, clonorchiasis, and viral hepatitis (especially type C). According to their growth pattern, ICCs can be classified into three types: mass-forming, periductal-infiltrating, or intraductal-growing cholangiocarcinoma. Imaging plays the most important role in preoperative characterization of ICC with mass-forming type presenting as lobulated hypovascular lesions causing retraction of liver capsule and peripheral bile duct dilatation. Periductal-infiltrating type is very difficult for timely diagnosis and

J. Kovač (✉)
Center for Radiology and Magnetic Resonance Imaging, Clinical Center of Serbia, Belgrade, Serbia

© Springer Nature Switzerland AG 2021
E. Quaia (ed.), *Imaging of the Liver and Intra-hepatic Biliary Tract*,
Medical Radiology Diagnostic Imaging, https://doi.org/10.1007/978-3-030-39021-1_6

is usually discovered in follow-up of PSC patients as worsening of dominant stricture. Intraductal-growing cholangiocarcinoma is the rarest type of ICC with much better outcome than other ICC forms. It presents usually as polypoid lesion filling the bile ducts with proximal biliary dilatation.

1 Introduction

Intrahepatic cholangiocarcinoma (ICC) represents the second most common primary liver tumor after hepatocellular carcinoma (Choi et al. 2004a). These tumors arise from the bile duct epithelium, peripheral to the secondary bifurcation of the left or right hepatic duct (Lazaridis and Gores 2005). Similarly to the other types of cholangiocarcinomas, intrahepatic form usually occurs in elderly population with a slight male predilection (men to women ratio of approximately 1.2–1.5) (Shaib and El-Serag 2004). Although most cholangiocarcinomas occur sporadically, the disease incidence is higher, and it develops earlier in the patients with primary sclerosing cholangitis (PSC), choledochal cyst, Caroli disease, clonorchiasis, and viral hepatitis (especially type C) (Lazaridis and Gores 2005; Shaib and El-Serag 2004; Shaib et al. 2007; Kim et al. 2006; Choi et al. 2004b).

According to their growth pattern, ICCs can be classified into three types: mass-forming, periductal-infiltrating, or intraductal-growing cholangiocarcinoma (Lim 2003). Precise preoperative characterization of the growth type is important for optimal treatment planning and prognosis, as mass-forming and periductal-infiltrating types have generally unfavorable course, while intraductal-growing tumors have much better outcome (Isaji et al. 1999; Sasaki et al. 1998; Yamamoto et al. 1998). Additionally, a combination of growth patterns can frequently occur. Thus, periductal-infiltrating type is rarely seen as the only growth pattern and in most cases it is encountered together with mass-forming cholangiocarcinoma (Lazaridis and Gores 2005). On the other hand, association of intraductal-growing cholangiocarcinoma and periductal-infiltrating type is not frequently present (Choi et al. 1995).

2 Mass-Forming Intrahepatic Cholangiocarcinoma

Mass forming type is the most common among ICCs, accounting for 80% of all cases (Lim 2003). These tumors usually present as large, lobulated, irregular lesions with well-defined borders (Choi et al. 2004a). Since it arises from the epithelium of small bile ducts, symptoms are rare early in the course of the disease. Moreover, laboratory and clinical findings are quite unspecific leading to delay in diagnosis (Isaji et al. 1999). Therefore, imaging procedures have important role in early detection, staging, and evaluation for surgical resectability (Lazaridis and Gores 2005).

2.1 Imaging Findings

Mass-forming ICCs are tumors characterized by rich fibrous stroma which determines their imaging appearance (Jhaveri and Hosseini-Nik 2015). On ultrasound examination, these lesions usually present as heterogeneous lesions with intermediate to increased echogenicity, while smaller tumors appears as iso- to hypoechoic lesions (Fig. 1a) (Chung et al. 2009). A hypoechoic halo, seen in about 15% of tumors, represents a rim of proliferating viable tumor cells in combination with compressed adjacent liver parenchyma. In general, there are no specific features on US examination which allow differentiation from the other more common entities, such as liver metastases, except the fact that cholangiocarcinoma is more likely associated with bile duct dilatation and capsular retraction (Wibulpolprasert and Dhiensiri 1992).

Further evaluation with CT typically demonstrates large, irregular, hypoattenuating mass with incomplete peripheral enhancement on arterial and progressive enhancement on delayed phases (Fig. 1b, c) (Han et al. 2002). In general, this vascular profile reflects pathohistological composition of the tumor, with the periphery composed of active tumor cells, and the center rich with desmoplastic stroma, necrotic tissue, or mucin (Fujita et al. 2017). Therefore, progressive enhancement could be explained by slow diffu-

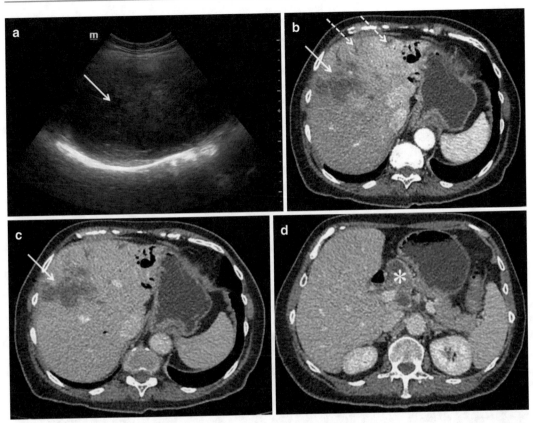

Fig. 1 Mass-forming intrahepatic cholangiocarcinoma in 67-year-old male patient. (**a**) Transverse sonogram shows a heterogeneous irregular hyperechoic mass in subcapsular location (*solid arrow*). (**b**) Arterial dominant phase CT image depicts a centrally hypoattenuated mass with only slight peripheral enhancement in liver segment IV (*solid arrow*). A dilated left intrahepatic bile ducts are seen (*dotted arrow*). Pneumobilia due to previous ERCP procedure is also visible. (**c**) Portal phase CT image demonstrates slight progressive enhancement (*solid arrow*) with persistent central hypodensity and dilatation of intrahepatic bile ducts in the left lateral segments of the liver. (**d**) Axial section at the level of liver hilum shows multiple centrally necrotic lymph nodes (*asterisk*)

sion of contrast material into the interstitial spaces of tumor which contains abundant fibrotic tissue (Fujita et al. 2017; Maetani et al. 2001; Valls et al. 2000). In cases of necrotic or mucin-producing tumors, the center of the lesion does not enhance and remains hypodense even in delayed phase (Choi et al. 1995; Sainani et al. 2008). Recent studies have shown that the degree of intralesional fibrosis may have prognostic implications. Thus, ICCs which are hypovascular in the hepatic arterial phase are more likely to demonstrate lymphatic, perineural, and biliary invasion (Valls et al. 2000; Sainani et al. 2008). On the other hand, hypervascularity may serve as an independent preoperative prognostic factor for better outcome (Fujita et al. 2017). Additional CT findings of mass-forming ICCs include cap-

sular retraction, peripheral biliary dilatation, satellite nodules, intralesional calcifications, vascular encasement, lobar atrophy, and lymphadenopathy (Fig. 1) (Valls et al. 2000). Since these tumors arise from bile duct epithelium, some degree of obstruction and peripheral bile duct dilatation is invariably seen, unless the tumor is subcapsullary located (Maetani et al. 2001; Manfredi et al. 2004). Capsular retraction is considered to be pathognomonic sign of mass-forming ICC. Nevertheless, this finding could also be seen in other tumors, such as metastatic colon carcinoma, scirrhous hepatocellular carcinoma (HCC), hemangioendothelioma, and other tumors with marked desmoplastic reaction (Soyer et al. 1994). However, in association with other MRI findings, and the absence of primary tumor elsewhere, capsular retraction is highly suggestive of mass-forming ICC (Kovač et al. 2017). Vascular encasement leading to lobar or segmental parenchymal atrophy is also frequently observed in mass-forming ICC, but unlike HCC, ICCs rarely lead to tumor thrombus formation (Han et al. 2002). In these cases, lobar or segmental atrophy secondary to vascular involvement must be distinguished from capsular retraction (Soyer et al. 1994). As a consequence of portal vein invasion, perfusion abnormalities in affected segments are seen in terms of arterial hypervascularity, together with persistent enhancement in portal venous phase. In addition, infiltration of peripheral portal vein branches, which occur in 10–20% of cases, leads to formation of satellite lesions around the main tumor (Manfredi et al. 2004). Lymphadenopathy in porta hepatis and hepatoduodenal ligament are nonspecific findings, present in up to 73% of cases (Valls et al. 2000).

MRI characteristics of mass-forming ICCs vary depending on the proportion of fibrosis, mucin production, and necrosis (Jhaveri and Hosseini-Nik 2015). The tumors are typically nonencapsulated T1-weighted hypointense lesions, while appearance on T2-weighted images range from hypointensity in highly fibrotic lesions to hyperintensity in cases of necrotic or mucin-rich tumors (Fig. 2) (Maetani et al. 2001). Central T2-weighted hypointensity corresponding to fibrosis is considered characteristic MRI feature of ICC (Valls et al. 2000). Nevertheless, this sign can also be seen in some colorectal metastases, due to the presence of coagulative necrosis inside the lesion (Outwater

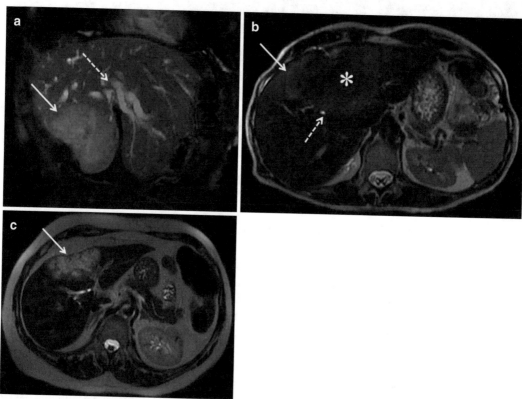

Fig. 2 Varying appearance of mass-forming intrahepatic cholangiocarcinoma on MRI. (**a**) Coronal fat-saturated T2-weighted image shows moderately hyperintense mass in segment IV (*solid arrow*) causing capsular retraction and marked peripheral bile duct dilatation (*dotted arrow*). (**b**) Axial T2-weighted image in another patient reveals a large liver mass (*solid arrow*) predominantly located in liver segment IV (*solid arrow*) with capsular retraction and central hypointensity reflecting rich fibrous stroma within the lesion (*asterisk*). Slight biliary dilatation is also seen (*dotted arrow*). (**c**) Axial T2-weighted image in third patient shows high signal intensity of the lesion corresponding to increased mucin content which is characteristic for biliary adenocarcinomas (*solid arrow*)

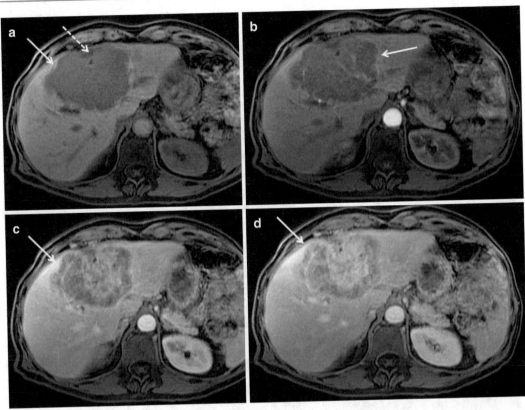

Fig. 3 Dynamic MRI findings of mass-forming intrahepatic cholangiocarcinoma in 73-year-old male. (**a**) Unenhanced T1-weighted image shows a hypointense mass with an irregular margin (*solid arrow*) in the left lobe of the liver. Note also capsular retraction (*dotted arrow*). (**b**) On the arterial phase image, the mass shows only slight enhancement along the periphery (*solid arrow*). (**c**) On the portal venous phase image, the tumor (*solid arrow*) shows progressive and concentric filling of contrast material with further enhancement on the delayed phase image (**d**)

et al. 1991). Similarly to CT, the most common postcontrast behavior, using conventional gadolinium-based extracellular contrast agents, is minimal to moderate peripheral rimlike enhancement on hepatic arterial phases, followed by progressive centripetal enhancement in late phases (Fig. 3) (Manfredi et al. 2004). Both peripheral and centripetal enhancement are better depicted on MR imaging in comparison to CT. In highly fibrotic lesions, postcontrast enhancement could sometimes be seen only in the delayed phase (Kim et al. 2011). In some cases, central parts may remain hypointense even on delayed images, due to internal necrosis (Fig. 4). However, opacification of the viable tumor on the periphery of the lesion is clue for differential diagnosis with hepatic abscess (Maetani et al. 2001). A few recent studies have pointed out the usefulness of gadolinium ethoxybenzyl-diethylenetriamine pentaacetic acid (Gd-EOB-DTPA) in characterization of mass-forming ICC (Kim et al. 2016; Jeong et al. 2013). Similarly to other focal liver lesions without functional hepatocytes, ICCs become increasingly conspicuous on delayed phase, appearing as hypointense lesions with a sharp contrast between the lesion and the background liver parenchyma (Jeong et al. 2013). Therefore, tumor extension as well as the presence of associated satellite nodules could be more precisely assessed on hepatobiliary phase in comparison to the use of conventional extracellular contrast (Kim et al. 2012a). In addition, mass-forming ICCs commonly show multilayered enhancement on the hepatobiliary phase, seen as cloudlike high signal intensity in the central part and a hypointense peripheral rim (Kim

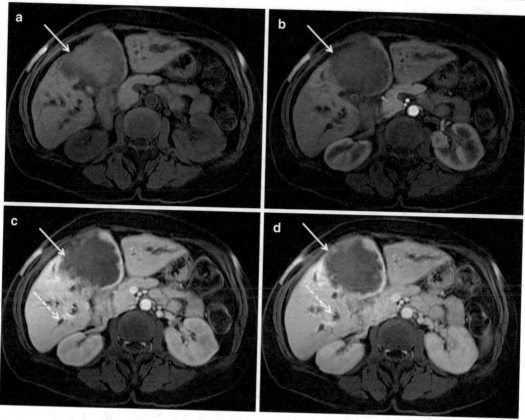

Fig. 4 Dynamic MR findings of mass-forming intrahepatic cholangiocarcinoma in 63-year-old male. (**a**) Unenhanced T1-weighted image shows a large hypointense mass occupying segment IV with slight central hyperintensity corresponding to necrotic and/or mucinous content (*solid arrow*). (**b**) On the arterial phase image no enhancement is seen inside the lesion (*solid arrow*). Portal venous phase (**c**) and delayed phase image (**d**) shows slight progressive opacification of the peripheral part of the lesion while central portion remains hypointense due to internal necrosis. Note also capsular retraction and peripheral biliary dilatation (*dotted arrow*)

et al. 2016; Feng et al. 2015). This appearance is closely related with pathological features of these tumors, since central fibrosis and necrosis are surrounded by highly cellular and vascular tumor cells (Jeong et al. 2013). As on CT, ancillary imaging features of mass-forming ICCs on MRI are vascular encasement, biliary obstruction, lobar atrophy, capsular retraction, and lymphadenopathy (Manfredi et al. 2004).

2.2 Differential Diagnosis

The differential diagnosis for mass-forming ICCs includes HCC, metastatic adenocarcinoma (especially from colorectal, breast, and pancreatic cancer), inflammatory pseudotumor, and angiosarcoma (Chung et al. 2009). HCC is the most common primary hepatic tumor and should be differentiated from mass-forming cholangiocarcinoma, because of different prognosis and treatment (Park et al. 2013). The typical vascular profile consisting of early arterial enhancement and washout in portal venous phase is the main feature of HCC, especially in the setting of cirrhotic liver (Lee et al. 2001). On the other hand, early peripheral enhancement which progresses centripetally on delayed phases, in association with capsular retraction and peripheral bile duct dilatation, favors the diagnosis of mass-forming ICC (Lee et al. 2001). Nevertheless, besides the typical enhancement pattern described for larger mass-forming ICCs, smaller lesions could display atypical vascular characteristics (Fig. 5)

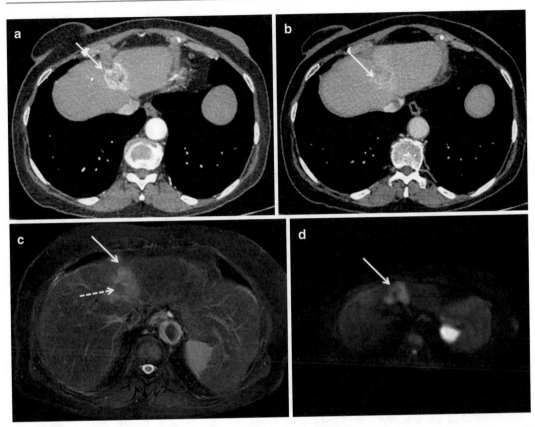

Fig. 5 Mass-forming intrahepatic cholangiocarcinoma in 69-year-old female patient with cirrhosis. (**a**) Contrast-enhanced CT in arterial phase shows heterogeneous hypervascular lesion in liver segment II (*solid arrow*). (**b**) Portal venous phase reveals slight "washout" with persistent peripheral enhancement (*solid arrow*). (**c**) On T2-weighted MR image the lesion (*solid arrow*) has moderate hyperintensity and irregular margins with high signal intensity on diffusion-weighted image (**d**). Note also small area of T2-weighted hypointensity within the lesion corresponding to rich fibrous stroma (*dotted arrow*) on **c**

(Kim et al. 2012a; Vilana et al. 2010). Homogeneous hypervascular enhancement on arterial phase has been demonstrated in 12.5–47% of ICCs in previous studies (Kim et al. 2011, 2012a). This behavior is mainly seen in smaller lesions and could be explained by abundant tumor vasculature in fibrotic stroma, less intratumoral fibrosis, and higher cellularity (Outwater et al. 1991; Lee et al. 2001). These tumors usually appear in the setting of cirrhotic liver and are discovered early due to surveillance protocol, which makes differential diagnosis with hepatocellular carcinoma very difficult (Rimola et al. 2009). In such cases, the absence of washout and the presence of progressive enhancement instead is suggestive of cholangiocellular carcinoma, rather than HCC (Vilana et al. 2010). Conversely,

in the study by Kim et al. all hypervascular ICC showed washout in portal phase (Kim et al. 2011). In this regard, additional findings such as EOB-cloud appearance in the hepatobiliary phase, and capsular retraction, could be helpful in differentiation from HCC (Manfredi et al. 2004; Kim et al. 2012a). However, scirrhous HCC may strongly mimic mass-forming ICC on imaging, and their differentiation may only be possible histopathologically (Park et al. 2013).

Solitary hypovascular metastases may closely resemble mass-forming ICC (Al Ansari et al. 2014). Besides enhancement pattern, these lesions can display some of the typical ICC features such as central T2-weighted hypointensity or peripheral intrahepatic bile duct dilatation (Al Ansari et al. 2014). Several other imaging features could be

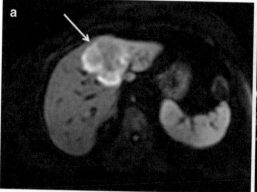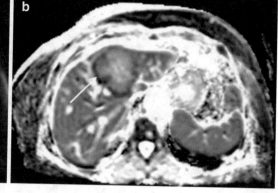

Fig. 6 Diffusion-weighted characteristics of mass-forming ICC. (**a**) Axial DWI image shows target appearance of the lesion (*solid arrow*) with central hypointense area surrounded by high signal intensity rim, corresponding to viable cells on the periphery and central fibrous stroma, respectively. (**b**) Target sign is also depicted on ADC map, as peripheral ringlike hypointensity and central hyperintensity (*solid arrow*)

useful for distinction among mass-forming ICCs and solitary hypovascular metastases, such as shape of the lesion, capsular retraction, segmental bile duct dilatation, and portal lymphadenopathy (Kovač et al. 2017). Recently, target sign defined as a central hypointensity with a peripheral hyperintense rim on diffusion-weighted images (DWI) was proposed as a characteristic finding of mass-forming ICC (Fig. 6) (Park et al. 2013). In this context Park et al. found target sign to be significant predictor of IMC, as it was present in 75% of mass-forming ICC patients (Park et al. 2013). Similarly, in another study target sign was found in 93.5% of ICCs, while only 4.5% of solitary hypovascular liver metastases showed this feature (Kovač et al. 2017). Nevertheless, the differential diagnosis between these two entities can be difficult even at histopathology and requires special immunohistochemistry studies. In conclusion, since both imaging and pathohistological features of mass-forming ICC and liver metastases significantly overlap, the first step in diagnosis of mass-forming ICC should be exclusion of extrahepatic primary malignancies, especially colorectal carcinoma.

3 Periductal-Infiltrating Type

Periductal-infiltrating type is the most common type of hilar cholangiocarcinoma, but is a rare manifestation of intrahepatic cholangiocarcinoma (Lee et al. 2001). This tumor is characterized by longitudinal growth along the bile duct wall, resulting in concentric thickening and irregular narrowing of the lumen with subsequent peripheral biliary dilatation (Lim 2003). In the later stage, the tumor may transform into exophytic cholangiocarcinoma and invade the hepatic parenchyma (Lee et al. 2001).

3.1 Imaging Findings

On US, segmental bile duct wall thickening with or without obliteration of the bile duct lumen can be found (Mittelstaedt 1997). However, lobar or segmental intrahepatic bile duct dilatation could be the only finding without obvious cause of obstruction. Further CT and MR examination may show mural thickening with increased enhancement of the bile duct wall at the level of irregularly narrowed duct, associated with upstream biliary dilatation (Lee et al. 2001). Prominent delayed phase enhancement is seen in up to 80% of periductal ICC, due to their sclerosing histology, and is considered to be pathognomonic finding for these tumors. Similarly to CT, periductal-infiltrating ICC manifests as periductal thickening at the level of biliary obstruction on MRI (Fig. 7). Lesions are mostly T1-weighted hypointense, whereas T2-weighted signal inten-

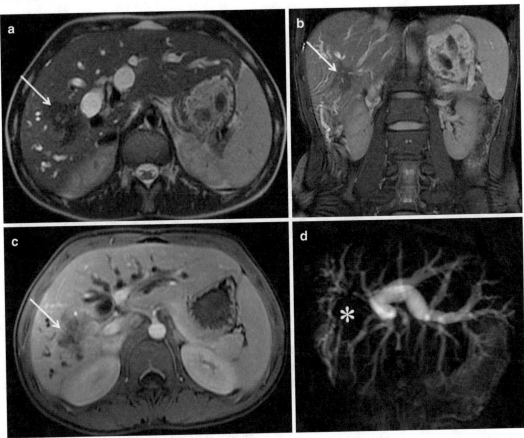

Fig. 7 Periductal-infiltrating ICC in 36-year-old women with long-standing PSC. (**a**) Irregular T2-weighted hypointense lesion is seen surrounding bile ducts in right posterior liver segments with subsequent peripheral biliary dilatation (*solid arrow*). In addition, bile duct dilatation is also observed in left liver lobe due to tumor propagation on primary biliary confluence. (**b**) Coronal T2-weighted image shows branching pattern of hypoin- tense lesion growing along bile duct wall (*solid arrow*). (**c**) Axial T1-weighted image in portal venous phase shows hypovascularity of the lesion, representing scle- rotic nature of the lesion (*solid arrow*). (**d**) MRCP shows loss of visualization of bile ducts in right posterior liver segments due to tumor infiltration (*asterisk*) with periph- eral bile duct dilatation. Note also marked biliary dilata- tion in left liver lobe

sity varies from hypo- to hyperintense, depend- ing on the amount of associated sclerosis or fibrosis. Prominent enhancement of the lesion is seen in the delayed phase, with variable degrees of arterial and venous phase enhancement (Maetani et al. 2001). It has been previously shown that the degree of enhancement strongly correlates with periductal and perineural spread (Ayuso et al. 2013). Additional MRCP examina- tion allows accurate assessment of the longitudi- nal extent of lesion, thus providing useful information regarding resectability of the tumor (Kim et al. 2007).

3.2 Differential Diagnosis

The early diagnosis of periductal-infiltrating cholangiocarcinoma is very challenging, since this tumor may resemble to benign strictures (Kim et al. 2007). Findings of a long-segmental stricture with an irregular margin, asymmetric luminal narrowing, increased bile duct wall enhancement, hilar lymphadenopathy, and a peri- ductal soft tissue lesion favor the diagnosis of malignant stricture (Katabathina et al. 2014). Rigorous follow-up must be performed in all cases where correct diagnosis cannot be made. If there is a progression of bile duct dilatation due to advanced stricture, diagnosis of periductal-infiltrating ICC is highly suspected.

4 Intraductal-Growing Type

Intraductal cholangiocarcinoma is a rare type, representing 8–18% of all ICCs, with a variety of imaging features and a better prognosis than other types of cholangiocarcinoma (Han et al. 2002; Lim et al. 2002). Most of these tumors are small, sessile, polypoid, or papillary lesions which grow slowly toward the lumen with intact bile duct wall. Occasionally, this type of cholangiocarcinoma spread superficially along the mucosa, resulting in multiple tumors (papillomatosis) along different segments of bile ducts (Han et al. 2002; Lim et al. 2002). However, if left untreated, tumor may infiltrate the surrounding liver parenchyma. In such cases, it might be difficult to differentiate the mass-forming type from the advanced intraductal-growing type of ICC with stromal invasion (Lim et al. 2002).

4.1 Imaging Findings

Currently, five distinct imaging patterns have been described: (1) diffuse and marked bile duct dilatation with a grossly visible intraductal mass (45.4%), (2) diffuse and marked biliary dilatation without a visible mass (23.7%), (3) an intraductal papillary mass with localized duct dilation (19.6%), (4) intraductal cast-like lesions within a moderately dilated duct (4.1%), and (5) focal stricture-like lesion with mild proximal duct dilation (7.2%) (Chung et al. 2009; Lim et al. 2002; Kim et al. 2012b). First type is the most common type and is characterized by diffuse biliary dilatation with multifocal superficial papillary or plaquelike lesions within the bile ducts (Fig. 8) (Kawakatsu et al. 1997). In contrast to other types of cholangiocarcinoma, where only upstream biliary dilatation is present, in this type of intraductal cholangiocellular carcinoma dilatation of the downstream bile ducts is also seen. This find-

ing is considered to be highly specific for intraductal-growing ICC. In addition, bile ducts are usually disproportionately dilated, being most prominent in branches containing tumors (Kim et al. 2012b; Kawakatsu et al. 1997; Lim et al. 2008). US can show biliary dilatation, but it can detect a low-echoic mass in less than 50% of patients (Lee et al. 2004). Endoscopic ultrasonography (EUS) and intraductal ultrasonography (IDUS) are useful imaging modalities for evaluation of the depth of invasion and involvement of the lymph nodes, even in the presence of thick mucin (Tsuyuguchi et al. 2010). CT examination demonstrates diffuse biliary dilatation and intraductal papillary lesions if larger than 1 cm (Yoon et al. 2000). Since these tumors are usually suspended on small fibrovascular stalks, washout is frequently seen, rather than progressive enhancement observed in conventional cholangiocarcinoma (Lee et al. 2000). MR with MRCP provides even better visualization of the tumor with multiple polypoid or papillary moderately T2-weighted hyperintense lesions within the lumen of bile ducts (Kim et al. 1998, 2010).

The second pattern of intraductal cholangiocarcinoma is characterized by diffuse and marked duct ectasia, but without a visible mass on CT, MRI, or even gross examination (Jhaveri and Hosseini-Nik 2015). These findings could be explained with micropapillary nature of the tumor and a high mucin production which leads to bile duct dilatation without visible tumor mass (Lim et al. 2004). Mucin is usually not visible on CT and MRI, because it shows attenuation and signal intensity same as the surrounding bile. Recently, a thread sign, described as linear or curvilinear hypointense striations within dilated bile ducts, was described as novel and characteristic MRCP finding of intraductal mucin-producing tumor (Hong et al. 2016). If MR with MRCP is not sufficient for definitive diagnosis, further work-up with endoscopic retrograde cholangioscopy (ERCP) should be performed. On ERCP mucin can be seen as amorphous, elongated cordlike filling defect in a bile duct filled with contrast medium (Tsuyuguchi et al. 2010). This mismatch between ERCP and MRCP

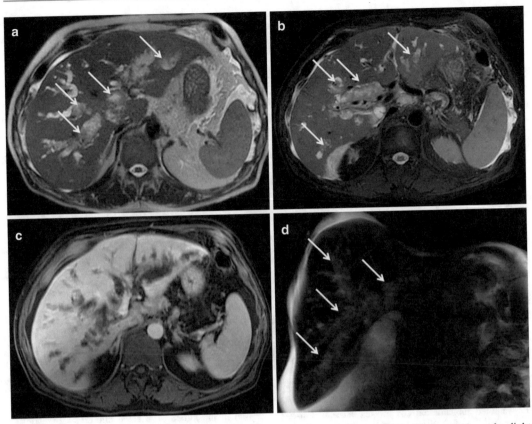

Fig. 8 Intraductal-growing intrahepatic cholangiocarci-noma in 73-year-old man. Axial T2-weighted (**a**) and T2-weighted fat-saturated (**b**) images show multiple pol-ypoid soft tissue lesions along diffusely dilated intrahe-patic bile ducts (*solid arrows*). (**c**) Axial T1-weighted image in portal venous phase demonstrates only slight enhancement of intraductal lesions. (**d**) Coronal MRCP image clearly depicts papillary feature of intraductal lesions (*solid arrows*) which are present in whole intrahe-patic biliary tree

findings indicates the presence of mucin. Moreover, ERCP can show hypersecretion of mucin draining through the ampulla (Tsuyuguchi et al. 2010). However, ERCP has a few draw-backs. An excessive amount of mucin within bile ducts and obstruction by the tumor may prevent opacification of the entire biliary system. Furthermore, cholangiography cannot detect multiple small tumors or lesions confined to mucosa, and it can be hard to distinguish tumors from stones or benign strictures. In certain diffi-cult cases, cholangioscopy with direct visualiza-tion of bile ducts is suggested.

Third type of intraductal-growing ICCs, with localized ductal dilatation and intraductal polyp-oid mass, is usually not difficult to diagnose (Lim et al. 2008). In this type mucin secretion is not remarkable; thus only bile ducts proximal to the tumor are dilated (Lim et al. 2008; Kim et al. 1998). Intraductal papillary mass is nicely depicted on T2-weighted images owing to the high contrast between the background bile and the tumor. This subtype usually shows enhance-ment equivalent to that of the hepatic parenchyma in the arterial phase of contrast enhanced CT or MRI. Persistent, intense enhancement on delayed phase is rarely seen, since fibrous stroma is scarce in these lesion, in contrast to other types of chol-angiocarcinoma (Chung et al. 2009).

Intraductal cast-like lesion is the rarest type of intraductal-growing ICC. It presents as dilated lobar or segmental bile ducts filled with soft tis-

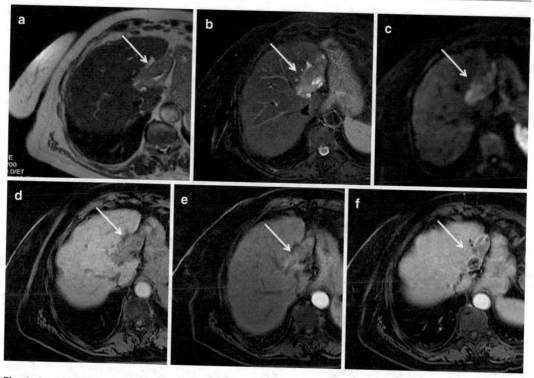

Fig. 9 Intraductal-growing intrahepatic cholangiocarcinoma in 65-year-old women. Axial T2-weighted (**a**) and T2-weighted fat-saturated (**b**) images show a cast-like tumor (*solid arrow*) filling bile ducts in left lateral segments associated with parenchymal atrophy. (**c**) On DWI tumor presents as hyperintense lesion in left lateral segments (*solid arrow*). (**d**) Unenhanced transverse fat-saturated T1-weighted shows a hypointense mass (*solid arrow*) in the lumen of affected bile ducts. (**e**) Arterial phase T1-weighted image shows hypervascularity of the lesion with washout on portal venous phase (**f**)

sue material, seen as heteroechogenic content within ducts on US examination (Chung et al. 2009). The characteristic CT finding is increased attenuation of the dilated ducts caused by diffuse superficial spread of the papillary tumor. On MRI, these tumors are seen as moderately hyperintense lesions with branching pattern, filling lobar or segmental bile ducts. Parenchymal atrophy of affected segments is almost always present. The enhancement pattern of a tumor is related to its pathohistological composition. Since these lesions are usually confined to the mucosa of the bile duct with a high blood flow and small amount stromal space, washout in portal venous phase is almost always observed (Fig. 9) (Lim et al. 2003). Loss of visualization of bile ducts filled with tumor, together with peripheral bile duct dilatation, is seen on MRCP (Fig. 10).

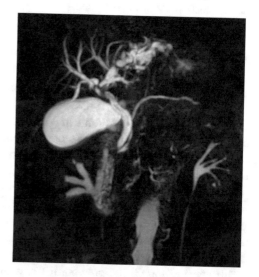

Fig. 10 Intraductal-growing intrahepatic cholangiocarcinoma in 65-year-old women. MRCP shows a central defect in the left lateral lobe corresponding to cast-like tumor with proximal biliary dilatation

4.2 Differential Diagnosis

The differential diagnosis of intraductal-growing ICC includes intrahepatic lithiasis, biliary cystadenoma/cystadenocarcinoma, HCC with intra-bile duct growth, and intraductal metastases (Lim et al. 2003; Rocha et al. 2012; Kojiro et al. 1982; Kim and Jeong 2016). The absence of calcifications and postcontrast enhancement within intraductal mass favors the diagnosis of intraductal cholangiocarcinoma (Lim et al. 2003). However, the presence of stones does not exclude the diagnosis of tumor. It is well known that long-standing intrahepatic lithiasis is predisposing factor to carcinogenesis (Rocha et al. 2012). Thus, all patients with this condition should be thoroughly examined on regular follow-up. Rarely, HCC can invade bile ducts leading to CT and/or MRI detection of soft tissue mass within the lumen of the duct (Kojiro et al. 1982). However, differential diagnosis is not difficult since intraductal part of the tumor shows typical enhancement pattern and is frequently accompanied by a parenchymal mass. Biliary cystadenoma and cystadenocarcinoma are cystic lesion with papillary soft tissue mass inside the cyst, mimicking intraductal cholangiocarcinoma (Arnaoutakis et al. 2014). These tumors occur mainly in females, and ovarian-like stroma is the pathognomonic microscopic finding (Arnaoutakis et al. 2014). The absence of communication with bile ducts is a clue for diagnosis, as it is always present in cystic forms of intraductal-growing ICC. Moreover, bile duct dilatation in intraductal cholangiocarcinoma is rarely such prominent to resemble cystic lesions, like biliary cystadenocarcinoma (Arnaoutakis et al. 2014). Intraductal metastasis from other primary malignancies could also mimic intraductal cholangiocarcinoma (Kim and Jeong 2016). However, these lesions are usually associated with a contiguous parenchymal mass in patients with a history of primary malignancy, particularly colorectal cancer (Kim and Jeong 2016).

5 Intraductal Papillary Neoplasm of Bile Ducts

Recently, the new clinical entity called intraductal papillary neoplasm of the bile duct (IPNB), including majority of intraductal papillary cholangiocarcinoma, and its precursor lesions, was added to the 2010 World Health Organization (WHO) classification (Bosman et al. 2010). These lesions are characterized predominantly by intraductal papillary growth, occasionally multifocal, with macroscopically visible mucin secretion present in one-third of cases (Wan et al. 2013). This entity includes lesions of any type of pathological transformation, from low-grade dysplasia to invasive carcinoma (Nakanuma et al. 2017). Many terms have previously been used to describe this condition, such as biliary papillomatosis, mucin-producing cholangiocarcinoma, mucin-hypersecreting bile duct tumor, and biliary intraductal papillary mucinous neoplasm (Wan et al. 2013). Histologically, IPNB is defined as tumor which shows papillary proliferation of neoplastic biliary epithelial cells with fibrovascular stalks within the bile duct, macroscopic or microscopic existence of mucin, and dilatation of the proximal or remote bile duct (Kim et al. 2012b; Nakanuma et al. 2017). Currently, IPNB is considered to be counterpart of more common similar lesion in pancreas, intraductal papillary mucinous neoplasm of the pancreas (IPMN) (Rocha et al. 2012; Kloppel and Kosmahl 2006). In contrast to IPMN, the most cases of IPNB are high-grade dysplastic and invasive neoplasms, while low-grade IPNB is rare (Nakanuma et al. 2014). Additionally, mucin secretion is present in one-third of patients while it is invariably seen in IPMN lesions (Kloppel and Kosmahl 2006). In recent literature, there has been some confusion regarding the relation between intraductal-growing ICC and IPNB, since both entities share many common features. In this regard, study by Nakanuma et al. has shown that a majority of intraductal-growing ICCs were found to belong to an IPNB spectrum of disease, while a minority of them showed other types of malignant lesions, such as poorly differentiated adenocarcinoma, tubular adenocarcinoma, carcinosarcoma, cholangiocarcinoma component of combined HCC-CCC, and other malignant neoplasms (Nakanuma et al. 2014).

The most common clinical manifestations of patients with IPNB are recurrent episodes of acute cholangitis and obstructive jaundice (Kim et al. 2012b; Lee et al. 2004). Intermittent biliary obstruction can be the consequence of detached tumor emboli, abundant mucin discharge into the bile ducts, or, rarely, concomitant biliary stones (Hayashi et al. 1996; Bennett et al. 2015). These intermittent nature of symptoms is pathognomonic for IPNB lesions (Lee et al. 2004). Almost all patients have an elevated level of alkaline phosphatase. Nevertheless, despite massive ductal dilatation, clinical jaundice is relatively rare (Kubota et al. 2014). This discrepancy between a marked dilatation and a normal to slightly elevated level of serum bilirubin, especially with an elevated carcinoembryonic antigen level, may suggest the diagnosis of this rare entity (Choi et al. 1995; Han et al. 2002; Kim and Jeong 2016).

6 Preoperative Staging and Management

Cholangiocarcinomas have overall a poor prognosis with 5-year survival rate of approximately 1% (Lazaridis and Gores 2005; Isaji et al. 1999). The only curative treatment is surgical resection which can prolong survival (5-year survival rate of approximately 10–30%) (Isaji et al. 1999). Hepatic resection is contraindicated in the presence of severe comorbidities, metastases, distant lymph node involvement, and/or advanced underlying liver disease (Doherty et al. 2017). Moreover, specific contraindications include diffuse bilobar involvement and/or future liver remnant less than 25% in the otherwise healthy liver (Doherty et al. 2017). Besides tumor characterization, in patients with ICC, CT or MRI report must include preoperative assessment of tumor relationship with major blood vessels (Choi et al. 2004a). Vascular involvement should be suspected when nonenhancing or stenotic vessel is seen, ipsilateral hepatic atrophy, contour deformity of vessel, or tumor-vessel contact more than half of the circumference (Han et al. 2002; Fujita et al. 2017; Maetani et al. 2001; Hennedige et al. 2014). Liver transplantation is not recommended in patients with unresectable ICC due to high risk of recurrence.

7 Combined Hepatocellular Carcinoma and Cholangiocarcinoma

Combined or biphenotypic HCC-CCC (cHC) are rare tumors and represent less than 1% of all liver carcinomas, with worse prognosis in comparison to pure HCC (Taguchi et al. 1996). The pathogenesis of cHC is still unclear, although recent studies have proposed the concept that cHC originates from hepatic progenitor stem cells. cHC has been classified into three categories: (1) double cancer representing tumors in which areas of HCC and CCC coexist separately, (2) combined type where both components are present adjacent each other and mixed together, and (3) mixed type in which both components are intimately mixed (Allen and Lisa 1949; Yeh 2010). However, this classification has its drawbacks as it is often very difficult to distinguish mixed and combined types. To date, there are only a few studies describing the radiological characteristics of cHC, which depend on the proportion of each tumor within the lesion (Sasaki et al. 2015; Lee et al. 2006; De Campos et al. 2012; Nishie et al. 2005; Aoki et al. 1993). The combined cHC usually presents as solitary heterogeneous mass, with variable hyperintensity on T2-weighted image (Fig. 11) (Hashimoto et al. 1994; Schiettecatte et al. 2008). De Campos et al. have shown that early ring enhancement with progressive enhancement in later phases is the most common vascular pattern (De Campos et al. 2012). The presence of washout in part of the lesion may favor the diagnosis of cHC, but is rarely seen. Enhancement pattern may also be geographic with parts of the lesion exhibiting typical vascular profile of HCC and other parts showing progressive enhancement (Fowler et al. 2013). Moreover, lesions may show arterial hypervascularity characteristic for HCC without subsequent washout (Fig. 11) (Willekens et al. 2009). In those cases the use of hepatospecific contrast agents together with tumor characteristics on T1- and T2-weighted images and epidemiological data allows differentiation from FNH. However, the preoperative diagnosis of

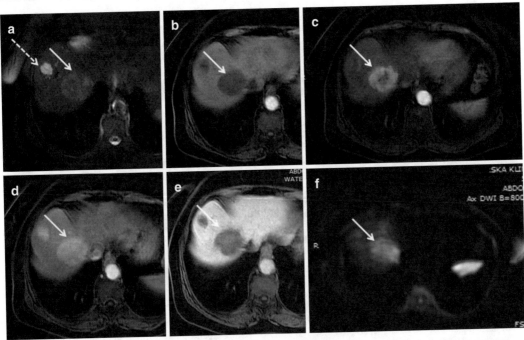

Fig. 11 Combined hepatocellular carcinoma and cholangiocarcinoma in 65-year-old woman without chronic liver disease. (**a**) Axial T2-weighted image shows lobulated heterogeneous mass located centrally in segments VII and VIII (*solid arrow*). Note also small hemangioma (*dotted arrow*). The tumor is hypointense on T1-weghted fat-saturated image (**b**), with thick rim of enhancement on arterial phase (**c**) and progressive enhancement on portal venous phase (**d**). The lesion is hypointense on hepatobiliary phase (**e**) with restricted diffusion on diffusion-weighted image (**f**) (*solid arrows*)

cHC is very difficult, since the imaging features overlap with both HCC and CCC, and in majority of cases it is established on histopathology (Lee et al. 2006).

References

Al Ansari N, Kim BS, Srirattanapong S et al (2014) Mass-forming cholangiocarcinoma and adenocarcinoma of unknown primary: can they be distinguished on liver MRI? Abdom Imaging 39:1228–1240

Allen RA, Lisa JR (1949) Combined liver cell and bile duct carcinoma. Am J Pathol 25:647–655

Aoki K, Takayasu K, Kawano T et al (1993) Combined hepatocellular carcinoma and cholangiocarcinoma: clinical features and computed tomographic findings. Hepatology 18:1090–1095

Arnaoutakis DJ, Kamel I, Anders R et al (2014) Cystic neoplasms of the liver: biliary cystadenoma and cystadenocarcinoma. J Am Coll Surg 218(1): 119–128

Ayuso JR, Pagés M, Darnell A (2013) Imaging bile duct tumors: staging. Abdom Imaging 38:1071–1081

Bennett S, Marginean EC, Paquin-Gobeil M et al (2015) Clinical and pathological features of intraductal papillary neoplasm of the biliary tract and gallbladder. HPB (Oxford) 17(9):811–818

Bosman FT, Carneiro F, Hruban RH et al (2010) WHO classification of tumours of the digestive system. 4th ed. Lyon: IARC, p 417

Choi BI, Han JK, Shin YM et al (1995) Peripheral cholangiocarcinoma: comparison of MRI with CT. Abdom Imaging 20:357–360

Choi BI, Lee JM, Han JK (2004a) Imaging of intrahepatic and hilar cholangiocarcinoma. Abdom Imaging 29:548–557

Choi D, Lim JH, Hong ST (2004b) Relation of cholangiocarcinomas to clonorchiasis and bile duct stones. Abdom Imaging 29(5):590–597

Chung YE, Kim MJ, Park YN et al (2009) Varying appearances of cholangiocarcinoma: radiologic-pathologic correlation. Radiographics 29:683–700

De Campos P, Semelka RC, Azevedo RM et al (2012) Combined hepatocellular carcinoma-cholangiocarcinoma: report of MR appearance in eleven patients. J Magn Reson Imaging 36(5):1139–1147

Doherty B, Nambudiri VE, Palmer WC (2017) Update on the diagnosis and treatment of cholangiocarcinoma. Curr Gastroenterol Rep 19(1):2

Feng ST, Wu L, Cai H et al (2015) Cholangiocarcinoma: spectrum of appearances on Gd-EOB-DTPA-enhanced MR imaging and the effect of biliary function on signal intensity. BMC Cancer 15:38

Fowler KJ, Sheybani A, Parker RA 3rd et al (2013) Combined hepatocellular and cholangiocarcinoma (biphenotypic) tumors: imaging features and diagnostic accuracy of contrast-enhanced CT and MRI. AJR Am J Roentgenol 201:332–339

Fujita N, Asayama Y, Nishie A et al (2017) Mass-forming intrahepatic cholangiocarcinoma: enhancement patterns in the arterial phase of dynamic hepatic CT—correlation with clinicopathological findings. Eur Radiol 27:498–506

Han JK, Choi BI, Kim AY et al (2002) Cholangiocarcinoma: pictorial essay of CT and cholangiographic findings. Radiographics 22:173–187

Hashimoto T, Nakamura H, Hori S et al (1994) MR imaging of mixed hepatocellular and cholangiocellular carcinoma. Abdom Imaging 19:430–432

Hayashi M, Matsui O, Ueda K et al (1996) Imaging findings of mucinous type of cholangiocellular carcinoma. J Comput Assist Tomogr 20:386–389

Hennedige TP, Neo WT, Venkatesh SK (2014) Imaging of malignancies of the biliary tract- an update. Cancer Imaging 14(14)

Hong GS, Byun JH, Kim JH et al (2016) Thread sign in biliary intraductal papillary mucinous neoplasm: a novel specific finding for MRI. Eur Radiol 26:3112–3120

Isaji S, Kawarada Y, Taoka H et al (1999) Clinicopathological features and outcome of hepatic resection for intrahepatic cholangiocarcinoma in Japan. J Hepatobil Pancreat Surg 6:108–116

Jeong HT, Kim MJ, Chung YE et al (2013) Gadoxetate disodium-enhanced MRI of mass-forming intrahepatic cholangiocarcinomas: imaging-histologic correlation. AJR Am J Roentgenol 201:W603–W611

Jhaveri KS, Hosseini-Nik H (2015) MRI of cholangiocarcinoma. J Magn Reson Imaging 42(5):1165–1179

Katabathina VS, Dasyam AK, Dasyam N et al (2014) Adult bile duct strictures: role of MR imaging and MR cholangiopancreatography in characterization. Radiographics 34(3):565–586

Kawakatsu M, Vilgrain V, Zins M (1997) Radiologic features of papillary adenoma and papillomatosis of the biliary tract. Abdom Imaging 22(1):87–90

Kim AY, Jeong WK (2016) Intraductal malignant tumors in the liver mimicking cholangiocarcinoma: imaging features for differential diagnosis. Clin Mol Hepatol 22:192–197

Kim YS, Myung ST, Kim SY et al (1998) Biliary papillomatosis: clinical, cholangiographic and cholangioscopic findings. Endoscopy 30:763–767

Kim JH, Kim TK, Eun HW et al (2006) CT findings of cholangiocarcinoma associated with recurrent pyogenic cholangitis. AJR Am J Roentgenol 187(6):1571–1577

Kim JY, Lee JM, Han JK et al (2007) Contrast-enhanced MRI combined with MR cholangiopancreatography for the evaluation of patients with biliary strictures: differentiation of malignant from benign bile duct strictures. J Magn Reson Imaging 26(2):304–312

Kim JE, Lee JM, Kim SH et al (2010) Differentiation of intraductal growing-type cholangiocarcinomas from nodular-type cholangiocarcinomas at biliary MR imaging with MR cholangiography. Radiology 257:364–372

Kim SA, Lee JM, Lee KB et al (2011) Intrahepatic mass-forming cholangiocarcinomas: enhancement patterns at multiphasic CT, with special emphasis on arterial enhancement pattern--correlation with clinicopathologic findings. Radiology 260:148–157

Kim SH, Lee CH, Kim BH et al (2012a) Typical and atypical imaging findings of intrahepatic Cholangiocarcinoma using gadolinium Ethoxybenzyl Diethylenetriamine Pentaacetic acid–enhanced magnetic resonance imaging. J Comput Assist Tomogr 36(6):704–709

Kim KM, Lee JK, Shin JU et al (2012b) Clinicopathologic features of intraductal papillary neoplasm of the bile duct according to histologic subtype. Am J Gastroenterol 107:118–125

Kim R, Lee JM, Shin CI et al (2016) Differentiation of intrahepatic mass-forming cholangiocarcinoma from hepatocellular carcinoma on gadoxetic acid-enhanced liver MR imaging. Eur Radiol 26:1808–1817

Kloppel G, Kosmahl M (2006) Is the intraductal papillary mucinous neoplasia of the biliary tract a counterpart of pancreatic papillary mucinous neoplasm? J Hepatol 44(2):249–250

Kojiro M, Kawabata K, Kawano Y et al (1982) Hepatocellular carcinoma presenting as intrabile duct tumor growth: a clinicopathologic study of 24 cases. Cancer 49(10):2144–2147

Kovač JD, Galun D, Đurić-Stefanović A et al (2017) Intrahepatic mass-forming cholangiocarcinoma and solitary hypovascular liver metastases: is the differential diagnosis using diffusion-weighted MRI possible? Acta Radiol 58(12):1417–1426

Kubota K, Nakanuma Y, Kondo F et al (2014) Clinicopathological features and prognosis of mucin-producing bile duct tumor and mucinous cystic tumor of the liver: a multi-institutional study by the Japan biliary association. J Hepatobiliary Pancreat Sci 21:176–185

Lazaridis KN, Gores GJ (2005) Cholangiocarcinoma. Gastroenterology 128(6):1655–1667

Lee JW, Han JK, Kim TK et al (2000) CT features of intraductal intrahepatic cholangiocarcinoma. AJR Am J Roentgenol 175:721–725

Lee WJ, Lim HK, Jang KM et al (2001) Radiologic spectrum of cholangiocarcinoma: emphasis on unusual manifestations and differential diagnoses. Radiographics 21:S97–S116

Lee SS, Kim MH, Lee SK et al (2004) Clinicopathologic review of 58 patients with biliary papillomatosis. Cancer 100:783–793

Lee WS, Lee KW, Heo JS et al (2006) Comparison of combined hepatocellular and cholangiocarcinoma with hepatocellular carcinoma and intrahepatic cholangiocarcinoma. Surg Today 36:892–897

Lim JH (2003) Cholangiocarcinoma: morphologic classification according to growth pattern and imaging findings. AJR Am J Roentgenol 181:819–827

Lim JH, Yi CA, Lim HK et al (2002) Radiological spectrum of intraductal papillary tumors of the bile ducts. Korean J Radiol 3(1):57–63

Lim JH, Kim MH, Kim TK et al (2003) Papillary neoplasms of the bile duct that mimic biliary stone disease. Radiographics 23(2):447–455

Lim JH, Yoon KH, Kim SH et al (2004) Intraductal papillary mucinous tumor of the bile ducts. Radiographics 24:53–66

Lim JH, Jang KT, Choi D (2008) Biliary intraductal papillary mucinous neoplasm manifesting only as dilatation of the hepatic lobar or segmental bile ducts: imaging features in six patients. AJR Am J Roentgenol 191:778–782

Maetani Y, Itoh K, Watanabe C et al (2001) MR imaging of intrahepatic cholangiocarcinoma with pathologic correlation. AJR Am J Roentgenol 176(6):1499–1507

Manfredi R, Barbaro B, Masselli G et al (2004) Magnetic resonance imaging of cholangiocarcinoma. Semin Liver Dis 24(2):155–164

Mittelstaedt CA (1997) Ultrasound of the bile ducts. Semin Roentgenol 32(3):161–171

Nakanuma Y, Sato Y, Ojima H et al (2014) Clinicopathological characterization of so-called "cholangiocarcinoma with intraductal papillary growth" with respect to "intraductal papillary neoplasm of bile duct (IPNB)". Int J Clin Exp Pathol 7(6):3112–3122

Nakanuma Y, Uesaka K, Miyayama S et al (2017) Intraductal neoplasms of the bile duct. A new challenge to biliary tract tumor pathology. Histol Histopathol 32(10):1001–1015

Nishie A, Yoshimitsu K, Asayama Y et al (2005) Detection of combined hepatocellular and cholangiocarcinomas on enhanced CT: comparison with histologic findings. AJR Am J Roentgenol 184:1157–1162

Outwater E, Tomaszewski JE, Daly JM et al (1991) Hepatic colorectal metastases: correlation of MR imaging and pathologic appearance. Radiology 180:327–332

Park HJ, Kim YK, Park MJ et al (2013) Small intrahepatic mass-forming cholangiocarcinoma: target sign on diffusion-weighted imaging for differentiation from hepatocellular carcinoma. Abdom Imaging 38:793–801

Rimola J, Forner A, Reig M et al (2009) Cholangiocarcinoma in cirrhosis: absence of contrast washout in delayed phase by magnetic resonance imaging avoids misdiagnosis of hepatocellular carcinoma. Hepatology 50:791–798

Rocha FG, Lee H, Katabi N et al (2012) Intraductal papillary neoplasm of the bile duct: a biliary equivalent to intraductal papillary mucinous neoplasm of the pancreas? Hepatology 56:1352–1360

Sainani NI, Catalano OA, Holalkere NS et al (2008) Cholangiocarcinoma: current and novel imaging techniques. Radiographics 28:1263–1287

Sasaki A, Aramaki M, Kawano K et al (1998) Intrahepatic peripheral cholangiocarcinoma: mode of spread and choice of surgical treatment. Br J Surg 85:1206–1209

Sasaki M, Sato H, Kakuda Y et al (2015) Clinicopathological significance of 'subtypes with stem-cell feature' in combined hepatocellular-cholangiocarcinoma. Liver Int 35:1024–1035

Schiettecatte A, Dujardin M, Beeck B et al (2008) Combined hepatocellular-cholangiocarcinoma: MR findings. Eur J Radiol Extra 67:e75–e77

Shaib Y, El-Serag HB (2004) The epidemiology of cholangiocarcinoma. Semin Liver Dis 24(2):115–125

Shaib YH, El-Serag HB, Nooka AK et al (2007) Risk factors for intrahepatic and extrahepatic cholangiocarcinoma: a hospital-based case-control study. Am J Gastroenterol 102(5):1016–1021

Soyer P, Bluemke DA, Vissuzaine C et al (1994) CT of hepatic tumors: prevalence and specificity of retraction of the adjacent capsule. AJR Am J Roentgenol 162:1119–1122

Taguchi J, Nakashima O, Tanaka M et al (1996) A clinicopathological study on combined hepatocellular and cholangiocarcinoma. J Gastroenterol Hepatol 11(8):758–764

Tsuyuguchi T, Sakai Y, Sugiyama H et al (2010) Endoscopic diagnosis of intraductal papillary mucinous neoplasm of the bile duct. J Hepatobiliary Pancreat Sci 17:230–235

Valls C, Guma A, Puig I et al (2000) Intrahepatic peripheral cholangiocarcinoma: CT evaluation. Abdom Imaging 25(5):490–496

Vilana R, Forner A, Bianchi L et al (2010) Intrahepatic peripheral cholangiocarcinoma in cirrhosis patients may display a vascular pattern similar to hepatocellular carcinoma on contrast-enhanced ultrasound. Hepatology 51:2020–2029

Wan XS, Xu YY, Qian JY et al (2013) Intraductal papillary neoplasm of the bile duct. World J Gastroenterol 19(46):8595–8604

Wibulpolprasert B, Dhiensiri T (1992) Peripheral cholangiocarcinoma: sonographic evaluation. J Clin Ultrasound 20(5):303–314

Willekens I, Hoorens A, Geers C et al (2009) Combined hepatocellular and cholangiocellular carcinoma presenting with radiological characteristics of focal nodular hyperplasia. World J Gastroenterol 15:3940–3943

Yamamoto M, Takasaki K, Yoshikawa T et al (1998) Does gross appearance indicate prognosis in intrahepatic cholangiocarcinoma. J Surg Oncol 69:162–167

Yeh MM (2010) Pathology of combined hepatocellular-cholangiocarcinoma. J Gastroenterol Hepatol 25:1485–1492

Yoon KH, Han HK, Kim CG et al (2000) Malignant papillary neoplasms of intrahepatic bile ducts: CT and histopathologic features. AJR Am J Roentgenol 175:1135–1139

Liver Metastases

Martina Scharitzer, Helmut Kopf,
and Wolfgang Schima

Contents

M. Scharitzer (✉)
Department of Biomedical Imaging and
Image-Guided Therapy, Medical University
of Vienna, Vienna, Austria
e-mail: martina.scharitzer@meduniwien.ac.at

H. Kopf · W. Schima
Department of Diagnostic and Interventional
Radiology, Goettlicher Heiland Krankenhaus,
Barmherzige Schwestern Krankenhaus, St. Josef
Krankenhaus, Vinzenzgruppe, Vienna, Austria
e-mail: helmut.kopf@khgh.at;
wolfgang.schima@khgh.at

Abstract

Liver metastases are the most common malignant hepatic lesions. Their accurate and early detection is crucial to select the most appropriate therapeutic strategy. Advances in the treatment of metastatic liver disease have been shown to improve significantly the survival of affected patients. Radiological diagnostic modalities play a major role in the workup and selection of appropriate treatment planning. An exact knowledge of lesion number, size, and distribution within the liver parenchyma, as well as volumetric and functional information about residual liver parenchyma, are essential for the optimal selection of patients who will benefit from individually planned resection. The detection of small focal liver lesions, in particular, remains a diagnostic challenge. The development of new imaging modalities, functional imaging, the availability of novel contrast agents, and the discussion about alternative tumor response criteria have further improved the radiological role in lesion detection, characterization, and assessment of treatment response. In addition to the typical imaging pattern of hepatic metastases, unusual radiological findings, uncommon response patterns, complications, and therapeutic toxicities should be known by radiologists to guide proper patient management.

1 Introduction, Epidemiology, Pathophysiology

The liver parenchyma is a common site for metastatic disease from a large variety of primary tumors, partly due to the double blood supply by the portal vein and the hepatic artery and partly due to the specific hepatic microenvironment, also called the "seed-and-soil" hypothesis (Paget 1989). Metastases do not contain functioning hepatocytes and biliary ducts and show variable vascularity and tissue composition, depending on the primary tumor. A nationwide analysis of pathology reports of liver biopsies revealed carcinomas as the most frequent tumor type at 92% (with the following primary origin in decreasing order: adenocarcinoma (75%) of colorectal, pancreatic, or breast origin, small cell carcinoma, neuroendocrine carcinoma, large cell carcinoma, and squamous cell carcinoma, followed by melanoma in 2.4% and sarcoma in 1% (de Ridder et al. 2016)). The last several years have seen a paradigm shift in the management of hepatic metastases, leading to a significant increase in

patients' survival. This is the result of the development of new chemotherapeutic regimens that include the use of new molecular target agents (antiangiogenesis drugs and immunomodulators). In addition, in several types of cancer, the presence of hepatic metastases does not preclude a curative approach, and a wider access to individually planned resection in patients with oligometastatic liver disease has demonstrated improved long-term survival, reaching 5-year survival rates of up to 50–60% (Kopetz and Vauthey 2008) after potentially curative resection of colorectal liver metastases.

2 Indications for Imaging

Diagnostic imaging plays a crucial role in selecting the most appropriate therapy for patients with hepatic metastases. Radiologists are integrated in the decisions on treatment, beginning after detection of the primary malignancy as part of the global staging, the more detailed assessment for the evaluation of suspected liver metastases, and presurgical planning before resection, as well as post-therapeutic follow-up, in particular cases over years. This includes accurate lesion detection, characterization, determination of resectability, and assessment of treatment response. Although radiologists are also an integral part of local specific interventional therapy to increase the number of surgical candidates, provide curative treatment options for nonsurgical patients, or improve survival in a palliative setting, the interventional radiological approaches will not be part of this chapter. The incidence of liver metastases at time of the initial presentation of the primary malignancy has been correlated with tumor type, location of the primary tumor, degree of differentiation, T and N staging, and other factors. Studies have shown that, even in patients with an underlying malignancy, small liver lesions (≤ 1 cm) are much more often found to be benign: only 11.6% of lesions too-small-to-characterize at CT were found to be malignant at follow-up (Schwartz et al. 1999). Therefore, accurate characterization of focal hepatic abnormalities is an important radiological task.

3 Imaging Modalities

Various imaging modalities are available for the detection of hepatic metastases. MRI and multiphasic CT are the primary imaging modalities for the assessment of liver metastases, with PET/CT and ultrasound as complementary methods. Many noninvasive diagnostic methods exist comprising certain advantages and disadvantages over others. Nevertheless, despite the high accuracy for the detection and follow-up of liver metastases, optimal, generally valid imaging strategies for patients with liver metastases are still lacking.

3.1 Transabdominal Sonography

Transabdominal sonography (US), an inexpensive and readily available method, is widely used as a primary imaging modality with which to assess the liver parenchyma, but has several limitations: variability in operator expertise and patient's habitus; less than ideal patients' cooperation; the presence of interfering bowel gas, or moderate results in patients with chemotherapy, such as induced fatty infiltration of the liver.

Ambiguity in segmental localization may be another drawback for surgical planning. Isoechoic lesions with an acoustic impedance similar to that of the liver parenchyma and hyperechoic lesions that resemble hemangiomas are difficult to detect and differentiate. Sonography is also a helpful guide for percutaneous biopsy of suspicious liver lesions if the lesion is easily visible and accessible by ultrasound.

Use of *contrast-enhanced sonography* (CE-US) is a safe, relatively inexpensive, and widely available possibility with which to increase the diagnostic capability for detection and characterization of focal liver lesions. Metastases may show a wide range of imaging appearances at gray-scale US. By intravenous application of contrast medium-containing microbubbles and the use of dedicated ultrasound sequences, dynamic real-time imaging with high temporal and spatial resolution is possible. In a large multicenter study, the addition of contrast-enhanced ultrasound increased the sensitivity for the detection of metastases on a per-lesion basis from 71% with standard US to 87% with CEUS (Albrecht et al. 2003). Lesions that are not or barely detectable on gray-scale ultrasound are distinctly visible with CEUS (Fig. 1). Due to the lack of

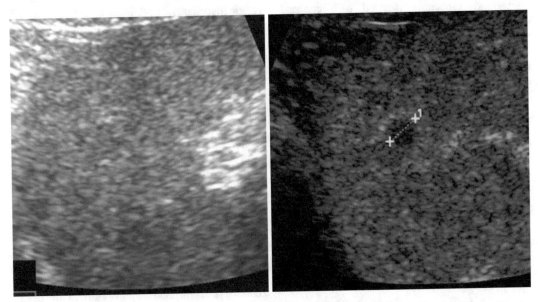

Fig. 1 CEUS of a small, singular colorectal liver metastasis. In gray-scale ultrasound (left), the lesion is not visible, but in the portal venous phase of CEUS (right), the metastasis in segment 4A is clearly detectable as a hypoenhancing focus

possible nephrotoxic complications, CEUS represents a valuable alternative to CECT and CEMRI in patients with renal insufficiency or with a known allergy to CT or MR contrast agents. In addition, in inconclusive lesions on CECT or CEMRI, CEUS can be used as a problem-solving tool. The efficacy of CEUS for the detection of liver metastases has been included in recent international guidelines (Claudon et al. 2013). CEUS has shown variable reports in the literature, ranging from 64.5% (Vialle et al. 2016) to a high diagnostic accuracy of up to 93% when assessing all vascular phases for the differentiation of benign from malignant liver lesions (Nicolau et al. 2006). Similar results have been found when comparing CEUS to CEMRI with gadoxetic acid (Shiozawa et al. 2017). Fusion imaging of CEUS with CECT or CEMRI (Bo et al. 2017), as well as quantitative dynamic CEUS (Krix 2005) and three-dimensional imaging (El Kaffas et al. 2017), are promising future tools for the detection of changes in tumor perfusion after stereotactic radiotherapy or chemotherapy and prediction of treatment response.

Intraoperative sonography has emerged as a valuable tool, showing higher sensitivities and specificities than conventional transabdominal ultrasound, especially if used with contrast-enhanced intraoperative ultrasound. Studies suggest that up to 32–57% of patients who are undergoing surgery have non-recognized hepatic metastases. IOUS may show liver metastases not detected by prior contrast-enhanced CT in up to 14% (Ellebæk et al. 2017). However, in this systematic review, no comparison between CE-MRI and IOUS could be performed. Since laparoscopic surgery of liver metastases is becoming increasingly important, laparoscopic ultrasound, although not routinely performed, may represent a helpful alternative imaging modality in the operating theater.

3.2 Computed Tomography

Computed tomography has been the most widely used imaging modality for the assessment of hepatic metastases due to the high speed of image acquisition, relatively inexpensive cost, and its ability to assess extrahepatic sites of metastatic disease as well. Volumetric acquisitions with isotropic voxels allow the reconstruction of high-quality reformatted images in various planes for the assessment of small lesions and exact segmental localization. Depending on various enhancement patterns, the portal venous phase or recently called "hepatic venous phase" (60–70 s after intravenous contrast medium administration) is the most reliable phase, with a detection rate of 85% and a positive predictive value of 96% (Soyer et al. 2004). The benefit of adding an arterial phase 15–18 s after the intravenous administration of contrast medium has been shown, with increasing detection rates of up to 8–13% (Silverman 2006). This is especially important for hypervascular tumors, including neuroendocrine tumors, melanoma, sarcoma, carcinoid, renal cell, thyroid, and choriocarcinoma. An equilibrium phase (>100 s after i.v. contrast injection) adds no significant value and is not routinely recommended. The use of non-contrast-enhanced CT is still under debate, but studies have shown only a small value to CECT (Sadigh et al. 2014). When using dual-energy CT, virtual non-contrast images may be occasionally helpful for the detection of calcified or hemorrhagic metastases. In addition, after liver-directed therapy, such as chemoembolization or radioembolization, differentiation from injected high-attenuation lipiodol and viable tumor can be facilitated. Nevertheless, in patients of younger age and potentially curative disease, radiation exposure should be kept in mind. The diagnostic accuracy of CT can be reduced by chemotherapy, which induces steatohepatitis or sinusoidal injury, resulting in decreased attenuation values of the liver parenchyma.

With regard to the amount of intravenous *contrast medium* for standard 64-slice CT, an iodine dose of 0.6 g/kg body weight is recommended, with a high flow rate ranging between 3 and 5 mL/s. For excellent arterial phase enhancement, the iodine delivery rate (iodine administered per second) is essential. An appropriate iodine delivery rate can be equally achieved by higher iodine concentrations (400 mg I/mL) and lower flow rates as well as by lower iodine concentrations

(300 mg/mL) with higher flow rates. The total amount of iodine administered largely rules the hepatic enhancement in the portal venous phase. However, higher amounts of iodine have the disadvantage of increasing the risk of contrast-induced nephropathy, which is related to the total quantity of iodine in patients with renal insufficiency. Reduction of tube kilovoltage results in decreased radiation dose and allows a reduction of iodine-contrast material dosage, but increases image noise, and therefore, reduces image quality. A relatively new algorithm, the "iterative reconstruction algorithm," enables the generation of images of comparable quality despite reduced contrast dose (Buls et al. 2015). The use of thinner reconstructed images over thicker ones improves lesion detection (Weg et al. 1998); therefore, slice thickness for reconstruction of axial acquired series should not exceed 3 mm.

CT texture analysis, a technique that shows spatial heterogeneity beyond visual perception, has been tested for non-contrast imaging (Ganeshan et al. 2009) and portal venous phase imaging (Miles et al. 2009), and showed promising results for the assessment of occult micrometastases.

3.3 Magnetic Resonance Imaging

During the past decade, MRI has emerged as the leading imaging modality for the assessment of focal liver lesions. Technical advances have enabled routine implementation of new MR sequences, such as 3D T1-weighted fast-spoiled gradient echo (GRE) and diffusion-weighted imaging (DWI). The unique, high, intrinsic soft tissue contrast between normal liver parenchyma and liver lesions on MR imaging can further be enhanced with the help of intravenous, nonspecific (extracellular) and liver-specific (hepatobiliary) gadolinium-based contrast agents, enabling morphological and functional assessment as well. Disadvantages include a higher susceptibility to motion artifacts, longer duration of a liver MR examination, and recently reported concerns about gadolinium deposition in human tissue. A multichannel phased array coil in combination with table-embedded spine coils are preferred whenever possible. A field strength of at least 1.5 T is required, but it has been shown that contrast-enhanced 3D-GE imaging at 3 T provides higher image quality (Ramalho et al. 2009).

3.3.1 Contrast Media

For dynamic phase imaging, all non-blood pool gadolinium-based contrast agents (GBCAs) are suitable, with distribution in the extracellular space within and outside the vessels comparable to the iodinated contrast media used in CT. However, due to possible gadolinium retention in a number of tissues, such as bone, skin, and brain, macrocyclic GBCAs should be used in favor of linear GBCAs (McDonald et al. 2018). A weight-based dosage of 0.1 mmol/kg is recommended at a rate of 1–2 mL/s, followed by a 20-mL saline flush at 1–2 mL/s using a power injector.

Hepatobiliary contrast agents represent a group of paramagnetic molecules that are taken up by hepatocytes and excreted into the bile, delineating lesions without functioning hepatocytes as hypointense to a normal-enhancing liver parenchyma in the hepatobiliary phase. Gadobenate dimeglumine (formerly known as Gd-BOPTA, MultiHance®, Bracco) and gadoxetic acid (formerly known as Gd-EOB-DTPA; Primovist® or Eovist®, Bayer Healthcare) show a biphasic liver enhancement and are eliminated by renal and hepatic excretion pathways as well, allowing assessment of early perfusion information about the renal elimination pathway and hepatocyte-specific information about the hepatic excretion pathway. There are only few currently available studies comparing both liver-specific contrast agents, indicating no diagnostic superiority of one agent when comparing the hepatobiliary phase (Gupta et al. 2012; Park et al. 2010), although gadoxetic acid provides the highest hepatocyte enhancement (Kim et al. 2013). Dosing is 0.025 mmol/kg bodyweight for gadoxetic acid and 0.1 mmol/kg gadobenate dimeglumine with a flow rate of 1 mL/s, followed by a sodium chloride flush. Respiratory artifacts during the arterial phase after injection of gadoxetic acid have been observed (Davenport et al. 2013; Motosugi et al. 2016; Luetkens et al. 2015).

However, fewer artifacts were reported with the use of a diluted power-injected protocol or a special 3D gradient-echo (GRE) pulse sequence with incomplete interpolated k-space filling and a parallel imaging technique (Polanec et al. 2017; Gruber et al. 2018).

A manganese-based liver-specific agent, mangafodipir trisodium, could not be administered as a bolus, and thus, the assessment capabilities of vascular structures were limited, although, for characterization of hepatocellular lesions, good accuracy has been shown (Scharitzer et al. 2005). Mangafodipir trisodium has been withdrawn from the market for some years, but, given the discussion about gadolinium-based MR contrast agents, it may reappear as a generic agent in the future. Reticuloendothelial system agents (RES) are superparamagnetic iron oxide-based (SPIO) contrast agents that are taken up by RES cells of the normal hepatic parenchyma, the spleen, and lymph nodes. By shortening T2 and T2* relaxation times, a loss of signal intensity has been observed in the normal liver parenchyma, delineating hyperintense malignant liver lesions without RES cells. Although a high accuracy for detection of liver metastases has been reported (del Frate et al. 2002; Ward et al. 2005), these agents have been taken off the market in Europe and the United States. A comparison of CE-CT, CE-US, SPIO-MRI, and gadoxetic acid-enhanced MRI in patients with colorectal liver metastases showed the highest sensitivities for MRI with the superiority of gadoxetic acid-enhanced MRI to SPIO-MRI for lesions smaller ≤10 mm (Muhi et al. 2011).

3.3.2 MRI Sequences

The European Society of Gastrointestinal and Abdominal Radiology (ESGAR) formed a multinational European panel of experts and provided updated recommendations on the methodology and clinical indications of MRI with liver-specific contrast agents (Neri et al. 2016), including MR sequences for the workup of focal liver lesions:

- Axial breath-hold, heavily T2-weighted, half-Fourier, single-shot turbo spin-echo (TSE) sequence.

- Navigator-triggered, intermediate T2-weighted TSE sequence.
- Breath-hold T1-weighted 2D GRE in-phase and opposed-phase sequence.
- Dynamic contrast-enhanced, fat-suppressed, 3D T1w GRE breath-hold sequence, acquired before and during the late arterial, portal venous, and equilibrium phase after IV administration of gadolinium chelate.
- Diffusion-weighted imaging (DWI) using low, intermediate, and high b-values should be implemented, with an ADC map included.
- If a liver-specific agent is administered: hepatocyte-specific imaging, with an additional hepatobiliary phase 20 min or 60–120 min post (depending on the contrast agent).

To shorten acquisition time, T2w and DWI sequences can be performed after completion of the late dynamic phase, if a hepatobiliary contrast agent is used. A slice thickness maximum of 5 mm for 2D sequences and 3 mm for 3D sequences should be used. In general, DWI pulse sequences are used for metastasis detection. The diffusion coefficient of lesions is related to lesion cellularity and the size of the extracellular space. Metastases show restricted diffusion, which results in high SI on DW images and lower ADC values than those of the surrounding liver parenchyma, which aids in detection (Taouli and Koh 2010). But, some benign lesions, such as hepatocellular adenoma or focal nodular hyperplasia, may show lower ADC values than malignant lesions and abscesses (Miller et al. 2010). Attempts to use DWI sequences alone as a reliable sequence for the preoperative detection of liver metastases have demonstrated good diagnostic performance, with a sensitivity of 87% and a specificity of 90%, comparable to CE-MRI, but diagnostic accuracy can be increased if DWI is combined with CE-MRI (Wu et al. 2013). A recent meta-analysis showed that the combination of gadoxetic acid-enhanced MRI and DWI is superior to gadoxetic acid–enhanced MRI or DWI alone. The combination of both techniques reaches a sensitivity of 95% for the detection of metastases (Vilgrain et al. 2016a).

A drawback of dynamic contrast-enhanced acquisitions is the presence of motion artifacts in patients who have difficulty holding their breath. Yoon et al. have studied the image quality of respiratory-triggered 3D T1W-GRE sequences compared to standard breath-hold T1W-GRE for hepatobiliary phase imaging. In noncooperative patients, respiratory-triggered 3D T1W-GRE imaging showed better image quality, with better diagnostic performance (Yoon et al. 2015). This was also true for patients with sufficient breath-holding capacities.

Routine T2-weighted sequences (TE around 90 ms) show a markedly increased signal intensity of benign lesions, such as cysts and hemangiomas, and a moderately increased signal intensity of malignant lesions. When echo time is increased (TE >160 ms), malignant lesions show less signal intensity and may appear isointense to the liver parenchyma. New quantitative functional imaging parameters have been developed and tested for the investigation of liver lesions. By measuring the hemodynamic response in mice, pathological changes in liver perfusion during CO_2 inhalation demonstrated better sensitivities for small metastases compared to CE-MRI (Edrei et al. 2014).

3.4 Hybrid Imaging

Fluorodeoxyglucose-positron emission tomography (18FDG-PET) combined with CT (PET-CT) includes molecular and metabolic mapping of glucose uptake, combined with the high spatial resolution of CT. In a meta-analysis and systematic review by Maffione (Maffione et al. 2015), FDG PET/CT was less sensitive, but more specific, compared to MRI and CT, with the added advantage of delineating extrahepatic disease. In other studies, PET showed no significant influence on survival if added to the regular diagnostic workup (Moulton et al. 2014); however, PET/CT performed better than other modalities in patients with CRLM (Mainenti et al. 2010). Due to the high cost and additional exposure to radiation, the application of PET/CT is reserved for suspected extrahepatic disease in candidates for liver surgery (Ruers et al. 2009). Possible applications include investigations of patients with an unexplained rise in CEA without identifiable metastatic lesions on conventional CT or MRI (Giacomobono et al. 2013) and metabolic monitoring to assess tumor response (Storto et al. 2009).

Recently, a fully integrated PET/MR imaging system that can acquire complementary anatomic and metabolic information was introduced to oncologic imaging. For the detection of liver metastases, recent studies have evaluated the performance, with results comparable to (Drzezga et al. 2012; Quick et al. 2013), or even better (Kershah et al. 2013) than, PET/CT. No significant difference in diagnostic performance compared to MR with liver-specific contrast medium was found by Lee (Lee et al. 2016), whereas Kirchner et al. reported an increased diagnostic accuracy of liver-specific contrast phase 18F-FDG PET/MRI compared to liver-specific MRI alone or PET/MRI without liver-specific contrast agent (Kirchner et al. 2017). Recent studies have investigated its possible role in assessing enhanced metabolism to show therapeutic response after ablation (Nielsen et al. 2014).

4 Imaging Features

Liver metastases usually present as multifocal lesions, sometimes as a single metastasis or a confluent mass with variable sizes (Silva et al. 2009). Various patterns at sonography and CT/MRI can be observed, which helps to distinguish benign and malign lesions and search for an unknown primary.

4.1 Sonographic Pattern

Most common, metastatic liver lesions are hypoechoic, and less commonly, hyperechoic (from colorectal, renal carcinoma, choriocarcinoma, liposarcoma, Kaposi sarcoma, or neuroendocrine tumors). A peripheral halo sign, also called a target or "bull's eye" sign is common in many metastases and is a concerning feature

(Fig. 2). This sign can help to distinguish a hyperechoic metastasis from benign lesions like hemangiomas (Fig. 3). Additional sonographic patterns include cystic lesions, as seen in patients with squamous cell carcinoma, ovarian, pancreatic, or colorectal cancer, and a calcific or mixed echogenic appearance. Infiltrative, poorly defined

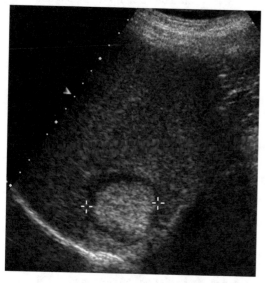

Fig. 2 Hyperechoic metastasis of a liposarcoma in the dorsal part of the right liver lobe. The hypoechoic halo around the lesion is highly suspicious for malignancy ("bull's eye lesion")

metastases are caused by melanoma, breast cancer, or lung cancer. Associated intrahepatic biliary dilation is seen in patients with colorectal carcinoma.

Similar to contrast-enhanced dynamic CT and MRI, different focal liver lesions show quite characteristic enhancement features. Metastases are either hypoechoic or hyperechoic in the arterial phase and usually show washout to hypoechogenicity in the portal venous and the delayed vascular phases (Fig. 4). Contrary to CECT and CEMRI, hypoenhancing metastases on single portal venous phase imaging show a transiently hypervascular enhancement on CEUS due to continuous recording of tumor angiogenesis during the early arterial phase and marked washout during late-phase imaging (Durot et al. 2018). Washout begins early, showing punched-out "black foci" demarcated from the homogeneously enhancing liver parenchyma (Claudon et al. 2013). Additional features include complete enhancement during the arterial phase or nonenhancing intralesional regions. Rare, false-positive results can be observed in small abscesses or necrotic lesions, as well as granulomas or inflammatory pseudotumors (Claudon et al. 2013). Cystic metastases may show vascular flow in thickened cystic walls or solid mural nodules (Larsen 2010).

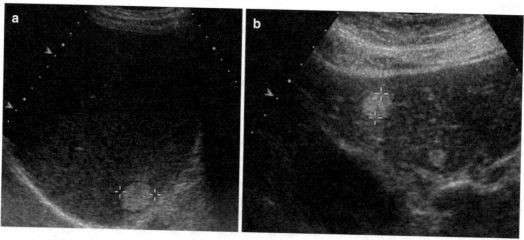

Fig. 3 Differentiation from benign hyperechoic lesion. (**a**) A small hyperechoic metastasis with a very subtle halo sign. The thin dark rim around the lesion helps to distinguish it from a benign hyperechoic lesion, such as a hemangioma (**b**)

CEUS is especially convenient when performing an ultrasound-guided biopsy of liver lesions. Indications for a CEUS-guided biopsy are a target lesion not visible on non-enhanced US (27.2%); improvement of conspicuity of the target (33%); and to choose a non-necrotic area inside the target lesion (39.8%), especially in a previously nondiagnostic cytohistological examination (Fig. 5). The diagnostic accuracy of the technique is 99% (Francica et al. 2017). In case of tumor ablation, CEUS, as a "real-time dynamic assessment method," can be very helpful in monitoring the ablation process (Dietrich et al. 2015), (Fig. 6).

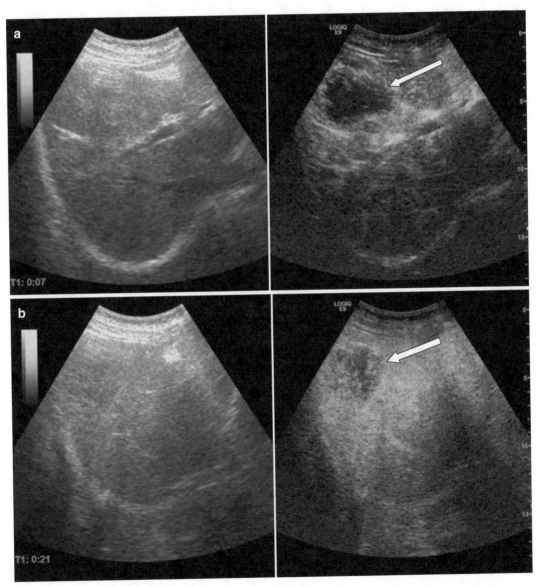

Fig. 4 CEUS of a colorectal liver metastasis shows the enhancement typical for malignancy: (**a**) early arterial phase with rim enhancement (arrow); (**b**) almost complete enhancement of the tumor in the late arterial phase (arrow); and (**c**) washout in the portal venous phase (arrow)

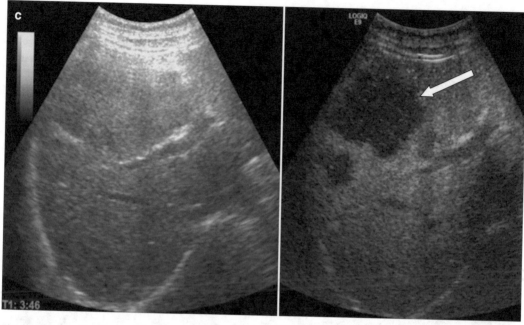

Fig. 4 (continued)

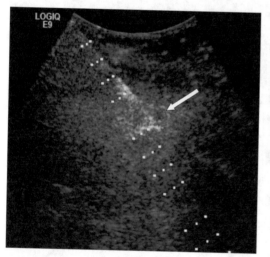

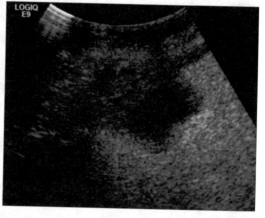

Fig. 5 US-targeted biopsy of a small subcapsular colorectal liver metastases. The metastasis was not visible on unenhanced CT (not shown). CEUS shows a small hypoenhancing lesion for about 2 min in the portal venous phase (arrow). In this time window, the CEUS-guided biopsy can be performed

Fig. 6 CEUS of tumor ablation (RFA) of a small colorectal liver metastasis. Peri-interventional monitoring with CEUS shows a well-circumscribed ablation zone. There are no microbubbles inside the ablation zone, which indicates complete necrosis

4.2 Imaging Pattern on CT and MRI

On precontrast CT, liver metastases are usually hypodense, and hypointense on T1-weighted images, with the exception of melanoma or hemorrhagic metastases, which may be T1-hyperintense (because of the paramagnetic properties of melanin (Fig. 7) and methemoglobin) (Fig. 8). On T2-weighted images, metastases are typically moderately hyperintense (Fig. 9), with very high signal observed in cystic or mucinous metastases (Fig. 10).

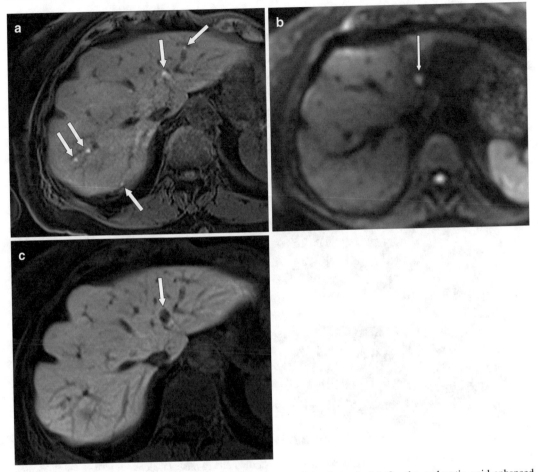

Fig. 7 Hyperintensity on T1: melanin-containing metastases (**a**) Multiple small lesions (arrows), which are hyperintense on the T1w fat-suppressed GRE image. (**b**) DW image (*B* = 400) shows only the larger metastasis in the left lobe (arrow). (**c**) On the gadoxetic acid-enhanced image the larger metastasis is clearly seen (arrow). The small metastases blend in with the enhanced parenchyma and are only faintly seen

Hemorrhagic metastases may show fluid–fluid levels (Fig. 8c). Typically, metastatic lesions are poorly circumscribed. On postcontrast images, small lesions show homogeneous enhancement versus large lesions with heterogeneous contrast uptake, with further various enhancement patterns that can be discriminated:

- *Hypoenhancing metastases:* These demonstrate lesser enhancement than the surrounding liver parenchyma and appear, therefore, hypodense/hypointense on contrast-enhanced images. Most primary tumors that demonstrate this pattern are adenocarcinoma (gastro-intestinal tract), squamous cell cancer, acinar cell cancer (prostate), or transitional cell carcinoma (Fig. 11). Sometimes, hypoenhancing lesions may be visible only in the early enhancing phase as areas of reduced enhancement, with enhancement similar to the liver parenchyma in the delayed phase.

- *Hyperenhancing metastases:* Common primary tumors leading to an enhancement greater than the liver parenchyma in the arterial phase are neuroendocrine tumors, renal cell carcinoma, melanoma, thyroid, and, sometimes, breast cancer (Fig. 12). Although termed hyperenhancing, these lesions may appear isodense or hypodense to the liver

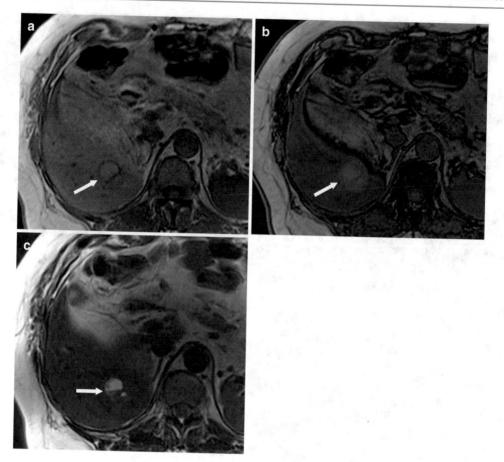

Fig. 8 Hyperintensity on T1: hemorrhagic metastasis in renal cell cancer. (**a**) The lesion shows a bright signal on T1w in-phase (arrow) and (**b**) opposed-phase images (arrow) due to methemoglobin. (**c**) There are fluid–fluid levels on the T2w TSE image (arrow)

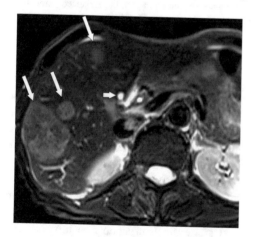

Fig. 9 Moderate hyperintensity on T2. MRI shows mild high signal intensity on transverse fat-suppressed T2-weighted images (arrows) in comparison to a very high signal intensity of a small intrahepatic cystic lesion (short arrow)

parenchyma on arterial and portal venous phases as well, emphasizing the need for multiphase imaging. Often, there is a washout of contrast material to hypointensity/hypodensity in the venous or delayed phase, which facilitates differentiation from a flash-filling hemangioma (which would display contrast pooling).

- *Cystic/necrotic metastases:* A minority of liver metastases may show a cystic pattern, with the risk of misinterpretation as more common benign lesions. Two different pathological mechanisms can be found (Mortele and Ros 2001): rarely, gastrointestinal stromal tumors and cancer of the ovary may result in cystic hepatic metastases (Fig. 13). More often, central cystic degeneration and

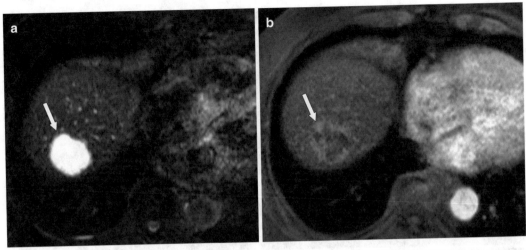

Fig. 10 Marked hyperintensity on T2: mucinous metastasis. (**a**) T2-weighted fat-suppressed image of a mucinous tumor (arrow) may approach the T2 signal intensity of a hemangioma. (**b**) However, thick irregular enhancement during the arterial phase (arrow) is suspicious of malignancy

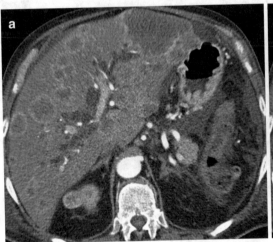
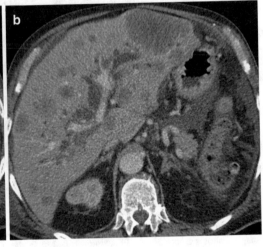

Fig. 11 Hypoenhancing metastases. (**a**) CT imaging in the arterial phase shows multiple hypodense metastases from an adenocarcinoma of the GI tract with less enhancement than the surrounding liver parenchyma and a thin rim enhancement. (**b**) During portal venous phase, lesions remain hypodense to normal hepatic tissue

necrosis are caused by a rapid growth in hypervascular metastases (Fig. 14). This increased growth in relation to the lesion's blood supply can be found in metastases of neuroendocrine tumors, melanoma, GIST, and certain subtypes of lung and breast cancer. Knowing the primary tumor and the clinical history, with rim enhancement on imaging, indistinct margins in the interstitial phase, size reduction, and multiple occurrences, can facilitate correct diagnosis.

Secondary cystic changes can also be seen after treatment, complicating the differentiation between active and inactive metastases. A PET scan can be used to show an increased FDG uptake and to enable differentiation between cystic metastases and benign hepatic lesions.

- *Peripherally enhancing metastases:* In the early phase after intravenous contrast administration, peripheral early enhancement with or without subsequent centripetal filling

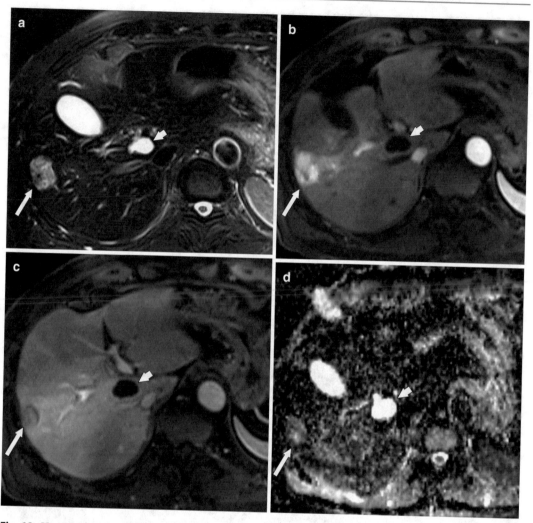

Fig. 12 Hyperenhancing metastases. (**a**) In this patient with a neuroendocrine tumor, T2-weighted fat-suppressed imaging shows a moderately hyperintense lesion in the right hepatic lobe (arrow) and a small markedly hyperintense lesion (short arrow). (**b**) After administration of gadolinium, marked uptake of contrast material can be seen within the metastasis (arrow) as opposed to the liver cyst (short arrow). (**c**) Portal venous phase shows a significant washout of contrast material in the metastatic lesion (arrow). (**d**) ADC helps in differentiating both lesions with decreased signal on ADC map of the metastasis (arrow), consistent with restricted diffusion, and high signal in the cyst due to a T2-shine through effect (short arrow)

in the delayed phase can be observed in hyper- and hypovascular metastases, a highly positive predictive finding for malignancy (Fig. 15). Studies have shown a histopathologic correlation with a thick tumor border containing a peritumoral desmoplastic reaction and compact tumor cells in the periphery of the metastases (Danet et al. 2003). This sign (also called the "halo" sign) must be distinguished from parenchymal enhancement around the lesion due to inflammatory cell infiltration or arterio-portal shunting in the compressed liver parenchyma, also seen in benign lesions, such as hemangiomas (Semelka et al. 2000).

- *Calcified metastases:* Eleven percent of liver metastases are calcified at initial presentation, most often as fine calcifications with a variable distribution (Hale et al. 1998). During chemotherapy, central calcifications may develop or

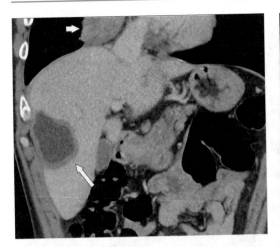

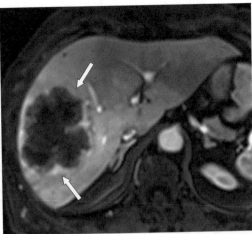

Fig. 13 Cystic metastases. In a patient with lung cancer (right lower lobe, short arrow), a thick-walled cystic metastasis (arrow) could be confused with an abscess. However, there are no signs of perifocal edema and the patient did not show clinical signs of sepsis

Fig. 15 Peripherally enhancing metastases. MRI imaging in a patient with renal cell cancer in the arterial phase after administration of gadolinium shows a large metastatic lesion with early peripheral rim enhancement (arrows), also called "halo sign," caused by the avid vascularized outer periphery of the metastasis

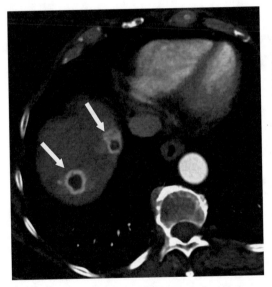

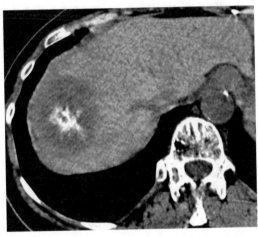

Fig. 16 Value of unenhanced CT for detecting calcified metastases. The unenhanced CT scan in this patient with colorectal cancer clearly shows a centrally hyperattenuating portion of the metastasis due to calcification

Fig. 14 Central necrosis. CT in the arterial phase shows two metastatic lesions in a patient with renal cell cancer in the superior aspect of the right lobe of the liver with avid peripheral rim enhancement and central hypodense attenuation due to necrosis (arrows)

change, without any prognostic correlation (Fig. 16).

- *Hemorrhagic metastases:* Hepatic metastases from pulmonary, renal, testicular, or melanoma primaries are the most frequent types that cause hepatic bleeding and show hyperintense

signal intensities on T1-weighted imaging (Fig. 8a). Hemoperitoneum has been reported in very few case reports (Casillas et al. 2000).

- *Fat-containing metastases:* These are uncommon and can be found in patients with a liposarcoma and a malignant germ cell tumor as primary. Although clear-cell renal cell carcinoma is the most likely fat-containing

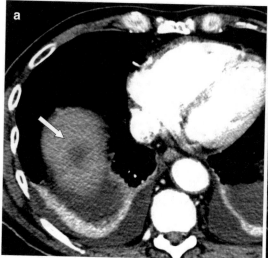

Fig. 17 Doughnut sign. (**a**) CT imaging in a patient with bronchial carcinoma in the arterial phase showing a hypodense round lesion in the right liver lobe (arrow) with a low signal intensity rim around a more hypodense center. (**b**) This "doughnut sign" is better depicted on portal venous phase imaging (arrow)

primary malignancy with liver metastases, fat is seldom proven on chemical-shift MRI in clear-cell RCC metastases (Costa et al. 2018). The visualization of intratumoral fat deposition in colorectal liver metastases has also been described by Nakai et al. 2018) in more than 50% of patients after chemotherapy on dual-echo GRE MR imaging and was an independent predictor of unfavorable overall survival in their study (Nakai et al. 2018).

- *"Doughnut" sign:* This sign shows a low-signal intensity rim around an irregular center of even lower signal intensity on T1-weighted imaging in some liver metastases (Fig. 17) (Wittenberg et al. 1988).

- *"Target" sign:* Lesions from breast carcinoma and gastrointestinal adenocarcinoma may demonstrate a peripheral rim enhancement with an inner ring of enhancement that simulates a target pattern on arterial and early portal venous phase imaging (Fig. 18).

- *"Peripheral washout" sign:* This is the same as the peripheral low-density/intensity area sign. It is seen in hyper- and hypovascular metastases during the portal venous phase and equilibrium phase (Fig. 19). The sign is defined by an enhancing liver lesion and a

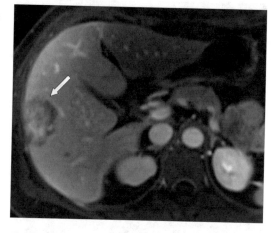

Fig. 18 Target sign. MR imaging in this patient with breast cancer in the portal venous phase after administration of gadolinium shows a lesion with a triple-layered appearance: a thin peripheral rim enhancement, a dark middle ring, and a bright center due to contrast uptake in the central fibrosis, mimicking a target pattern (arrow)

peripheral hypodense/hypointense rim, caused by the growing peripheral tumor margin and the center-containing necrotic areas. The sign is associated with malignancy, with a sensitivity of 24.5% and a specificity of 100%, but also includes other malignant hepatic lesions, such as hepato-

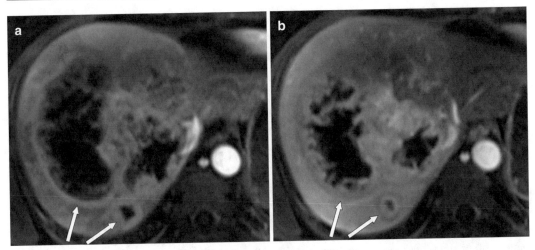

Fig. 19 Peripheral washout sign. (**a**) Axial T1-weighted MR image in the arterial phase after gadolinium administration shows hypoattenuating lesions with thick irregular peripheral enhancement (arrows). (**b**) In the equilibrium phase, there is washout of contrast in the periphery of the vital tumor, which results in a dark outer rim (arrows), indicating malignancy in this patient with breast cancer

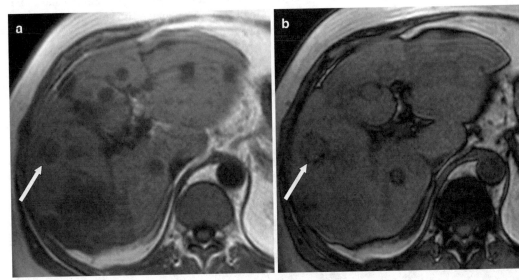

Fig. 20 Metastases of insulinoma. (**a**) T1-weighted unenhanced in-phase imaging shows multiple hypointense liver lesions (arrow). (**b**) Some of them show a peripheral signal loss on opposed-phase imaging due to a perilesional fat deposition caused by local insulin production (arrow)

cellular carcinoma and cholangiocarcinoma (Mahfouz et al. 1994).

A perilesional fat deposition with a bright signal on T1-weighted imaging can occasionally be found in metastases from pancreatic insulinoma caused by local insulin production as an inhibitor of fatty acid oxidation and accumulation of lipid in hepatocytes adjacent to the metastasis (Sohn et al. 2001), or, in lesions that occlude the segmental portal or hepatic venous blood flow (Fig. 20). A pseudocapsule is not found in metastases, which is helpful for the discrimination from hepatocellular carcinoma.

4.3 Treated Metastases

After beginning chemotherapy, there is a less aggressive enhancement of hypervascular liver metastases that mimics hemangiomas. This is due to therapy-associated antiangiogenesis with altered vascularity, which results in early peripheral enhancement and retention of contrast material on a 10-min delayed phase due to an enlarged extracellular space or decreased venous drainage (Semelka et al. 1999). In contrast to a discontinuous enhancement rim of hemangiomas, treated metastases show an early, intact peripheral enhancement. A hypointense pattern of surrounding liver parenchyma in the hepatobiliary phase, also called focal hepatopathy, has been reported by Han et al. (2014) as a potential pitfall of liver-specific contrast agents in patients who received oxaliplatin as part of their chemotherapy regimen. Specifically, in these patients, due to the sinusoidal obstruction syndrome, the morphologic pattern of the focal hepatopathy at the hepatobiliary phase with ill-defined margins may help to avoid this potential pitfall (Han et al. 2014).

Calcification of colorectal metastases (Fig. 16) can also be found in patients enrolled in chemotherapeutic therapy regimens. The presence of calcification has been correlated to an improved survival, as stated by Easson et al. (Easson et al. 1996). Abscess formation (Fig. 21) is an unusual complication after hepatic transarterial chemoembolization with a reported frequency of up to 2% of procedures (Kim et al. 2001). In patients with bilioenteric anastomosis, retrograde colonization with intestinal flora may lead to biliary necrosis after chemoembolization.

4.3.1 The Disappearing Metastasis after Preoperative Chemotherapy

"Disappearing liver metastases," which mimic a complete response after neoadjuvant chemotherapy, may cause a mismatch between the radiological diagnosis and the true histologic response. Since only a very small percentage of patients have a complete response of all liver metastases on imaging, surgery remains an important therapeutic tool (Kuhlmann et al. 2016). But, as shown in a study by Benoist et al., the majority of disap-

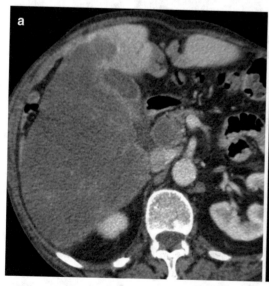
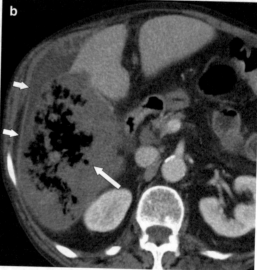

Fig. 21 Abscess formation. (**a**) Patient with large colorectal metastases in the right liver lobe diagnosed on CT at portal venous phase. (**b**) After chemotherapy, CT demonstrates air within the shrinking metastases, consistent with intralesional abscess formation (arrow) with inflammatory enhancement of the peritoneum and perihepatic fluid collection (short arrows)

pearing liver metastases (up to 83%), as assessed by CT, showed viable tumor cells by histopathology or recurrence in situ (Benoist et al. 2006). Factors that lead to underestimation on imaging include reduced uptake of contrast media of ill-defined and very small lesions, increasing intralesional fat content, and reduced attenuation difference between the liver parenchyma and metastases on CT after chemotherapy (Park et al. 2017). MRI with hepatobiliary contrast agents appears to be the most appropriate imaging method (van Kessel et al. 2012) compared to the

more false-positive complete imaging responses reported with CT and PET-CT (Auer et al. 2010). Disappearing colorectal liver metastases on gadoxetic acid-enhanced liver MRI and DWI show low recurrence rates, except in patients with reticular hypointensity of the liver parenchyma on hepatobiliary phase imaging, indicative of chemotherapy-induced sinusoidal obstruction syndrome, and warranting special care during follow-up (Kim et al. 2017), (Fig. 22).

Other predictive factors for a true complete response are the use of hepatic arterial infusion

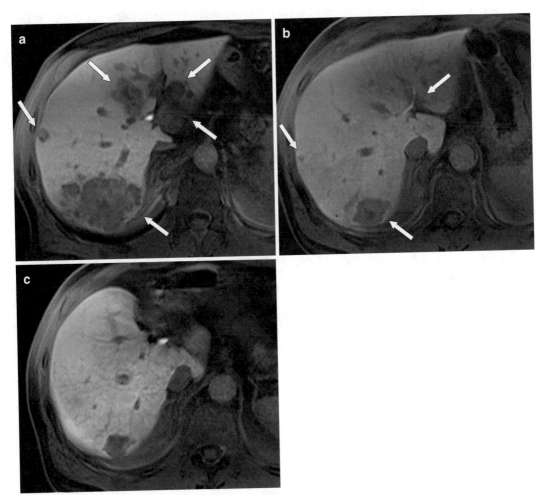

Fig. 22 Disappearing metastases after chemotherapy in a patient with colorectal cancer. (**a**) Gadoxetic acid–enhanced staging MRI shows multiple hypointense metastases (arrows). (**b**) After chemotherapy there is considerable shrinkage of metastases (arrows). Patients were scheduled for two-staged liver surgery, with left hepatectomy first, followed by atypical resection of right-sided metastases. (**c**) Follow-up after left hepatectomy shows further size reduction of lesion in S7, the small metastasis in S8 has disappeared

chemotherapy and normalization of serum carcinoembryonic antigen levels, as shown by Auer et al. (2010). After local or systemic therapy, a slight increase in size may be misinterpreted as tumor progression, even though it is caused by an early response to antiangiogenic treatment, also called "pseudo-progression." This increase in size at CT is combined with a reduction of attenuation due to edema within the lesion and decreasing tumor markers (Chung et al. 2012).

5 Algorithms for Imaging

Multiphasic CT or MR imaging should be the preferred diagnostic tests, depending on the clinical setting (such as follow-up examination or presurgical planning). The choice of these tests can vary depending on local radiological expertise and available equipment. In addition, patient-related factors, such as renal function, known contrast allergy, cardiac pacemakers, and others affect the choice of imaging modality. A meta-analysis comparing the diagnostic performance values of CT, MR, FDG-PET, and FDG PET/CT in studies published between 1990 and 2010 showed that MRI should be the first-line investigation method for the detection of hepatic metastases (Niekel et al. 2010).

The detection of lesions smaller than 1 cm at CT, in particular, has a lower sensitivity compared to MRI with hepatocyte-specific contrast medium (Scharitzer et al. 2013). This was confirmed in a meta-analysis by Vreugdenburg et al. (2016), which showed higher sensitivities for gadoxetic acid-enhanced MRI compared to CECT for the detection of liver metastases, especially for lesions smaller than 10 mm (sensitivity ratio 2.21), with a decrease in specificity (specificity ratio 0.92). The International Hepato-Pancreato-Biliary Association (IHPBA) stated in their consensus that MRI, using gadoxetic acid and DWI imaging, have the best performance characteristics for the evaluation of liver metastases, especially for small lesions and preexisting steatosis (Adams et al. 2013), which was subsequently confirmed by a large meta-analysis by Vilgrain (Vilgrain et al. 2016a).

The direct relationship between the incidence of hepatic metastases and the histological type and stage of the primary tumor should be considered when planning the type of diagnostic test. According to the ACR Appropriateness Criteria® (Expert Panel on Gastrointestinal Imaging 2017), the appropriateness of imaging depends on specific clinical scenarios:

Initial imaging test following newly diagnosed primary tumor

Consensus recommendations of the Expert Group of OncoSurgery Management of Liver Metastases agree that an initial CT should be performed, including injection of iodine contrast for primary staging (Adams et al. 2015). Contrast-enhanced CT phases should include an arterial and venous phase for the initial examination in patients with or suspicion of liver metastases, which will also enable an evaluation of extrahepatic disease. But, CECT may miss up to 25% of liver metastases, especially in patients with hepatic steatosis (Berger-Kulemann et al. 2012). Multiparametric MRI, including DWI and hepatobiliary-phase imaging, is an excellent modality for the assessment of liver metastases, but is limited by scan time, susceptibility to motion artifacts, economic factors, and availability. Han et al. tested the additional impact of liver MRI in newly diagnosed patients with colorectal cancer by dividing three groups according to CT results and concluded that MRI is beneficial for patients with suspicious or not-too-small-to-characterize indeterminate lesions, but adds no benefit for patients with diminutive lesions or patients with no metastases found at CT (Han et al. 2015). Regardless of the technique, a high-quality baseline investigation should be performed before any chemotherapeutic treatment is started since lesions can be more easily detected before treatment.

The sensitivities for ultrasonographic detection of metastases are reportedly low and variable, with sensitivities ranging from 50 to 76% (Cantisani et al. 2014), thus limiting its use as a staging modality. Recommendations of recent international guidelines for the use of CEUS include: (1) characterization of indeterminate lesions at MRI/CT; (2) as an alternative when CT and MRI contrast are contraindicated; and (3) surveillance of oncological patients if CEUS has been useful before (Claudon et al. 2013). FDG-PET/CT is recommended as an initial staging method for several primary tumors, such as lung, esophageal, head and neck cancer, or lymphoma. For the assessment of malignant disease that commonly spreads to the liver, the role of CEUS has not yet been established (Brush et al. 2011).

Assessment before surgery: the incremental value of MRI

Since unnecessary hepatectomies should be avoided, a combined diagnostic approach that includes CT and multiparametric liver MRI is generally optimal. The ESMO consensus guidelines favor MRI with a hepatobiliary contrast agent to identify resectable/unresectable disease, especially for lesions <10 mm (Van Cutsem et al. 2016). This was confirmed in a study by Ko et al., which showed an overall sensitivity of preoperative CT imaging of 8% for a nodule size of 1–5 mm and a sensitivity of 23.5% for a nodule size of 6–10 mm (Ko et al. 2017). When comparing patients with synchronous colorectal liver metastases, who were undergoing preoperative CT only, to patients with an additional MRI, a significantly higher 5-year survival rate was found in the group who underwent both (Kim et al. 2018). The use of gadoxetic acid-enhanced MRI decreased the need for further imaging studies, increased confidence in the diagnosis, and altered surgical plans in a significant number of patients in the preoperative setting, because MRI showed additional metastases in 21–30% of patients (Kim et al. 2015) (Fig. 23).

CE-CT and CE-MRI angiography have shown similar results for the assessment of vascular anatomy before surgery (Sahani et al. 2004), although CT has some advantages, such as rapid acquisition, less susceptibility to motion artifacts, and thin collimation. If synchronous liver metastases are initially resectable, liver MRI can be performed according to availability and local expertise. The role of PET-CT, when added to

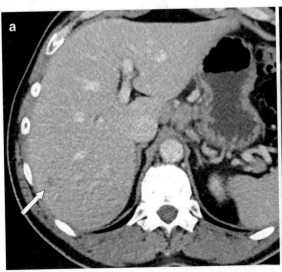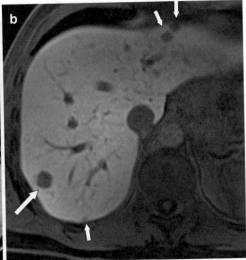

Fig. 23 Incremental value of MRI. (**a**) Portal venous phase CT shows only one lesion (arrow), suspicious of hepatic metastasis in this patient with colorectal cancer. (**b**) Gadoxetic acid-enhanced MRI (T1-weighted VIBE, hepatobiliary phase) shows another three subcapsular lesions of non-hepatocellular origin that could be assigned with high confidence (short arrows)

cross-sectional imaging, has to be further assessed, although it is helpful for the assessment of extrahepatic disease (Adams et al. 2015). Intraoperative ultrasound combined with surgical exploration is the method of choice. This was shown in a systematic review by Ellebæk and colleagues, who reported a detection rate of 32–57% additional liver metastases compared to preoperative imaging modalities, especially for liver metastases <10 mm in diameter (Ellebæk et al. 2017).

Surveillance following treatment of primary tumor

Intervals for surveillance imaging depend on individual risk factors and the therapeutic possibilities to find a curable recurrence as soon as possible. CT is commonly recommended as a standardized screening tool after therapy of the primary malignancy since liver metastases are not the only clinical question for surveillance. Nevertheless, whole-body MRI may represent a valid alternative, with the benefit of no radiation. After chemotherapy, CE-MRI should be the preferred method over CT and PET/CT, because chemotherapy-induced liver steatosis reduces liver-to-lesion contrast on CT. In general, for follow-up, identical CT examination protocols, as well as comparable MR sequences, timing, and contrast agents, should ideally be used, and measurements should be made on the same sequence for each time point.

Patients with severe steatosis

In cases of severe steatosis already visible on CT, an additionally performed MRI should be considered, even if no suspect lesions are detected on CT. When comparing the diagnostic value of gadoxetic acid-enhanced MRI at 3 T with 64-row MDCT in the detection of colorectal liver metastases in diffuse fatty infiltration of the liver, MRI was significantly superior to MDCT in detecting metastases ≤1 cm (detection rate of 93% compared to 42% by MDCT) (Berger-Kulemann et al. 2012). The addition of fat suppression to

T2-weighted images and the use of diffusion-weighted images are very important since small lesions can easily be missed due to the relatively increased signal intensity of the liver parenchyma (Fig. 24).

Indeterminate liver lesions on CT

For the differentiation of indeterminate liver lesions on CT, the use of different MR contrast agents should depend on the primary clinical question: when distinguishing between small hemangiomas versus metastases, the use of a nonspecific (extracellular) MR contrast agent is recommended. When the differential diagnosis is primarily either a solid benign lesion or metastasis, liver-specific contrast agents should be used, due to the ability to diagnose FNH with high confidence (Neri et al. 2016).

Lesions too small to characterize (TSTC)

Small hepatic lesions (≤15 mm) can be found in a large number of patients undergoing abdominal CT (17%), more than 80% of them with an underlying malignant disease (Jones et al. 1992). But, even in these patients, these lesions are highly likely to be benign. In 93–97% of women with breast cancer, TSTC hepatic lesions at initial CT presented as benign findings (Khalil et al. 2005). In a study of patients with gastric and colorectal cancer, 25.5% had TSTC lesions (Jang et al. 2002). Diagnostic clues for a malignant classification were the synchronous finding of larger metastases, indistinct margins, and higher intralesional attenuation. In addition, the percentage of malignancy largely depends on the known primary tumor, with the highest probabilities in patients with breast cancer (Schwartz et al. 1999). This is in accordance with the fact that primary tumors, such as colorectal cancer and lymphoma, have a tendency to cause solitary or a few larger hepatic metastases. Thus, in patients with a known malignancy, a single TSTC lesion can be assumed to be benign. In multiple TSTCs, the risk of malignancy is low, especially if lesions are sharply defined and hypodense.

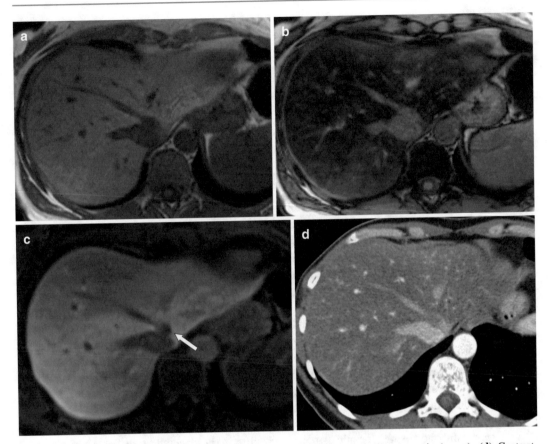

Fig. 24 Liver metastases in hepatic steatosis. T1-weighted in-phase (**a**) and opposed phase (**b**) GRE images demonstrate a significant signal intensity loss of liver background in the opposed phase due to marked fat content of the liver parenchyma. (**c**) Gadoxetic acid-enhanced T1-weighted GRE imaging in the hepatobiliary phase shows a small metastasis (arrow). (**d**) Contrast-enhanced MDCT in the portal venous phase performed on the same day for pulmonary staging does not show the liver metastasis due to the marked hypoattenuation of the liver parenchyma

6 Preoperative Assessment

A surgical approach is the leading treatment for a curative attempt in patients with hepatic metastases. The criteria for anatomic operability are continuously evolving, since modern multidisciplinary decisions are predominantly based on the fact that the tumors can be resected completely (R0) while maintaining enough functioning residual liver volume (Mattar et al. 2016). The selection criteria for chemotherapy and surgery are continuously expanding and the combination of chemotherapy and biological agents has been increasingly used for conversion from an unresectable to a resectable situation (Fiorentini et al. 2017). In addition to patient factors, such as med-ical comorbidity, tumor factors, including biology of the tumor, as well as anatomic factors, are crucial for operability. However, no international guidelines have been published about preoperative imaging, although meta-analyses and reviews have been found (Mainenti et al. 2015, Matos et al. 2015, van Kessel et al. 2012). Several scores have tried to develop predictive factors for optimal patient selection for surgery. Thus, no single scoring system has shown excellent predictive results, and should, therefore, not replace individual patient selection. Optimal management should be tailored to each patient and decided by a multidisciplinary team that consists of different disciplines, such as oncology, surgery, radiology, and radiotherapy.

Radiological preoperative assessment in candidates for surgery includes an exact definition of number, size (in mm) of the largest metastases, and the location of hepatic metastases. In addition, specification about the location of metastases in relation to the main portal veins and hepatic veins should be included to facilitate decisions about the technical resectability and the type of operation method. Although nomenclatures concerning hepatic territories remain heterogeneous and the portal venous branching pattern includes more branches than generally assumed, the well-established Couinaud system is commonly used as the most surgically relevant anatomic classification system (Fasel and Schenk 2013). Unaffected segments should be mentioned in the report, which is important information for surgical planning.

The viability of the remaining liver after individual resection depends on adequate inflow (hepatic arteries and portal vein) and hepatic outflow (hepatic veins and bile ducts), assessable by CT and MRI. Any observed anatomical variants should be noted in the report since detailed knowledge of liver angioarchitecture is crucial to ensure successful and safe hepatic surgery. Radiological signs of portal hypertension, such as splenomegaly or abdominal varices, should be reported due to the increased risk of perioperative coagulopathy and hemorrhage in patients with portal hypertension. The functional capacity of the remaining liver, as well as the surgical outcome, are directly related to its volume. In normal liver parenchyma, the future liver remnant should be at least 20–25% to avoid liver failure, which is the most common cause of perioperative mortality. However, in diseased liver parenchyma, the liver remnant percentage should be at least 40% (Pawlik et al. 2004). Three-dimensional CT volumetry can be used to estimate the remaining liver parenchyma after the proposed resection. Quality of liver parenchyma (e.g., cirrhosis, steatosis, etc.) is another relevant factor for postoperative morbidity. To assess chronic liver disease, MR imaging with diffusion-weighted imaging, the use of hepatobiliary contrast, MR perfusion, and MR elastography is a promising method for the noninvasive grading of fibrosis and chronic damage to the liver parenchyma of the individual patient. Moreover, variants of vascular structures, such as hepatic arteries, the portal venous system, and the biliary tree, have to be described to prevent unexpected surgical complications (Catalano et al. 2008).

7 Post-Therapeutic Assessment and Prognostic Factors

The detection of the therapeutic effects of systemic and local therapies at an early stage is relevant to stop inappropriate therapeutic regimens, to avoid unnecessary side effects, and to initiate alternative treatment methods. Radiological measurements are important to objectively prove the early effectiveness of anticancer therapy. In addition to the comparison of existing lesions regarding size, a visible residual tumor within or immediately adjacent to the ablation zone within a time interval of 6 months after ablation is suggestive of local tumor progression.

The Response Evaluation Criteria in Solid Tumors (RECIST) provide simplified standardized criteria depending on mono-dimensional change in tumor size, i.e., the sum of the longest tumor diameters (Eisenhauer et al. 2009). But, although a change in size is a key indicator of treatment response, a lack of association between outcome and radiological response based on the RECIST criteria has been observed, which has led to a search for alternative parameters. Especially in patients treated with a regimen that includes biological agents, such as antiangiogenic monoclonal antibodies, the comparison of size is a poor predictor for prognosis, compared to other parameters. Morphological, but non-size-based criteria, have been developed at the MD Anderson Cancer Center (Chun et al. 2009) to predict response and survival after chemotherapy. Since tumor response in CRLM is based on fibrous replacement and not tumor necrosis (Rubbia-Brandt et al. 2007), these authors showed a better correlation to clinical outcome when using morphological changes based on tumor attenuation and normal liver–tumor interface analysis. They achieved this by differentiating lesions into three groups, one with homogenous attenuation and thin, well-defined edges, one with heterogeneous attenuation with thick, poorly defined edges, and a third group with not-assignable lesions. Optimal therapeutic response included a change from heterogeneous, poorly defined to homogeneous, well-defined lesions (Chun et al. 2009).

Two other methods of categorizing the morphological changes of liver metastases are early tumor shrinkage, defined as a ≥20% decrease in size from baseline to first restaging, and depth of response, defined as the percentage of shrinkage observed at the nadir size compared with baseline (Mazard et al. 2018). This was supported by a recent study that showed a significant correlation between increased attenuation of colorectal liver metastases in baseline portal–venous phase CT when defining a threshold of ≥61.62 HU, early tumor shrinkage, and increased depth of response, with prolonged overall survival (Froelich et al. 2018).

Therefore, alternative morphological criteria for changes in size of hepatic metastases should be considered as an early marker of treatment efficacy in addition to the preexisting RECIST criteria.

In addition to changes in tumor size and morphologic changes unrelated to size, additional functional parameters are useful for the assessment of early therapeutic effectiveness. Angiogenesis with intralesional blood flow and mean vessel density, in particular, has been shown to correlate with tumoral invasive potential (Meyers and Watson 2003). Kannan et al. demonstrated that MRI biomarkers of vascular function, such as the volume transfer constant or the initial area-under-the-curve of contrast uptake up to the first 90 s after injection, reflect vessel morphology depending on vascularity and anti-angiogenic therapy (Kannan et al. 2018). Treatment-related changes in tumor perfusion can also be assessed by CEUS, and arterial perfusion of liver metastases is better reflected by low-mechanical index CEUS than by CECT (Krix 2005). In addition, changes in liver hemodynamics, with an increase of arterial blood flow and a decrease of portal venous flow, may indicate occult liver metastases or predict the development of metastases, as first described by Breedis

(Breedis and Young 1954). Attempts have been made to show this change in perfusion index by ultrasound (Kopljar et al. 2014) and DCE-MRI (De Bruyne et al. 2012).

With regard to the value of hybrid imaging for the follow-up of liver metastases, a meta-analysis comparing 18F-FDG PET/CT and CT for the detection of disease progression after ablation therapy showed a higher sensitivity of PET/CT compared to CT and a specificity and diagnostic accuracy comparable to MR (Samim et al. 2017). Initial results have shown a significant relationship between the degree of FDG uptake on PET-MR images and recurrence-free survival.

8 Pitfalls in Imaging of Liver Metastases

- Most hepatic *arterial hyperenhancing lesions* are hepatocellular carcinomas or benign lesions, such as focal nodular hyperplasia, adenoma, or nodular regenerative hyperplasia. Other differential diagnoses for hypervascular metastases include hepatic arterioportal shunts due to communication between the small hepatic artery and the portal vein branches. Clues to a correct diagnosis include the peripheral localization and wedge-shaped configuration, the normal vascularization on portal venous- or delayed-phase imaging, and no abnormal signal intensity on nonenhanced imaging. In atypical cases, gadoxetic acid–enhanced MRI may help in the differential diagnosis, because arterioportal shunts will show a normal uptake of liver-specific contrast in the hepatobiliary phase (Motosugi et al. 2010).
- *Discrimination between intrahepatic and extrahepatic lesions*: Especially in patients with gynecologic malignancies, peritoneal carcinomatous seeding as soft-attenuating plaques or masses may mimic hepatic disease. Ascites, peritoneal implants in other locations, a distinctly distinguishable lesion-liver interface, and a small fatty layer can help in the exact local assignment of lesions.
- *Pseudolesions around the falciform ligament*: These small hypodense or hypointense lesions are typically found in segment IV in up to

20% of patients (Genchellac et al. 2007) (Fig. 25). Although their development has been attributed to the local accumulation of fat, pseudolesions probably evolve due to anomalous venous drainage, such as an inferior vein of Sappey (Genchellac et al. 2007). The distinction of a peritoneal metastatic lesion within the falciform ligament may be a diagnostic challenge (Fig. 26).

• *Pseudolesions in the posterior part of segment IV* may be due to focal fatty sparing or focal deposits of fat. Recent studies suggest the "insulin theory" as a cause for these pseudolesions. Reportedly, aberrant gastric veins with low insulin concentration may drain directly into segment IV, which results in focal fatty sparing; however, aberrant duodenopancreatic collaterals with high insulin concentrations result in focal fatty steatosis (Vilgrain et al. 2016b), possibly mimicking malignant hepatic lesions. Further workup with MRI, including in-phase and opposed-phase imaging can

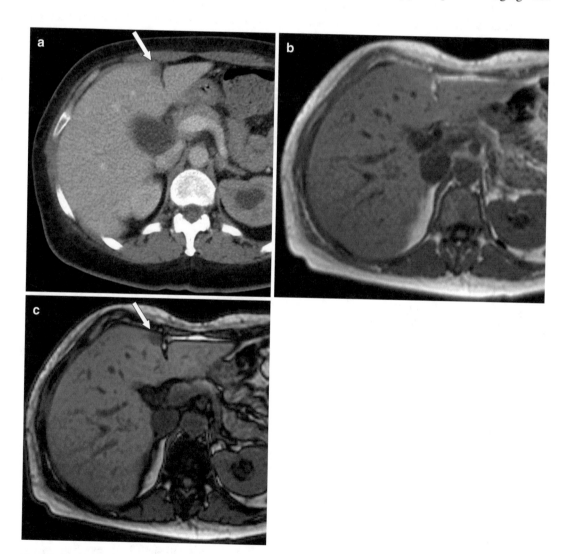

Fig. 25 Pseudolesion around the falciform ligament. (**a**) CT imaging in the portal venous phase shows a small liver lesion (arrow) in segment 4 of the liver in this patient with a gynecological cancer. (**b**) T1-weighted in-phase imaging typically shows no correlate to the CT finding, but (**c**) opposed-phase imaging confirms geographic fatty change of the liver with significant signal drop (arrow) in the typical location along the falciform ligament

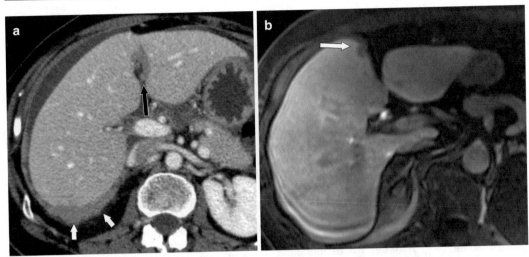

Fig. 26 Differentiation of peritoneal and hepatic metastases. (**a**) Ovarian cancer patient with peritoneal carcinomatosis (short arrows) and a soft-attenuating plaque-like lesion in the fissure, causing indentation of liver parenchyma, indicative of capsular implant (arrow). Clues to the diagnosis are preservation of the liver–lesion border, presence of other peritoneal implants and ascites. (**b**) A different patient with a hypointense round lesion in the hepatobiliary phase after gadoxetic-enhanced MR imaging (arrow) in a patient with adenocarcinoma of the GI tract, suggestive of intraparenchymal metastatic disease

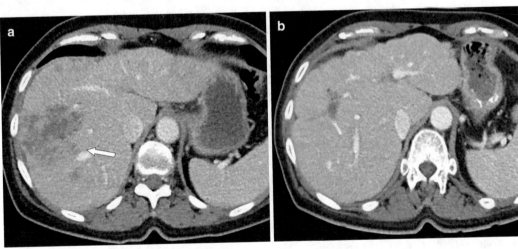

Fig. 27 Pseudocirrhosis. (**a**) Initial staging CT in a patient with breast cancer shows large indistinct metastases in the right lobe (arrow). (**b**) After 6 months of chemotherapy, the lesions have virtually disappeared, but there are fibrotic strands with liver deformation and capsular retraction, mimicking cirrhosis. Pseudocirrhosis is quite common after chemotherapy of breast cancer metastases

detect steatosis with the chemical shift technique.

- *Pseudocirrhosis* (also called "hepar lobatum") is a finding in patients with liver metastases and is characterized by segmental atrophy with enlargement of the caudate lobe and nodular liver surface. Although the exact mechanisms are not known yet, tumor shrinkage with desmoplastic fibrosis around the metastases or nodular regenerative hyperplasia is presumed (Battisti et al. 2014). This type of tumor response is most often found in patients with breast cancer (Fig. 27). Knowledge of prior chemotherapy and regular liver imaging prior to therapy are the clues to correct interpretation and possibility to modify or interrupt therapy.

- *Multiple pseudotumors that mimic metastastic disease*: Rarely, pseudotumoral nodular steatosis is described as multiple lesions in both lobes, which are hypodense during all CT phases and show enhancement parallel to the regular liver parenchyma. A pathognomonic finding is a signal drop on opposed-phase imaging and a fatty rim at the lesion periphery (Vilgrain et al. 2013). Another rare differential diagnosis includes granulomatous liver lesions in tuberculosis, sarcoidosis, and brucellosis, with a military, nodular, or multinodular appearance (Vilgrain et al. 2016b).

9   Conclusion

The absence of well-defined, generally applicable imaging protocols for liver metastases is partly due to the rapidly evolving technological and pharmacological developments that continuously improve radiological imaging. Contrast-enhanced CT is the preferred imaging modality for initial staging and follow-up. MRI provides additional information in indeterminate lesions, in the detection of small lesions, in the presence of hepatic steatosis, or for liver evaluation post chemotherapy. In candidates for surgery, multiparametric MRI adds important morphologic and functional information for optimal patient selection. Hybrid imaging (^{18}F-PET-MRI) may represent a future tool for the assessment of liver metastases and extrahepatic disease as well. A multidisciplinary approach with close collaboration between medical and radiation oncologists, hepatobiliary surgeons, radiologists, pathologists, and nursing staff is mandatory to select optimal surgical candidates and plan individual oncological treatment for patients with liver metastases.

References

Adam R, de Gramont A, Figueras J, Kokudo N, Kunstlinger F, Loyer E, Poston G, Rougier P, Rubbia-Brandt L, Sobrero A, Teh C, Tejpar S, Van Cutsem E, Vauthey J-N, Påhlman L, (2015) Managing synchronous liver metastases from colorectal cancer: A multidisciplinary international consensus. Cancer Treatment Reviews 41(9):729–741

Adams RB, Aloia TA, Loyer E, Pawlik TM, Taouli B, Vauthey JN, Americas Hepato-Pancreato-Biliary A, Society of Surgical O, Society for Surgery of the Alimentary T (2013) Selection for hepatic resection of colorectal liver metastases: expert consensus statement. HPB (Oxford) 15(2):91–103. https://doi.org/10.1111/j.1477-2574.2012.00557.x

Albrecht T, Blomley MJ, Burns PN, Wilson S, Harvey CJ, Leen E, Claudon M, Calliada F, Correas JM, LaFortune M, Campani R, Hoffmann CW, Cosgrove DO, LeFevre F (2003) Improved detection of hepatic metastases with pulse-inversion US during the liver-specific phase of SHU 508A: multicenter study. Radiology 227(2):361–370. https://doi.org/10.1148/radiol.2272011833

Auer RC, White RR, Kemeny NE, Schwartz LH, Shia J, Blumgart LH, Dematteo RP, Fong Y, Jarnagin WR, D'Angelica MI (2010) Predictors of a true complete response among disappearing liver metastases from colorectal cancer after chemotherapy. Cancer 116(6):1502–1509. https://doi.org/10.1002/cncr.24912

Battisti S, Guida FM, Pagliara E, Tonini G, Zobel BB, Santini D (2014) Pseudocirrhosis after anti-EGFR-based neoadjuvant therapy for hepatic metastasis from colon cancer: a different point of view. Clin Colorectal Cancer 13(3):e13–e15. https://doi.org/10.1016/j.clcc.2014.06.003

Benoist S, Brouquet A, Penna C, Julie C, El Hajjam M, Chagnon S, Mitry E, Rougier P, Nordlinger B (2006) Complete response of colorectal liver metastases after chemotherapy: does it mean cure? J Clin Oncol 24(24):3939–3945. https://doi.org/10.1200/JCO.2006.05.8727

Berger-Kulemann V, Schima W, Baroud S, Koelblinger C, Kaczirek K, Gruenberger T, Schindl M, Maresch J, Weber M, Ba-Ssalamah A (2012) Gadoxetic acid-enhanced 3.0 T MR imaging versus multidetector-row CT in the detection of colorectal metastases in fatty liver using intraoperative ultrasound and histopathology as a standard of reference. Eur J Surg Oncol 38(8):670–676. https://doi.org/10.1016/j.ejso.2012.05.004

Bo XW, Xu HX, Guo LH, Sun LP, Li XL, Zhao CK, He YP, Liu BJ, Li DD, Zhang K, Wang D (2017) Ablative safety margin depicted by fusion imaging with post-treatment contrast-enhanced ultrasound and pre-treatment CECT/CEMRI after radiofrequency ablation for liver cancers. Br J Radiol 90(1078):20170063. https://doi.org/10.1259/bjr.20170063

Breedis C, Young G (1954) The blood supply of neoplasms in the liver. Am J Pathol 30(5):969–977

Brush J, Boyd K, Chappell F, Crawford F, Dozier M, Fenwick E, Glanville J, McIntosh H, Renehan A, Weller D, Dunlop M (2011) The value of FDG positron emission tomography/computerised tomography (PET/CT) in pre-operative staging of colorectal cancer: a systematic review and economic evaluation. Health Technol Assess 15(35):1–192., iii-iv. https://doi.org/10.3310/hta15350

Buls N, Van Gompel G, Van Cauteren T, Nieboer K, Willekens I, Verfaillie G, Evans P, Macholl S, Newton B, de Mey J (2015) Contrast agent and radiation dose reduction in abdominal CT by a combination of low tube voltage and advanced image reconstruction algorithms. Eur Radiol 25(4):1023–1031. https://doi.org/10.1007/s00330-014-3510-5

Cantisani V, Grazhdani H, Fioravanti C, Rosignuolo M, Calliada F, Messineo D, Bernieri MG, Redler A, Catalano C, D'Ambrosio F (2014) Liver metastases: contrast-enhanced ultrasound compared with computed tomography and magnetic resonance. World J Gastroenterol 20(29):9998–10007. https://doi.org/10.3748/wjg.v20.i29.9998

Casillas VJ, Amendola MA, Gascue A, Pinnar N, Levi JU, Perez JM (2000) Imaging of nontraumatic hemorrhagic hepatic lesions. Radiographics 20(2):367–378. https://doi.org/10.1148/radiographics.20.2.g00mc10367

Catalano OA, Singh AH, Uppot RN, Hahn PF, Ferrone CR, Sahani DV (2008) Vascular and biliary variants in the liver: implications for liver surgery. Radiographics 28(2):359–378. https://doi.org/10.1148/rg.282075099

Chun YS, Vauthey JN, Boonsirikamchai P, Maru DM, Kopetz S, Palavecino M, Curley SA, Abdalla EK, Kaur H, Charnsangavej C, Loyer EM (2009) Association of computed tomography morphologic criteria with pathologic response and survival in patients treated with bevacizumab for colorectal liver metastases. JAMA 302(21):2338–2344. https://doi.org/10.1001/jama.2009.1755

Chung WS, Park MS, Shin SJ, Baek SE, Kim YE, Choi JY, Kim MJ (2012) Response evaluation in patients with colorectal liver metastases: RECIST version 1.1 versus modified CT criteria. AJR Am J Roentgenol 199(4):809–815. https://doi.org/10.2214/AJR.11.7910

Claudon M, Dietrich CF, Choi BI, Cosgrove DO, Kudo M, Nolsoe CP, Piscaglia F, Wilson SR, Barr RG, Chammas MC, Chaubal NG, Chen MH, Clevert DA, Correas JM, Ding H, Forsberg F, Fowlkes JB, Gibson RN, Goldberg BB, Lassau N, Leen EL, Mattrey RF, Moriyasu F, Solbiati L, Weskott HP, Xu HX, World Federation for Ultrasound in M, European Federation of Societies for U (2013) Guidelines and good clinical practice recommendations for Contrast Enhanced Ultrasound (CEUS) in the liver - update 2012: a WFUMB-EFSUMB initiative in cooperation with representatives of AFSUMB, AIUM, ASUM, FLAUS and ICUS. Ultrasound Med Biol 39(2):187–210. https://doi.org/10.1016/j.ultrasmedbio.2012.09.002

Costa AF, Thipphavong S, Arnason T, Stueck AE, Clarke SE (2018) Fat-containing liver lesions on imaging: detection and differential diagnosis. AJR Am J Roentgenol 210(1):68–77. https://doi.org/10.2214/AJR.17.18136

Danet IM, Semelka RC, Leonardou P, Braga L, Vaidean G, Woosley JT, Kanematsu M (2003) Spectrum of MRI appearances of untreated metastases of the liver. AJR Am J Roentgenol 181(3):809–817. https://doi.org/10.2214/ajr.181.3.1810809

Davenport MS, Viglianti BL, Al-Hawary MM, Caoili EM, Kaza RK, Liu PS, Maturen KE, Chenevert TL, Hussain HK (2013) Comparison of acute transient dyspnea after intravenous administration of gadoxetate disodium and gadobenate dimeglumine: effect on arterial phase image quality. Radiology 266(2):452–461. https://doi.org/10.1148/radiol.12120826

De Bruyne S, Van Damme N, Smeets P, Ferdinande L, Ceelen W, Mertens J, Van de Wiele C, Troisi R, Libbrecht L, Laurent S, Geboes K, Peeters M (2012) Value of DCE-MRI and FDG-PET/CT in the prediction of response to preoperative chemotherapy with bevacizumab for colorectal liver metastases. Br J Cancer 106(12):1926–1933. https://doi.org/10.1038/bjc.2012.184

Dietrich CF, Cui SW, Chiorean L, Appelbaum L, Leen E, Ignee A (2015) Local ablative procedures of the liver. Z Gastroenterol 53(6):579–590. https://doi.org/10.1055/s-0034-1399446

Drzezga A, Souvatzoglou M, Eiber M, Beer AJ, Furst S, Martinez-Moller A, Nekolla SG, Ziegler S, Ganter C, Rummeny EJ, Schwaiger M (2012) First clinical experience with integrated whole-body PET/MR: comparison to PET/CT in patients with oncologic diagnoses. J Nucl Med 53(6):845–855. https://doi.org/10.2967/jnumed.111.098608

Durot I, Wilson SR, Willmann JK (2018) Contrast-enhanced ultrasound of malignant liver lesions. Abdom Radiol (NY) 43(4):819–847. https://doi.org/10.1007/s00261-017-1360-8

Easson AM, Barron PT, Cripps C, Hill G, Guindi M, Michaud C (1996) Calcification in colorectal hepatic metastases correlates with longer survival. J Surg Oncol 63(4):221–225. https://doi.org/10.1002/(SICI)1096-9098(199612)63:4<221::AID-JSO2>3.0.CO;2-E

Edrei Y, Freiman M, Sklair-Levy M, Tsarfaty G, Gross E, Joskowicz L, Abramovitch R (2014) Quantitative functional MRI biomarkers improved early detection of colorectal liver metastases. J Magn Reson Imaging 39(5):1246–1253. https://doi.org/10.1002/jmri.24270

Eisenhauer EA, Therasse P, Bogaerts J, Schwartz LH, Sargent D, Ford R, Dancey J, Arbuck S, Gwyther S, Mooney M, Rubinstein L, Shankar L, Dodd L, Kaplan R, Lacombe D, Verweij J (2009) New response evaluation criteria in solid tumours: revised RECIST guideline (version 1.1). Eur J Cancer 45(2):228–247. https://doi.org/10.1016/j.ejca.2008.10.026

El Kaffas A, Sigrist RMS, Fisher G, Bachawal S, Liau J, Wang H, Karanany A, Durot I, Rosenberg J, Hristov D, Willmann JK (2017) Quantitative three-dimensional dynamic contrast-enhanced ultrasound imaging: first-in-human pilot study in patients with liver metastases. Theranostics 7(15):3745–3758. https://doi.org/10.7150/thno.20329

Ellebæk SB, Fristrup CW, Mortensen MB (2017) Intraoperative ultrasound as a screening modality for the detection of liver metastases during resection of primary colorectal cancer - a systematic review. Ultrasound Int Open 3(2):E60–E68. https://doi.org/10.1055/s-0043-100503

Expert Panel on Gastrointestinal I, Kaur H, Hindman NM, Al-Refaie WB, Arif-Tiwari H, Cash BD, Chernyak V, Farrell J, Grajo JR, Horowitz JM, MM MN, Noto RB, Qayyum A, Lalani T, Kamel IR (2017) ACR appropriateness criteria((R)) suspected liver metastases. J Am Coll Radiol 14(5S):S314–S325. https://doi.org/10.1016/j.jacr.2017.01.037

Fasel JH, Schenk A (2013) Concepts for liver segment classification: neither old ones nor new ones, but a comprehensive one. J Clin Imaging Sci 3:48. https://doi.org/10.4103/2156-7514.120803

Fiorentini G, Sarti D, Aliberti C, Carandina R, Mambrini A, Guadagni S (2017) Multidisciplinary approach of colorectal cancer liver metastases. World J Clin Oncol 8(3):190–202. https://doi.org/10.5306/wjco.v8.i3.190

Francica G, Meloni MF, de Sio I, Terracciano F, Caturelli E, Riccardi L, Roselli P, Iadevaia MD, Scaglione M, Lenna G, Chiang J, Pompili M (2017) Biopsy of liver target lesions under contrast-enhanced ultrasound guidance – a multi-center study. Ultraschall Med 39(4):448–453. https://doi.org/10.1055/s-0043-122496

del Frate C, Bazzocchi M, Mortele KJ, Zuiani C, Londero V, Como G, Zanardi R, Ros PR (2002) Detection of liver metastases: comparison of gadobenate dimeglumine-enhanced and ferumoxides-enhanced MR imaging examinations. Radiology 225(3):766–772. https://doi.org/10.1148/radiol.2253011854

Froelich MF, Heinemann V, Sommer WH, Holch JW, Schoeppe F, Hesse N, Baumann AB, Kunz WG, Reiser MF, Ricke J, D'Anastasi M, Stintzing S, Modest DP, Kazmierczak PM, Hofmann FO (2018) CT attenuation of liver metastases before targeted therapy is a prognostic factor of overall survival in colorectal cancer patients. Results from the randomised, open-label FIRE-3/AIO KRK0306 trial. Eur Radiol. https://doi.org/10.1007/s00330-018-5454-7

Ganeshan B, Miles KA, Young RC, Chatwin CR (2009) Texture analysis in non-contrast enhanced CT: impact of malignancy on texture in apparently disease-free areas of the liver. Eur J Radiol 70(1):101–110. https://doi.org/10.1016/j.ejrad.2007.12.005

Genchellac H, Yilmaz S, Ucar A, Dursun M, Demir MK, Yekeler E (2007) Hepatic pseudolesion around the falciform ligament: prevalence, aberrant venous supply, and fatty infiltration evaluated by multidetector computed tomography and magnetic resonance imaging. J Comput Assist Tomogr 31(4):526–533. https://doi.org/10.1097/01.rct.0000284387.68449.ec

Giacomobono S, Gallicchio R, Capacchione D, Nardelli A, Gattozzi D, Lettini G, Molinari L, Mainenti P, Cammarota A, Storto G (2013) F-18 FDG PET/CT in the assessment of patients with unexplained CEA

rise after surgical curative resection for colorectal cancer. Int J Color Dis 28(12):1699–1705. https://doi.org/10.1007/s00384-013-1747-0

Gruber L, Rainer V, Plaikner M, Kremser C, Jaschke W, Henninger B (2018) CAIPIRINHA-Dixon-TWIST (CDT)-VIBE MR imaging of the liver at 3.0T with gadoxetate disodium: a solution for transient arterial-phase respiratory motion-related artifacts? Eur Radiol 28(5):2013–2021. https://doi.org/10.1007/s00330-017-5210-4

Gupta RT, Iseman CM, Leyendecker JR, Shyknevsky I, Merkle EM, Taouli B (2012) Diagnosis of focal nodular hyperplasia with MRI: multicenter retrospective study comparing gadobenate dimeglumine to gadoxetate disodium. AJR Am J Roentgenol 199(1):35–43. https://doi.org/10.2214/AJR.11.7757

Hale HL, Husband JE, Gossios K, Norman AR, Cunningham D (1998) CT of calcified liver metastases in colorectal carcinoma. Clin Radiol 53(10):735–741

Han NY, Park BJ, Sung DJ, Kim MJ, Cho SB, Lee CH, Jang YJ, Kim SY, Kim DS, Um SH, Won NH, Yang KS (2014) Chemotherapy-induced focal hepatopathy in patients with gastrointestinal malignancy: gadoxetic acid--enhanced and diffusion-weighted MR imaging with clinical-pathologic correlation. Radiology 271(2):416–425. https://doi.org/10.1148/radiol.13131810

Han K, Park SH, Kim KW, Kim HJ, Lee SS, Kim JC, Yu CS, Lim SB, Joo YS, Kim AY, Ha HK (2015) Use of liver magnetic resonance imaging after standard staging abdominopelvic computed tomography to evaluate newly diagnosed colorectal cancer patients. Ann Surg 261(3):480–486. https://doi.org/10.1097/SLA.0000000000000708

Jang HJ, Lim HK, Lee WJ, Lee SJ, Yun JY, Choi D (2002) Small Hypoattenuating Lesions in the Liver on Single-phase Helical CT in Preoperative Patients With Gastric and Colorectal Cancer: Prevalence, Significance, and Differentiating Features. Journal of Computer Assisted Tomography 26(5):718–724

Jones EC, Chezmar JL, Nelson RC, Bernardino ME (1992) The frequency and significance of small (less than or equal to 15 mm) hepatic lesions detected by CT. AJR Am J Roentgenol 158(3):535–539. https://doi.org/10.2214/ajr.158.3.1738990

Kannan P, Kretzschmar WW, Winter H, Warren D, Bates R, Allen PD, Syed N, Irving B, Papiez BW, Kaeppler J, Markelc B, Kinchesh P, Gilchrist S, Smart S, Schnabel JA, Maughan T, Harris AL, Muschel RJ, Partridge M, Sharma RA, Kersemans V (2018) Functional parameters derived from magnetic resonance imaging reflect vascular morphology in preclinical tumors and in human liver metastases. Clin Cancer Res 24(19):4694–4704. https://doi.org/10.1158/1078-0432.CCR-18-0033

Kershah S, Partovi S, Traughber BJ, Muzic RF Jr, Schluchter MD, O'Donnell JK, Faulhaber P (2013) Comparison of standardized uptake values in normal structures between PET/CT and PET/MRI in an oncology patient population. Mol Imaging Biol 15(6):776–785. https://doi.org/10.1007/s11307-013-0629-8

van Kessel CS, Buckens CF, van den Bosch MA, van Leeuwen MS, van Hillegersberg R, Verkooijen HM (2012) Preoperative imaging of colorectal liver metastases after neoadjuvant chemotherapy: a meta-analysis. Ann Surg Oncol 19(9):2805–2813. https://doi.org/10.1245/s10434-012-2300-z

Khalil HI, Patterson SA, Panicek DM (2005) Hepatic lesions deemed too small to characterize at CT: prevalence and importance in women with breast cancer. Radiology 235(3):872–878. https://doi.org/10.1148/radiol.2353041099

Kim W, Clark TW, Baum RA, Soulen MC (2001) Risk factors for liver abscess formation after hepatic chemoembolization. J Vasc Interv Radiol 12(8):965–968

Kim MJ, Kim SH, Kim HJ, Kim BS, Hernandes M, Semelka RC (2013) Enhancement of liver and pancreas on late hepatic arterial phase imaging: quantitative comparison among multiple gadolinium-based contrast agents at 1.5 tesla MRI. J Magn Reson Imaging 38(1):102–108. https://doi.org/10.1002/jmri.23934

Kim HJ, Lee SS, Byun JH, Kim JC, Yu CS, Park SH, Kim AY, Ha HK (2015) Incremental value of liver MR imaging in patients with potentially curable colorectal hepatic metastasis detected at CT: a prospective comparison of diffusion-weighted imaging, gadoxetic acid-enhanced MR imaging, and a combination of both MR techniques. Radiology 274(3):712–722. https://doi.org/10.1148/radiol.14140390

Kim SS, Song KD, Kim YK, Kim HC, Huh JW, Park YS, Park JO, Kim ST (2017) Disappearing or residual tiny (</=5 mm) colorectal liver metastases after chemotherapy on gadoxetic acid-enhanced liver MRI and diffusion-weighted imaging: is local treatment required? Eur Radiol 27(7):3088–3096. https://doi.org/10.1007/s00330-016-4644-4

Kim C, Kim SY, Kim MJ, Yoon YS, Kim CW, Lee JH, Kim KP, Lee SS, Park SH, Lee MG (2018) Clinical impact of preoperative liver MRI in the evaluation of synchronous liver metastasis of colon cancer. Eur Radiol 28(19):4234–4242. https://doi.org/10.1007/s00330-018-5422-2

Kirchner J, Sawicki LM, Deuschl C, Gruneisen J, Beiderwellen K, Lauenstein TC, Herrmann K, Forsting M, Heusch P, Umutlu L (2017) 18 F-FDG PET/MR imaging in patients with suspected liver lesions: value of liver-specific contrast agent Gadobenate dimeglumine. PLoS One 12(7):e0180349. https://doi.org/10.1371/journal.pone.0180349

Ko Y, Kim J, Park JK-H, Kim H, Cho JY, Kang S-Bk Ahn S, Lee KJ, Lee KH (2017) Limited detection of small (≤10mm) colorectal liver metastasis at preoperative CT in patients undergoing liver resection. PLoS One 12(12):e0189797. https://doi.org/10.1371/journal.pone.0189797

Kopetz S, Vauthey JN (2008) Perioperative chemotherapy for resectable hepatic metastases. Lancet 371(9617):963–965. https://doi.org/10.1016/S0140-6736(08)60429-8

Kopljar M, Patrlj L, Busic Z, Kolovrat M, Rakic M, Klicek R, Zidak M, Stipancic I (2014) Potential use of Doppler perfusion index in detection of occult liver metastases from colorectal cancer. Hepatobiliary Surg Nutr 3(5):259–267. https://doi.org/10.3978/j.issn.2304-3881.2014.09.04

Krix M (2005) Quantification of enhancement in contrast ultrasound: a tool for monitoring of therapies in liver metastases. Eur Radiol 15(Suppl 5):E104–E108

Kuhlmann K, van Hilst J, Fisher S, Poston G (2016) Management of disappearing colorectal liver metastases. Eur J Surg Oncol 42(12):1798–1805. https://doi.org/10.1016/j.ejso.2016.05.005

Larsen LP (2010) Role of contrast enhanced ultrasonography in the assessment of hepatic metastases: a review. World J Hepatol 2(1):8–15. https://doi.org/10.4254/wjh.v2.i1.8

Lee DH, Lee JM, Hur BY, Joo I, Yi NJ, Suh KS, Kang KW, Han JK (2016) Colorectal Cancer liver metastases: diagnostic performance and prognostic value of PET/MR imaging. Radiology 280(3):782–792. https://doi.org/10.1148/radiol.2016151975

Luetkens JA, Kupczyk PA, Doerner J, Fimmers R, Willinek WA, Schild HH, Kukuk GM (2015) Respiratory motion artefacts in dynamic liver MRI: a comparison using gadoxetate disodium and gadobutrol. Eur Radiol 25(11):3207–3213. https://doi.org/10.1007/s00330-015-3736-x

Maffione AM, Lopci E, Bluemel C, Giammarile F, Herrmann K, Rubello D (2015) Diagnostic accuracy and impact on management of (18)F-FDG PET and PET/CT in colorectal liver metastasis: a meta-analysis and systematic review. Eur J Nucl Med Mol Imaging 42(1):152–163. https://doi.org/10.1007/s00259-014-2930-4

Mahfouz AE, Hamm B, Wolf KJ (1994) Peripheral washout: a sign of malignancy on dynamic gadolinium-enhanced MR images of focal liver lesions. Radiology 190(1):49–52. https://doi.org/10.1148/radiology.190.1.8259426

Mainenti PP (2015) Non-invasive diagnostic imaging of colorectal liver metastases. World J Radiol 7(7):157

Mainenti PP, Mancini M, Mainolfi C, Camera L, Maurea S, Manchia A, Tanga M, Persico F, Addeo P, D'Antonio D, Speranza A, Bucci L, Persico G, Pace L, Salvatore M (2010) Detection of colorectal liver metastases: prospective comparison of contrast enhanced US, multidetector CT, PET/CT, and 1.5 Tesla MR with extracellular and reticulo-endothelial cell specific contrast agents. Abdom Imaging 35(5):511–521. https://doi.org/10.1007/s00261-009-9555-2

Matos AP, Altun E, Ramalho M, Velloni F, AlObaidy M, Semelka RC (2015) An overview of imaging techniques for liver metastases management. Expert Rev

Gastroenterol Hepatol 9(12):1561–1576. https://doi.org/10.1586/17474124.2015.1092873

Mattar RE, Al-Alem F, Simoneau E, Hassanain M (2016) Preoperative selection of patients with colorectal cancer liver metastasis for hepatic resection. World J Gastroenterol 22(2):567–581. https://doi.org/10.3748/wjg.v22.i2.567

Mazard T, Boonsirikamchai P, Overman MJ, Asran MA, Choi H, Herron D, Eng C, Maru DM, Ychou M, Vauthey JN, Loyer EM, Kopetz S (2018) Comparison of early radiological predictors of outcome in patients with colorectal cancer with unresectable hepatic metastases treated with bevacizumab. Gut 67(6):1095–1102. https://doi.org/10.1136/gutjnl-2017-313786

McDonald RJ, Levine D, Weinreb J, Kanal E, Davenport MS, Ellis JH, Jacobs PM, Lenkinski RE, Maravilla KR, Prince MR, Rowley HA, Tweedle MF, Kressel HY (2018) Gadolinium retention: a research roadmap from the 2018 NIH/ACR/RSNA workshop on gadolinium chelates. Radiology 289(2):517–534. https://doi.org/10.1148/radiol.2018181151

Meyers MO, Watson JC (2003) Angiogenesis and hepatic colorectal metastases. Surg Oncol Clin N Am 12(1):151–163

Miles KA, Ganeshan B, Griffiths MR, Young RC, Chatwin CR (2009) Colorectal cancer: texture analysis of portal phase hepatic CT images as a potential marker of survival. Radiology 250(2):444–452. https://doi.org/10.1148/radiol.2502071879

Miller FH, Hammond N, Siddiqi AJ, Shroff S, Khatri G, Wang Y, Merrick LB, Nikolaidis P (2010) Utility of diffusion-weighted MRI in distinguishing benign and malign hepatic lesions. J Magn Reson Imaging 32(1):138–147. https://doi.org/10.1002/jmri.22235

Mortele KJ, Ros PR (2001) Cystic focal liver lesions in the adult: differential CT and MR imaging features. Radiographics 21(4):895–910. https://doi.org/10.1148/radiographics.21.4.g01jl16895

Motosugi U, Ichikawa T, Sou H, Sano K, Tominaga L, Muhi A, Araki T (2010) Distinguishing hypervascular pseudolesions of the liver from hypervascular hepatocellular carcinomas with gadoxetic acid-enhanced MR imaging. Radiology 256(1):151–158. https://doi.org/10.1148/radiol.10091885

Motosugi U, Bannas P, Bookwalter CA, Sano K, Reeder SB (2016) An investigation of transient severe motion related to gadoxetic acid-enhanced MR imaging. Radiology 279(19):93–102. https://doi.org/10.1148/radiol.2015150642

Moulton CA, Gu CS, Law CH, Tandan VR, Hart R, Quan D, Fairfull Smith RJ, Jalink DW, Husien M, Serrano PE, Hendler AL, Haider MA, Ruo L, Gulenchyn KY, Finch T, Julian JA, Levine MN, Gallinger S (2014) Effect of PET before liver resection on surgical management for colorectal adenocarcinoma metastases: a randomized clinical trial. JAMA 311(18):1863–1869. https://doi.org/10.1001/jama.2014.3740

Muhi A, Ichikawa T, Motosugi U, Sou H, Nakajima H, Sano K, Sano M, Kato S, Kitamura T, Fatima Z, Fukushima K, Iino H, Mori Y, Fujii H, Araki T (2011)

Diagnosis of colorectal hepatic metastases: comparison of contrast-enhanced CT, contrast-enhanced US, superparamagnetic iron oxide-enhanced MRI, and gadoxetic acid-enhanced MRI. J Magn Reson Imaging 34(2):326–335. https://doi.org/10.1002/jmri.22613

Nakai Y, Gonoi W, Hagiwara A, Nishioka Y, Abe H, Shindoh J, Hasegawa K, (2018) MRI Detection of Intratumoral Fat in Colorectal Liver Metastases After Preoperative Chemotherapy. Am J Roentgenology 210(5):W196–W204

Neri E, Bali MA, Ba-Ssalamah A, Boraschi P, Brancatelli G, Alves FC, Grazioli L, Helmberger T, Lee JM, Manfredi R, Marti-Bonmati L, Matos C, Merkle EM, Op De Beeck B, Schima W, Skehan S, Vilgrain V, Zech C, Bartolozzi C (2016) ESGAR consensus statement on liver MR imaging and clinical use of liver-specific contrast agents. Eur Radiol 26(4):921–931. https://doi.org/10.1007/s00330-015-3900-3

Nicolau C, Vilana R, Catala V, Bianchi L, Gilabert R, Garcia A, Bru C (2006) Importance of evaluating all vascular phases on contrast-enhanced sonography in the differentiation of benign from malignant focal liver lesions. AJR Am J Roentgenol 186(1):158–167. https://doi.org/10.2214/AJR.04.1009

Niekel MC, Bipat S, Stoker J (2010) Diagnostic imaging of colorectal liver metastases with CT, MR imaging, FDG PET, and/or FDG PET/CT: a meta-analysis of prospective studies including patients who have not previously undergone treatment. Radiology 257(3):674–684. https://doi.org/10.1148/radiol.10100729

Nielsen K, Scheffer HJ, Pieters IC, van Tilborg AA, van Waesberghe JH, Oprea-Lager DE, Meijerink MR, Kazemier G, Hoekstra OS, Schreurs HW, Sietses C, Meijer S, Comans EF, van den Tol PM (2014) The use of PET-MRI in the follow-up after radiofrequency- and microwave ablation of colorectal liver metastases. BMC Med Imaging 14:27. https://doi.org/10.1186/1471-2342-14-27

Paget S (1989) The distribution of secondary growths in cancer of the breast. 1889. Cancer Metastasis Rev 8(2):98–101

Park Y, Kim SH, Kim SH, Jeon YH, Lee J, Kim MJ, Choi D, Lee WJ, Kim H, Koo JH, Lim HK (2010) Gadoxetic acid (Gd-EOB-DTPA)-enhanced MRI versus gadobenate dimeglumine (Gd-BOPTA)-enhanced MRI for preoperatively detecting hepatocellular carcinoma: an initial experience. Korean J Radiol 11(4):433–440. https://doi.org/10.3348/kjr.2010.11.4.433

Park MJ, Hong N, Han K, Kim MJ, Lee YJ, Park YS, Rha SE, Park S, Lee WJ, Park SH, Lee CH, Nam CM, An C, Kim HJ, Kim H, Park MS (2017) Use of imaging to predict complete response of colorectal liver metastases after chemotherapy: MR imaging versus CT imaging. Radiology 284(2):423–431. https://doi.org/10.1148/radiol.2017161619

Pawlik TM, Scoggins CR, Thomas MB, Vauthey JN (2004) Advances in the surgical management of liver malignancies. Cancer J 10(2):74–87

Polanec SH, Bickel H, Baltzer PAT, Thurner P, Gittler F, Hodge JC, Bashir MR, Ba-Ssalamah A (2017) Respiratory motion artifacts during arterial phase imaging with gadoxetic acid: can the injection protocol minimize this drawback? J Magn Reson Imaging 46(4):1107–1114. https://doi.org/10.1002/jmri.25657

Quick HH, von Gall C, Zeilinger M, Wiesmuller M, Braun H, Ziegler S, Kuwert T, Uder M, Dorfler A, Kalender WA, Lell M (2013) Integrated whole-body PET/MR hybrid imaging: clinical experience. Investig Radiol 48(5):280–289. https://doi.org/10.1097/RLI.0b013e3182845a08

Ramalho M, Heredia V, Tsurusaki M, Altun E, Semelka RC (2009) Quantitative and qualitative comparison of 1.5 and 3.0 tesla MRI in patients with chronic liver diseases. J Magn Reson Imaging 29(4):869–879. https://doi.org/10.1002/jmri.21719

de Ridder J, de Wilt JH, Simmer F, Overbeek L, Lemmens V, Nagtegaal I (2016) Incidence and origin of histologically confirmed liver metastases: an explorative case-study of 23,154 patients. Oncotarget 7(34):55368–55376. https://doi.org/10.18632/oncotarget.10552

Rubbia-Brandt L, Giostra E, Brezault C, Roth AD, Andres A, Audard V, Sartoretti P, Dousset B, Majno PE, Soubrane O, Chaussade S, Mentha G, Terris B (2007) Importance of histological tumor response assessment in predicting the outcome in patients with colorectal liver metastases treated with neo-adjuvant chemotherapy followed by liver surgery. Ann Oncol 18(2):299–304. https://doi.org/10.1093/annonc/mdl386

Ruers TJ, Wiering B, van der Sijp JR, Roumen RM, de Jong KP, Comans EF, Pruim J, Dekker HM, Krabbe PF, Oyen WJ (2009) Improved selection of patients for hepatic surgery of colorectal liver metastases with (18)F-FDG PET: a randomized study. J Nucl Med 50(7):1036–1041. https://doi.org/10.2967/jnumed.109.063040

Sadigh G, Applegate KE, Baumgarten DA (2014) Comparative accuracy of intravenous contrast-enhanced CT versus noncontrast CT plus intravenous contrast-enhanced CT in the detection and characterization of patients with hypervascular liver metastases: a critically appraised topic. Acad Radiol 21(1):113–125. https://doi.org/10.1016/j.acra.2013.08.023

Sahani D, Mehta A, Blake M, Prasad S, Harris G, Saini S (2004) Preoperative hepatic vascular evaluation with CT and MR angiography: implications for surgery. Radiographics 24(5):1367–1380. https://doi.org/10.1148/rg.245035224

Samim M, Molenaar IQ, Seesing MF, van Rossum PS, van den Bosch MA, Ruers TJ, Borel Rinkes IH, van Hillegersberg R, Lam MG, Verkooijen HM (2017) The diagnostic performance of (18)F-FDG PET/CT, CT and MRI in the treatment evaluation of ablation therapy for colorectal liver metastases: a systematic review and meta-analysis. Surg Oncol 26(1):37–45. https://doi.org/10.1016/j.suronc.2016.12.006

Scharitzer M, Schima W, Schober E, Reimer P, Helmberger TK, Holzknecht N, Stadler A, Ba-Ssalamah A, Weber M, Wrba F (2005) Characterization of hepatocellular tumors: value of mangafodipir-enhanced magnetic resonance imaging. J Comput Assist Tomogr 29(2):181–190

Scharitzer M, Ba-Ssalamah A, Ringl H, Kolblinger C, Grunberger T, Weber M, Schima W (2013) Preoperative evaluation of colorectal liver metastases: comparison between gadoxetic acid-enhanced 3.0-T MRI and contrast-enhanced MDCT with histopathological correlation. Eur Radiol 23(8):2187–2196. https://doi.org/10.1007/s00330-013-2824-z

Schwartz LH, Gandras EJ, Colangelo SM, Ercolani MC, Panicek DM (1999) Prevalence and importance of small hepatic lesions found at CT in patients with cancer. Radiology 210(1):71–74. https://doi.org/10.1148/radiology.210.1.r99ja0371

Semelka RC, Worawattanakul S, Noone TC, Burdeny DA, Kelekis NL, Woosley JT, Lee JK (1999) Chemotherapy-treated liver metastases mimicking hemangiomas on MR images. Abdom Imaging 24(4):378–382

Semelka RC, Hussain SM, Marcos HB, Woosley JT (2000) Perilesional enhancement of hepatic metastases: correlation between MR imaging and histopathologic findings-initial observations. Radiology 215(1):89–94. https://doi.org/10.1148/radiology.215.1.r00mr2989

Shiozawa K, Watanabe M, Ikehara T, Matsukiyo Y, Kogame M, Kikuchi Y, Otsuka Y, Kaneko H, Igarashi Y, Sumino Y (2017) Comparison of contrast-enhanced ultrasonograpy with Gd-EOB-DTPA-enhanced MRI in the diagnosis of liver metastasis from colorectal cancer. J Clin Ultrasound 45(3):138–144. https://doi.org/10.1002/jcu.22421

Silva AC, Evans JM, McCullough AE, Jatoi MA, Vargas HE, Hara AK (2009) MR imaging of hypervascular liver masses: a review of current techniques. Radiographics 29(2):385–402. https://doi.org/10.1148/rg.292085123

Silverman PM (2006) Liver metastases: imaging considerations for protocol development with multislice CT (MSCT). Cancer Imaging 6:175–181. https://doi.org/10.1102/1470-7330.2006.0024

Sohn J, Siegelman E, Osiason A (2001) Unusual patterns of hepatic steatosis caused by the local effect of insulin revealed on chemical shift MR imaging. AJR Am J Roentgenol 176(2):471–474. https://doi.org/10.2214/ajr.176.2.1760471

Soyer P, Poccard M, Boudiaf M, Abitbol M, Hamzi L, Panis Y, Valleur P, Rymer R (2004) Detection of hypovascular hepatic metastases at triple-phase helical CT: sensitivity of phases and comparison with surgical and histopathologic findings. Radiology 231(2):413–420. https://doi.org/10.1148/radiol.2312021639

Storto G, Nicolai E, Salvatore M (2009) [18F]FDG-PET-CT for early monitoring of tumor response: when and why. Q J Nucl Med Mol Imaging 53(2):167–180

Taouli B, Koh DM (2010) Diffusion-weighted MR imaging of the liver. Radiology 254(1):47–66. https://doi.org/10.1148/radiol.09090021

Van Cutsem E, Cervantes A, Adam R, Sobrero A, Van Krieken JH, Aderka D, Aranda Aguilar E, Bardelli A, Benson A, Bodoky G, Ciardiello F, D'Hoore A, Diaz-Rubio E, Douillard JY, Ducreux M, Falcone A, Grothey A, Gruenberger T, Haustermans K, Heinemann V, Hoff P, Kohne CH, Labianca R, Laurent-Puig P, Ma B, Maughan T, Muro K, Normanno N, Osterlund P, Oyen WJ, Papamichael D, Pentheroudakis G, Pfeiffer P, Price TJ, Punt C, Ricke J, Roth A, Salazar R, Scheithauer W, Schmoll HJ, Tabernero J, Taieb J, Tejpar S, Wasan H, Yoshino T, Zaanan A, Arnold D (2016) ESMO consensus guidelines for the management of patients with metastatic colorectal cancer. Ann Oncol 27(8):1386–1422. https://doi.org/10.1093/annonc/mdw235

Vialle R, Boucebci S, Richer JP, Velasco S, Herpe G, Vesselle G, Ingrand P, Tasu JP (2016) Preoperative detection of hepatic metastases from colorectal cancer: prospective comparison of contrast-enhanced ultrasound and multidetector-row computed tomography (MDCT). Diagn Interv Imaging 97(9):851–855. https://doi.org/10.1016/j.diii.2015.11.017

Vilgrain V, Ronot M, Abdel-Rehim M, Zappa M, d'Assignies G, Bruno O, Vullierme MP (2013) Hepatic steatosis: a major trap in liver imaging. Diagn Interv Imaging 94(7–8):713–727. https://doi.org/10.1016/j.diii.2013.03.010

Vilgrain V, Esvan M, Ronot M, Caumont-Prim A, Aubé C, Chatellier vG (2016a) A meta-analysis of diffusion-weighted and gadoxetic acid-enhanced MR imaging for the detection of liver metastases. Eur Radiol 26:4595–4615. https://doi.org/10.1007/s00330-016-4250-5

Vilgrain V, Lagadec M, Ronot M (2016b) Pitfalls in liver imaging. Radiology 278(1):34–51. https://doi.org/10.1148/radiol.2015142576

Vreugdenburg TD, Ma N, Duncan JK, Riitano D, Cameron AL, Maddern GJ (2016) Comparative diagnostic accuracy of hepatocyte-specific gadoxetic acid (Gd-EOB-DTPA) enhanced MR imaging and contrast enhanced CT for the detection of liver metastases: a systematic review and meta-analysis. Int J Color Dis 31(11):1739–1749. https://doi.org/10.1007/s00384-016-2664-9

Ward J, Robinson PJ, Guthrie JA, Downing S, Wilson D, Lodge JP, Prasad KR, Toogood GJ, Wyatt JI (2005) Liver metastases in candidates for hepatic resection: comparison of helical CT and gadolinium- and SPIO-enhanced MR imaging. Radiology 237(1):170–180. https://doi.org/10.1148/radiol.2371041444

Weg N, Scheer MR, Gabor MP (1998) Liver lesions: improved detection with dual-detector-array CT and routine 2.5-mm thin collimation. Radiology 209(2):417–426. https://doi.org/10.1148/radiology.209.2.9807568

Wittenberg J, Stark DD, Forman BH, Hahn PF, Saini S, Weissleder R, Rummeny E, Ferrucci JT (1988) Differentiation of hepatic metastases from hepatic hemangiomas and cysts by using MR imaging. Am J Roentgenol 151(1):79 84

Wu LM, Hu J, Gu HY, Hua J, Xu JR (2013) Can diffusion-weighted magnetic resonance imaging (DW-MRI) alone be used as a reliable sequence for the preoperative detection and characterisation of hepatic metastases? A meta-analysis. Eur J Cancer 49(3):572–584. https://doi.org/10.1016/j.ejca.2012.08.021

Yoon JH, Lee JM, Lee ES, Baek J, Lee S, Iwadate Y, Han JK, Choi BI (2015) Navigated three-dimensional T1-weighted gradient-echo sequence for gadoxetic acid liver magnetic resonance imaging in patients with limited breath-holding capacity. Abdom Imaging 40(2):278–288. https://doi.org/10.1007/s00261-014-0214-x

Part II

Hepatic Tumoral Pathology: Chronic Liver Disease and Liver Cirrhosis

Hepatocellular Carcinoma: Diagnostic Imaging Criteria

Alessandro Furlan and Roberto Cannella

Contents

Abstract

The diagnosis of hepatocellular carcinoma (HCC) can be reached noninvasively on imaging in patients at high risk as discussed in chapter "Hepatocellular carcinoma: Diagnostic Guidelines." In this chapter, we describe the CT and MR imaging criteria more commonly used in the guidelines for the diagnosis and management of patients with HCC, including arterial phase hyperenhancement, washout, capsule, growth, and hypointensity on hepatobiliary phase MR imaging. The provided definitions are based on the latest version (v2018) of the liver imaging reporting and data system (LI-RADS) document (American College of Radiology 2018, https://www.acr.org/Clinical-Resources/Reporting-and-Data-Systems/LI-RADS).

A. Furlan (✉)
Department of Radiology, University of Pittsburgh Medical Center, Pittsburgh, PA, USA

R. Cannella
Section of Radiology—BiND, University Hospital "Paolo Giaccone", Palermo, Italy

1 Arterial Phase Hyperenhancement

Arterial phase hyperenhancement (APHE) is defined as enhancement of the lesion on the hepatic arterial phase images significantly higher than the surrounding liver parenchyma (American College of Radiology 2018) (Fig. 1).

E. Quaia (ed.), *Imaging of the Liver and Intra-hepatic Biliary Tract*,
Medical Radiology Diagnostic Imaging, https://doi.org/10.1007/978-3-030-39021-1_8

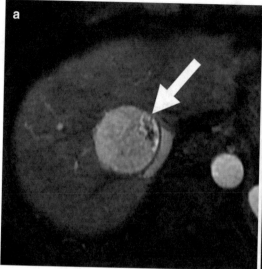
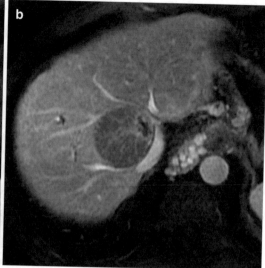

Fig. 1 53-year-old male with history of chronic hepatitis C and cirrhosis. MR imaging obtained after injection of Gd-BOPTA shows a 5.4 cm mass with arterial phase hyperenhancement (APHE) (arrow, **a**) and washout on portal venous phase (**b**) consistent with hepatocellular carcinoma (HCC). The combination of APHE and washout is considered the typical presentation of HCC and it is included in all imaging guidelines for the diagnosis and management of HCC

The sign reflects the neoangiogenesis occurring during the hepatocarcinogenetic process (Tang et al. 2018). While dysplastic nodule and early HCC may appear hypoenhancing because of an initial reduction in arterial flow due to the overall decrease in the number of portal triads, the presence of new unpaired (non-triadal) arteries is typically seen in progressed HCC and it is eventually responsible for APHE (Park et al. 1998). The sign is a key component of all available imaging guidelines and has a high sensitivity for the detection of progressed HCC (Tang et al. 2018). The per nodule sensitivity for multiphasic contrast-enhanced CT ranges 65–87% (Oliver et al. 1996; Laghi et al. 2003; Pitton et al. 2009; Sangiovanni et al. 2010) and for gadolinium-enhanced MRI 66–98% (Pitton et al. 2009; Sangiovanni et al. 2010; Kim et al. 2011; An et al. 2013; Cerny et al. 2018a). The sensitivity is not 100% because some small and well-differentiated tumors may present as hypovascular lesions. In the study by Takayasu et al. including 4474 patients with a solitary HCC < 3 cm, 18% of the tumors were hypovascular (Takayasu et al. 2013). In this study, most hypovascular HCC developed arterial phase hyperenhancement when they grew over 1.5 cm. Poorly differentiated tumors may also appear hypovascular because of the progressive decrease in blood flow in these lesions. Moreover, in diffuse HCC, because of the presence of multiple small tumor nodules spread through a large portion of the hepatic parenchyma, the resulting imaging appearance is an infiltrating lesion which is usually less conspicuous on the arterial phase images compared to a tumor presenting as a well-defined nodule (Reynolds et al. 2015). In diffuse HCC, tumor conspicuity may be higher on T2-weighted and diffusion-weighted MR images (Reynolds et al. 2015) compared to the dynamic study (Fig. 2).

The specificity of APHE is limited (62–97%) (Sangiovanni et al. 2010; Kim et al. 2011; An

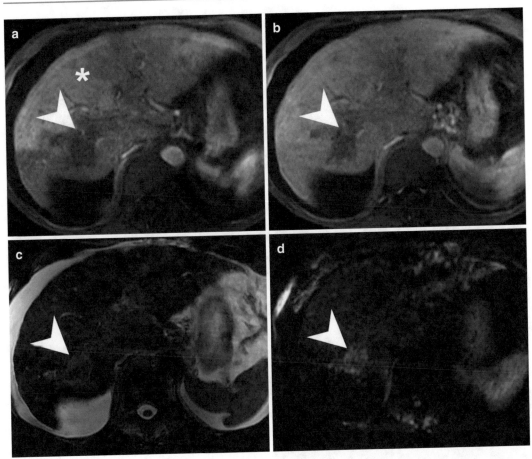

Fig. 2 55-year-old man with cirrhosis and elevated alpha-fetoprotein (247 ng/mL). Gd-BOPTA-enhanced MRI shows an ill-defined mass in the right hepatic lobe only minimally hyperenhancing on the arterial phase (asterisk, **a**) and with minimal washout on the portal venous phase (**b**). The mass appears more conspicuous on the T2-weighted (**c**) and diffusion-weighted (**d**) images where it is mildly hyperintense with an infiltrative appearance. The imaging appearance is compatible with a diffuse-type hepatocellular carcinoma (HCC), also referred to as infiltrative HCC. Note also the presence of tumor in vein in the right lobe (arrowhead, **a–d**)

et al. 2013) because multiple other lesions in cirrhosis can show APHE including hemangioma, small intrahepatic cholangiocarcinoma (ICC), vascular shunt, and dysplastic nodule (Galia et al. 2014).

A small percentage of HCCs, 5% in Choi et al. (2017), can present enhancement more pronounced at the periphery of the lesion. In the LI-RADS system (American College of Radiology 2018), the presence of rim-APHE is enough to classify a lesion in the LR-M group. The LR-M category includes observations probably or definitely malignant but with imaging features not specific for HCC. The rim-APHE appearance is more common in other primary hepatic malignancies, such as ICC and combined hepatocellular-cholangiocarcinoma (cHCC-CCA) (Fig. 3). When rim-APHE is present, the diagnosis of HCC may be suggested by the detection of other features such as intralesional fat favoring a hepatocellular origin (American College of Radiology 2018; Choi et al. 2017) (Fig. 4).

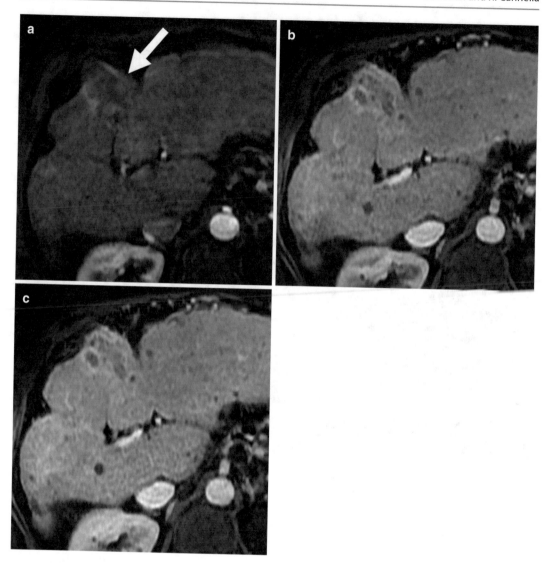

Fig. 3 Combined hepatocellular-cholangiocarcinoma (cHCC-CCA) presenting as a LR-M observation. A partially exophytic mass arising from segment 5 of a cirrhotic liver (arrow, **a**) shows rim hyperenhancement on arterial phase (**a**) and progressive centripetal enhancement on portal venous (**b**) and delayed (**c**) phase. The mass was classified as LR-M and proven a cHCC-CCA at ultrasound-guided percutaneous biopsy

2 Washout

Washout (or washout appearance) is defined as temporal reduction in enhancement from an earlier arterial to a later phase resulting into lesion hypoenhancement to the surrounding liver parenchyma on the images acquired during the portal venous and/or delayed phase (American College of Radiology 2018) (Fig. 5).

The exact nature of this sign is not yet completely understood. It is likely the result of a combination of tumor de-enhancement from venous drainage and progressive enhancement of the surrounding liver parenchyma from retention of contrast in fibrosis and interstitial space (Choi et al. 2014). The per-nodule specificity ranges 62–100% (Sangiovanni et al. 2010; Kim et al. 2011; Cerny et al. 2018a) while the

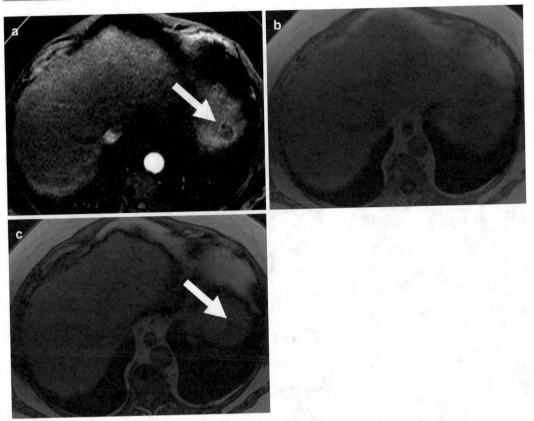

Fig. 4 Atypical presentation of hepatocellular carcinoma (HCC). Gd-BOPTA-enhanced MR image obtained during the arterial phase shows a rim-enhancing lesion (arrow, **a**) in the left lobe of a cirrhotic liver. Compared to the T1-weighted gradient-recalled echo image obained in-phase (**b**), signal drop of the lesion on image obtained opposed-phase (arrow, **c**) is compatible with intralesional fat, thus indicating a hepatocellular origin. HCC was confirmed at laparoscopic biopsy

per-nodule sensitivity ranges 53–79% (Sangiovanni et al. 2010; Kim et al. 2011; Cerny et al. 2018a). Up to one-third of HCCs, prevalently small and well-differentiated tumors do not show washout (Kim et al. 2011; Lee et al. 2012; Yoon et al. 2009; Luca et al. 2010). On contrast-enhanced CT, washout may be more conspicuous on the images acquired during the delayed phase rather than portal venous phase (Furlan et al. 2011) (Fig. 5). On gadolinium-enhanced MRI, washout is to be evaluated during the extracellular phases, i.e., the portal venous and delayed (3–5 min post-contrast administration) phase, when using a purely or prevalently extracellular contrast agent (e.g., Gd-BOPTA), and only during the portal venous phase when using the hepatobiliary contrast agent Gd-EOB-DTPA (American College of Radiology 2018). The uptake of Gd-EOB-DTPA into the hepatocytes may occur as soon as 90 seconds post-contrast administration (Vogl et al. 1996). Therefore, the hypointensity of the lesion on the images acquired between the portal venous and the hepatobiliary phase (i.e., transitional phase) may be due to the relatively increased signal intensity of the surrounding parenchyma and not to washout. It has been shown that considering lesion hypointensity on transitional phase as washout while increasing sensitivity (from 70.9 to 86.6%) reduces the specificity (from 97.7 to 86.3%) for the diagnosis of HCC (Joo et al. 2015).

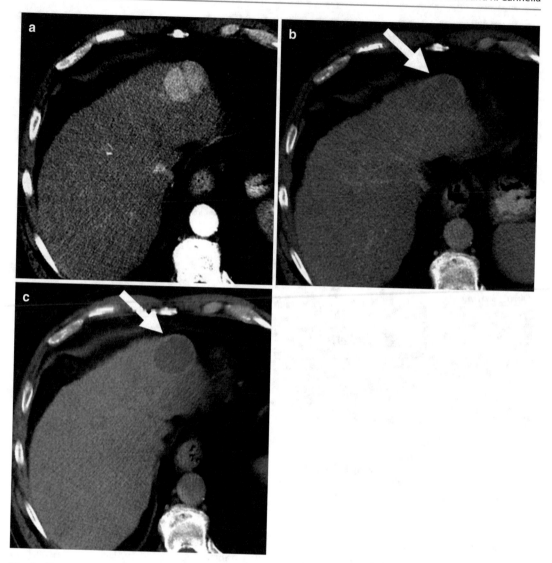

Fig. 5 69-year-old male with history of NASH cirrhosis. Contrast-enhanced CT shows a 4.4 cm lesion with arterial phase hyperenhancement (**a**) and washout on portal venous (arrow, **b**) and delayed (arrow, **c**) phase, typical of hepatocellular carcinoma

Washout is included in all available guidelines for the noninvasive diagnosis of HCC along with APHE. The combination of APHE and washout in a cirrhotic liver is considered the typical enhancement pattern of HCC (Figs. 1, 5, 6, 7, 8). This combination of imaging findings has a sensitivity of 43–98% and a specificity of 81–100% for the diagnosis of HCC (Sangiovanni et al. 2010; Luca et al. 2010; Marrero et al. 2005; Forner et al. 2008; Sersté et al. 2012; Jang et al. 2013; Rimola et al. 2012).

3 Capsule

Capsule is defined as a smooth rim of enhancement detected on the contrast-enhanced CT and MR images acquired during the portal venous and/or delayed phase images (American College of Radiology 2018) (Fig. 6). In the hepatocarcinogenesis process, capsule formation is related to the expansive growth of a progressed HCC. At histology, this feature may correspond to a true, histologic fibrous capsule

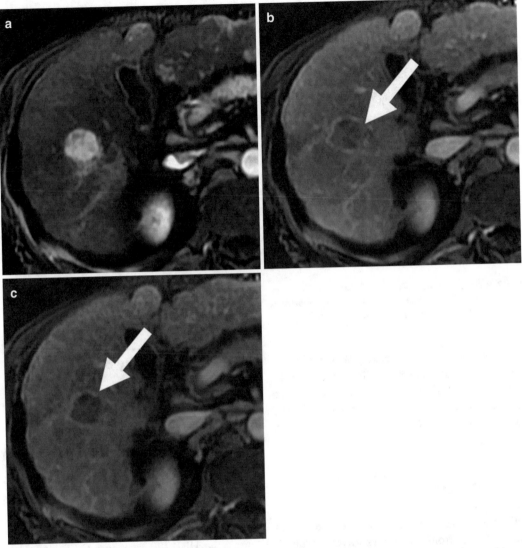

Fig. 6 72-year-old female with NASH cirrhosis. Gd-BOPTA-enhanced MR imaging shows a 2.2 cm arterial phase hyperenhancing lesion (**a**), with washout and capsule visible on both portal venous (arrow, **b**) and delayed (arrow, **c**) phase, consistent with hepatocellular carcinoma

or a pseudocapsule made of a combination of compressed parenchyma, prominent sinusoid, and peritumoral fibrosis (Ishigami et al. 2009). Imaging cannot distinguish a true capsule from a pseudocapsule (perilesional, compressed parenchyma). While the sensitivity is low (33–34%) especially for lesion <2 cm (Cerny et al. 2018a; Khan et al. 2010), the specificity is very high 86–99% (Cerny et al. 2018a; Rimola et al. 2012; Khan et al. 2010) making it a very helpful sign to distinguish HCC from other hepatic malignancies such as ICC (Tang et al. 2018; Choi et al. 2017).

Capsule needs to be differentiated from other perilesional enhancements such as rim-APHE and corona enhancement. Corona enhancement is defined as an ill-defined perilesional area of hyperenhancement visualized on the arterial phase images and fading on portal venous and delayed phase images (Cerny et al. 2018b). Although infrequently detected, corona enhancement is a feature indicative of progressed HCC

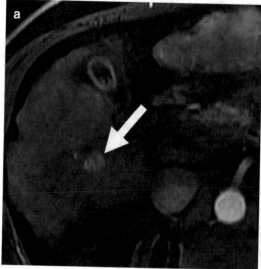
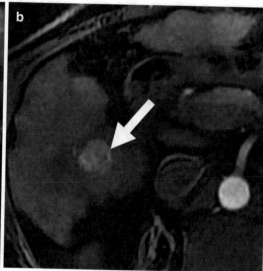

Fig. 7 62-year-old male with chronic hepatitis C and cirrhosis. Gd BOPTA-enhanced MR imaging demonstrates a 1.2 cm arterial phase hyperenhancing lesion (arrow, **a**) measuring 2.2 cm at 6 months imaging follow-up (arrow, **b**) compatible with threshold growth (i.e., >50% within 6 months) according to the LI-RADS guidelines

reflecting the contrast drainage from the tumor to the peritumoral sinusoids (Choi et al. 2014). While rim-APHE and corona enhancement are appreciated on the arterial phase images, capsule appears on the images acquired during the portal venous and delayed phases.

4 Growth

HCC has a large range of tumor volume doubling time (TVDT) from a few days to years with an estimated median of 178 days (Tang et al. 2018). In cirrhosis, the growth of a nodule is not highly specific for HCC, since other malignancies can grow. The growth rate is associated with the degree of tumor differentiation being slower in well-differentiated tumors and faster in poorly differentiated tumors. Based on the available evidences, the LI-RADS v2018 set the threshold growth as an increase in diameter of a mass by at least 50% in less than 6 months (minimum of 5 mm change) (American College of Radiology 2018) (Fig. 7). In Cerny et al. (2018a), the presence of threshold tumor growth had a sensitivity of 41.6% and a specificity of 83.2% for the diagnosis of HCC.

5 Hypointensity on HBP

The uptake of Gd-EOB-DTPA (gadoxetate disodium) into the hepatocytes is regulated by the membranous transporter organic anion transporting polypeptide 1B1/3 (OATP1B1/3). The expression of this transporter progressively decreases during hepatocarcinogenesis. Progressed HCC typically lacks the ability of incorporating Gd-EOB-DTPA, thus generally appearing hypointense on the images acquired during the HBP (20 min post Gd-EOB-DTPA contrast administration) (Choi et al. 2014) (Fig. 8). The use of Gd-EOB-DTPA increases the sensitivity for the detection of HCC (85–87%) compared to the use of extracellular contrast agents (61–77%) (Hanna et al. 2016; Roberts et al. 2018). However, lesion hypointensity on HBP is not a specific feature of HCC (Joo et al. 2015). False-positive lesions in cirrhosis, i.e., lesions that are hypointense on HBP but are not HCC, include hemangioma, confluent fibrosis, dysplastic nodule, ICC (Fig. 9), and cHCC-CCA (Choi et al. 2014). Finally, 5–12% of HCCs appear iso- or hyperintense on HBP images given the preserved expression of the OATP transporter (Fig. 10) (Kitao et al. 2010).

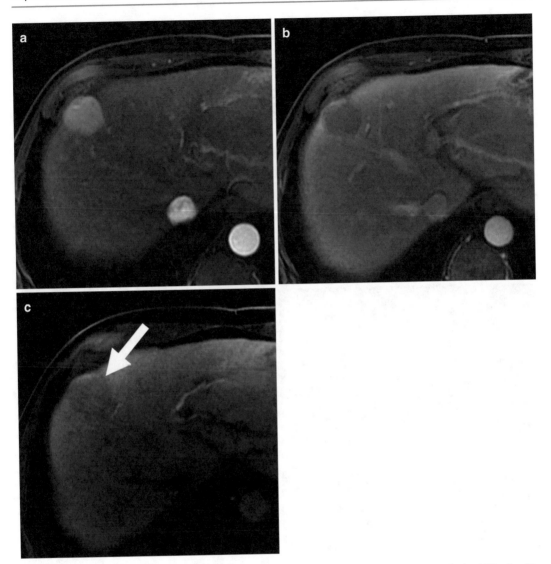

Fig. 8 53-year-old male with chronic hepatitis C and cirrhosis. Gd-EOB-DTPA-enhanced MR imaging shows a 3.0 cm lesion with arterial phase hyperenhancement (**a**), washout on portal venous phase (**b**), and hypointensity on the hepatobiliary phase (arrow, **c**) obtained 20 min after contrast administration. The imaging appearance is typical for a progressed hepatocellular carcinoma

6 Summary

APHE, washout, capsule, and growth are CT and MR imaging features commonly used in imaging guidelines for the noninvasive diagnosis of HCC. The combination of APHE and washout has high specificity although limited sensitivity. The use of Gd-EOB-DTPA and the evaluation of lesion hypointensity on the HBP images while increasing sensitivity may decrease specificity for the diagnosis of HCC.

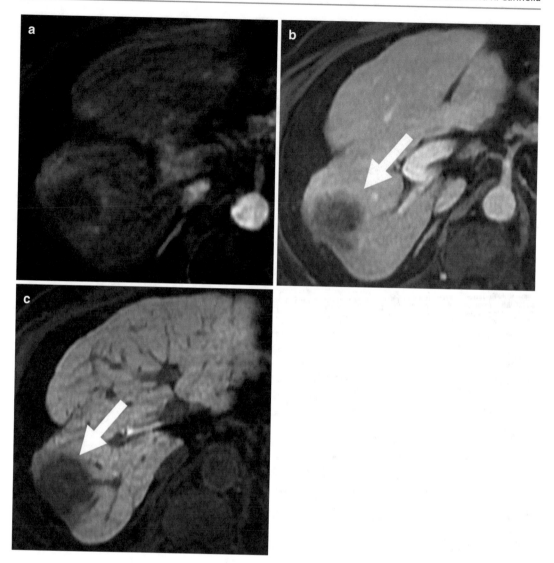

Fig. 9 70-year-old male with alcohol-induced cirrhosis. Gd-EOB-DTPA MR imaging shows a 4.8 cm mass with rim arterial phase hyperenhancement (arrow, **a**), centripetal enhancement on portal venous phase (arrow, **b**), and hypointensity on hepatobiliary phase (arrow, **c**). The lesion was classified as LR-M and biopsy-proven intrahepatic cholangiocarcinoma

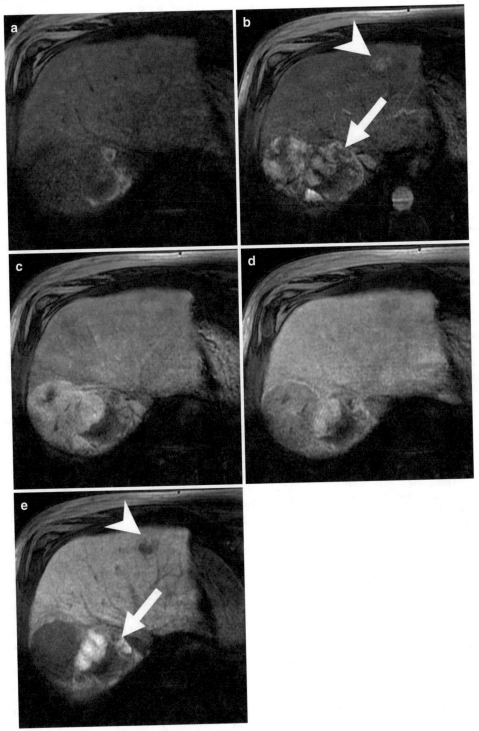

Fig. 10 65-year-old man with hepatocellular carcinoma (HCC). MR imaging obtained before (**a**) and after (**b–e**) the intravenous administration of Gd-EOB-DTPA. A large, complex mass in segment 7 shows hyperintensity on arterial phase (arrow, **b**) and lack of definitive washout on portal venous phase (**c**). While the lesion appears mainly iso- to hypointense on the transitional phase (**d**), a central component appears hyperintense on the hepatobiliary phase (arrow, **e**). Of note, the mass is mainly hypointense on the pre-contrast image (**a**). These images show also a small HCC presenting with arterial phase hyperenhancement (arrowhead, **b**) and hypointensity on hepatobiliary phase (arrowhead, **e**) (Case courtesy of Dr. Antonino Vallone, Ospedale Garibaldi Nesima, Catania, Italia)

References

American College of Radiology. Liver imaging reporting and data system. https://www.acr.org/Clinical-Resources/Reporting-and-Data-Systems/LI-RADS. Accessed on December 2018

An C, Park MS, Kim D et al (2013) Added value of subtraction imaging in detecting arterial enhancement in small (<3 cm) hepatic nodules on dynamic contrast-enhanced MRI in patients at high risk of hepatocellular carcinoma. Eur Radiol 4:924–930

Cerny M, Chernyak V, Olivié D (2018a) LI-RADS version 2018 ancillary features at MRI. Radiographics 38(7):1973–2001

Cerny M, Bergeron C, Billiard JS et al (2018b) LI-RADS for MR imaging diagnosis of hepatocellular carcinoma: performance of major and ancillary features. Radiology 288(1):118–128

Choi JY, Lee JM, Sirlin CB (2014) CT and MR imaging diagnosis and staging of hepatocellular carcinoma: part II. Extracellular agents, hepatobiliary agents, and ancillary imaging features. Radiology 273(1):30–50

Choi S, Lee SS, Kim SY et al (2017) Intrahepatic cholangiocarcinoma in patients with cirrhosis: differentiation from hepatocellular carcinoma by using gadoxetic acid-enhanced MR imaging and CT. Radiology 3:771–781

Forner A, Vilana R, Ayuso C et al (2008) Diagnosis of hepatic nodules 20 mm or smaller in cirrhosis: prospective validation of the non-invasive diagnostic criteria for hepatocellular carcinoma. Hepatology 1:97–104

Furlan A, Marin D, Vanzulli A et al (2011) Hepatocellular carcinoma in cirrhotic patients at multidetector CT: hepatic venous phase versus delayed phase for the detection of tumour washout. Br J Radiol 84(1001):403–412

Galia M, Taibbi A, Marin D et al (2014) Focal lesions in cirrhotic liver: what else beyond hepatocellular carcinoma? Diagn Interv Radiol 20(3):222–228

Hanna RF, Miloushev VZ, Tang A et al (2016) Comparative 13-year meta-analysis of the sensitivity and positive predictive value of ultrasound, CT, and MRI for detecting hepatocellular carcinoma. Abdom Radiol (NY) 41(1):71–90

Ishigami K, Yoshimitsu K, Nishihara Y et al (2009) Hepatocellular carcinoma with a pseudocapsule on gadolinium-enhanced MR images: correlation with histopathologic findings. Radiology 2:435–443

Jang HJ, Kim TK, Khalili K et al (2013) Characterization of 1- to 2-cm liver nodules detected on HCC surveillance ultrasound according to the criteria of the American Association for the Study of Liver Disease: is quadriphasic CT necessary? AJR Am J Roentgenol 201(2):314–321

Joo I, Lee JM, Lee DH et al (2015) Noninvasive diagnosis of hepatocellular carcinoma on gadoxetic acid-enhanced MRI: can hypointensity on the hepatobiliary phase be used as an alternative to washout? Eur Radiol 25(10):2859–2868

Khan AS, Hussain HK, Johnson TD et al (2010) Value of delayed hypointensity and delayed enhancing rim in magnetic resonance imaging diagnosis of small hepatocellular carcinoma in the cirrhotic liver. J Magn Reson Imaging 2:360–366

Kim TK, Lee KH, Jang HJ et al (2011) Analysis of gadobenate dimeglumine-enhanced MR findings for characterizing small (1-2 cm) hepatic nodules in patients at high risk for hepatocellular carcinoma. Radiology 259(3):730–738

Kitao A, Zen Y, Matsui O, Gabata T et al (2010) Hepatocellular carcinoma: signal intensity at gadoxetic acid-enhanced MR imaging—correlation with molecular transporters and histopathologic features. Radiology 256(3):817–826

Laghi A, Iannaccone R, Rossi P et al (2003) Hepatocellular carcinoma: detection with triple-phase multi-detector row helical CT in patients with chronic hepatitis. Radiology 226(2):543–549

Lee JH, Lee JM, Kim SJ et al (2012) Enhancement patterns of hepatocellular carcinomas on multiphasic multidetector row CT: comparison with pathological differentiation. Br J Radiol 85(1017):e573–e583

Luca A, Caruso S, Milazzo M et al (2010) Multidetector-row computed tomography (MDCT) for the diagnosis of hepatocellular carcinoma in cirrhotic candidates for liver transplantation: prevalence of radiological vascular patterns and histological correlation with liver explants. Eur Radiol 20(4):898–907

Marrero JA, Hissain HK, Nghiem HV et al (2005) Improving the prediction of hepatocellular carcinoma in cirrhotic patients with an arterially-enhancing liver mass. Liver Transpl 11(3):281–289

Oliver JH 3rd, Baron RL, Federle MP, Rockette HEJ (1996) Detecting hepatocellular carcinoma: value of unenhanced or arterial phase CT imaging or both used in conjunction with conventional portal venous phase contrast-enhanced CT imaging. AJR Am J Roentgenol 167(1):71–77

Park YN, Yang CP, Fernandez GJ et al (1998) Neoangiogenesis and sinusoidal "capillarization" in dysplastic nodules of the liver. Am J Surg Pathol 22(6):656–662

Pitton MB, Kloeckner R, Herber S et al (2009) MRI versus 64-row MDCT for diagnosis of hepatocellular carcinoma. World J Gastroenterol 28(48):6044–6051

Reynolds AR, Furlan A, Fetzer DT et al (2015) Infiltrative hepatocellular carcinoma: what radiologists need to know. Radiographics 35(2):371–386

Rimola J, Forner A, Tremosini S et al (2012) Non-invasive diagnosis of hepatocellular carcinoma ≤2 cm in cirrhosis. Diagnostic accuracy assessing fat, capsule and signal intensity at dynamic MRI. J Hepatol 56(6):1317–1323

Roberts LR, Sirlin CB, Zaiem F et al (2018) Imaging for the diagnosis of hepatocellular carcinoma: a systematic review and meta-analysis. Hepatology 67(1):401–421

Sangiovanni A, Manini MA, Iavarone M et al (2010) The diagnostic and economic impact of contrast imaging techniques in the diagnosis of small hepatocellular carcinoma in cirrhosis. Gut 59(5):638–644

Sersté T, Barrau V, Ozenne V et al (2012) Accuracy and disagreement of computed tomography and magnetic resonance imaging for the diagnosis of small hepatocellular carcinoma and dysplastic nodules: role of biopsy. Hepatology 55(3):800–806

Takayasu K, Arii S, Sakamoto M et al (2013) Clinical implication of hypovascular hepatocellular carcinoma studies in 4,474 patients with solitary tumour equal or less than 3 cm. Liver Int 33(5):762–770

Tang A, Bashir MR, Corwin MT et al (2018) Evidence supporting LI-RADS major features for CT- and MR imaging-based diagnosis of hepatocellular carcinoma: a systematic review. Radiology 286(1):29–48

Vogl TJ, Kümmel S, Hammerstingl R et al (1996) Liver tumors: comparison of MR imaging with Gd-EOB-DTPA and Gd-DTPA. Radiology 200:59–67

Yoon SH, Lee JM, So YH et al (2009) Multiphasic MDCT enhancement pattern of hepatocellular carcinoma smaller than 3 cm in diameter: tumor size and cellular differentiation. AJR Am J Roentgenol 6:W482–W489

Hepatocellular Carcinoma: Diagnostic Guidelines

Luis Martí-Bonmatí and Asunción Torregrosa

Contents

L. Martí-Bonmatí (✉) · A. Torregrosa
Department of Radiology and Biomedical Imaging
Research Group (GIBI230), Hospital Universitario y
Politécnico La Fe and Instituto de Investigación
Sanitaria La Fe, Valencia, Spain
e-mail: marti_lui@gva.es

Abstract

Imaging is used to screen, detect, characterized, grade, stage and follow-up hepatocellular carcinoma lesions and to evaluate the severity of the underlying liver disease. In this chapter, we will summarize the different worldwide diagnostic guidelines assisting

© Springer Nature Switzerland AG 2021
E. Quaia (ed.), *Imaging of the Liver and Intra-hepatic Biliary Tract*,
Medical Radiology Diagnostic Imaging, https://doi.org/10.1007/978-3-030-39021-1_9

decisions to be taken in the process of hepato-carcinogenesis with a deep insight into similarities and differences. The differences in modalities, protocols, dynamic and intracellular contrast-enhanced approaches, main and secondary criteria, vocabulary, ontology, terminology and pitfalls will be discus and highlighted. The structured standardized radiology reporting and radiomics quantitative information will be also highlighted.

1 Introduction

Radiology plays a crucial central role in the evaluation of malignant liver lesions in patients with chronic liver diseases. Different imaging modalities are used in the surveillance of patients at risk, aiming to detect, establish the diagnosis of, and stage hepatocellular carcinoma (HCC) lesions. Imaging also informs on the prognosis and guides treatment decisions, including transplantation, being able to assess treatment response. Imaging is also employed to evaluate the severity of the underlying liver disease.

The clinical pathways to properly perform all these important items are summarized under different diagnostic guidelines, considered as evidence-based statements assisting decisions to be taken in the process of hepatocarcinogenesis. There are many guidelines trying to facilitate and unify HCC management in imaging studies. Since 2001, these diagnostic systems have been proposed by different worldwide-based scientific organizations and societies, the published guidelines having clear similarities but also important dissimilarities (Tang et al. 2018; Yoon et al. 2016; Song et al. 2017; Cruite et al. 2013).

In this chapter, we will try to summarize these aspects related to tumor screening and imaging diagnostic criteria by the comparison of the main and most recently updated published guidelines, considering also a balanced geographical distribution. They are those currently endorsed by the Liver Cancer Study Group of Japan (LCSGJ 2014) (Kudo et al. 2014), Korean Liver Cancer Study Group-National Cancer Center (KLCSG-NCC, 2014) (Lee et al. 2014; Korean Liver Cancer Study Group and National Cancer Center

Korea 2015), European Society of Gastrointestinal and Abdominal Radiology (ESGAR 2016) (Neri et al. 2016), Asian Pacific Association for the Study of the Liver (APASL 2017) (Omata et al. 2017), National Health and Family Planning Commission of the People's Republic of China (NHFPC-PRCh 2018) (Zhou et al. 2018), American Association for the Study of Liver Diseases (AASLD and LI-RADS, 2018) (Marrero et al. 2018), and European Association for the Study of the Liver (EASL 2018) (Galle et al. 2018). The differences in ontology and terminology will be also highlighted.

2 Diagnostic Guidelines

Clinical diagnostic guidelines are considered systematically developed statements that are periodically updated and published to assist practitioner and patients to take decisions about appropriate healthcare for specific clinical circumstances. These recommendations are specifically devoted to efficaciously support clinical practice and improve quality of care through a standardized and evidence-based process. Guidelines should not be considered as rigid protocols but a basis on which clinicians can clearly consider the available options within the best level of confirmation and recommendation.

Clinicians dealing with HCC diagnosis need diagnostic guidelines to decrease unnecessary biopsies, decrease the false-positive and false-negative imaging reports, and facilitate access of patients to the best therapeutic options as soon as feasible. Since the expert consensus achieved in the 2000 Barcelona EASL Conference (Bruix et al. 2001), different guidelines have been published by scientific organizations and societies worldwide, assigning similar but also slightly different HCC imaging criteria as well as surveillance, follow-up, and treatment policies. The goal of diagnostic guidelines is not only to positively screen and precisely diagnose these patients but also to differentiate HCC from other lesions that can also occur in screened patient, such as benign biliary cysts, hemangiomas, FNH (focal nodular hyperplasia)-like lesions, sinusoid congestion, portal vein abnormalities and thrombosis with parenchyma pseudo-lesions, arterio-portal shunts, parasitic third flow, peliosis and telangiectasia, fibrotic changes and collapse, focal steatonecrosis, intrahepatic cholangiocarcinoma (ICC), and metastases.

Appropriate patient diagnosis and staging is currently based on the known carcinogenesis process and natural history of HCC, available diagnostic criteria, defined prognostic grades, agreed staging categories, and available treatment options. All these aspects are evaluated in most guidelines. As the etiology of the underlying liver disease differs in Europe, the United States, and Asia, guidelines might be different regarding the different tumor incidence, expression, and phenotyping. The influence of geographical distribution on the guidelines is mainly based on the a priori probability of HCC and the availability of some diagnostic techniques, such as contrast-enhanced ultrasonography (CE-US) with Sonazoid® which is only available, nowadays, in some Asiatic countries (Kudo et al. 2014; Omata et al. 2017). The real influence of geographical distribution on the guidelines has not been fully evaluated.

3   Risk Factors

Hepatocellular carcinoma is one of the most prevalent malignant tumors around the world, with a high overall incidence rate and cancer-related deaths. Around 850,000 new cases a year of HCC and 800,000 HCC-related deaths a year were reported from 2015 to 2018 (Global Burden of Disease Liver Cancer Collaboration 2017; Bray et al. 2018). Although the etiologic factors are multiple and highly based on the geographic location, 90% of HCC cases have a recognizable cause which converts it into a preventable tumor if we are able to avoid the risk factors that promote its development. This known multifactorial etiology also allows the development of screening programs.

Patients with chronic liver disease and cirrhosis are prone to carcinogenesis development in a complex and multistep process, involving the accumulation of both epigenetic and genetic events. The pathway initiates from the persis-

tently diseased liver microenvironment leading to the occurrence of hyperplastic and dysplastic nodules, ultimately inducting the cancerous process. Among the etiologic factors, the most frequently identified are the infection by hepatitis C virus (HCV) and hepatitis B virus (HBV), alcohol abuse, and other diffuse liver diseases, such as metabolic syndrome with non-alcoholic fatty liver disease (NAFLD), non-alcoholic steatohepatitis (NASH), and iron overload. The role of fatty liver as an HCC risk factor is probably underestimated, and its increasingly high prevalence should be seriously taken into consideration (Omata et al. 2017; Zhou et al. 2018; Marrero et al. 2018). Globally, HBV infection was the most common cause of incident cases and HCC-related deaths, particularly in East Asian countries, followed by alcohol and HCV infection in recent years (Marrero et al. 2018; Galle et al. 2018; Global Burden of Disease Liver Cancer Collaboration 2017). Also to be considered, different risk factors frequently co-exist in the same patient, further increasing the risk of HCC development. Regardless of the different causes, liver cirrhosis is the main factor in HCC development, being chronic viral infection the main single risk condition. It must be stated that also the frequency of ICC and combined HCC/CC is increased in patients with cirrhosis (Kudo et al. 2014; Marrero et al. 2018; Galle et al. 2018; Bruix et al. 2001; Global Burden of Disease Liver Cancer Collaboration 2017).

Primary prevention strategies are mandatory in all guidelines to reduce HCC incidence. Infant vaccination against HBV significantly decreases new infection cases, while the new direct antiviral agents for HCV, educational policies to reduce alcohol consumption, encouraging healthy eating, and fighting the sedentary way of life associated with metabolic syndrome are extremely important targets in the primary prevention of HCC (Korean Liver Cancer Study Group and National Cancer Center Korea 2015; Omata et al. 2017; Marrero et al. 2018; Galle et al. 2018).

Secondary prevention screening strategies, such as active surveillance of HCC risk patients, have shown their usefulness for the early detection of focal liver lesions that could be HCC in an early tumor stage, in which case curative or survival-increasing therapies are applicable. Active surveillance programs with liver ultrasonography (US) performed by well-experienced professionals every 6 months on patients suffering from HCC high-risk factors aim to detect small and early liver tumors. All the main guidelines establish this minimum time of every 6 months for the follow-up exam in the high-risk population (Kudo et al. 2014; Korean Liver Cancer Study Group and National Cancer Center Korea 2015; Omata et al. 2017; Zhou et al. 2018; Marrero et al. 2018; Galle et al. 2018).

Although most HCCs do not produce symptoms per se, they can be diagnosed at an early stage in economically developed countries where risk factors are present, and the prevalence of HCC allows the healthcare system to establish target screening programs. These programs are implemented in patients with chronic HCV and HBV infection and cirrhosis of all causes. Currently, active surveillance includes both Child-Pugh A and B patients for whom therapies that improve overall survival could be applicable. On the contrary, Child-Pugh C and decompensated patients with hepatorenal syndrome or clinical jaundice should not be screened as there is not effective HCC therapy in these situations. Patients waiting for a liver transplant for whom HCC detection would modify their waiting list allocation should be also screened (Marrero et al. 2018; Galle et al. 2018). Although patients with severe fibrosis, confirmed by either biopsy or elastography, should be included in an HCC active surveillance program, evidence is needed to consistently include patients with HBV infection, NAFLD, or diffuse liver diseases without advanced fibrosis or cirrhosis (Omata et al. 2017; Marrero et al. 2018; Galle et al. 2018). Patients with NASH are also considered as high-risk population for screening in China (Zhou et al. 2018). This Chinese guideline includes a family history of liver cancer, men older than 40 years with long-term alcohol abuse, or those who consume aflatoxin-contaminated food, and these items are generally not considered per se in Western guidelines. Imaging guidelines are usually not applied to young patients under 18 years of age, patients with cirrhosis due to congenital hepatic

fibrosis, and patients with cirrhosis due to vascular disorders such as Budd-Chiari (Elsayes et al. 2018). The Japan Society of Hepatology (JSH) guidelines (Kudo et al. 2014) divided the risk population into super-high-risk (HBV- and HCV-related liver cirrhosis) and high-risk (active chronic hepatitis B or C and non-viral etiology of liver cirrhosis) population, the first one being evaluated every 3–4 months.

In Europe and Western countries, alpha-fetoprotein (AFP) is not recommended during surveillance because the aim is to detect early HCC, which usually does not overproduce AFP, and exacerbation of the underlying liver inflammation might increase AFP levels (Marrero et al. 2018; Galle et al. 2018). However, AFP can be helpful to increase confidence in the positive identification of a nodule as HCC when the level is high ($\geq$20 ng/mL) (Omata et al. 2017). Even more, longitudinal changes in AFP may increase sensitivity and specificity (Marrero et al. 2018). In this sense, the KLCSG states that HCC nodules <1 cm can be diagnosed if typical features are seen in dynamic contrast-enhanced (DCE) exams with a continuously rising AFP with hepatitis activity under control (Yoon et al. 2016; Korean Liver Cancer Study Group and National Cancer Center Korea 2015). As a result, some guidelines include AFP in their routine surveillance in combination with liver US to improve accuracy (Kudo et al. 2014; Lee et al. 2014; Korean Liver Cancer Study Group and National Cancer Center Korea 2015; Omata et al. 2017; Zhou et al. 2018; Marrero et al. 2018). Nevertheless, Asia Pacific guidelines propose to raise AFP level until 200 ng/mL as cutoff value in order to increase specificity (Omata et al. 2017). Other liquid biopsy HCC markers under research evaluation, but not validated, include AFP-L3 (*Lens culinaris* agglutinin fraction of alpha-fetoprotein), DCP (des-γ-carboxy prothrombin), CTC (circulating tumor cells), NLR (neutrophil-to-lymphocyte ratio), OPN (osteopontin), and cfDNA (cell-free DNA). These biomarkers are only recommended in Japan (Amado et al. 2018). Up till now, serum tumor biomarkers are still considered suboptimal by most guidelines in terms of cost-effectiveness (Omata et al. 2017; Marrero et al. 2018; Galle et al. 2018).

4 Imaging Modalities and Techniques

Imaging plays a crucial role in the diagnostic process. Periodic liver US is considered, by all the guidelines, as the imaging modality of choice for HCC surveillance based on its acceptable accuracy, ease of use, availability and moderate cost, lack of ionizing radiation, and convenience. US also allows to depict subclinical complications such as ascites or portal vein thrombosis (Galle et al. 2018). The exam has to be performed by trained operators, allowing the depiction of small early tumors and their relationship with vessels. US elastography can also be performed at the same time, giving information on the parenchyma stiffness and, therefore, the fibrosis stage of the liver parenchyma.

Multiphase contrast-enhanced CT and MR imaging have more sensitivity than US exams but are more expensive and might have false-positive findings. Their use is usually restricted to those patients with a positive finding in US or in patients with a high risk of developing HCC even with a negative or technically suboptimal US study (Kudo et al. 2014; Korean Liver Cancer Study Group and National Cancer Center Korea 2015; Zhou et al. 2018; Marrero et al. 2018; Galle et al. 2018). Contrast-enhanced CT capability to detect and diagnose small liver tumor is slightly inferior to that of MR imaging, mainly due to the higher tissue contrast obtained with the different MR sequences and weightings. The multiparametric approach of MR imaging is obtained with the use of different sequences, such as T1-weighted (T1W), T2-weighted (T2W), diffusion-weighted (DW), and dynamic contrast-enhanced (DCE) images. Even more, the MR detection rate and differential diagnoses for small malignant lesions (≤ 1 cm) are improved with the added acquisition of the hepatobiliary phase after hepatocyte-specific contrast agent administration.

CT radiation exposure and MR higher cost are limitations of these techniques for screening purposes. CT is usually restricted to second-line modality when MR is not available or contraindicated. Only the KLCSG states that CT is essential for diagnosis and follow-up in HCC patients (Yoon et al. 2016; Korean Liver Cancer Study Group and National Cancer Center Korea 2015). However, CT is usually recommendable for presurgical patient evaluation (measurements of liver and tumor volume) and to rule out the presence of distant metastasis, mainly lung, adrenal, and bone metastases, in order to allocate the more appropriate treatment. Although 2 cm nodule diameter is well known as a cutoff beyond microvascular invasion and satellite nodules can appear (Galle et al. 2018), none of the main guidelines focuses on size-based criteria for chest, abdomen, and pelvis CT exam recommendation because extrahepatic spread would contraindicate surgical or liver transplantation as curative therapies. Patients with extrahepatic metastases had more advanced intrahepatic tumors at the first diagnosis, most metastases occurring from T3 or T4 tumors (Natsuizaka et al. 2005). Selective use of bone scan is indicated when skeletal symptoms are present at initial diagnosis of HCC and for monitoring disease while on the transplant waiting list or during or after treatment for response assessment. Regional metastatic lymph nodes are also associated with a higher probability of other metastatic sites. DCE studies might differentiate metastatic from benign lymphadenopathy when arterial enhancement is seen (Natsuizaka et al. 2005).

If a focal liver lesion is detected in liver US examination, HCC diagnosis should be confirmed with a dynamic imaging technique after a bolus contrast media administration to demonstrate the wash-in and wash-out signs, noninvasive criteria adopted by consensus at the EASL Conference as an imaging diagnostic hallmark due to their high specificity (Bruix et al. 2001). This pivotal role of imaging is unique in oncology as, even though many other tumors might have very specific radiological features, such as pancreatic adenocarcinoma, it is considered mandatory to obtain a histological sample before starting any oncologic treatment. However, in cirrhotic patients with a focal liver lesion having wash-in and wash-out in the multiphase DCE study, biopsy is not considered necessary due to the high specificity and positive predictive value of these noninvasive perfusion diagnostic criteria and the high pretest probability of HCC. All guidelines consider biopsy only in those cases without the typical radiological behavior and the lesion appearance is not typically benign. Also, biopsy is mandatory in cases suspicious of HCC in patients with non-cirrhotic or non-chronic liver disease. Importantly, a negative biopsy result does not exclude the possibility of liver cancer.

HCC tumor allows for a noninvasive diagnosis without histologic confirmation with nearly perfect specificity and positive predictive value in cirrhosis. All guidelines allow a positive HCC diagnosis if the lesion shows hyperenhancement on the late arterial phase (wash-in) and hypoenhancement on the venous or delayed phases (wash-out) in the dynamic examination. When a lesion is depicted on US, dynamic studies must be performed. In this setting, it is generally appreciated that DCE-MRI has a higher overall accuracy than DCE-CT and DCE-US. Most guidelines accept CT and MR as diagnostic examinations, while only some recognize the contribution of DCE-US (Omata et al. 2017). Vascularity is mandatory in HCC depiction as vascular supply change in the hepatocarcinogenesis process from the normal dual portal and arterial supply to lesion hypovascularity and then neoangiogenesis where new immature blood arterial vessels are formed. On pathological analysis, neoangiogenesis with increased arterial supply and diminished or absent portal flow are clear hallmarks of HCC development (Tochio and Kudo 2008).

However, other pathological hallmarks can be found in HCC carcinogenesis, including clear cell and fatty metamorphosis, increased cell density, pseudocapsule appearance formation, mosaic pattern, and biliary impairment. These other changes can be depicted with other techniques, including chemical shift, DW and hepatobiliary phase (HBP) MR imaging after hepatobiliary contrast media (HBCM) administration. Therefore, some guidelines also allow the diagnosis to be carried out on a less strict way, as a hypoenhanced lesion on the arterial phase having other typical features on the liver imaging reporting and data system (LI-RADS) stratification or hypointensity and defect on the HBP or the Kupffer phase on CE-US with Sonazoid®

(Omata et al. 2017; Chernyak et al. 2018). Considering that pathologically and phenotypically different HCC might have different dynamic imaging findings due to the lack of new arterialized neovascularization to produce hyperenhancement on the late arterial phase, especially in early small lesions detected in surveillance programs, and the enlarged interstitial space showing contrast enhancement with isointensity on the venous and/or equilibrium phases, it was crucial for some guidelines to include other complementary noninvasive diagnostic criteria. These differences between guidelines are also due to difference in prevalence, risk factors, and treatment strategies depending on the geographical distribution of the target population (Tang et al. 2018; Song et al. 2017).

There are also differences in the worldwide contrast agent's availability. Intravenous administered contrast media distribute within the intravascular and extracellular spaces, some of them also reaching the intracellular space for partial biliary excretion. In this chapter, contrast media will be classified regarding the differential pharmacokinetic distribution as intravascular (IVCM), extracellular (ECCM), and hepatobiliary contrast media (HBCM). In this sense, CT iodine- and MR gadolinium-based agents are considered ECCM. Gadobenate dimeglumine (Gd-BOPTA) has a large ECCM component with a small (close to 5%) but clinically relevant HBCM, while gadoxetic acid (Gd-EOB-DTPA) has similar ECCM and HBCM components (Kitao et al. 2011; Kogita et al. 2010; Gatto et al. 2013; Hope et al. 2015; Kim et al. 2013).

As dynamic phases after contrast administration are key in the diagnosis and staging of HCC, we will define them here. For both CT and MR, the main phases are the late arterial, portal, venous, and equilibrium ones. The late arterial phase is defined when the contrast media is preferentially within the hepatic artery and liver capillaries, even with initial portal enhancement, but with no contrast media within the hepatic veins. This late arterial phase should be obtained approximately 12 seconds after the aortic enhancement (bolus tracking technique, 100 HU threshold). A multi-arterial phase MR imaging is recommended if available in order to ensure the detection of arterial vascularization in HCC nodules (Neri et al. 2016). The portal phase is reached when the portal flow has the highest contrast media, approximately 48 s after the bolus arrival time, while the equilibrium, 90 s after the aortic enhancement, and delayed phases, 180 s after bolus arrival, represent the same parallel enhancement profiles within the interstitial and vascular compartments, both at the arterial and venous system.

On the other hand, all the guidelines recommend dynamic CT or MR with extracellular contrast as the standard or first-line techniques, but not all of them include hepatobiliary contrast agents or ultrasound contrast. For the Gd-EOB-DTPA, the equilibrium and delayed phases are considered transitional phases as interstitial, vascular, and hepatocyte compartments have the contrast media. The hepatobiliary phase is obtained at 120 min after Gd-BOPTA administration but only 10–20 min after Gd-EOB-DTPA administration (Yoon et al. 2016; Kudo et al. 2014; Neri et al. 2016; Zhou et al. 2018).

Additionally, US IVCM have different time protocols for lesion characterization as an HCC after a DCE study, as wash-out is defined later, more than 60 seconds after the contrast administration, and of mild degree. On the other hand, the reticuloendothelial-specific US contrast agent Sonazoid® is considered only in those guidelines which come from geographic areas where this is commercially available. Lesions are shown as hypoechoic nodules at the Kupffer phase imaging, which last for at least 60 min that allows examining the entire liver, improving tumor depiction and characterization (Galle et al. 2018).

Although digital angiography and positron emission tomography (PET) have been used for HCC depiction, they are not usually considered as their accuracy and availability are lower. Angiography is used for local treatment, such as embolization of bleeding arteries or chemo- and radioembolization. PET with ^{18}F-FDG can be used for staging and response evaluation, but its use is limited to distant metastases in selected cases. This technique has a high rate of false-negative results for early diagnosis (Galle et al. 2018).

There are many different available therapeutic options to treat these tumors. Best treatment options mainly depend on availability, experience, tumor stage, and functional liver condition. Although surgical resection and liver transplantation are considered standard curative options, several locoregional therapies such as ablation, chemoembolization, radioembolization, and systemic medical therapies, alone or in combination, are frequently used. Importantly, most HCC guidelines are not only focused on tumor diagnosis but also on the more effective and available therapeutic choice.

In this sense, many tumor scoring systems have been developed to stratify patients with HCC, based on several imaging-related tumor parameters, liver function, and patient's status. The Barcelona Clinic Liver Cancer (EASL-BCLC) system provides treatment recommendations for each clinical stage, linking them with an expected prognosis (Faria et al. 2014). This system is being endorsed mainly by Western countries' guidelines, having other guidelines from different world regions some differences in their approach to treatment allocation. Also, diagnostic and staging systems might vary in the treatment response evaluation and in the terminology and ontology used for the description of the findings, limiting the proper scientific communication between radiologists, hepatologists, and hepatic surgeons. All these aspects will be highlighted in the following lines.

5 Imaging Criteria

Diagnostic systems and structured radiology reporting are advocated by several societies as they improve consistency in reporting and overall positive predictive value for HCC diagnosis (Elsayes et al. 2018). Main imaging criteria to be considered when reporting on CT or MR in patients showing a lesion in a cirrhotic liver are summarized in this section, trying to keep imaging terms with accepted imaging vocabulary and ontology.

5.1　Size

Reason: Most lesions below 1 cm in patients with chronic liver disease are benign regenerating nodules (Marrero et al. 2018; Galle et al. 2018). The larger the lesions, the higher the probability to be neoplastic.

Criteria: Most guidelines use 1 cm as the threshold limit to separate those lesions smaller than 1 cm that should be followed up from the larger ones that should be diagnosed. The EASL states that nodules <1 cm in diameter detected by US should be followed every 4 months, for the first year, and every 6 months thereafter (Galle et al. 2018). This guideline states that most of these lesions will be regenerating-dysplastic nodules and biopsy is not needed. The diagnosis of HCC for nodules of >1 cm in diameter should be attempted on noninvasive DCE criteria, either on CT or MR. The role of DCE-US with Sonazoid® is being considered in APASL guidelines (Omata et al. 2017). Biopsy confirmation is required in case of uncertainty or atypical imaging findings, being a second biopsy recommended in case of inconclusive pathologic findings, tumor growth, or lesion enhancement during follow-up exams. Importantly, key criteria used in all guidelines to improve diagnostic specificity-sensitivity relate to the presence of a mass lesion, although 10% of HCCs are infiltrative, mainly higher grades, without compression, distortion, or displacement of normal parenchymal structures. The presence of an infiltrative lesion fulfilling diagnostic criteria should not limit a diagnosis. The Chinese guideline uses 2 cm as the threshold for the number of examinations needed to establish a positive diagnosis, needing at least two exams (from DCE-MR, DCE-CT, DCE-US) but allowing a positive diagnosis even in lesions smaller than 1 cm (Zhou et al. 2018). The LCSGJ and KLCSG-NCC guidelines allow subcentimeter-sized HCCs to be diagnosed when the lesion has all of the following criteria: typical vascular features of HCC observed with one or two CE imaging modalities plus a progressive increase in serum AFP levels with suppressed hepatitis activity, respectively (Yoon et al. 2016; Kudo et al. 2014; Lee et al.

2014). The APASL also allows a subcentimeter diagnosis after Gd-EOB-DTPA DCE and hepatobiliary phase images or Kupffer phase defect is seen after Sonazoid® (Omata et al. 2017). AASLD/LI-RADS uses various cutoff points to assign diagnostic categories (<1, 1–2, and >2 cm) depending on the presence of non-rim arterial hyperenhancement and additional major features (wash-out, capsule appearance, growth) (Marrero et al. 2018). Although lesions smaller than 1 cm cannot be classified as LR-5, those showing hypervascularity and one finding among wash-out, capsule, or threshold growth can be scored as probably HCC (LR-4) (Elsayes et al. 2018).

Pitfalls: As measurements have variability and inaccuracies, the closest the lesion size is to 1 cm, the less important should size threshold be considered as a limitation to the positive diagnosis of HCC. Also, even small lesions can be HCC and, therefore, should be either followed up or treated if imaging criteria are clearly positive for malignancy. In this sense, high-resolution images are improving the small lesion characterization rates. Of relevance, Japan and APASL guidelines do not consider size a limiting variable for HCC diagnosis if AFP is elevated and HBCM or Kupffer phase CE-US studies are available (Song et al. 2017).

5.2　Hypervascularity in the Late Arterial Phase

Reason: Tumor neoangiogenesis is a pathological hallmark of HCC. During carcinogenesis, the natural vessels are being substituted by abnormal arterial feeding vessels that generate a vivid arterial vascular supply to the tumor.

Criteria: Typical hallmark of HCC is the hypervascularity of the liver mass in the arterial phase, sometimes named the wash-in phenomena. Most tumors (>85%) will show a strong, fast, and homogeneous enhancement on the late arterial phase (Figs. 1 and 2). Ring annular and stable enhancement is not considered typical for HCC, and ICC or metastases should be considered in these cases, being biopsy mandatory (Marrero et al. 2018).

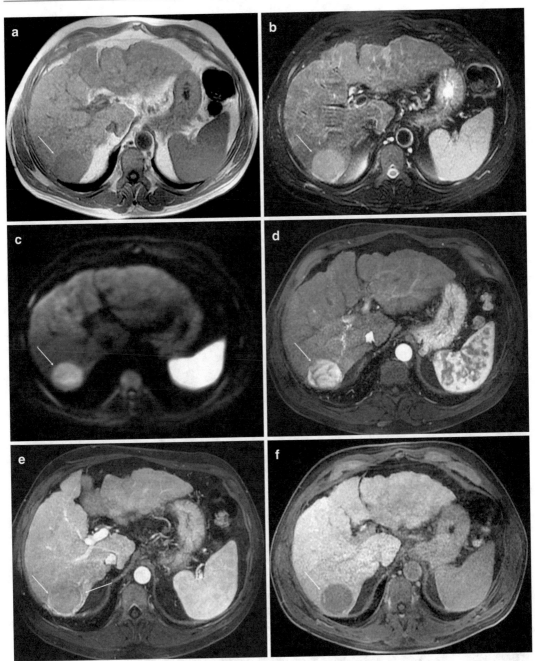

Fig. 1 Typical features of HCC in a cirrhotic patient. In-phase gradient echo T1W (**a**) and fat-suppressed T2W (**b**) images showing a hypointense (**a**) and hyperintense (**b**) liver nodule regarding the liver parenchyma. On the DW image (**c**), the lesion has an unequivocal signal hyperintensity due to restriction. After Gd-BOPTA administration, 3D fat-suppressed gradient echo T1W arterial (**d**) and portal (**e**) phase images demonstrate a hyperenhancement (**d**) and wash-out (**e**) regarding the liver parenchyma. Note the mosaic architecture with internal septa in the arterial phase and the capsule appearance in the portal venous phase. The hepatobiliary phase obtained 120 min after contrast administration (**f**) shows the nodule is hypointense to surrounding liver parenchyma

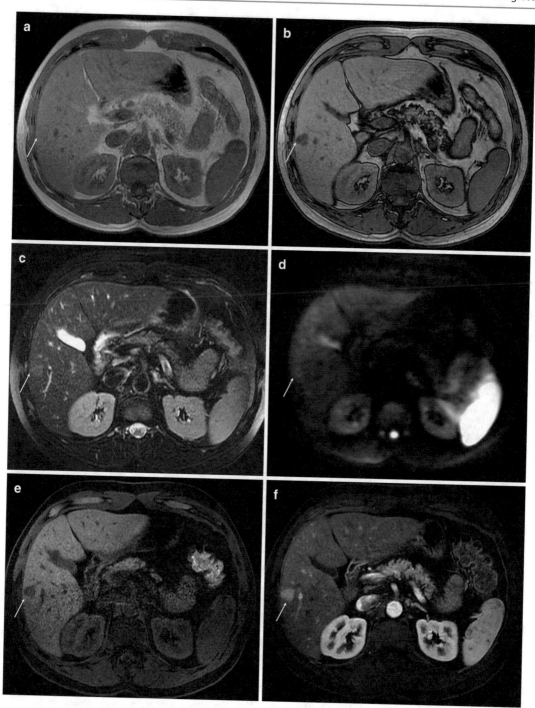

Fig. 2 Small HCC. In-phase (**a**) and opposed-phase (**b**) gradient echo T1W images show the nodule signal drop (**b**) due to the presence of fat and water within the same voxel. A mild hyperintensity occurs on T2W (**c**) and DW (**d**) images. Fatty metamorphosis is also shown as signal drop in pre-contrast fat-suppressed gradient echo T1W image (**e**). Post-contrast late arterial phase (**f**) and portal venous phase (**g**) T1W images show arterial hyper- and portal hypoenhancement regarding the liver parenchyma, respectively. In the hepatobiliary phase, the nodule is seen lacking HBCM uptake (**h**)

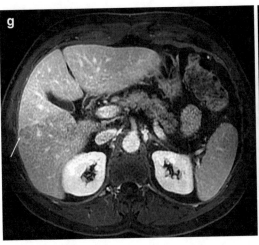
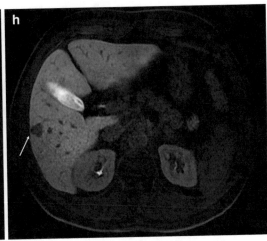

Fig. 2 (continued)

Pitfalls: In the early process of tumor development, neoangiogenesis might not be present. Low- and high-grade dysplastic nodules, early HCCs, and well-differentiated HCCs might be hypovascular (Yoon et al. 2016; Omata et al. 2017). In this sense, close to 15% of HCCs are hypovascular, and other imaging findings are needed to establish a confident diagnosis of HCC. Before hypovascularity is considered in a mass lesion, bolus arrival time and short plateau duration biases should be excluded. These relate to the fact that some modalities, such as CT and MR, do not sample the liver with the needed temporal resolution and nodules with a short hyperenhancement can be overlooked (Neri et al. 2016).

5.3 Wash-Out After the Late Arterial Phase

Reason: Most HCC lesions, mainly those more advanced in their oncologic progression, have internal vascular derangements, lacking internal portal veins and showing much less enhancement than the liver parenchyma in the portal and equilibrium phases after contrast administration.

Criteria: Wash-out is defined in CT and MR as lesion hypointensity in the portal venous (ECCM/HBCM) or delayed (ECCM) phases. Peripheral wash-out should not be considered typical for HCC (Marrero et al. 2018). It is mandatory in all guidelines that the mass exhibits wash-out in the portal phase (Figs. 1 and 2). When using ECCM, the equilibrium or delayed phases can also be used to define lesion hypointensity. If hepatobiliary contrast agents are being used in MR, such as gadoxetic acid (Gd-EOB-DTPA), the wash-out phase is mainly limited to the portal phase as some hepatocyte uptake is already present at the equilibrium phase, which can be confusing. The wash-out is defined on DCE-US as late onset (after 60 s) and of mild intensity (Galle et al. 2018).

Pitfalls: Close to 20% of HCC lesions are isointense to the liver parenchyma. The higher liver enhancement related to the degree of inflammation and fibrosis that is shown in the delayed phases could contribute to consider a wash-out as a dynamic criterion instead of a contrast intensity regarding the background liver. After Gd-EOB-DTPA, wash-out can only be defined as lesion hypointensity in the portal phase, as the equilibrium and delayed phases have a contribution of hepatocyte cellular enhancement, severely limiting accuracy.

5.4 Hypointensity in the Hepatobiliary Phase

Reason: When HBCM are used, those lesions without an appropriate active transport mechanism will be seen as hypointense nodules on the hepatobiliary phase. Most HCCs (80–90%) are hypointense in the HBP, helping to increase HCC depiction and differentiation from benign nodules developed on chronic liver diseases. Loosing OATP8 expression is one of the earliest changes associated with HCC (Yoon et al. 2016; Kudo et al. 2014; Omata et al. 2017).

Criteria: HBCM are uptake by the hepatocytes and export to the biliary channel through OATP8 and MRP2 export cell transporters, whose expression decreases in the hepatocarcinogenesis process even before the neoangiogenesis has been enough to produce hyperenhancement in the arterial phase (Kitao et al. 2011; Kogita et al. 2010). In the process from dysplastic nodule to HCC in a cirrhotic liver, the HBCM uptake by the nodule, relative to the hepatic parenchyma, decreases. Even though an overlapping is possible, it is well known that the majority of HCC and many high-grade dysplastic nodules have a hypointense appearance with regard to the liver surrounding parenchyma (Figs. 1 and 2). On the other hand, low-grade dysplastic nodules show iso- or hyperintense appearance on hepatobiliary phase (Gatto et al. 2013). Even more, hypointense solid nodules on the HBP have a higher risk of progression to typical HCC than iso- or hyperintense nodules (Kudo et al. 2014; Omata et al. 2017; Galle et al. 2018).

Pitfalls: Some of the commonest focal liver lesions such as flash-filling hemangiomas that typically have an arterial hyperenhancement and other malignancies will be hypointense on the hepatobiliary phase. Also to be considered, 10–20% of well-differentiated HCC will show uptake on this hepatobiliary phase due to an overexpression of OATP8 (Omata et al. 2017). In that case, the presence of a hypointense rim on the hepatobiliary phase would suggest HCC in an appropriate background (Hope et al. 2015). Moreover, radiologists should be aware of the appropriateness of the hepatobiliary phase in patients with liver functional damage in whom the hepatic enhancement and the conspicuity of the HCC may be impaired (Kim et al. 2013).

5.5 Tumor Capsule

Reason: There are few lesions with an external thick layer. Liver cell adenoma, hydatid cyst, and a few metastases can have this appearance. Capsule is the liver fibrotic reaction to lesion enlargement by expansion.

Criteria: A well-defined thick peripheral structure having well-defined both inner and outer borders and prolonged enhancement after contrast administration (Fig. 1). The signal intensity is slightly hypointense on T1W images and hyper- or isointense on T2W images. Sometimes, a double appearance can be seen, with a higher signal-intensity external layer on the T2W images. As fibrosis is the predominant histologic component, tumor capsule enhancement is seen at the portal phase, being prolonged on the equilibrium/delayed phases, being this finding the most important diagnostic criteria.

Pitfalls: Although unspecific, lesion capsule can be present in other liver lesions. However, a solid tumor with a peripheral thick capsule in a cirrhotic liver can be considered an HCC, as adenomas are not recognized in this setting, and hydatid cysts are non-enhancing lesions with a completely different appearance. Tumor capsule must be differentiated from distinctive peripheral rims, being smooth border with different signal intensity but without the typical contrast enhancement of the pseudocapsule. These distinctive rims are considered ancillary findings favoring malignancy, although they are not specific for HCC. Also, hypointense rim on transitional phase should not be regarded as capsule appearance but discrete rim, which is ancillary finding according to LI-RADS (Hope et al. 2015).

5.6 Tumor Growth

Reason: The rate of tumor growth is an important criterion that supports malignancy. In general terms, malignant lesions grow faster than benign due to the cellular duplication and neoangiogenesis. It is well known that hypervascular nodules and those in which portal blood flow is reduced in cirrhotic liver have a short doubling time and a high risk to become an HCC (Tochio and Kudo 2008).

Criteria: Tumor growth, mainly considered as mean tumor volume doubling time shorter than 86 days, is a relevant criterion. However, most guidelines do not consider a threshold growth as an HCC diagnostic criterion. Actually, they only include the enlargement of the lesion in the follow-up as a condition to proceed with corresponding diagnostic procedures when a detected nodule does not fit the typical noninvasive criteria. On the contrary, LI-RADS advocates the threshold growth as a major criterion. LI-RADS 2018 defines growth as an increase of at least 50% in 6 months or less. Former definitions of threshold growth such as a new observation of at least 10 mm in less than 24 months or an increase larger than 100% in more than 6 months are considered a subthreshold growth in the current version (Elsayes et al. 2018).

Pitfalls: It is mandatory to have previous examinations to include the tumor growth in the radiological evaluation. It is important to measure the lesion in the same plane and sequence trying to avoid the arterial phase in order to not include some peritumoral enhancement that could appear in this phase. Moreover, we should avoid measuring the lesion on DWI due to the possible image distortion.

5.7 Mild-Moderate T2 Hyperintensity

Reason: Most HCCs show intracellular and interstitial edema with high T2W signal intensity. Most regenerative and dysplastic nodes do not show this hyperintensity. ICC also shows hyperintensity, but usually as an outer hyperintense ring or a target appearance.

Criteria: Hyperintensity is mainly either homogeneous or with a mosaic appearance, some large homogeneous areas showing hyperintensity, while others are isointense (Figs. 1 and 2). Hyperintensity should not be seen as a peripheral ring or annular structure, as this finding is atypical in HCC and quite typical of ICC. Lesion hyperintensity must be differentiated from peripheral bad-defined edema, which, although unusual in HCC, can be found in case of fast-growing aggressive tumors. Sometimes, a nodule-within-a-nodule appearance is seen as a central small hyperintense region within an isointense tumor. This central hyperintensity, which usually suffers from different perfusion characteristics, should be considered an early HCC degeneration within a premalignant nodule.

Pitfalls: Other lesions in cirrhotic livers can be hyperintense. Hemangiomas and cysts are typically much brighter than HCC, with a completely different dynamic perfusion behavior.

5.8 Restricted Diffusion

Reason: Malignant tumors show hypercellularity with a decreased interstitial space, restricting the diffusion of water within the voxels. Lesion restriction favors malignancy, as most benign nodules do not show hyperintensity in the high b-value images. Regenerative and dysplastic nodules do not show restriction on the DW images.

Criteria: Hyperintensity on high b-value DW images should be either homogeneous or with a mosaic appearance (Fig. 1). Peripheral annular restriction is mainly typical for ICC.

Pitfalls: Restricted diffusion on the high b-value DW images can be misleading, as 25–85% of small HCC will not show a clear signal difference with the liver parenchyma as restriction is observed in those cases when the Child-Pugh score is high (Fig. 2). Liver restriction in chronic liver disease is probably related to the inflammatory activity and the increased sinusoidal deposits. Some hemangiomas might be hyperintense due to the T2 shine-through effect, which is easily excluded by the evaluation of the T2W images and the calculation of the ADC values of the lesion.

5.9 Corona Enhancement

Reason: This peripheral area of early enhancement after contrast media administration is due to the early drainage of the contrast material from hypervascular HCC into surrounding sinusoids.

Criteria: Peripheral area or even rim of transitional enhancement observed in the late arterial phase (Fig. 3), but sometimes extending also to the early portal phase, occurring in HCC with arterial hyperenhancement.

Pitfalls: Other hypervascular tumors might also have corona enhancement. It seems to be associated with microvascular invasion at the parenchyma close to the main tumor.

5.10 Portal Vein Thrombosis

Reason: Large HCC tumors have a tendency to disseminate through macrovascular vein invasion, which can also be seen in small tumors, being a major bad prognostic factor.

Criteria: Non-enhancement and absent flow within the main or intrahepatic portal veins in any CE study (CT, MR, US). Neither Doppler spectra nor color Doppler signal and increased luminal echogenicity are shown in US.

Pitfalls: Other lesions such as ICC and metastases might have portal vein thrombosis. Even more, portal vein thrombosis might also be present as a complication in cirrhotic livers without HCC. CE images can distinguish tumoral from non-tumoral portal vein thrombosis with high accuracy when arterial enhancement is seen within the obstructed vessel. On high b-value diffusion-weighted MR images, tumor thrombi have hyperintensity due to diffusion restriction.

5.11 Mosaic Architecture

Reason: The mosaic architecture is considered an ancillary feature that may favor HCC diagnosis.

Criteria: Some HCCs, particularly those >3 cm in diameter, have a heterogeneous hyperenhancement on arterial phase with fibrous septa that separate different parts into the nodule with different imaging features (enhancement, intensity, or attenuation) called mosaic architecture (Fig. 1). Probably, this reflects various stages of hepatocarcinogenesis and components in the same nodule (Neri et al. 2016). Mosaic is characteristic of large HCC, being useful to differentiate them from ICC.

Pitfalls: Small HCCs, usually, have a homogeneous hyperenhancement and mosaic architecture appearance being unusual to behave. In order to measure appropriately an HCC with a mosaic architecture, it is important to include all internal nodules that make up the lesion.

5.12 Intralesional Fat

Reason: Some HCC might show internal fatty metamorphosis. Clear cell microscopic transformation in HCC is mainly related to well-differentiated tumors.

Criteria: A signal intensity drop in the T1W opposed-phase gradient echo (GRE) images in comparison with the in-phase images is characteristic of the presence of both fat and water components within the same voxel. This microscopic fat deposition within the cytoplasm of malignant hepatocytes is extremely characteristic of HCC (Fig. 2).

Pitfalls: Other liver tumors with inner fat are adenomas and FNH. Adenomas are considered a well-differentiated HCC in patients with chronic liver disease and therefore are not a differential diagnosis in this setting. FNH with steatosis is unusual and has been reported in normal livers. Metastases from liposarcoma are secondary to a known primary extrahepatic fatty tumor.

5.13 Intralesional Blood Products

Reason: The presence of hemorrhage into or surrounding a lesion helps to diagnose a nodule as HCC in a cirrhotic liver. Actually, this sign is

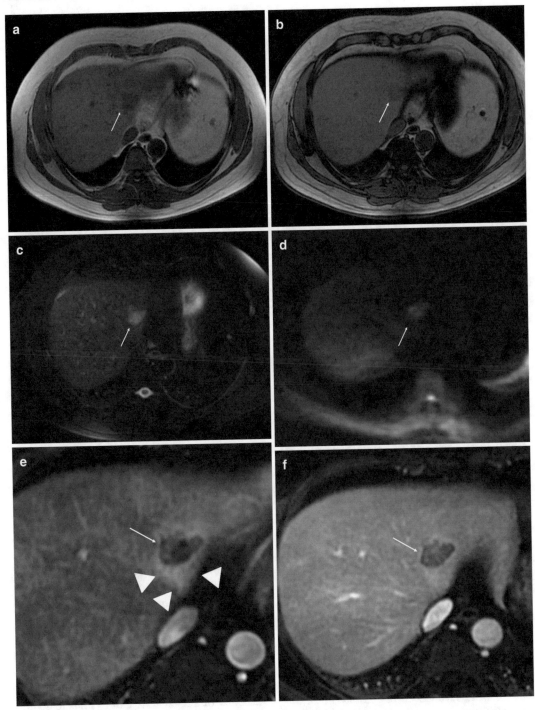

Fig. 3 Atypical HCC in HCV-infected patient. In-phase (**a**) and opposed-phase (**b**) gradient echo T1W images show a hypointense focal liver lesion that behaves as hyperintense on fat-suppressed T2W (**c**) and DW (**d**) images. On the dynamic contrast-enhanced images, the nodule is hypovascular in the arterial (**e**), portal (**f**), and delayed (**g**) phases. Corona enhancement surrounding the lesion is seen as a bad-defined hyperenhanced area in the arterial phase (arrowhead). The lesion is hypointense in the hepatobiliary phase (**h**). Pathologic specimen showed an undifferentiated hepatocellular carcinoma

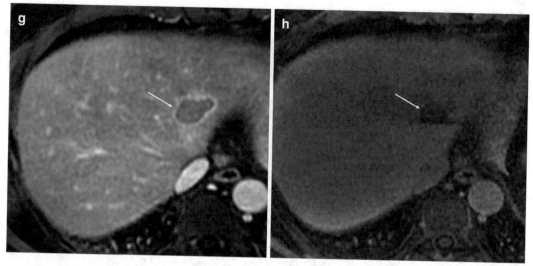

Fig. 3 (continued)

considered as an ancillary criterion for HCC in LI-RADS guidelines in absence of trauma, biopsy, or treatment.

Criteria: The presence of blood products into some focal liver lesions is more frequent in those hypervascularized lesions with arterial hyperenhancement such as HCC and hepatic adenoma. It is well known the risk of hemorrhage of these lesions and their clinical presentation with hemoperitoneum due to spontaneous bleeding.

The MR appearance depends on the stage of blood, with hyperintensity on T1W images in case of acute or subacute bleeding. On the other hand, the CT appearance of a hemorrhagic nodule can be hyperattenuated in all phases.

Pitfalls: We should be aware of the particular appearance of the different stages of blood products in MR sequences. It could be mandatory to perform subtraction imaging to detect enhancement on T1W images in a hemorrhagic nodule. The same in case of CT images, in which the intranodular hemorrhage can mimic hyperenhancement if unenhanced images are not available. Moreover, the nodular size reduction due to the blood product involution does not favor benignity.

5.14 Lesional Fat or Iron Sparing

Reason: Both lesional fat and iron sparing in a fatty liver or iron-overloaded liver background are characteristics that support malignancy. As a diffuse liver disease that involves the whole liver, a growing nodule that does not contain neither fat nor iron is suspicious of malignancy.

Criteria: Although fat content into a suspicious nodule supports HCC diagnosis, the lesional fat sparing in fatty liver is an ancillary feature that favors malignancy, not specifically HCC, but this diagnosis can be considered in the cirrhosis background if more specific HCC criteria are present, particularly with any dynamic criteria. The nodule will show higher signal intensity in whole or in part than the low signal surrounding liver parenchyma on out-phase T1W images.

Iron sparing in a solid mass is defined as the loose of iron in a nodule that grows with regard to the surrounding iron-overloaded liver or in the center of a regenerative or dysplastic nodule that cumulates iron. It can be attributed to growing iron resistance cells often malignant (Chernyak et al. 2018). It shows higher signal intensity than the surrounding nodule or liver parenchyma on in-phase chemical shift T1W and T2*W images. Both features can be also evaluated on CT images based on decreased or increased liver attenuation in fat or iron deposition, respectively.

Pitfalls: As fat sparing liver parenchyma with associated alteration of perfusion is relatively frequent in liver diseases, it is important to take into consideration fat sparing feature only in case of a solid mass that shows enhancement alteration at least in one dynamic phase. In case of iron sparing, radiologists should be aware of confluent fibrosis that can mimic a lesional iron sparing.

6 Multivariable Tumor Definition

Reason: All guidelines use the wash-in/wash-out main criteria for HCC diagnosis. However, some HCCs will be either hypovascular at the late arterial phase or have no clear hypointensity at the portal or equilibrium phases in the CE studies (Fig. 3). Therefore, some ancillary findings might be used to increase sensitivity and specificity, avoiding the use of biopsy if proven accurate. Although ancillary findings might be most valuable in nodules <2 cm in diameter, any liver lesion in a cirrhotic liver without the typical CE dynamic behavior will benefit from a positive accurate diagnosis. Somewhat, a nodule should not be defined as hypovascular before another dynamic technique is performed, including CE-US (Bota et al. 2012). Strategies suggested to improve diagnostic accuracy with the incorporation of ancillary findings are gaining interest. The certainty of diagnosis and effectiveness of therapy represent a high priority of this approach.

Criteria: The AASLD guideline endorsed the LI-RADS reporting system (Marrero et al. 2018). The LI-RADS also uses imaging features as criteria for HCC, including enhancing capsule and threshold growth (Elsayes et al.

2018; Kitao et al. 2011). Other ancillary features favoring HCC but not being able to provide a definitively positive diagnosis are enhancing T2W hyperintensity, diffusion restriction, hepatobiliary phase hypointensity, corona enhancement, mosaic architecture, nodule-in-nodule appearance, lesional fat or hemorrhage, and lesional fat or iron sparing. LI-RADS establishes diagnostic categories, from definitive and probably benign HCC (LI-RADS 1 and 2), low probability and probable HCC (LI-RADS 3 and 4), and definite HCC (LI-RADS 5). LI-RADS M is assigned to any malignant lesions not being specific for HCC, including features characteristic of ICC such as rim arterial hyperenhancement, peripheral wash-out, delayed central enhancement, or targetoid appearance at the diffusion or HBP images. Overall probability of HCC in LI-RADS 5 lesions is quite high (95–99%) (Marrero et al. 2018; Elsayes et al. 2018).

The ESGAR guideline states that if either one of the major vascular criteria (wash-in/wash-out) is lacking, hypointensity on the HBP plus restricted diffusion on high b-values or hyperintensity on T2W images is highly suspicious for HCC (Neri et al. 2016). Inclusion of these additional features increased sensitivity from 78 to 88% and decreased specificity from 80 to 75%, resulting in higher accuracy (84%) and larger area under the curve (AUC) (81.5). Although the differences were not statistically significant, the sensitivity, specificity, accuracy, and overall diagnostic ability of LI-RADS criteria were slightly higher than with the ESGAR criteria (Rosiak et al. 2018).

The APASL guideline (Omata et al. 2017) also states that the combined interpretation of DCE and hepatobiliary phase images after Gd-EOB-DTPA administration together with diffusion-weighted images improves the diagnostic accuracy of MR, but only for detection purposes.

The JSH states that hypovascular nodules that are also hypointense in the hepatobiliary phase and hypoechoic in the Kupffer phase of Sonazoid® CE-US can be diagnosed as early HCC even without biopsy (Kudo et al. 2014).

The criteria developed in our own facility use the two major vascular hallmarks and seven minor complementary criteria, including pseudo-capsule, fatty metamorphosis, T2W and T1W hyperintensity, mosaic pattern, vascular invasion, and diffusion restriction with hyperintensity on high b-value images. A positive imaging diagnosis of HCC is stablished with at least one major finding plus at least two minor criteria. The called VLC-MV is a very accurate classification system with 98.5% of positive predictive value, higher than LI-RADS and EASL guidelines (Marti-Bonmati et al. 2017).

Pitfalls: The increased positive diagnosis has to be balanced with an increased false-positive rate (Yoon et al. 2016; Omata et al. 2017). In this sense, a recent study using CT showed a higher diagnostic performance and sensitivity, with the same specificity that guidelines using only the vascular hallmark (wash-in/wash-out) criteria compared to LI-RADS (Seo et al. 2019). On the other hand, none of the cited guidelines state how to differentiate between dysplastic nodules, especially high-grade ones, and HCC. Also, as patients with history of HCC have greatest risk of tumor recurrence (Lee et al. 2014; Korean Liver Cancer Study Group and National Cancer Center Korea 2015), lesions <1 cm should be clearly considered HCC if typical hallmarks are found, mainly if minor findings are also present.

7 Structured Report

Standardized diagnostic and reporting systems have improved the communication between radiologists and clinicians, favoring to take the right decisions on the multidisciplinary meetings. Although most guidelines do not consider the use of structured report (SR) in their implementation, this tool is extremely helpful in the clinical setting.

To be useful, SR items should be defined after a comprehensive literature review with an in-depth decision in a multidisciplinary committee, consisting of radiologists, hepatologists, surgeons, and pathologists, all of them specialists in primary liver tumors. Most SR are based on HTML format and are compatible with Management of Radiology Report Templates (MRRT), and SR includes mainly customized checkbox for each item to be defined on the radiology report, most of them being drop-down lists. Web-based platforms allow the construction and progressive filling of the generated information on a centralized database. All data is finally stored for further analysis and research. In our institution, the following sections are included: (1) technique (CT/MR, field strength, contrast media type and dose, sequences and phases, hepatocellular phase, and technical limitations); (2) morphologic criteria of cirrhosis hallmarks (portal hypertension, splenomegaly, varices, shunts, thrombosis); (3) untreated lesions (number, location, size, LI-RADS diagnosis); (4) treated lesions (response criteria: mRECIST); and (5) other organ lesions (pancreas, adrenals, kidneys, and lymph nodes). Then, the report finalized with a staging classification and a proposed treatment to be considered by the multidisciplinary committee. The Milan criteria and any other local relevant information are also provided (Fig. 4). The final diagnosis can be adjusted to any (or different) guideline.

SR developments allow to incorporate radiomics quantitative information related with the digital analysis and processing of the data from the acquired images to accurately and precisely describe the biological properties and behavior of tissues by means of radiomics characteristics and dynamic parameters (Martí-Bonmatí et al. 2018).

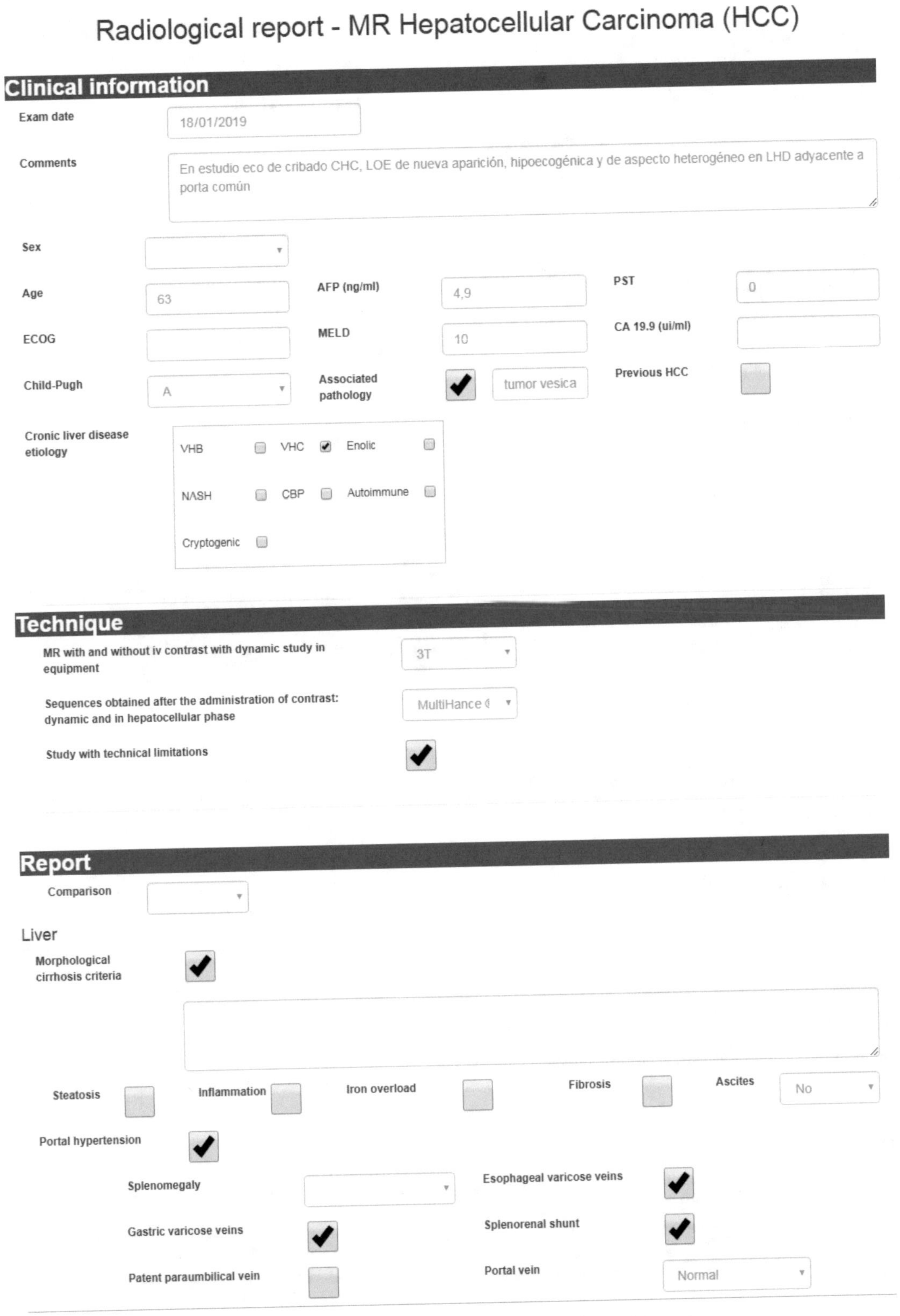

Radiological report - MR Hepatocellular Carcinoma (HCC)

Clinical information

Exam date
18/01/2019

Comments
En estudio eco de cribado CHC, LOE de nueva aparición, hipoecogénica y de aspecto heterogéneo en LHD adyacente a porta común

Sex

Age 63 **AFP (ng/ml)** 4,9 **PST** 0

ECOG **MELD** 10 **CA 19.9 (ui/ml)**

Child-Pugh A **Associated pathology** ✔ tumor vesica **Previous HCC** ☐

Cronic liver disease etiology

VHB ☐ VHC ☐ Enolic ✔

NASH ☐ CBP ☐ Autoimmune ☐

Cryptogenic ☐

Technique

MR with and without iv contrast with dynamic study in equipment 3T

Sequences obtained after the administration of contrast: dynamic and in hepatocellular phase MultiHance ◊

Study with technical limitations ✔

Report

Comparison

Liver

Morphological cirrhosis criteria ✔

Steatosis ☐ **Inflammation** ☐ **Iron overload** ☐ **Fibrosis** ☐ **Ascites** No

Portal hypertension ✔

Splenomegaly Esophageal varicose veins ✔

Gastric varicose veins ✔ Splenorenal shunt ✔

Patent paraumbilical vein ☐ Portal vein Normal

Fig. 4 Hepatocellular carcinoma structured report at Hospital Universitario y Politécnico La Fe

Lesions

Number of treated lesions [ ]

Number of untreated lesions [2]

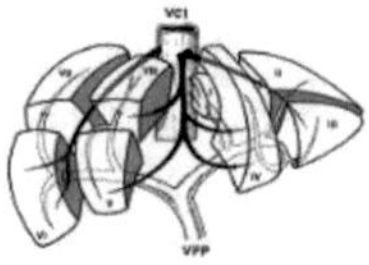

Number of untreated lesions	Segment	Diameter (mm)	HUPLF - ACIM diagnosis [?]	LI/RADS diagnosis [?]	
L1	8	21	Yes	LR-5	Definitely HCC

Multifocal [ ]   **Infiltrative** [ ]

Major HCC criteria

Hypervascular [✔]   Washout [?] [✔]

Minor HCC criteria

Mild hyperintensity in T2 [✔]	Intratumoral bleeding [ ]	Nodule-in-nodule [ ]
Mosaic pattern [ ]	Diffusion restriction [✔]	Hypointensity in hepatobiliary phase [✔]
Macrovascular invasion [ ]	Microvascular invasion [ ]	Intraperitoneal rupture [ ]
Direct invasion of adjacent organs [ ]		

Intrahepatic Cholangiocarcinoma criteria

Consider CCC / HCC-CCC [ ]

Other findings

Dudoso trombo mural en la unión portomesentérica

Extrahepatic metastasis in the visualized structures [ ]

Incidental findings not related to the hepatic tumour

Benign hepatic lesions [ ]

Other organs

Pancreas [Normal]   Adrenal glands [Normal]

Kidneys [Normal]   Lymph nodes [Normal]

Other [ ]

Fig. 4 (continued)

Staging

EASL-HUPLF staging and management strategies

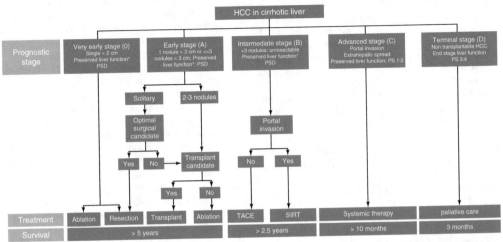

*Preserved liver function = Child-Pugh A without ascites

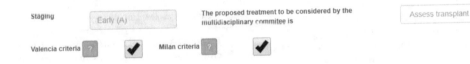

SUMMARY

TECHNIQUE

MR with and without iv contrast with dynamic study in equipment 3T
Sequences obtained after the administration of contrast: dynamic and in hepatocellular phase: MultiHance ®
Study with technical limitations.

REPORT

Liver

Morphological cirrhosis criteria:
It is observed: portal hypertensionsplenomegaly moderada (12 cm - 19 cm), gastric varicose veins, esophageal varicose veins, splenorenal shunt and portal vein normal

Lesions

- Untreated lesions: 2

- Lesion in segment 8 with a diameter of 21 mm
HCC diagnosis according to HUPLF-ACIM criteria: Yes
LI-RADS diagnosis: LR-5

- Lesion in segment 6 with a diameter of 23 mm
HCC diagnosis according to HUPLF-ACIM criteria: Yes
LI-RADS diagnosis: LR-4

Other findings

Dudoso trombo mural en la unión portomesentérica

Other organs

Pancreas - Normal
Adrenal glands - Normal
Kidneys - Normal
Lymph nodes - Normal

CONCLUSION

Staging: Early (A)
The proposed treatment to be considered by the multidisciplinary commitee is: Assess transplant
It meets the Milan criteria
It meets the Valencia criteria

Fig. 4 (continued)

References

Amado V, Rodríguez-Perálvarez M, Ferrín G, De la Mata M (2018) Selecting patients with hepatocellular carcinoma for liver transplantation: incorporating tumor biology criteria. J Hepatocell Carcinoma 21(6):1–10

Bota S, Piscaglia F, Marinelli S, Pecorelli A, Terzi E, Bolondi L (2012) Comparison of international guidelines for noninvasive diagnosis of hepatocellular carcinoma. Liver Cancer 1:190–200

Bray F, Ferlay J, Soerjomataram I, Siegel R, Torre L, Jemal A (2018) Global Cancer Statistics 2018: GLOBOCAN estimates of incidence and mortality worldwide for 36 cancers in 185 countries. Cancer J Clin 68:394–424

Bruix J, Sherman M, Llovet JM, Beaugrand M, Lencioni R, Burroughs AK et al (2001) Clinical management of hepatocellular carcinoma. Conclusions of the Barcelona-2000 EASL conference. J Hepatol 35:421–430

Chernyak V, Tang A, Flusberg M, Papadatos D, Bijan B, Kono Y et al (2018) LI-RADS® ancillary features on CT and MRI. Abdom Radiol (NY) 43 82 100

Cruite I, Tang A, Sirlin CB (2013) Imaging-based diagnostic systems for hepatocellular carcinoma. AJR Am J Roentgenol 201(1):41–55

Elsayes KM, Kielar AZ, Elmohr MM et al (2018) White paper of the Society of Abdominal Radiology hepatocellular carcinoma diagnosis disease-focused panel on LI-RADS v2018 for CT and MRI. Abdom Radiol (NY) 43(10):2625–2642

Faria SC, Szklaruk J, Kaseb AO, Hassabo HM, Elsayes KM (2014) TNM/Okuda/Barcelona/UNOS/CLIP international multidisciplinary classification of hepatocellular carcinoma: concepts, perspectives, and radiologic implications. Abdom Imaging 39:1070–1087

Galle PR, Forner A, Llovet JM, Mazzaferro V, Piscaglia F, Raoul JL et al (2018) EASL clinical practice guidelines: management of hepatocellular carcinoma. J Hepatol 69:182–236

Gatto A, De Gaetano AM, Giuga M, Ciresa M, Siciliani L, Miele L et al (2013) Differentiating hepatocellular carcinoma from dysplastic nodules at gadobenate dimeglumine-enhanced hepatobiliary-phase magnetic resonance imaging. Abdom Imaging 38:736–744

Global Burden of Disease Liver Cancer Collaboration, et al (2017) The burden of primary liver cancer and underlying etiologies from 1990 to 2015 at the global, regional, and national level results from the global burden of disease study 2015. JAMA Oncol 3(12):1683–1691

Hope TA, Fowler KJ, Sirlin CB, Costa EAC, Yee J, Yeh BM et al (2015) Hepatobiliary agents and their role in LI-RADS. Abdom Imaging 40:613–625

Kim JY, Lee SS, Byun JH, Kim SY, Park SH, Shin YM et al (2013) Biologic factors affecting HCC conspicuity in hepatobiliary phase imaging with liver-specific contrast agents. AJR Am J Roentgenol 201:322–331

Kitao A, Matsui O, Yoneda N, Kozaka K, Shinmura R, Koda W et al (2011) The uptake transporter OATP8 expression decreases during multistep hepatocarcinogenesis: correlation with gadoxetic acid enhanced MR imaging. Eur Radiol 21:2056–2066

Kogita S, Imai Y, Okada M, Kim T, Onishi H, Takamura M et al (2010) Gd-EOB-DTPA-enhanced magnetic resonance images of hepatocellular carcinoma: correlation with histological grading and portal blood flow. Eur Radiol 20:2405–2413

Korean Liver Cancer Study Group (KLCSG) National Cancer Center Korea (NCC) (2015) 2014 KLCSG-NCC Korea practice guideline for the management of hepatocellular carcinoma. Gut Liver 9(3):267–317

Kudo M, Matsui O, Izumi N, Iijima H, Kadoya M, Imai Y et al (2014) JSH consensus-based clinical practice guidelines for the management of hepatocellular carcinoma: 2014 update by the Liver Cancer Study Group of Japan. Liver Cancer 3:458–468

Lee ML, Park JW, Choi BI (2014) 2014 KLCSG-NCC Korea practice guidelines for the management of hepatocellular carcinoma: HCC diagnostic algorithm. Dig Dis 32:764–777

Marrero JA, Kulik LM, Sirlin CB, Zhu AX, Finn RS, Abecassis MM et al (2018) Diagnosis, staging, and management of hepatocellular carcinoma: 2018 practice guidance by the American Association for the Study of Liver Diseases. Hepatology 68:723–750

Marti-Bonmati L, Torregrosa A, Navarro V, Rubin A, Breso L (2017) Magnetic resonance widened diagnostic criteria for hepatocellular carcinoma. Hellenic J Radiol 2(4):19–26

Martí-Bonmatí L, Ruiz-Martínez E, Ten A, Alberich-Bayarri A (2018) How to integrate quantitative information into imaging reports for oncologic patients. Radiologia 60(Suppl 1):43–52

Natsuizaka M, Omura T, Akaike T et al (2005) Clinical features of hepatocellular carcinoma with extrahepatic metastases. J Gastroenterol Hepatol 20:1781–1787

Neri E, Bali MA, Ba-Ssalamah A, Boraschi P, Brancatelli G, Caseiro-Alves F et al (2016) ESGAR consensus statement on liver MR imaging and clinical use of liver-specific contrast agents. Eur Radiol 26:921–931

Omata M, Cheng AL, Kokudo N, Kudo M, Lee JM, Jia J et al (2017) Asia-Pacific clinical practice guidelines on the management of hepatocellular carcinoma: a 2017 update. Hepatol Int 11:317–370

Rosiak G, Podgorska J, Rosiak E, Cieszanowski A (2018) Comparison of LI-RADS v.2017 and ESGAR guidelines imaging criteria in HCC diagnosis using MRI with hepatobiliary contrast agents. Biomed Res Int:7465126

Seo N, Kim MS, Park MS et al (2019) Optimal criteria for hepatocellular carcinoma diagnosis using CT in patients undergoing liver transplantation. Eur Radiol 29(2):1022–1031

Song P, Cai Y, Tang H, Li C, Huang J (2017) The clinical management of hepatocellular carcinoma worldwide: a concise review and comparison of current guidelines from 2001 to 2017. Biosci Trends 11(4):389–398

Tang A, Cruite I, Mitchell DG, Sirlin CB (2018) Hepatocellular carcinoma imaging systems: why they exist, how they have evolved, and how they differ. Abdom Radiol (NY) 43:3–12

Tochio H, Kudo M (2008) Intranodular blood supply correlates well with biological malignancy grade determined by tumor growth rate in pathologically proven hepatocellular carcinoma. Oncology 75:55–64

Yoon JH, Park JW, Lee JM (2016) Noninvasive diagnosis of hepatocellular carcinoma: elaboration on Korean Liver Cancer Study Group-National Cancer Center Korea practice guidelines compared with other guidelines and remaining issues. Korean J Radiol 17(1):7–24

Zhou J, Sun HC, Wang Z et al (2018) Guidelines for diagnosis and treatment of primary liver cancer in China (2017 edition). Liver Cancer 7(3):235–260

Benign Lesions in Cirrhosis

Roberta Catania, Amir A. Borhani,
and Alessandro Furlan

Contents

Abstract

The accurate diagnosis of benign lesions in a cirrhotic liver is clearly important to avoid misdiagnosis of hepatocellular carcinoma (HCC) or other malignancies and to direct the patient toward the most appropriate management. In this chapter we review the appearance of the most common benign lesions encountered on CT and MR imaging of a cirrhotic liver. The lesions are divided into two main groups depending on the histological composition as non-hepatocellular lesions (i.e., cysts and peribiliary cysts, hemangiomas, pseudolesions) and hepatocellular lesions (i.e., nonmalignant cirrhosis-associated nodules, focal nodular hyperplasia like nodules, and hepatobiliary hypointense nodules without arterial phase hyperenhancement).

R. Catania
Department of Radiology, University of Pittsburgh Medical Center, Pittsburgh, PA, USA

Department of Radiology, University of Pavia, Pavia, Italy

A. A. Borhani · A. Furlan (✉)
Department of Radiology, University of Pittsburgh Medical Center, Pittsburgh, PA, USA

© Springer Nature Switzerland AG 2021
E. Quaia (ed.), *Imaging of the Liver and Intra-hepatic Biliary Tract*,
Medical Radiology Diagnostic Imaging, https://doi.org/10.1007/978-3-030-39021-1_10

1 Non-hepatocellular Lesions

1.1 Peribiliary Cysts and Hepatic Cysts

Peribiliary cysts result from dilatation of obstructed periductal glands and have a prevalence of 9% in cirrhotic patients (Baron et al. 1994; Bazerbachi et al. 2018). They are usually multiple and seen along the portal triads in the hilum and central part of liver (Elsayes et al. 2018; Ronot et al. 2017). Peribiliary cysts do not communicate with the bile ducts but may mimic biliary ductal dilatation (Baron et al. 1994). Their presence on both sides of portal vein without upstream biliary dilatation is key finding for a proper diagnosis (Ronot et al. 2017) (Fig. 1). When the diagnosis is unclear on contrast-enhanced CT or MR cholangiography, injection of a hepatobiliary contrast agent (i.e., Gd-EOB-DTPA or Gd-BOPTA) may be considered to differentiate the contrast-enhanced bile ducts from the unenhanced peribiliary cysts on hepatobiliary phase (Bazerbachi et al. 2018; Ronot et al. 2017). Size progression of peribiliary cysts has been reported with worsening of the liver disease and rarely results in biliary obstruction (Bazerbachi et al. 2018).

Hepatic cysts in cirrhosis do not usually represent a diagnostic challenge as they maintain the same imaging appearance as in non-cirrhotic livers (Ronot et al. 2017). The lack of enhancement and the bright signal intensity on T2-weighted MR images are key features for a confident diagnosis.

1.2 Hemangiomas

Hemangiomas are among the most common benign lesions, but are less frequently encountered in cirrhotic patients (Dodd et al. 1999; Duran et al. 2015). In the early stages of hepatic fibrosis hemangiomas show a classic appearance including peripheral nodular and progressive enhancement that remains isoattenuating/isointense to blood pool, as well as high signal intensity on T2-weighted MR images (Brancatelli et al. 2001) (Fig. 2). As fibrosis progresses, hemangiomas become smaller and may lack the

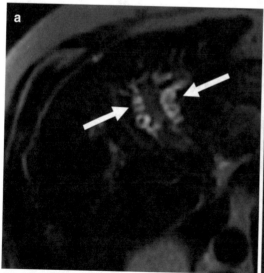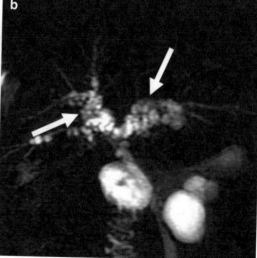

Fig. 1 Axial T2-weighted MR image (**a**) in a 63-year-old man with cirrhosis and para-coronal thick slab MR cholangiography image (**b**) in a 78-year-old man with cirrhosis show multiple small cystic lesions (arrows in **a**, **b**) compatible with peribiliary cysts. The location of the cysts on both sides of the portal vein and the lack of upstream biliary ductal dilatation are key features for a proper diagnosis

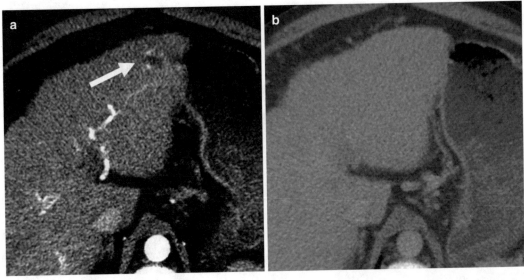

Fig. 2 Axial contrast-enhanced CT images in a 53-year-old-male with history of alcoholic cirrhosis show a small hypodense nodule with peripheral nodular enhancement (arrow) on the image obtained during the arterial phase (**a**). The nodule is isoattenuating on the image obtained during the portal venous phase (**b**). The diagnosis of hemangioma was pathologically proven at fine needle biopsy

typical imaging features, thus making it difficult to characterize radiologically (Brancatelli et al. 2001). Additionally, regressing hemangiomas may show capsular retraction further complicating the differential diagnosis with other lesions in cirrhosis. In such cases, other imaging features may help in the differential diagnosis with HCC, including the low signal intensity on diffusion weighted images and the evolution over time from prior studies. More recently, Duran et al. (Duran et al. 2015) found no significant difference in the rate of typical enhancement pattern on MR images for hemangiomas arising in a normal liver compared to those arising in a fibrotic or cirrhotic liver.

The radiologists using Gd-EOB-DTPA-enhanced MR for the surveillance of HCC in cirrhotic patients should be aware of an important diagnostic pitfall related to the diagnosis of hemangiomas. Flash-filling hemangiomas are usually hypointense on hepatobiliary phase images and may appear hypointense also on the images acquired during the transitional phase (i.e., delay of at least 120 seconds post-contrast). The phe-

nomenon, referred as "pseudo-washout," is due to the rapid uptake of contrast agent in the surrounding liver after the extracellular phase and may result in misdiagnosis of HCC (Chernyak et al. 2019; Doo et al. 2009). This phenomenon emphasizes that washout for the diagnosis of HCC should only be assessed during the portal venous phase, when using Gd-EOB-DTPA as the contrast agent, in order to reduce the number of false-positive diagnoses (Joo et al. 2015).

1.3 Pseudolesions

Pseudolesions are observations only detected on imaging in absence of a true pathological lesion (Papadatos et al. 2018). Vascular pseudolesions are usually due to arterioportal shunting, as a consequence of the altered microcirculation in cirrhosis (American College of Radiology 2018). They classically appear as triangular-shaped, subcapsular, hyperenhancing areas visible only on the images obtained during the arterial phase (Fig. 3). When they appear round,

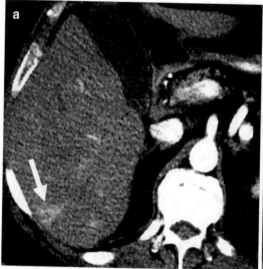

Fig. 3 Axial contrast-enhanced CT image obtained during the arterial phase (**a**) shows a triangular-shaped, subcapsular hyperenhancing "lesion" (arrow) lacking washout on the corresponding image obtained during the portal venous phase (**b**). The combination of imaging features and enhancement pattern is most compatible with a pseudolesion, such as arterioportal shunt in cirrhosis

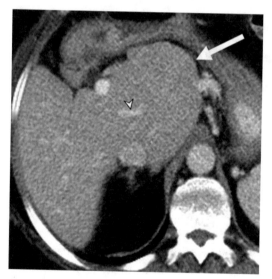

Fig. 4 Axial contrast-enhanced CT image obtained during the portal venous phase shows a hypertrophic caudate lobe (arrow) simulating a liver mass. The "lesion" iso-attenuation to the background liver parenchyma and the lack of mass effect on vessels (arrowhead) are key imaging features to exclude malignancy

the isodensity/isointensity to the background liver on all other phases and sequences and the lack of mass effect on vascular and biliary structures are clues to differentiate them from HCC (Murakami and Tsurusaki 2014). Other pseudolesions that can be encountered in cirrhosis include a hypertrophic pseudomass and confluent hepatic fibrosis (Papadatos et al. 2018; Elsayes et al. 2018). A hypertrophic pseudomass is a hypertrophic area of liver surrounded by fibrosis mimicking a mass on imaging (Fig. 4). A hypertrophic pseudomass can be differentiated from HCC or other malignancies on the basis of iso-enhancement to the background parenchyma and lack of mass effect on vessels or bile ducts. Confluent hepatic fibrosis (or focal parenchymal extinction) is a focal or regional area of marked increased fibrosis and parenchymal loss compared to the surrounding liver parenchyma (Wanless et al. 1995). On imaging, confluent hepatic fibrosis typically appears as wedge-shaped observations, peripherally located most often in segments 4, 5, and 8 and associated with liver surface retraction and delayed enhancement (Ohtomo et al. 1993) (Fig. 5). The morphology and the typical location as well as the progressive contraction at imaging follow-up are key features for a correct diagnosis (Elsayes et al. 2018).

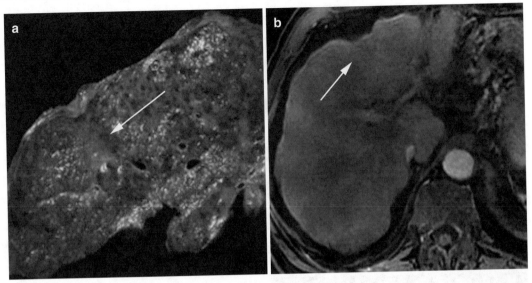

Fig. 5 Gross pathology specimen (**a**) demonstrating cirrhosis and confluent hepatic fibrosis (arrow). Axial T1-weighted MR images obtained during the delayed phase postinjection of Gd-BOPTA (**b**) demonstrate wedge-shaped area of delayed enhancement with capsular retraction (arrow) compatible with confluent hepatic fibrosis

2 Hepatocellular Lesions

2.1 Regenerative and Dysplastic Nodules

Cirrhosis is the endpoint of a long-standing fibrotic repair process in response to repetitive injuries (Papadatos et al. 2018). The key pathologic features of cirrhosis are bridging fibrosis surrounding regenerative nodules (RN), also called cirrhotic nodules. RNs are composed of nonneoplastic hepatocytes and are histologically and radiologically identical to the background liver. On contrast-enhanced cross-sectional imaging, RNs are not hypervascular and mostly appear isointense compared to the surrounding liver on all MR sequences, including the images obtained during the hepatobiliary phase (American College of Radiology 2018; Ronot et al. 2017) (Fig. 6). Dysplastic nodules are caused by clonal expansion of a certain cell lineage and are typically distinct from the background parenchyma. They may have a higher content of fat and iron compared to the surrounding liver which may result in intrinsic hyperintensity on T1-weighted imaging (American College of Radiology—LI-RADS 2018). Based on the presence and degree of atypia DNs are further classified into low-grade and high-grade subtypes (Ronot et al. 2017). Low-grade DNs are histologically benign although they have the potential to become neoplastic due to presence of molecularly aberrant cells (American College of Radiology—LI-RADS 2018). High-grade DNs are the last step in the hepatocarcinogenetic process (premalignant nodules) before early and progressed HCC. High-grade DNs show cellular and architectural atypia without stromal invasion or other malignant features (Choi et al. 2015). They may show changes in their blood supply resulting in imaging features commonly described in HCC, such as arterial phase hyperenhancement because of arterial neo-angiogenesis and hypointensity on the hepatobiliary phase after injection of Gd-EOB-DTPA because of reduced expression of the organic anion transporter (OATP), the peptide responsible for the intracellular accumulation of Gd-EOB-DTPA (Motosugi et al. 2015) (Fig. 7).

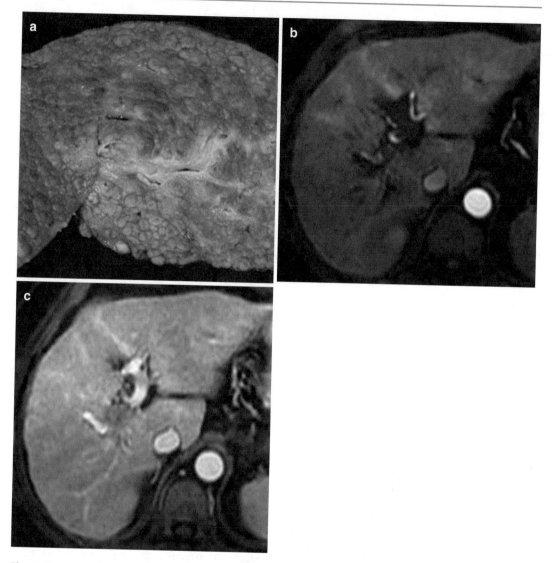

Fig. 6 Gross pathology specimen (**a**) of a cirrhotic liver shows innumerable tan, regenerative nodules delineated by fibrous septa. On the axial T1-weighted MR images obtained during the arterial (**b**) and portal venous (**c**) phases after injection of Gd-BOPTA, the regenerative (cirrhotic) nodules are barely visible and only minimally hypoenhancing on the portal venous phase image

2.2 Focal Nodular Hyperplasia-Like Nodules

Focal nodular hyperplasia (FNH) is a benign hepatic lesion arising as a hyperplastic response to a congenital vascular malformation in an otherwise normal liver (Vilgrain et al. 1992). FNH-like lesions are microscopically, macroscopically, and immunohistochemically identical to FNH but occur in patients with liver diseases or hepatic vascular abnormalities (Yoneda et al. 2016; Vilgrain 2006). Although rare in cirrhosis, FNH-like nodules have been described more often when the etiology of liver disease is alcoholic with an incidence ranging from 3.4 to 8% (Quaglia et al. 2003; Libbrecht et al. 2006) (Fig. 8). In a cirrhotic background, these nodules likely arise from a hyperplastic hepatocellular response to a localized arterial over-inflow caused by focal angio-architectural

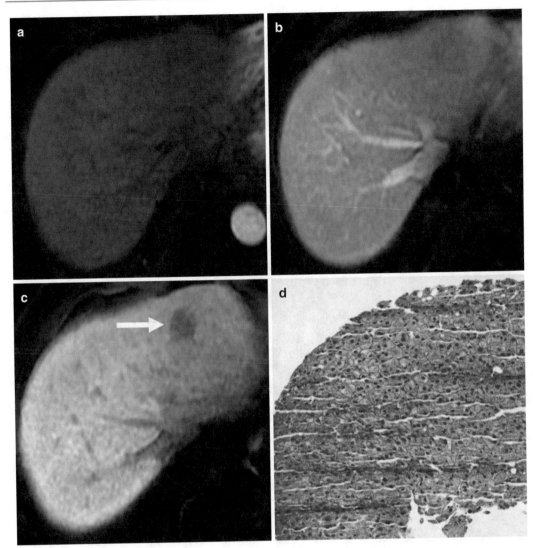

Fig. 7 Axial MR images of a cirrhotic liver obtained during the arterial (**a**), portal venous (**b**), and hepatobiliary phase (**c**) following injection of Gd-EOB-DTPA show a small hepatobiliary hypointense nodule (arrow in **c**) without arterial phase hyperenhancement. Hematoxylin and eosin staining of the specimen (**d**) obtained at ultrasound-guided core biopsy of the lesion shows areas of increased cellularity with hepatocytes displaying uniform hyperchromatic nuclei with slightly increased nuclear/cytoplasmic ratio and focal irregular nuclear contour, suggesting a dysplastic nodule. The lesion was monitored with repeated MR imaging studies and developed arterial phase hyperenhancement (arrow in **e**) and portal venous washout (arrow in **f**) 5 years later while maintaining hypointensity on hepatobiliary phase (arrow in **g**). The microscopic evaluation of the surgical specimen post resection (**h**) demonstrates hypercellular proliferation of hepatoid appearing cells in a trabecular pattern with pseudo-acini, bile production, and Mallory hyaline compatible with hepatocellular carcinoma. Unpaired (so-called aberrant) arteries were also identified (black arrows in **h**, inlet) (Images **d** and **h** are courtesy of Marta I. Minervini, MD, Department of Pathology, University of Pittsburgh)

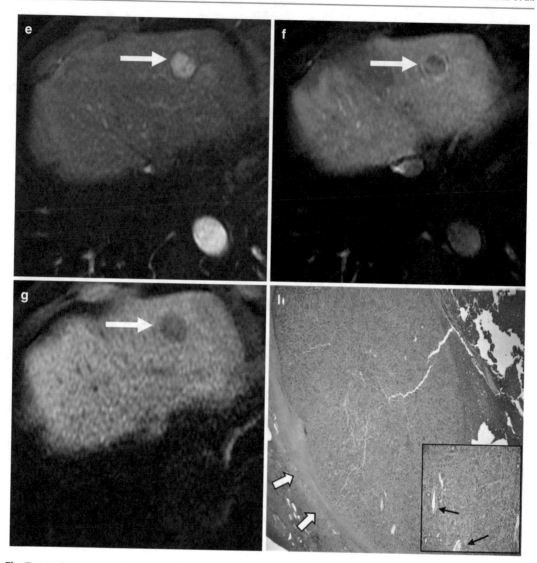

Fig. 7 (continued)

anomalies (Nakashima et al. 2004). Histologically, FNH-like lesions may show a modest increase in cell density with irregular trabecular pattern, unpaired arteries, and diffuse capillarization of the sinusoids similar to well-differentiated HCC. In such cases, immunohistochemistry is helpful, demonstrating increased staining for HSP70 GPC3 and glutamine synthetase in FNH-like lesions (Choi et al. 2011). On contrast-enhanced cross-sectional imaging FNH-like lesions generally present with brisk arterial phase hyperenhancement, lack of washout on the extracellular phase images, and iso- to hyperintensity on the images acquired during the hepatobiliary phase postinjection of Gd-BOPTA or Gd-EOB-DTPA (Figs. 9 and 10). The signal intensity on hepatobiliary phase images is key for differentiating FNH-like lesions from HCC. Most HCCs are hypointense on hepatobiliary phase images, although 10–15% of HCC have been reported to be iso- to hyperintense given the overexpression of OATP (also referred as "paradoxical uptake"). The most common appearance of both FNH-like lesions and HCCs with contrast uptake on hepatobiliary phase images is diffuse

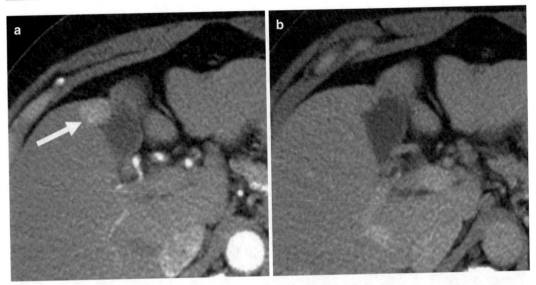

Fig. 8 Axial contrast-enhanced CT images in a 57-year-old male with history of alcoholic cirrhosis show a 2 cm lesion with homogeneous enhancement on the image obtained during the arterial phase (arrow in **a**) and lack of washout on the image obtained during the portal venous phase (**b**). A FNH-like nodule was pathologically proven at resection

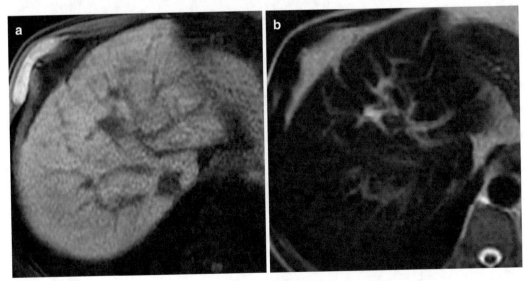

Fig. 9 Axial MR images obtained prior to (**a, b**) and following (**c–e**) the administration of Gd-EOB-DTPA in a 64-year-old male with history of cirrhosis. The image obtained during the hepatobiliary phase (**e**) shows multiple small hyperintense lesions (arrow) which appear iso-intense on pre-contrast T1- (**a**) and T2-weighted (**b**) and post-contrast images obtained during the arterial (**c**) and portal venous (**d**) phases. The pathological analysis of the specimen obtained via ultrasound-guided biopsy of the lesion reveals changes similar to those seen in FNH lesions. The immunohistochemistry for glutamine synthetase (**f**) shows increased diffuse positive hepatocyte uptake without a definite maplike pattern. The CD34 staining (**g**) demonstrates diffuse capillarization of the hepatic sinusoids (Images (**f, g**) are courtesy of Marta I. Minervini, MD, Department of Pathology, University of Pittsburgh)

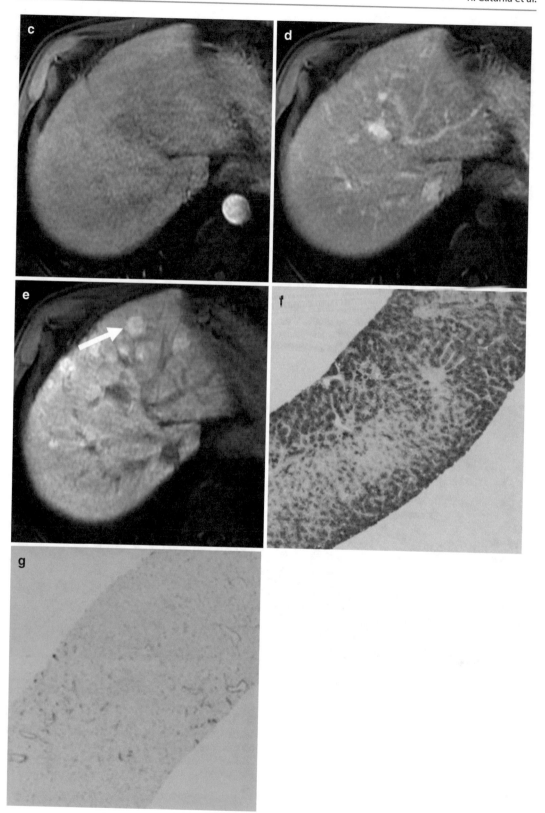

Fig. 9 (continued)

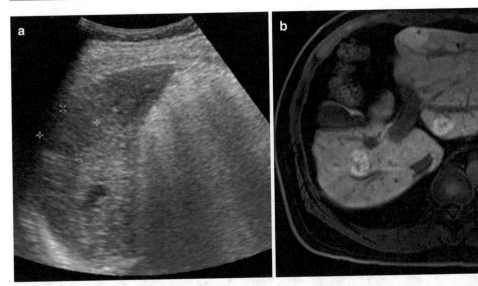

Fig. 10 Surveillance ultrasound (**a**) in a cirrhotic patient shows an ill-defined hypoechoic nodule prompting further evaluation with contrast-enhanced MR. Axial (**b**) Gd-EOB-DTPA-enhanced MR image obtained during the hepatobiliary phase shows several hyperintense lesions with central hypointense scar suggesting FNH-like lesions. At follow-up MR imaging studies (not shown), the lesions remained stable in size (Case courtesy of Dr. Jessica Yang, MD, Concord Repatriation General Hospital, Sydney, Australia)

homogeneous hyperintensity. Other patterns of signal distribution have also been described, which could help with the diagnosis. A mosaic pattern and a nodule-in-nodule appearance are typical of HCC while a doughnut pattern is more commonly seen in FNH-like nodule. Presence of washout, a low ADC value, and the absence of a central scar are other features helpful to differentiate HBP hyperintense HCC from FNH-like lesion (Kim et al. 2017; Kitao et al. 2018). Finally, longitudinal assessment of changes in lesion size is important because FNH-like lesions tend to show no change or decrease in size over time. Recently a new subset of FNH-like lesions has been described in alcoholic cirrhosis which shows strong immune-reactivity to serum amyloid A (SAA) with histologic features commonly seen in inflammatory adenomas including sinusoidal dilatation, ductular reaction, and inflammatory reaction (Yoneda et al. 2016). While FNH-like nodules are typically iso- to hyperintense on hepatobiliary phase images, SAA-positive nodules may appear hypointense (Yoneda et al. 2016; Sasaki et al. 2015).

2.3 Hepatobiliary Hypointense Nodules Without Arterial Phase Hyperenhancement

This is a separate group of hepatocellular nodules encountered in cirrhotic patients after injection of hepatobiliary contrast agent (Motosugi et al. 2015; Motosugi et al. 2018). Although discussed in this chapter, pathologically these lesions may represent either early HCC or high-grade DNs (Golfieri et al. 2011). The key element to differentiate early HCCs from dysplastic nodules on histologic examination is the presence of stromal invasion, a feature that is not possible to discern on imaging (American College of Radiology 2018; Motosugi et al. 2015). Early HCC is a well-differentiated tumor usually described as "vaguely nodular" (The international Consensus Group for Hepatocellular neoplasia 2009). On imaging, early HCCs typically lack the hallmark arterial phase hyperenhancement of progressed HCCs, given the combination of reduced number of portal triads and a not-yet-fully-developed arterial neo-angiogenesis. These lesions are typically hypovascular during the dynamic contrast-enhanced CT or Gd-enhanced MRI study and have reduced expression of OATP, thus resulting in hypointensity on hepatobiliary phase compared to the surrounding liver parenchyma after injection of Gd-EOB-DTPA. Hepatobiliary hypointense nodules without arterial phase hyperenhancement should be carefully evaluated because of the increased risk of progression to typical HCC (Motosugi et al. 2015). A recent meta-analysis showed that 18.3, 25.2, and 30.3% of these nodules develop arterial phase hyperenhancement at 1, 2, and 3 years, respectively (Fig. 7). In contrast, only less than 1% of hypovascular nodules isointense on hepatobiliary phase images develop arterial hyperenhancement on subsequent imaging (Suh et al. 2017) (Fig. 11).

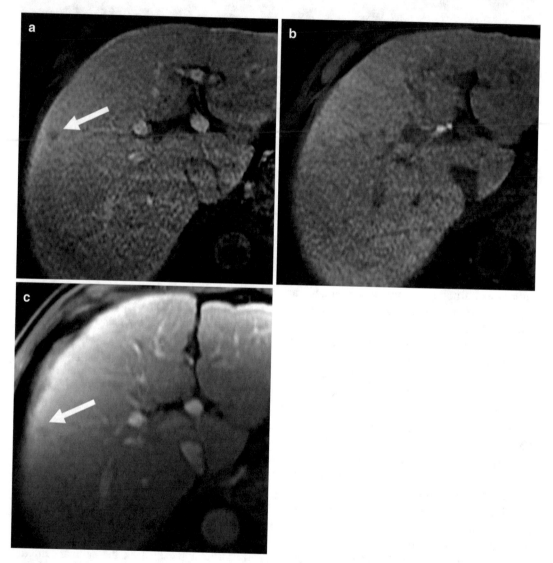

Fig. 11 Axial MR images of a cirrhotic liver obtained during the portal venous (**a**) and hepatobiliary (**b**) phases following injection of Gd-EOB-DTPA show a small hypoenhancing lesion (arrow in **a**), which is isointense compared to the surrounding liver on hepatobiliary phase. The lesion was monitored with MRI for years. In an MR imaging study obtained 7 years later, the lesion shows long-term size stability and hypovascular appearance on portal venous phase (**c**). Arterial phase images (not showed) also demonstrate lack of arterialization after 7 years

The risk of progression to arterial hyperenhancement is associated with the initial nodule size (i.e., higher risk for nodules larger than 9 mm), the presence of intralesional fat, and the high signal intensity on T2-weighted and diffusion-weighted images (Suh et al. 2017). Moreover, the presence of these nodules increases the risk of developing cancer elsewhere in the liver and the risk of recurrence of HCC after resection (Komatsu et al. 2014; Toyoda et al. 2013). The management of hepatobiliary hypointense nodules without arterial phase hyperenhancement is still controversial – options include (1) further evaluation with another imaging modality to assess arterial phase hyperenhancement (e.g., contrast-enhanced ultrasound), (2) imaging follow-up, and (3) biopsy.

3   Summary

Benign hepatic lesions may have imaging features overlapping with those of malignant lesions. Also, they frequently have atypical imaging features due to alteration in liver perfusion and architectural distortion in setting of cirrhosis. As such, radiologists have to be familiar with them in order to provide correct diagnosis and optimal care.

References

American College of Radiology. Liver imaging reporting and data system. https://www.acr.org/Clinical-Resources/Reporting-and-Data-Systems/LI-RADS. Accessed July 2018

Baron RL, Campbell WL, Dodd GD 3rd (1994) Peribiliary cysts associated with severe liver disease: imaging-pathologic correlation. AJR Am J Roentgenol 3:631–636

Bazerbachi F, Haffar S, Sugihara T et al (2018) Peribiliary cysts: a systematic review and proposal of a classification framework. BMJ Open Gastroenterol 5(1):e000204

Brancatelli G, Federle MP, Blachar A, Grazioli L (2001) Hemangioma in the cirrhotic liver: diagnosis and natural history. Radiology 219(1):69–74

Chernyak V, Fowler KJ, Heiken JP, Sirlin CB (2019) Use of gadoxetate disodium in patients with chronic liver disease and its implications for liver imaging reporting and data system (LI-RADS). J Magn Reson Imaging 49(5):1236–1252

Choi JY, Lee HC, Yim JH et al (2011) Focal nodular hyperplasia or focal nodular hyperplasia-like lesions of the liver: a special emphasis on diagnosis. J Gastroenterol Hepatol 26(6):1004–1009

Choi BI, Lee JM, Kim TK et al (2015) Diagnosing borderline hepatic nodules in hepatocarcinogenesis: imaging performance. AJR Am J Roentgenol 205(1):10–21

Dodd GD 3rd, Baron RL, Oliver JH 3rd, Federle MP (1999) Spectrum of imaging findings of the liver in end-stage cirrhosis: Part II, focal abnormalities. AJR Am J Roentgenol 173(5):1185–1192

Doo KW, Lee CH, Choi JW et al (2009) "Pseudo washout" sign in high-flow hepatic hemangioma on gadoxetic acid contrast-enhanced MRI mimicking hypervascular tumor. AJR Am J Roentgenol 193(6):W490–W496

Duran R, Ronot M, Di Renzo S et al (2015) Is magnetic resonance imaging of hepatic hemangioma any different in liver fibrosis and cirrhosis compared to normal liver? Eur J Radiol 84(5):816–822

Elsayes KM, Chernyak V, Morshid AI et al (2018) Spectrum of pitfalls, pseudolesions, and potential misdiagnoses in cirrhosis. AJR Am J Roentgenol 211(1):87–96

Golfieri R, Renzulli M, Lucidi V et al (2011) Contribution of the hepatobiliary phase of Gd-EOB-DTPA-enhanced MRI to dynamic MRI in the detection of hypovascular small ($\leq$ 2 cm) HCC in cirrhosis. Eur Radiol J 6:1233–1242

Joo I, Lee JM, Lee DH et al (2015) Noninvasive diagnosis of hepatocellular carcinoma on gadoxetic acid-enhanced MRI: can hypointensity on the hepatobiliary phase be used as an alternative to washout? Eur Radiol 25(10):2859–2868

Kim JW, Lee CH, Kim SB et al (2017) Washout appearance in Gd-EOB-DTPA-enhanced MR imaging: a differentiating feature between hepatocellular carcinoma with paradoxical uptake on the hepatobiliary phase and focal nodular hyperplasia-like nodules. J Magn Reson Imaging 45(6):1599–1608

Kitao A, Matsui O, Yoneda N et al (2018) Differentiation between hepatocellular carcinoma showing hyperintensity on the hepatobiliary phase of gadoxetic acid-enhanced MRI and focal nodular hyperplasia by CT and MRI. AJR Am J Roentgenol 21(2):347–357

Komatsu N, Motosugi U, Maekawa S et al (2014) Hepatocellular carcinoma risk assessment using gadoxetic acid-enhanced hepatocyte phase magnetic resonance imaging. Hepatol Res 44(13):1339–1346

Libbrecht L, Cassiman D, Verslype C et al (2006) Clinicopathological features of focal nodular hyperplasia-like nodules in 130 cirrhotic explant livers. Am J Gastroenterol 101(10):2341–2346

Motosugi U, Bannas P, Sano K, Reeder SB (2015) Hepatobiliary MR contrast agents in hypovascular hepatocellular carcinoma. J Magn Reson Imaging 41(2):251–265

Motosugi U, Murakami T, Lee JM et al (2018) LI-RADS HBA Working Group. Recommendation for terminology: nodules without arterial phase hyperenhancement and with hepatobiliary phase hypointensity in chronic liver disease. J Magn Reson Imaging 5:1169–1171

Murakami T, Tsurusaki M (2014) Hypervascular benign and malignant liver tumors that require differentiation from hepatocellular carcinoma: key points of imaging diagnosis. Liver Cancer 3(2):85–96

Nakashima O, Kurogi M, Yamaguchi R et al (2004) Unique hypervascular nodules in alcoholic liver cirrhosis: identical to focal nodular hyperplasia-like nodules? J Hepatol 41(6):992–998

Ohtomo K, Baron RL, Dodd GD 3rd et al (1993) Confluent hepatic fibrosis in advanced cirrhosis: appearance at CT. Radiology 188(1):31–35

Papadatos D, Fowler KJ, Kielar AZ et al (2018) Cirrhosis and LI-RADS. Abdom Radiol (NY) 43(1):26–40

Quaglia A, Tibballs J, Grasso A et al (2003) Focal nodular hyperplasia-like areas in cirrhosis. Histopathology 42(1):14–21

Ronot M, Dioguardi Burgio M, Purcell Y et al (2017) Focal lesions in cirrhosis: not always HCC. Eur J Radiol 93:157–168. https://doi.org/10.1016/j.ejrad.2017.05.040

Sasaki M, Yoneda N, Sawai Y et al (2015) Clinicopathological characteristics of serum amyloid A-positive hepatocellular neoplasms/nodules arising in alcoholic cirrhosis. Histopathology 66(6):836–845

Suh CH, Kim KW, Pyo J et al (2017) Hypervascular transformation of hypovascular hypointense nodules in the hepatobiliary phase of gadoxetic acid-enhanced MRI: a systematic review and meta-analysis. AJR Am J Roentgenol 209(4):781–789

The International Consensus Group for Hepatocellular Neoplasia (2009) Pathologic diagnosis of early hepatocellular carcinoma: a report of the international consensus group for hepatocellular neoplasia. Hepatology 49(2):658–664

Toyoda H, Kumada T, Tada T et al (2013) Non-hypervascular hypointense nodules detected by Gd-EOB-DTPA-enhanced MRI are a risk factor for recurrence of HCC after hepatectomy. J Hepatol 58(6):1174–1180

Vilgrain V, Fléjou JF, Arrivé L et al (1992) Focal nodular hyperplasia of the liver: MR imaging and pathologic correlation in 37 patients. Radiology 184(3):699–703

Vilgrain V (2006) Focal nodular hyperplasia. Eur J Radiol 2:236–245

Wanless IR, Wong F, Blendis LM (1995) Focal nodular hyperplasia of the liver: MR imaging and pathologic correlation in 37 patients. Radiology. Hepatic and portal vein thrombosis in cirrhosis: possible role in development of parenchymal extinction and portal hypertension. Hepatology 5:1238–1247

Yoneda N, Matsui O, Kitao A et al (2016) Benign hepatocellular nodules: hepatobiliary phase of gadoxetic acid-enhanced MR imaging based on molecular background. Radiographics 36(7):2010–2027

Pseudolesions in the Cirrhotic Liver

Rita Golfieri, Stefano Brocchi, Matteo Milandri, and Matteo Renzulli

Contents

Abstract

This chapter analyses the different benign liver lesions and pseudolesions occurring in cirrhotic livers, such as regenerative nodules (RNs), siderotic nodules (SNs), nodular regenerative hyperplasia (NRH), large regenerative nodules (LRNs), perfusion defects and transient hepatic attenuation difference (THAD)/ transient hepatic intensity difference (THID), hemangiomas in a cirrhotic liver, pseudomass in chronic portal vein thrombosis (PVT), confluent fibrosis and focal fatty changes, such as focal steatosis and fat sparing, focusing on imaging features helpful in achieving a correct diagnosis.

R. Golfieri (✉) · S. Brocchi · M. Milandri · M. Renzulli
Radiology Unit, Department of Experimental, Diagnostic and Speciality Medicine, Sant'Orsola Hospital, University of Bologna, Bologna, Italy
e-mail: rita.golfieri@unibo.it

© Springer Nature Switzerland AG 2021
E. Quaia (ed.), *Imaging of the Liver and Intra-hepatic Biliary Tract*,
Medical Radiology Diagnostic Imaging, https://doi.org/10.1007/978-3-030-39021-1_11

1 Introduction

Cirrhosis is end-stage chronic liver disease and is characterized pathologically by innumerable regenerative nodules separated by fibrous septa (Vilgrain et al. 2016). Cirrhosis is considered to be one of the leading causes of death having a 1-year mortality rate of up to 57% in cases of decompensated cirrhosis (D'Amico et al. 2006). Chronic hepatitis B or C virus infection, alcoholism and non-alcoholic fatty liver disease (NAFLD) are the most common causes of cirrhosis (Brancatelli et al. 2007).

Hepatocellular carcinoma (HCC) is the most common primary tumour in cirrhotic livers, the second leading cause of cancer-related mortality worldwide and the third most common cause of death in patients with cirrhosis (D'Amico et al. 2006; Mittal and El-Serag 2013). Unfortunately, HCC is not rare in cirrhotic patients, with a fairly constant rate of approximately 3% per year, regardless of the cirrhotic stage (D'Amico et al. 2006).

Nevertheless, several other benign and malignant lesions can occur in cirrhotic patients, they should be differentiated from HCC (Brancatelli et al. 2003) in order to minimize both false-negative and false-positive findings, to carry out the proper treatment and, therefore, to improve patient outcome (Galia et al. 2014). The treatment could be erroneously delayed in cases of undetected or misdiagnosed HCC. Misinterpretation of pseudolesions or benign liver lesions, such as HCC, may incorrectly increase the total tumour burden or even lead to the ineligibility of a patient for potentially curative treatment or the inappropriate assignment of increased priority scores for patients on the waiting list for liver transplantation (Galia et al. 2014).

In recent years, magnetic resonance imaging (MRI) has been confirmed to be the most accurate imaging method for the study of the liver. The introduction of hepatocyte-specific contrast agents in MRI, such as gadoxetic acid (Gd-EOB-DTPA, Primovist, Bayer-Schering Pharma, Berlin, Germany) and gadobenate dimeglumine (Gd-BOPTA, Multihance, Bracco Imaging, Milan, Italy), has added new diagnostic functional parameters to those obtained in the dynamic vascular phases by also evaluating the hepatobiliary (HB) phase of MRI and, therefore, the hepatocyte presence and activity. Moreover, the addition of diffusion-weighted imaging (DWI) sequences can additionally confirm or exclude malignancy in the majority of lesions.

Despite these recent technical innovations in liver imaging, there are still many challenges for radiologists in differentiating HCC from other hepatic lesions, particularly from benign ones and pseudolesions.

2 Technical Pitfalls

Hypervascular tumours, such as HCC, require adequate delivery of contrast media to create a satisfactory contrast between the tumour and the background liver parenchyma. The rate of contrast injection can affect the tumour-to-background contrast ratio; therefore, the use of an adequately high injection rate is important in order to avoid missing lesions. Moreover, correct acquisition during the late arterial phase is particularly important since this is a unique non-repeatable phase. The American College of Gastroenterology guidelines recommend a minimum flow rate of 4–6 cm^3/s to obtain a correct examination (Marrero et al. 2014). A slower rate of infusion of 2.5 cm^3/s may result in suboptimal enhancement, not useful in differentiating lesions from the surrounding hepatic parenchyma.

3 Regenerative Nodules and Siderotic Nodules

Liver cirrhosis is characterized by irreversible remodeling of the hepatic architecture with bridging fibrosis and a spectrum of hepatocellular nodules. Cirrhosis-associated hepatocellular nodules result from the localized proliferation of hepatocytes and their supporting stroma in response to liver injury (International Working Party 1995). The majority of hepatocellular nodules are benign regenerative nodules; however, regenerative nodules may progress along a well-described carcinogenic pathway to become low-grade and high-grade dysplastic nodules evolving into hepatocellular carcinoma (HCC) (Hanna et al. 2008).

Regenerative nodules (RNs) are classified, according to their size, as micronodules (<3 mm) and macronodules (≥3 mm) (International Working Party 1995; Hanna et al. 2008). On computed tomography (CT) and MRI, RNs typically appear isodense/isointense to the surrounding liver parenchyma without arterial phase enhancement or washout appearance and, therefore, they are identifiable due to the peripheral fibrosis which appears hypodense in the portal phase. On MRI, RNs can appear hypointense on T2-weighted images unlike HCC which classically appears moderately hyperintense on T2-weighted images (Elsayes and Shaaban 2015; Hussain et al. 2002).

Some RNs could demonstrate hyperintensity on T1-weighted images and iso- or hypointensity on T2-weighted images (Fig. 1) (Hanna et al. 2008; Martin et al. 2002). Although the reason for these signal intensity (SI) findings is not well understood, the presence of paramagnetic materials or glycogen in the nodule may contribute to T1 hyperintensity (Mathieu et al. 1997). Regenerative nodules may also contain some degree of lipid accumulation in the hepatocytes. Lipid-containing RNs display signal loss on out-of-phase T1-weighted images in comparison with in-phase images (Fig. 2). Steatotic RNs are usually multiple; a single fatty nodule is suggestive of a dysplastic or malignant process (Hanna et al. 2008).

Siderotic nodules (SNs) are iron-containing nodules which develop in a cirrhotic liver (Mitchell et al. 1991).

Even in the absence of systemic iron storage diseases such as hemochromatosis, iron can accumulate within regenerative or dysplastic nodules (DNs) in a cirrhotic liver (Zhang and Krinsky 2004). In systemic iron storage diseases, the mechanism of iron deposition (siderosis) within reticuloendothelial cells, mobilizing iron from damaged hepatocytes, has been identified; however, in a cirrhotic liver, the process of SN formation remains uncertain. Active viral replication and transferrin receptor abnormalities probably play a role. Although a small percentage of SNs are dysplastic, approximately 25% of all DNs are also SNs (Elsayes and Shaaban 2015; Terada and Nakanuma 1989). Moreover, dysplastic SNs are premalignant lesions while regenerative SNs are markers for severe viral or alcoholic cirrhosis. Therefore, the diagnosis of iron content is clinically important. The relationships between hepatic iron deposition and hepatic fibrosis, cirrhosis and neoplasia are also not fully understood (Krinsky et al. 2001; Breitkopf et al. 2009).

Magnetic resonance imaging is currently unable to differentiate siderotic RNs from siderotic DNs (Krinsky et al. 2000), and the association of SNs and malignancy remains controversial. According to some published series, patients with SNs do not show an increased risk of developing DNs or HCC (Zhang and Krinsky 2004; Krinsky et al. 2002), but other authors have reported that SN can be precursors of HCC in patients with chronic liver diseases (Terada et al. 1990; Siegelman et al. 1996; Ito et al. 1999) and that the incidence of HCC is higher in patients with iron-containing nodules than in those without (Krinsky et al. 2000). Whenever iron-free foci are found within an SN in liver cirrhosis, these foci should be considered as early HCCs or borderline lesions showing an expansive growth pattern (Zhang and Krinsky 2004); the finding of the displacement of iron within a nodule by focal tumour growth is a sentinel of HCC (Elsayes and Shaaban 2015; Krinsky et al. 2001; Sadek et al. 1995). Therefore, the diagnosis of SNs and iron-free nodules in the cirrhotic liver is clinically relevant for the early detection of HCC.

On CT, SNs occasionally show high attenuation on unenhanced images which can be misinterpreted on the arterial phase as lesion hyperenhancement. In these nodules, both arterial hyperenhancement and washout are absent. Therefore, only the combined evaluation of unenhanced images and post-contrast behaviour allows the proper characterization of SNs.

On MRI, SNs usually appear hypointense on T1-weighted images, depending on the degree of iron accumulation and the exact imaging parameters (Fig. 3) (Siegelman and Chauhan 2014). Furthermore, SNs have decreased SI in long-echo chemical-shift gradient-echo sequences. A pitfall of MRI is misinterpreting susceptibility from iron content within SNs as areas of washout appearance (Brancatelli et al. 2007): therefore, it is important to evaluate the unenhanced T1- and T2*-weighted images in which SNs appear hypointense. T2*-weighted imaging is

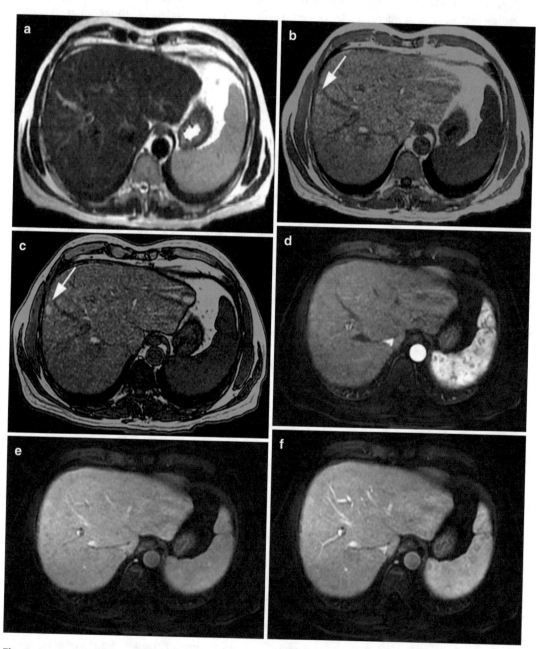

Fig. 1 Regenerative nodule with glycogen content on MRI. T2-weighted image (**a**) demonstrating the absence of focal lesions. T1-weighted "in-phase" (**b**) and "out-of-phase" (**c**) images showing a hyperintense nodule in liver segment VIII (arrows), as a result of the glycogen content, with no changes during arterial (**d**), portal (**e**), delayed (**f**) and hepatobiliary (**g**) phases. Diffusion-weighted image (**h**) revealing no diffusion restriction of the nodule

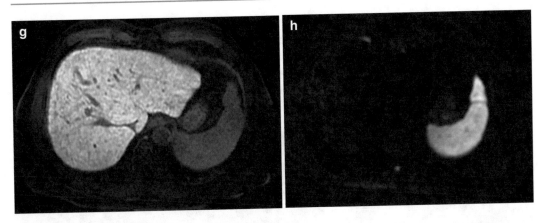

Fig. 1 (continued)

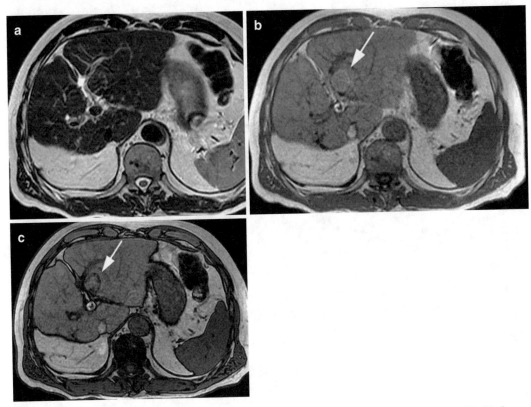

Fig. 2 Regenerative nodule with fat content on MRI. T2-weighted image (**a**) demonstrating a round isointense focal lesion in segment II. T1-weighted "in-phase" (**b**) and "out-of-phase" (**c**) images revealing a hyperintense nodule (arrows) at segment II with dropout in signal intensity in "out-of-phase" images, due to conspicuous fat content

currently the most sensitive MRI technique for detecting SN in the liver having a reported 80% sensitivity and 95% specificity. MRI is therefore helpful in the follow-up in monitoring the distribution and the amount of iron content over time: this could allow the detection of early HCC developing within a DN (Kudo 2009; Park and Kim 2011; Chen et al. 2012).

Severe long-standing portal deprivation with portal obliterative changes, as observed in chronic PVT, or in cases of venous outflow obstruction, such as in Budd–Chiari Syndrome, produce a progressive and reactive compensatory increase in hepatic arterial perfusion ("arterial buffer response"), causing the secondary onset of nodular regenerative hyperplasia (NRH) of the liver tissue (Cazals-Hatem et al. 2003) and large regenerative nodules (LRNs, also called focal

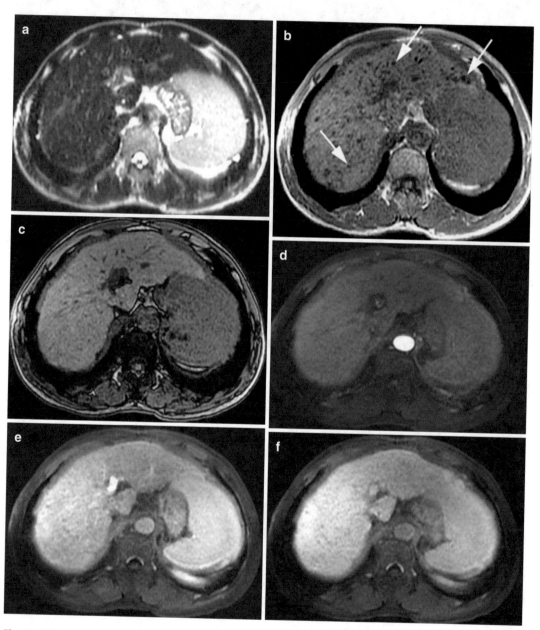

Fig. 3 Multiple siderotic nodules on MRI. T2-weighted image (**a**): no evidence of focal lesions. T1-weighted "in-phase" image (**b**) showing multiple tiny hypointense nodules (arrows) due to their siderotic content, appearing isointense on the T1-weighted "out-of-phase" image (**c**), with no changes during the arterial (**d**), portal (**e**), delayed (**f**) and hepatobiliary (**g**) phases. Diffusion-weighted image (**h**) revealing the absence of diffusion restriction of the nodules

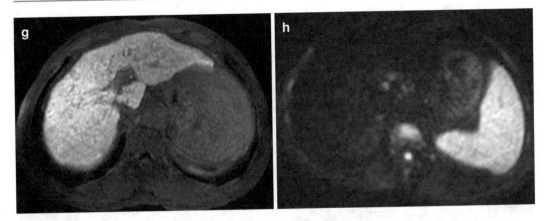

Fig. 3 (continued)

nodular hyperplasia (FNH)-like lesions (Kondo 2001; Brancatelli et al. 2002a, b). In the same liver, a continuous spectrum of nodular regenerative lesions, such as *NRH and LRNs* (Park and Kim 2011; De Sousa et al. 1991), always coexists. Their pathogenesis is similar to FNH development as proposed by Wanless et al. (1985) in livers with syndromic vascular malformations, leading to portal deprivation and subsequent enlargement of the hepatic artery. In support of the vascular pathogenetic hypothesis, Steiner et al. also noted that NRH is frequently associated with severe congestive heart failure, hypothesizing that patients with cardiovascular disease, especially right heart failure, could develop liver NRH as a consequence of venous outflow impairment, sinusoidal–portal flow reduction and compensatory increase in the hepatic arterial flow (Steiner 1959).

According to the International Working Party classification (International Working Party 1995), NRH is defined as monoacinar nodules, undetectable at imaging, unlike multiacinar nodules, such as LRNs, clearly identified on both CT and MRI.

Nodular regenerative hyperplasia is a benign liver disease, macroscopically characterized by multiple small regenerative nodules of variable dimensions, ranging from 1 to 15 mm. The main cause of NRH is a normal liver with blood flow disturbance (also due to myeloproliferative and rheumatologic disease, organ transplantation and classes of drugs). In patients with NRH, unlike LRNs, no enhancing liver lesions can be detected on imaging (Ames et al. 2009).

Large regenerative nodules are benign multiacinar regenerative nodules, usually multiple, containing more than one portal tract, located in a liver which is otherwise abnormal, either with cirrhosis or with severe portal vein disease, hepatic veins or sinusoids. Large regenerative nodules are distinctly larger than the majority of cirrhotic nodules in the same liver, at least 5 mm in diameter (International Working Party 1995). They are also associated with some systemic disease, such as chronic vascular disease (polyarteritis nodosa), rheumatologic disease (Felty syndrome, rheumatoid arthritis, scleroderma, telangiectasia), systemic lupus erythematosus, lymphoproliferative disorder (Hodgkin lymphoma and non-Hodgkin lymphoma, chronic lymphocytic leukemia), myeloproliferative disorder (polycythemia vera, chronic myeloid leukemia, myeloid metaplasia), hepatic vascular disease (Budd Chiari syndrome, sinusoidal obstruction syndrome) and drugs (steroids, chemotherapy, immunosuppressors and contraceptives) (Wanless 1990; Stromeyer and Ishak 1981). In contrast to NRH, LRNs are clearly depicted at imaging since, on MRI, they appear hyperintense to the liver in T1-weighted images due to the presence of copper within the nodules, and isointense or hypointense on T2-weighted images (Wanless et al. 1990). On post-contrast CT and MRI, LRNs typically enhance in the arterial phase and might potentially be misdiagnosed as HCCs; the differential diagnosis relies on the persistent enhancement in the portal and delayed phases with absent washout in LRN unlike HCC (Vilgrain et al. 1999; Takayasu et al. 1994). However, there is little evidence to suggest that LRNs are premalignant or evolve into HCC (Stromeyer and Ishak 1981). In the HB phase of MRI, hyperplastic hepatocytes, such as those in LRNs which often contain ductular proliferation (Tanaka and Wanless 1998), appear isointense or more often hyperintense as compared to the normal parenchyma, unlike HCC (Fig. 4) (Renzulli et al. 2011).

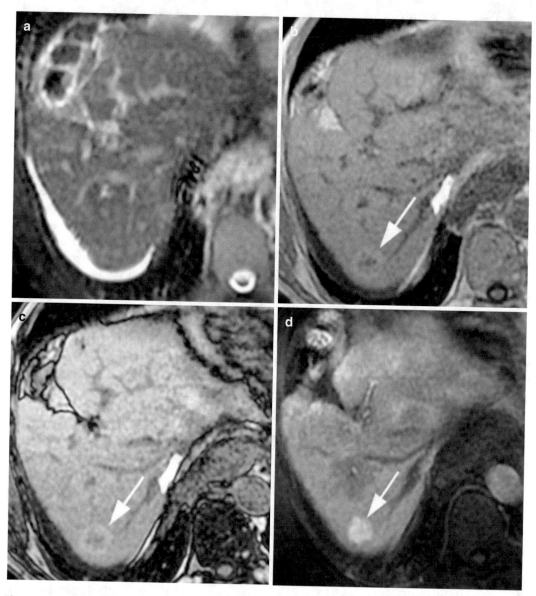

Fig. 4 Large regenerative nodule on MRI. T2-weighted image (**a**) demonstrating no hyperintense focal lesions. T1-weighted "in-phase" (**b**) and "out-of-phase" (**c**) images revealing a hyperintense nodule at segment VII (arrows). Arterial phase (**d**) showing nodule hyperenhancement, persistent (arrows) during the portal phase (**e**), additionally increasing in the hepatobiliary phase (arrow) (**f**)

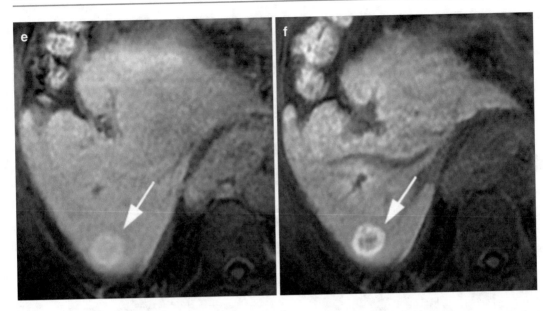

Fig. 4 (continued)

4 Perfusion Defects Due to Third Inflow

The third inflow is a non-portal blood venous system with hepatopetal flow. This system vascularizes some parenchymal regions of the liver and deprives these districts of the nutritional contents deriving from the absorption of the small intestine which characterizes the portal blood. The third inflow represents approximately 1–5% of the total liver inflow and includes the following veins (Fig. 5) (Itai and Matsui 1999; Couinaud 1988; Yoshimitzu et al. 2001; Kobayashi et al. 2010):

(a) Cholecystic vein branches which penetrate the hepatic parenchyma in segments IV and V and flow into the parabiliary system at the porta hepatis. They drain the gallbladder and extrahepatic bile ducts.

(b) Parabiliary venous system (Couinaud system) is a network of venules which goes up to the hepatic hilum, near the hepatoduodenal ligament and the main portal trunk, together with the biliary ducts and arterial branches. It originates from the pyloric–pancreatic–duodenal veins and penetrates the hepatic parenchyma of segments I and IV. It drains the gastric antrum, duodenum and pancreas.

(c) Sappey's aberrant right gastric vein which originates from the gastric antrum, runs within the hepatogastric ligament and enters the hepatic parenchyma at the hilum, anastomosing with the left portal branch, perfusing segments II, III and IV. It drains the stomach and the gastric antrum. In portal hypertension, the reduced portal inflow can cause the compensatory enlargement of this right gastric vein, with reversed flow.

(d) Paraumbilical veins, which originate in the abdominal wall around the umbilical region, run near the round ligament to drain into the left portal branch. In patients with portal hypertension (PH), these collaterals frequently dilate and become an efferent system with hepatofugal flow.

The blood coming from the third inflow enters the hepatic sinusoids at a different rate as compared to the portal blood flow, thus diluting the portal blood flow after contrast media administration, leading to potential *hypovascular or hypervascular pseudolesions*. *Hypovascular pseudolesions* are created by delayed, diluted or missed perfusion. *Hypervascular pseudolesions* are visible during the arterial phase as hyperdense/hyperintense on CT/MRI and as perfusion

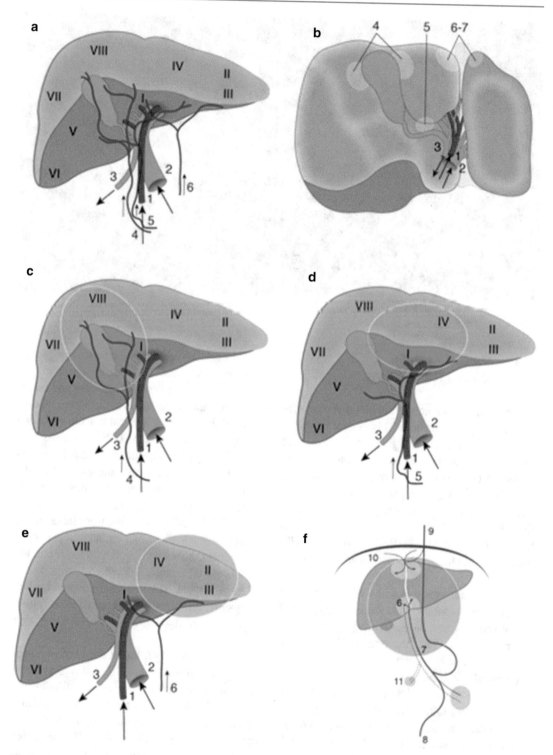

Fig. 5 Non-portal venous system: Third inflow (**a**) and liver portions involved in the corresponding perfusion defects (b; view from below). Drawing showing the hepatic segments drained by the cholecystic veins (**c**), the parabiliary venous system (Couinaud system) (**d**), the Sappey's aberrant right gastric vein (**e**) and the paraumbilical veins (**f**). Modified from Itai and Matsui 1999; Yoshimitzu et al. 2001; Kobayashi et al. 2010

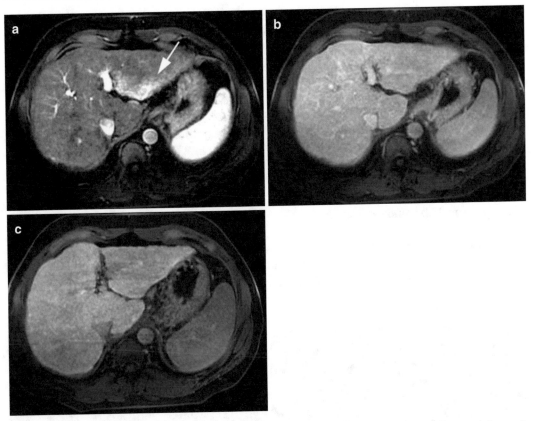

Fig. 6 THID due to third inflow venous system. Arterial phase image (**a**) shows a triangular area of enhancement involving the dorsal portion of segment III (arrow) due to the faster drainage of the Sappey's aberrant right gastric vein. The same area appears isointense in portal (**b**) and delayed (**c**) phase images

defects during the portal phase (because the drainage of the third inflow is faster than that of the portal flow) (Fig. 6).

Liver segments I and IV have a higher frequency of portal branch anomalies; during embryogenesis, these two segments have a later portal vein development (32–34th day of pregnancy) than the other segments (26–28th day of pregnancy).

Three main types of hepatic pseudolesions are directly correlated with the non-portal venous system (third inflow): THAD/THID, focal steatosis and focal fat sparing. Each of these hepatic pseudolesions is systematically analysed in the corresponding paragraph.

5 Transient Hepatic Attenuation Difference (THAD) and Transient Hepatic Intensity Difference (THID)

Transient hepatic attenuation differences (THADs) are areas of liver parenchymal enhancement during the arterial phase of multiphasic CT of the liver. It is a physiological phenomenon due to the dual supply of the liver, with a localized disparity in hepatic arterial (relatively increased) versus portal venous blood supply (decreased), thus giving a higher attenuation to the affected region. Transient hepatic intensity differences

(THIDs) are the corresponding findings during the arterial phase of dynamic MRI. Therefore, THADs/THIDs derive from regional variations in the portal and arterial supply, due to local *inflow and outflow disorders*.

5.1 Hepatic Inflow Disorders

These can be due to: (a) a reduction in portal blood inflow; (b) spontaneous or iatrogenic arterioportal shunts (APSs); (c) an increase in hepatic artery inflow and (d) outflow reduction.

5.1.1 Reduction of Portal Inflow

THIDs/THADs are due to intrinsic portal vein (PV) obstruction from extrinsic hepatic parenchymal compression and/or biliary obstruction.

Portal vein obstruction can be due to thrombosis from several causes, such as pylephlebitis, invasion/compression of the portal vein by tumours (HCC or cholangiocarcinoma), infection or surgical ligation. Portal vein obstruction is responsible for a physiological mechanism characterized by a compensatory increase in arterial flow ("arterial buffer response") (Fig. 7). After a reduction in PV inflow, hepatocytes secrete adenosine and vasopressin mediators which activate the local autonomic nervous system, with consequent vasodilation of the hepatic artery and increased arterial perfusion into the corresponding parenchyma. A 19% reduction in portal inflow induces a vasopressin-mediated increase in arterial flow of about 83%.

Liver parenchymal compression, by the ribs, diaphragm, expansive lesions, perihepatic

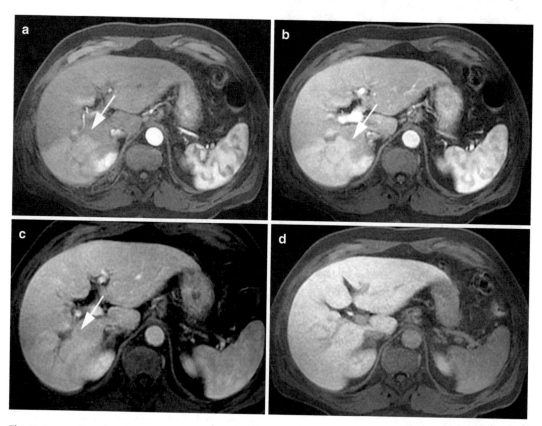

Fig. 7 Large triangular THID involving the entire segment VII (arrows) due to bland PVT. Arterial phase image (**a**) showing a large hyperintense wedge-shaped area with persistent enhancement (arrows) during the delayed arterial phase (**b**) and the portal phase (**c**) images (arrows). Delayed phase image (**d**) demonstrates the recovery of isointensity in the same area as compared to the adjacent parenchyma. Right portal branch thrombosis is evident in the portal phase image (**c**)

peritoneal collections or pseudomyxoma peritonei, can lead to a regional decrease in portal blood inflow since the portal system is a low-pressure system and is therefore susceptible to extrinsic compression and to local THAD and THID formation. In these cases, THADs/THIDs are reversible and disappear after the resolution of the compressive causes (Yoshimitsu et al. 1999).

Biliary obstruction may also result in decreased portal venous flow by means of obstruction of the peribiliary plexus and can cause THADs or THIDs (Itai and Matsui 1997).

5.1.2 Hepatic Arterioportal Shunt (APS) or Iatrogenic Fistula

Hepatic arterioportal shunt (APS) or iatrogenic fistula is the communication between a hepatic arterial branch and the portal venous system resulting in a redistribution of arterial flow in a parenchymal area usually perfused by portal blood flow. Arterioportal shunts can have an iatrogenic origin, occurring after liver biopsies (Fig. 8) or locoregional treatments (percutaneous ethanol injection, thermal ablation and intra-arterial treatments) (Fig. 9) and can also develop

as a consequence of tumours (especially HCC), cirrhosis or trauma.

Arterioportal shunts are usually undetected on grey scale ultrasound (US) but can be diagnosed at Doppler US as a reverse, hepatofugal flow in the portal branch involved parallel to the feeding artery.

Arterioportal shunts can occur through a macroscopic fistula between a large hepatic arterial branch and a large portal branch; they can be detected at contrast-enhanced CT/MRI imaging as the simultaneous opacification of arteries and portal branches during the arterial phase (Itai and Matsui 1997) (Fig. 8).

On dynamic CT/MRI, APSs are typically responsible for areas of parenchymal misperfusions appearing as homogeneously hyperdense/hyperintense during the arterial phase and isodense/isointense during the portal and delayed phases. These areas usually have sharp margins and have no mass effect on the hepatic structures (bile ducts or blood vessels); they are usually stable at imaging follow-up (Galia et al. 2014).

Low flow APSs can show a *"dot-like"* vascular structure consisting of a portal branch strongly

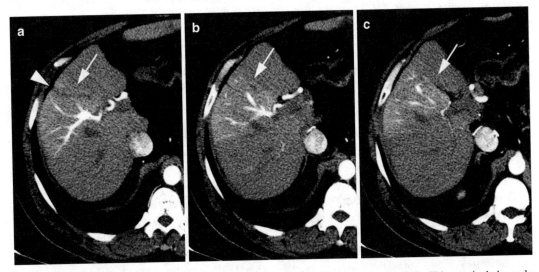

Fig. 8 Large iatrogenic fistula after liver biopsy and THADs. Arterial phase images (**a–c**) in different axial planes showing a large hyperenhancing triangular area involving segment V (arrows) with early enhancement of the corresponding portal branch. This area includes early retrograde enhancement of a large portal branch during the arterial phase of multiphasic CT. Note the hypodense line anterior to the THAD due to the biopsy (arrowhead)

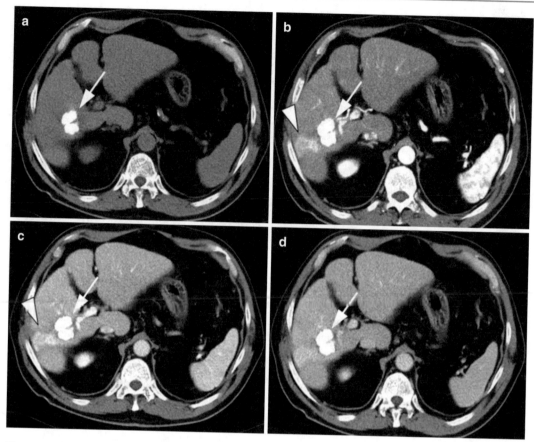

Fig. 9 THAD following trans-arterial chemoemboliza-tion (TACE). Unenhanced-CT image (**a**) demonstrating round, well-defined lipiodol accumulation in segment VI (arrows) as a result of previous TACE treatment. Arterial phase CT image (**b**) showing a hypervascular triangular area (arrowhead) downstream of the lipiodol accumula-tion, without mass effect and with persistent enhancement (arrowhead) during the portal phase image (**c**), recovering isodensity on the delayed phase (**d**)

enhancing during the arterial and venous phase in the middle of a parenchymal triangular-shaped hypervascular pseudolesion (Fig. 10) (Yu et al. 1997). Differentiation from a true malignant liver lesion, such as HCC, relies on the findings of the triangular appearance of the hypervascular area, the "sharp margin sign" and the absence of mass effect.

Depending on the size of an arterioportal fis-tula, the capacity of the draining portal vein can be worsened by the high-pressure hepatic artery inflow. In small arterioportal shunts, shunted hepatic artery blood joins the adjacent portal vein bloodstream without disturbing flow in the more proximal portal vein branches (Fig. 11). Conversely, inflow from a large arterioportal fis-tula can overload the capacity of the intrahe-patic portal venous system and precipitate hepatofugal flow in the main portal vein. In the latter case, shunted hepatic artery blood is divided between two routes: (a) the sinusoids, exiting via hepatic veins and (b) the portal vein with reversed flow, reaching the systemic circu-lation via portosystemic collateral vessels so that the liver is only perfused by arterial blood, and a condition of secondary portal hyperten-sion (PH) can be created (Wachsberg et al. 2002; Bookstein et al. 1982).

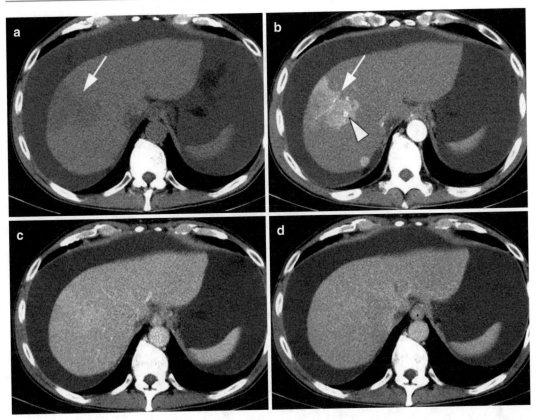

Fig. 10 Large THAD with the «dot sign». Unenhanced-CT (**a**) reveals a hypodense trapezoidal area in segment VIII with sharp margins (arrow). The arterial phase (**b**) shows a hyperattenuation of this area (arrow) with an internal round, well-defined more hypervascular spot (dot sign) (arrowhead), referring to the early enhancement of a peripheral portal vein. Portal (**c**) and delayed (**d**) phases reveal the restored parenchymal attenuation

In the presence of a liver tumour, the morphology of the fistula depends on the site of the tumour in relation to the portal system (Itai and Matsui 1997). When the tumour is located in the apex of the THADs/THIDs, the reduction of the portal flow is caused by portal compression and the THADs/THIDs have a trapezoidal or a fan shape (Fig. 12). When the tumour causes thrombosis of a proximal portal vein, THADs/THIDs are wedge-shaped, and the tumour is located within the perfusion defect ("Shaded area"), and is therefore partially hidden within the perfusion defect in the arterial phase of CT/MRI studies (Fig. 13). Therefore, THADs/THIDs can always be considered as possible sentinel signs of an underlying HCC (Itai and Matsui 1997; Chen et al. 1999a).

An APS can also occur through a trans-vessel shunt from neoplastic thrombus, due to the intra-tumoural neo-angiogenesis of the vasa vasorum, which is responsible for the typical aspect of the "thread and streaks sign" during the arterial phase on contrast-enhanced imaging (Itai and Matsui 1997).

The morphology of THADs/THIDs differs according to the modality of CT/MR reconstructions since, in the axial acquisitions, they can appear as round or oval lesions; therefore, the combined evaluation of 2D and 3D is mandatory (Fig. 14) (Itai and Matsui 1997). The differentiation of a round-shaped enhancing pseudolesion due to THADs/THIDs from hypervascular lesions, such as HCC, in a cirrhotic liver is mandatory. In fact, in cirrhotic

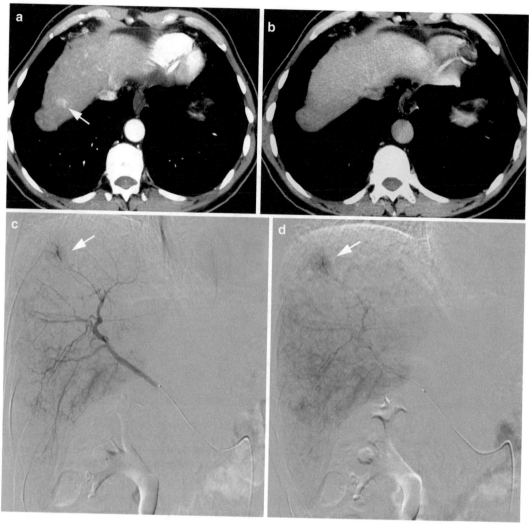

Fig. 11 Spontaneous arterioportal shunt (APS) in cirrhosis. CT shows a small hyperenhancing area in segment VIII (arrow) during the arterial phase (**a**), isodense to the adjacent parenchyma in the portal phase (**b**). The following angiography confirms the early enhancement of a peripheral portal branch (arrow) during the arterial phase (**c**) having a pseudonodular shape (arrow) in the parenchymal phase of the study (**d**), pathognomonic for APS

patients, a focal hypervascular finding has a 70% probability of being benign and the majority of these are THADs/THIDs due to APSs (Wachsberg et al. 2002; Yu et al. 2000; Shimizu et al. 2003; O'Malley et al. 2005; Kim et al. 2015). The clue to differentiating round-shaped enhancing pseudolesions due to THADs/THIDs from HCC is the absence of wash-out during the portal and delayed phases, without capsule appearance or mass effect on the liver struc-

tures. On MRI, HCC, unlike APSs, is usually slightly hypointense on T1-weighted images and mildly hyperintense on T2-weighted images, round-shaped and it has an evident mass effect on the adjacent liver structures (Vilgrain et al. 2016). Moreover, on MRI performed with HB contrast agents, THADs/THIDs due to APSs appear isointense to the liver parenchyma in the HB phase images, whereas HCC is markedly hypointense (Ronot

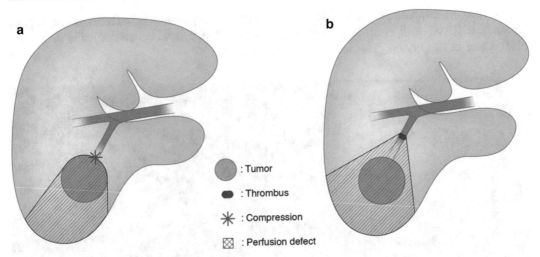

Fig. 12 Relationship between the morphology of the fistulae caused by a tumour and the site of the tumour in relation to the portal system. Drawing showing a trapezoidal- or fan-shaped THAD/THID when the tumour is located in the apex (**a**) or a wedge-shaped THAD/THID when the tumour causes proximal portal thrombosis and is located within the perfusion defect ("shaded area") (**b**). Modified from Itai Y, Radiology 1997

et al. 2017). In very few cases (5–15%), THADs/THIDs due to APSs appear slightly hypointense on the HB phase of MRI, but the level of SI is always higher than in HCCs (Sun et al. 2010; Motosugi et al. 2010).

Iatrogenic intrahepatic arterial–portal fistula is not a rare complication of liver puncture and transhepatic manipulative procedures, or also after percutaneous ablations or intra-arterial treatments (chemoembolization or radioembolization) of liver tumours (Figs. 8 and 9). It has been reported as a sequela of liver biopsy in about 5% of cases and after transhepatic cholangiography and biliary catheterization in up to 26% of cases (Okuda et al. 1978). However, APSs after biopsy tend to resolve spontaneously. Hellekant et al. reported that the frequency of finding APSs depends on the interval between biopsy and imaging detection; the incidence was as high as 50% in <1 week, dropping to 10% after 1 week (Hellekant 1976). Iatrogenic causes (e.g. percutaneous liver biopsy) represent more than 50% of published cases of APSs (Fig. 8). Similarly, after successful intra-arterial treatment, the necrotic tumoural area can induce direct communication between the arterial and the portal radicles at the

periphery of the treated area, creating an APS (Fig. 9). The majority of APSs resolve spontaneously within a few months as they are small and peripherally located. In rare instances, when APSs are centrally located, clinical symptoms develop (Lee et al. 1997). There have been 30 reported cases of symptomatic intrahepatic APSs following percutaneous liver biopsy. Hepatic arterioportal fistulae can result in portal hypertension secondary to arterial blood flowing directly into the portal vein, bypassing the hepatic sinusoids.

Iatrogenic APS is evident in contrast-enhanced imaging as a peripheral fan-shaped, sharply margined THAD/THID as previously described.

5.1.3 Increase in Hepatic Arterial Blood Flow

Increase in hepatic arterial blood flow can be caused by tumour or inflammation. Almost all hepatic tumours, including benign lesions such as hemangiomas, are vascularized by the hepatic artery (both hypervascular and hypovascular tumours). The increase in hepatic arterial flow to the tumour can also lead to an increase in arterial flow to the adjacent parenchyma ("steal phenomenon"), responsible for THAD/THID appearances (Gryspeerdt et al. 1997; Itai et al. 1995; Chen et al. 1999b). The most frequent inflammatory causes of increase in the hepatic arterial blood flow are cholecystitis or hepatic abscess.

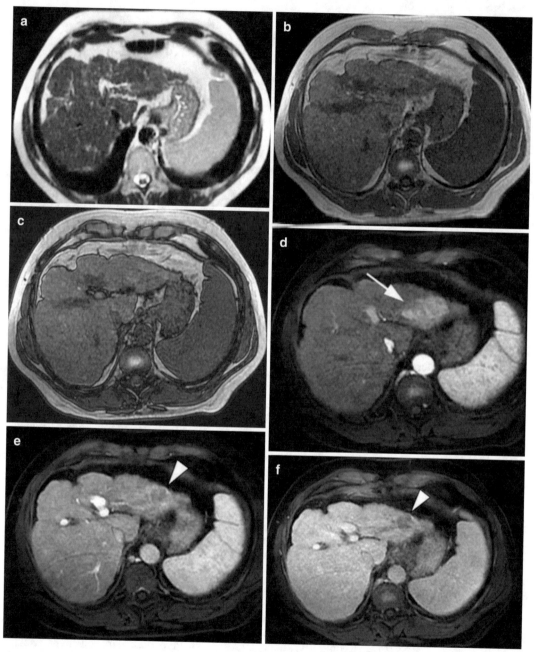

Fig. 13 THID and "shaded area" on MRI. T2-weighted (**a**) and T1-weighted "in-phase" (**b**) and "out-phase" (**c**) images demonstrating no definite focal lesions. The arterial phase image (**d**) shows a hyperenhancing wedge-shaped area (arrow), fully involving segment II. Within this area is included a nodular HCC (arrowhead) which is more evident only due to the washout on the portal and delayed phases (e–f) and due to hypointensity on the hepatobiliary phase image (arrowhead) (**g**). Diffusion-weighted image (**h**) reveals restriction (arrowhead) of the nodule

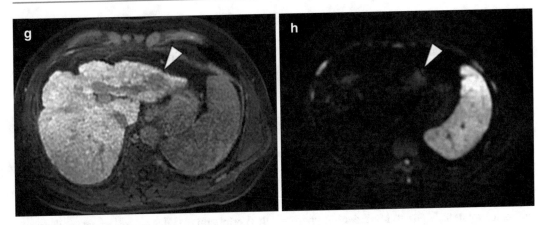

Fig. 13 (continued)

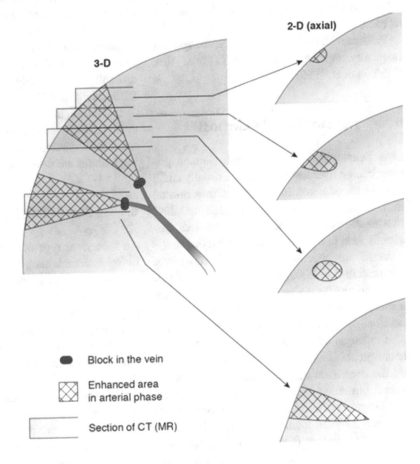

Fig. 14 Relationship between the appearance of a THAD/THID on CT/MRI and the modality of reconstructions; 2D or 3D. Modified from Itai Y, Radiology 1997

5.2 Hepatic Outflow Disorders

Outflow disorders inducing a reduction in hepatic vein flow can also be responsible for THIDs/THADs. The increase in sinusoidal pressure due to outflow blockade produces a portal flow reduction which becomes hepatofugal, and inversion of the pressure gradient between sinusoids and the portal vein system; sinusoidal stasis stimulates adenosine secretion from hepatocytes with subsequent arterial vasodilatation and an increase in the arterial flow (Murata et al.

1995). The main causes of outflow impairment can be functional, such as right heart failure, pulmonary hypertension, pericardial disease and mediastinal fibrosis, or organic, such as Budd–Chiari syndrome and sinusoidal obstruction syndrome (SOS). Complications of Budd–Chiari syndrome and SOS are hepatomegaly, portal hypertension, ascites, jaundice and then cirrhosis (DeLeve et al. 2002).

A pathognomonic CT/MRI pattern of the outflow disorders is heterogeneous enhancement after contrast media administration, with the typical "patchy pattern", due to hyperdense/hyperintense blood not diluted in the lobules and hypodensity/hypointensity surrounding the portal triad.

Patients with these hemodynamic changes can frequently develop benign LRNs over time (Vilgrain et al. 1999).

6 Hemangioma in Cirrhosis

Liver hemangiomas are the most common primary benign liver lesions; they are usually small and are encountered in patients with a normal liver, having an incidence as high as 20% (Karhunen 1986). Hemangiomas are less frequently seen in a cirrhotic background due to the distorted architecture of a fibrotic liver (Brancatelli et al. 2007, 2001; Duran et al. 2015). Some authors have also demonstrated that hemangiomas can become smaller in a liver which is developing cirrhosis (Duran et al. 2015; Mastropasqua et al. 2004). The hallmark of a hemangioma is excessive angiogenesis followed by the regression and inhibition of new blood vessel formation (Makhlouf and Ishak 2002). The diagnosis of a cavernous hemangioma can be obtained on MRI, identifying a very high SI on T2-weighted images (equal to that of gallbladder bile content or cerebrospinal fluid) combined with the typical vascular pattern at dynamic CT/MRI of discontinuous, peripheral, globular enhancement at initial imaging in the arterial phase, with progressive centripetal enhancement

in the portal and delayed phases (Fig. 15) (Brancatelli et al. 2007). In cirrhosis, larger hemangiomas maintain the typical peripheral, discontinuous nodular enhancement pattern and can be diagnosed confidently (Itai et al. 1995). In fact, Mastropasqua et al. (2004) have demonstrated that the hallmarks of hemangiomas did not differ in normal livers as compared to patients with chronic liver disease or cirrhosis. Therefore, the differentiation between hemangiomas and HCC, even in cirrhotic livers is relatively easy since dynamic contrast-enhanced imaging can show the peripheral nodular enhancement, with subsequent central fill-in and sustained enhancement of the delayed phases (Brannigan et al. 2004).

During the follow-up, in cirrhotic livers, hemangiomas can develop scarring, becoming more fibrotic; they usually decrease in size and can be difficult to correctly diagnose at imaging (Brancatelli et al. 2007; Itai et al. 1995).

Therefore, the characterization of a lesion in a cirrhotic liver, such as hemangiomas, should be made with caution and only when classic imaging features are detectable.

6.1 Fast-Filling Hemangiomas

An infrequent type of hemangioma is the "fast-filling hemangioma", also called "capillary" or "flash-filling" hemangioma. On imaging, unlike the cavernous type, it shows complete and homogeneous enhancement during the arterial phase without globular enhancement and without a central fill-in pattern. In these cases, the diagnosis can be uncertain and differentiating them from HCC can be challenging (Jang et al. 2003).

On grey scale US, hemangiomas are hyperechoic but, in rare cases, especially in patients with a fatty liver, they can appear isoechoic, hypoechoic or even with a mixed echogenicity (Yu et al. 2000).

The arterial phase of contrast-enhanced US (CEUS) can be useful in showing the real-time globular enhancement of fast-filling hemangiomas with very rapid central fill-in (Kim et al.

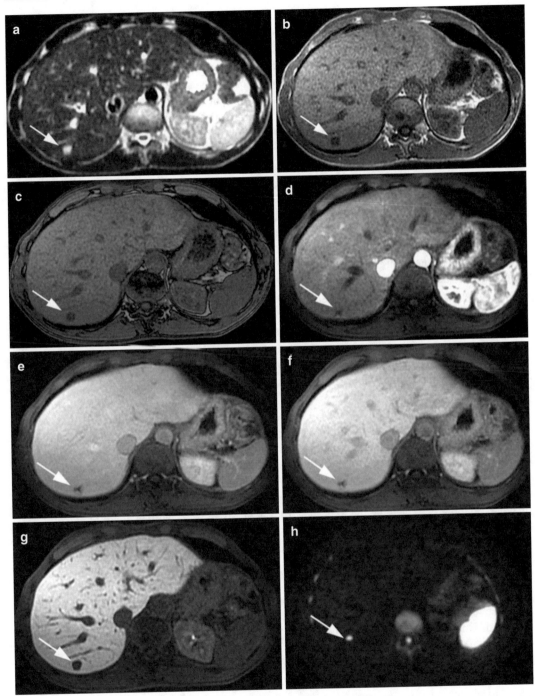

Fig. 15 Cavernous hemangioma on MRI. T2-weighted image (**a**) depicts a round strong hyperintense lesion at segment VII (arrow), hypointense on T1-weighted images (arrows) (**b**, **c**). Dynamic study after contrast administration shows the typical peripheral and globular enhance-ment (arrows) (**d**, **e**) followed by a central enhancement on the delayed phase (arrow) (**f**), with hypointensity during the hepatobiliary phase (arrow) (**g**). Diffusion-weighted image reveals evident diffusion restriction of the lesion (arrow)

2006; Jang et al. 2009a, b; Wilson et al. 2008). However, an important limitation of this technique is that sometimes these pseudolesions can show a mild washout during the portal or delayed phases, caused by microbubble destruction due to continuous ultrasound scanning (Bhayana et al. 2010).

On contrast-enhanced CT/MRI, both fast-filling hemangiomas and small HCCs show hypervascularity in the hepatic arterial phase. However, hemangiomas demonstrate a strong homogeneous enhancement analogous to that of the aorta or other arterial vessels in the arterial phase and similar to the portal vein during the portal phase. Conversely, HCC usually exhibits a milder enhancement during the arterial phase coupled with the typical wash out of contrast media during the portal and delayed phase images (Galia et al. 2014).

On MRI, a typical pattern of all hemangiomas is a strong hyperintensity on T2-weighted images (the "light bulb sign") useful in the differentiation with HCC, which usually shows only a mild hyperintensity (Tamada et al. 2011).

Therefore, the MRI key findings for the diagnosis of fast-filling hemangiomas are strong hyperintensity on T2-weighted images and enhancement parallel to that of the aorta in the arterial phase, with persistent enhancement in the delayed phase (Fig. 16) (Ronot et al. 2017). Other imaging features can include the presence of hepatic THIDs/THADs at its periphery due to the sump effect (Fig. 17).

Smaller, fast-filling hemangiomas can be difficult to differentiate from small HCC in the HB phase of MRI. (Doo et al. 2009; Goodwin et al. 2011; Francisco et al. 2014; Kim et al. 2016; Dioguardi Burgio et al. 2016) since hemangiomas can exhibit a "pseudo-washout" in the transitional and HB phases (20 min), with the lesion appearing hypointense relative to the surrounding parenchyma due to the rapid uptake of Gd-EOB-DTPA by the background parenchyma (Doo et al. 2009). Radiologists should be aware of this possibility while evaluating patients with

cirrhosis. However, the *"pseudo-washout"* phenomenon of a hemangioma is more gradual than the true washout in malignant tumours, and attenuation on CT images and SI on MRI typically parallels the enhancement of the blood pool in all phases of contrast enhancement, thus helping in differentiating between hemangiomas and HCC (Kim et al. 2016). The DWI sequences are also of great help; the majority of hemangiomas have the "T2 shine-through effect", which refers to a high signal on DWI which is not due to restricted diffusion, but rather to a high T2 signal which "shines through" to the DWI. The "T2 shine-through effect" occurs because of the long T2 decay time in some normal tissue. However, Duran et al. have shown that a T2 shine through effect is less common in flash-filling hemangiomas than in other hemangiomas (Duran et al. 2014).

6.2 Sclerosed Hemangiomas

Hemangiomas undergoing degeneration and fibrous replacement are called sclerosed hemangiomas (Brancatelli et al. 2009). Several imaging findings of sclerosed hemangiomas have been described in different series, such as the lack of early enhancement, gradual and persistent mild peripheral enhancement (Doo et al. 2009; Kim et al. 2016; Brancatelli et al. 2009; Itai and Saida 2002) and mild hyperintensity on T2-weighted images, much lower than typical hemangiomas (Brancatelli et al. 2009). Other imaging features include geographic margins, capsular retraction, decrease in size over time, presence of hepatic THIDs/THADs at their periphery and loss of previously seen regions of enhancement at follow-up (Goodwin et al. 2011). However, these imaging findings are non-specific and, therefore, correct differentiation from malignant tumours is difficult (Itai and Saida 2002); in the majority of cases, sclerosed hemangiomas are diagnosed only by pathologists after biopsy or surgical excision.

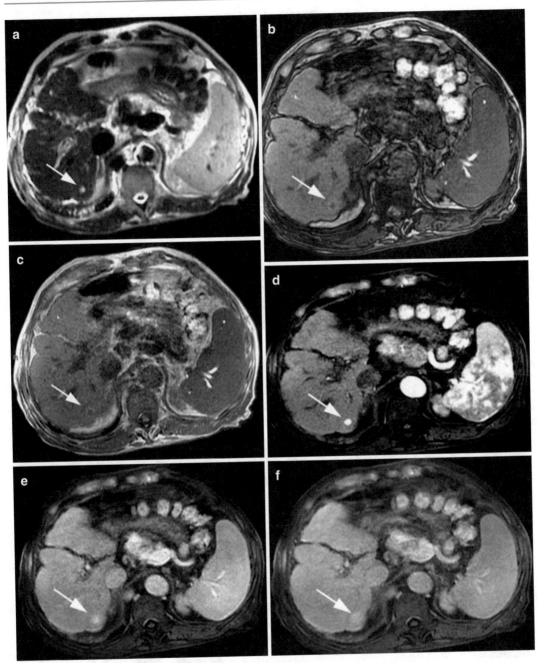

Fig. 16 Fast-filling hemangioma on MRI. T2-weighted image (**a**) depicts a small strong hyperintense lesion at segment VI (arrow), hypointense on T1-weighted images (arrows) (**b**, **c**). Dynamic study after contrast administration shows complete and rapid filling-in (arrow) during the arterial phase (**d**), persisting during the portal and delayed phases (arrows in **e**, **f**) and hypointensity on the hepatobiliary phase (arrow) (**g**). Diffusion-weighted image (**h**) confirms evident diffusion restriction of the lesion (arrow)

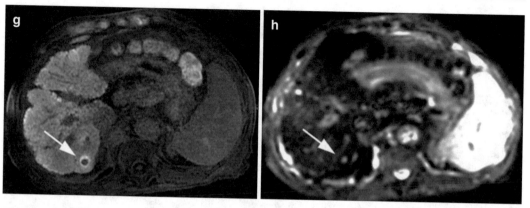

Fig. 16 (continued)

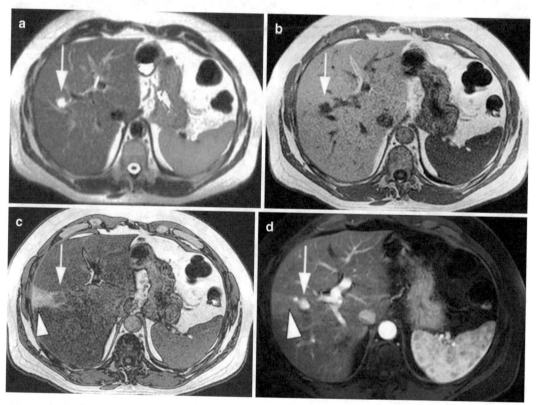

Fig. 17 Fast-filling (or capillary) hemangioma with peripheral THID and focal fat sparing area on MRI. T2-weighted image (**a**) shows a small strong hyperintense lesion in segment VIII (arrow), hypointense on T1-weighted images (arrows) (**b**, **c**), on the apex of a wedge-shaped area (arrowhead) hyperintense on the T1-weighted "out-of-phase" image (**c**) as compared to adjacent hypointense steatotic parenchyma, appearing isointense on the T1-weighted "in phase" image (**b**), characteristic of a hemangioma with a peripheral focal fat-sparing area. The dynamic study after contrast administration shows complete and rapid filling-in of the hemangioma (arrows) and hyperintensity of the peripheral THID (arrowhead) during the arterial phase (**d**), persisting during the portal and delayed phases (arrowheads) (**e**, **f**) with hypointensity of the hemangioma (arrow) on the hepatobiliary phase (**g**). Diffusion-weighted image (**h**) reveals strong diffusion restriction of the hemangioma (arrow)

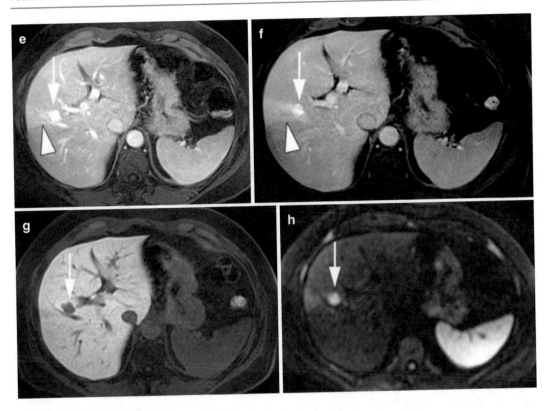

Fig. 17 (continued)

7 Pseudomass in Cirrhosis and Chronic Portal Vein Thrombosis (PVT)

When the main portal vein is obstructed by thrombosis, many collaterals are gradually hypertrophied in order to provide a compensatory liver inflow, forming the "cavernous transformation of the portal vein", also called "portal cavernoma" (Chen et al. 2017). In the case of PVT, the "central zone" of the liver parenchyma, close to the hepatic hilum, preferentially receives the residual portal venous flow by collaterals (via the parabiliary venous system, peribiliary plexus and proximal accessory branches of the main portal vein) as compared to the peripheral liver which is perfused to a lesser degree from a predominantly arterial supply, which is thought to occur via trans-sinusoidal arterioportal shunts ("*zonal perfusion*" theory). The central zone, including the caudate lobe and perihilar hepatic parenchyma gradually becomes relatively hypertrophic and may simulate a mass-like lesion. Conversely, the peripheral zone of the liver gradually becomes atrophic, despite the arterial compensation. The concept of "central" and "peripheral" zones may also be of value in explaining the deformity of a cirrhotic liver with portal hypertension since PH may induce hemodynamic changes of portal flow similar to those seen in portal cavernomas (Itai et al. 1994).

These hemodynamic and morphologic changes in chronic PVT determine the following typical appearances on contrast-enhanced CT-MRI imaging; the atrophic peripheral region of the liver shows hyperenhancement in the arterial phase, whereas the enlarged central zone displays hypoenhancement, mimicking a large mass. In the delayed phase, the central zone shows isoenhancement to the liver (Chen et al.

2017) helping in the differential diagnosis with true lesions. Magnetic resonance imaging with hepatospecific contrast media can help in the differential diagnosis of pseudomass in chronic PVT which is isointense to the surrounding liver in the HB phase as compared to true lesions, usually hypointense (Fig. 18).

8 Confluent Fibrosis

In cirrhotic livers, fibrosis can be diffusely or heterogeneously distributed (Galia et al. 2014). In some cases, fibrosis can become focal and confluent due to the coalescence of fibrous tissue, with consequent development of large fibrous scars (Ohtomo et al. 1993a, b). Confluent fibrosis is more frequent in alcoholic cirrhosis and less frequent in other etiologies, such as primary sclerosing cholangitis or autoimmune chronic hepatitis (Vilgrain et al. 2016).

Focal fibrosis is typically wedge-shaped, with the base on the subcapsular region, radiating from the porta hepatis, frequently involving segments IV, VII or VIII, and associated with capsular retraction or focal flattening (retraction) of the hepatic capsule (Ohtomo et al. 1993a, b) (Fig. 19). In approximately 15% of cases, the hepatic vessels can become part of ("trapped") the focal fibrosis, appearing irregular but patent (Brancatelli et al. 2009). The typical peripheral location of fibrosis can be explained by the zonal perfusion changes occurring in cirrhosis, as previously described (Breen et al. 2004).

Ultrasound is widely used as a first-line imaging modality in the evaluation of patients with cirrhosis. However, measurements of liver echogenicity have shown poor accuracy in diagnosing fibrosis (Mathiesen et al. 2002).

On CT, fibrosis appears as a wedge-shaped region of hypoattenuation on unenhanced images, persisting on the arterial and portal venous phases which may gradually enhance in the delayed phase. This feature is explained by the slow contrast accumulation in the extracellular compartment characteristic of the fibrous tissue (Décarie et al. 2011).

On MRI, fibrotic septa in cirrhotic livers include reticulations surrounding regenerative nodules leading to the typical "lace-lake pattern". These fibrous septa are hypointense on T1-weighted images and hyperintense on T2-weighted images and enhance at the equilibrium phase after gadolinium administration. Usually, on contrast-enhanced MRI with extracellular agents, unlike HCC, focal fibrosis does not enhance during the arterial phase but can slightly enhance during the portal phase and highly enhance during the delayed phase (Fig. 19) (Vilgrain et al. 2016).

In rare cases, focal confluent fibrosis can mimic the appearance of an infiltrative HCC (Ohtomo et al. 1993a, b) when it shows irregular margins and mild enhancement on the arterial phase of contrast-enhanced imaging. Enhancement during the arterial phase could be explained by the associated inflammation (Goodwin et al. 2011), especially in the early phase of its development in which confluent fibrosis might not be associated with capsular retraction (Fig. 20) (Galia et al. 2014; Francisco et al. 2014). However, progressive enhancement from the arterial to the delayed phases helps in differentiating focal confluent fibrosis from infiltrative HCC, which shows the typical washout pattern (Ohtomo et al. 1993a, b). Magnetic resonance imaging with HB agents is less useful than MRI with extracellular contrast media in the differential diagnosis of focal confluent fibrosis and infiltrative HCC since, during the transitional (at about 5 min from contrast media injection) and the HB (at about 20 min) phases, both focal confluent fibrosis and HCC are typically hypointense, the first due to the lack of hepatocytes and the second due to degenerated hepatocytes. Other MRI features could be helpful in differentiating confluent fibrosis from HCC: mild hyperintensity on T2-weighted images, although some HCCs can show the same feature (Ohtomo et al. 1993a, b), and a diffusion restriction in DWI, but with an apparent diffusion coefficient (ADC) slightly higher than that of HCC (Park et al. 2013).

Other imaging characteristics pointing towards infiltrating HCC are contour bulging, satellite nodules and neoplastic PVT (Dioguardi

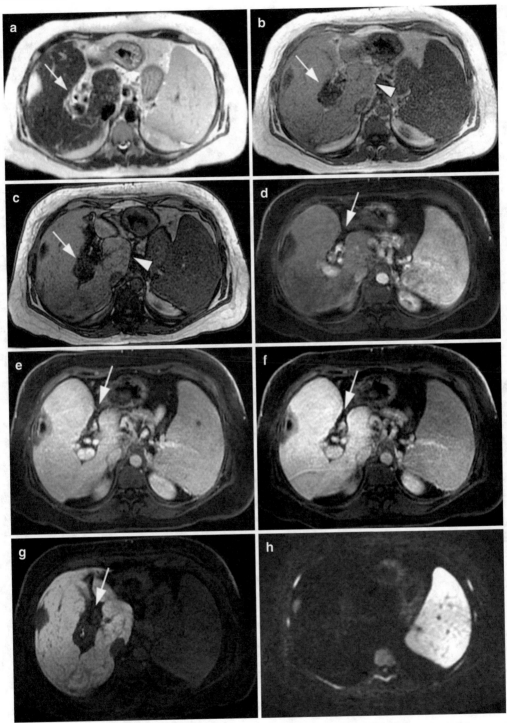

Fig. 18 Liver pseudomass in the presence of portal cavernoma on MRI. T2- and T1-weighted images demonstrating a pseudomass at the hepatic hilum (arrows), hyperintense on the T2-weighted image (**a**) and hypointense on T1-weighted images (**b**, **c**) with hypertrophy of segment I (arrowheads). The arterial (**d**), portal (**e**) and delayed (**f**) phases confirm the presence of multiple dilated vessels at the hepatic hilum (cavernous transformation of the portal vein (arrows). Hepatobiliary phase (**g**) revealing hypointensity of the pseudomass at the hepatic hilum (arrow) with no restriction on the diffusion-weighted image (**h**)

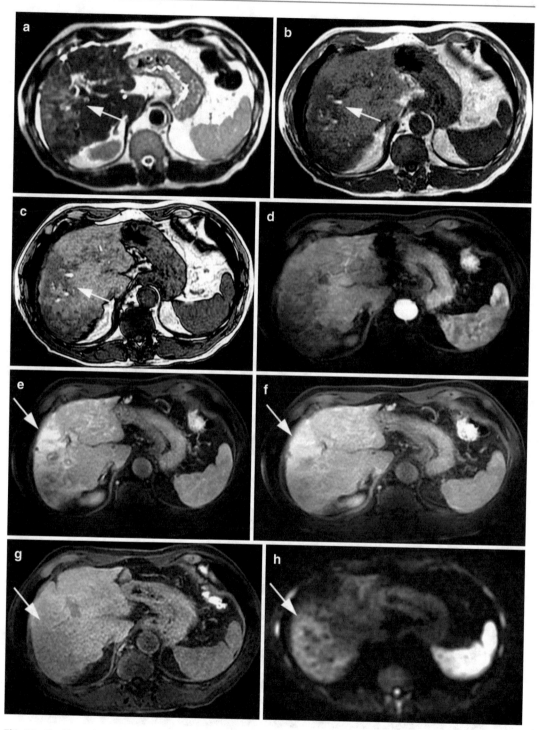

Fig. 19 Confluent fibrosis on MRI. T2-weighted image (**a**) shows an irregular peripheral hyperintense area (arrow) involving segments V and VI, hypointense on T1-weighted images (**b**, **c**, arrows). Arterial phase (**d**) showing no significant enhancement of this area, distorted vessels at its periphery, and late enhancement (arrows) in the portal–venous (**e**) and delayed (**f**) phases coupled with hypointensity (arrow) on the hepatobiliary phase (**g**). A typical mild restriction (arrow) of the entire area is shown in the diffusion-weighted image (**h**)

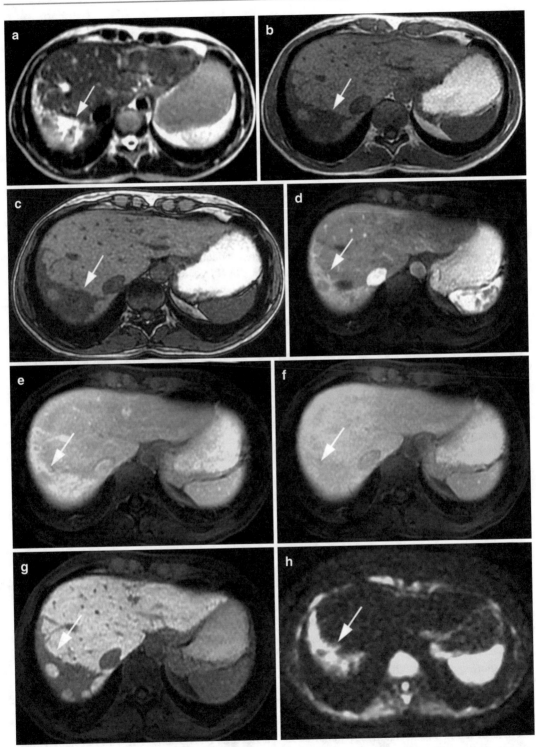

Fig. 20 Confluent fibrosis on MRI. T2-weighted images (**a**) demonstrating an irregular strongly hyperintense area largely involving segment VII (arrows), hypointense on T1-weighted images (**b**, **c**, arrows). The dynamic study shows hyperintensity of this area (arrows) during the arterial (**d**) and portal (**e**) phases, with isointensity (arrow) in the delayed (**f**) phase and hypointensity (arrow) during the hepatobiliary (**g**) phase. Diffusion-weighted image (**h**) reveals a strong diffusion restriction (arrow)

Burgio et al. 2016; Park et al. 2013), all absent in focal confluent fibrosis.

In the absence of these key features for differentiating confluent fibrosis from HCC and when the differential diagnosis remains uncertain, image-guided biopsy is mandatory (Vilgrain et al. 2016).

9 Focal Fatty Changes

Fatty liver disease is a pathological condition in which triglycerides accumulate within the cytoplasm of hepatocytes, due to an altered hepatocellular lipid metabolism and a defect in free fatty acid metabolic pathways (Brunt and Tiniakos 2002; Angulo 2002). Fatty liver disease usually does not get worse but, in the final evolution, it can cause scarring of the liver, which leads to cirrhosis.

Two main conditions are responsible for this aberrant fat accumulation: alcoholic liver disease and non-alcoholic fatty liver disease (NAFLD) related to insulin resistance and metabolic syndrome. Other less common causes of fat accumulation are viral hepatitis, drug overuse, dietary and nutritional abnormalities and congenital disorders.

Typically, lipid accumulation affects the centre of the hepatic lobule, near the central vein, and subsequently involves the peripheral zone, near the portal triads (Brunt and Tiniakos 2002) whereas, in advanced steatosis, the lipid accumulation involves the entire hepatic parenchyma (Scheuer and Lefkowitch 2000), frequently with inhomogeneous distribution, resulting in the formation of fat sparing areas (i.e. around the gallbladder, hepatic hilum, posterior edge of segment IV) (Matsui et al. 1995).

Fat-sparing areas in diffuse steatosis involve the same regions affected by *focal fat accumulation*: most frequently the perivascular and subcapsular regions, hepatic hilum and along the insertion of the falciform ligament (Hamer et al. 2006; Mathieu et al. 2001). This is explained by the different blood supply of these regions where portal flow is replaced by the third inflow (see corresponding paragraph) (Itai and Matsui 1999).

The third inflow causes local hemodynamic anomalies which produce focal tissue hypoxia; the high insulin content in the parabiliary venous system and right gastric vein predispose to the accumulation of fat into hepatocytes in the territories perfused by these aberrant veins (Fig. 21).

Focal fatty deposition is often a simple diagnosis, due to some key imaging features, such as fat content in characteristic areas, absence of mass effect on adjacent structures of the liver, contrast enhancement similar to those of the hepatic parenchyma, irregular margins and geographic rather than a round-shaped configuration. Fat sparing or local fat depositions are small areas which are rarely confluent (Angulo 2002).

On US, fat-sparing areas are usually homogenous hypoechoic zones within a bright liver background and colour Doppler can reveal a hepatopetal flow in the lesion. Contrast-enhanced ultrasound is helpful in confirming the benignity of these findings, showing normal arterial and portal perfusion in the surrounding parenchyma (Nicolau and Brú 2004) and an early opacification of small venous branches within the lesion, during the arterial phase, caused by aberrant splanchnic venous drainage. However, *focal fat depositions* are homogeneously hyperechoic on US, with normal arterial and portal perfusion as compared to the adjacent liver parenchyma on CEUS, as in fat-sparing areas.

On *unenhanced CT,* the diagnosis of a fatty liver is based on a liver density lower than 40 hounsfield units (HU) (Boyce et al. 2010) or an attenuation difference higher than 10 HU between the spleen and the liver (Alpern et al. 1986). Liver parenchyma hypoattenuation relative to the liver vasculature establishes the presence of moderate to severe fatty liver disease (Hamer et al. 2006). On portal phase contrast-enhanced CT, an attenuation difference greater than 25 HU between the spleen and the liver suggests fatty liver deposition (Fig. 22) (Alpern et al. 1986). However, *focal fat sparing* appears as a hyperdense area in a steatotic background, but with normal HU and with absent mass-effect on the adjacent vessels.

On MRI, focal fat sparing areas appear isointense to the liver parenchyma on "in-phase" T1-weighted images and hyperintense on

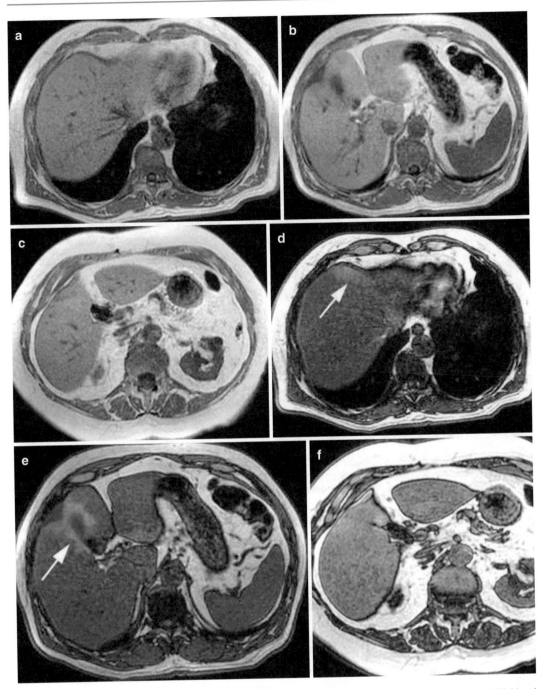

Fig. 21 Focal fat-sparing area on MRI. T1-weighted "in-phase" (**a–c**) and "out-phase" (**d–f**) images in different planes. In T1-weighted "out-of-phase" images (**d–f**), a hepatic dropout of signal intensity of the entire liver with a focal hyperintense area (arrows) in segments VIII, V and IV, characteristic of a focal fat sparing area adjacent to the gallbladder

"out-phase" T1-weighted images (Fig. 23). Nevertheless, *focal fat depositions* on T1-weighted images show a significant loss of SI on "out-phase" as compared to "in-phase" images, due to chemical shift artefacts (Hamer et al. 2006). Moreover, focal fat accumulation is

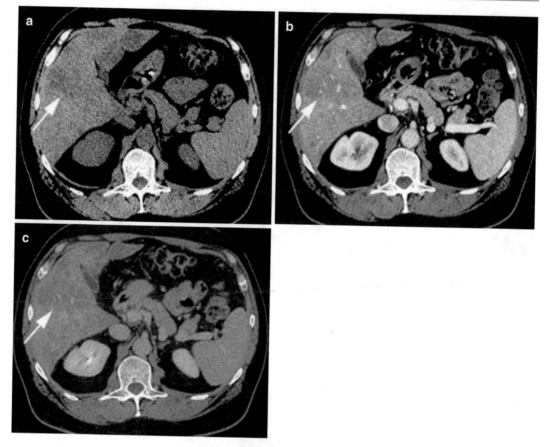

Fig. 22 Geographic steatosis on CT. Unenhanced CT (**a**) revealing geographic hypodense areas involving segments V, IV and III (arrow), with persistent mild hypodensity (arrows) during the portal (**b**) and delayed (**c**) phases, characteristic of geographic steatosis

not hyperintense on DWI, thus confirming its benignity (Fig. 24).

A rare pattern of fatty deposition is that, in the perivascular areas, surrounding vessels, such as portal vein branches or central hepatic venules, appear as tram-like or ring-like fatty lesions, depending on imaging plans. Ring-like fatty deposition can mimic metastases or HCC (Hamer et al. 2006). A diagnosis regarding the evaluation of T1-weighted "in-phase" and "out-phase" images can easily be achieved.

Another pattern is the subcapsular fat deposition which may appear as a confluent fat area confined in the peripheral zone or sometimes appearing as small fatty nodules (Hamer et al. 2006). The subcapsular pattern may be idiopathic or may be related to the use of insulin added to the peritoneal dialysate in patients with insulin-dependent diabetes and renal failure (Sohn et al. 2001; Khalili et al. 2003). In these patients, insulin promotes the esterification of free fatty acids into triglycerides, especially in subcapsular hepatocytes, because they are exposed to a higher insulin concentration. A patient's clinical history should be helpful in achieving a correct diagnosis.

The last rare pattern of fat deposition is multifocal fat infiltration, also known as "multinodular hepatic steatosis" (Prasad et al. 2005). Round foci of fat deposition are disseminated within the liver, also in atypical regions, mimicking true hepatic nodules (Kroncke et al. 2000; Kemper et al. 2002). A differential diagnosis can be challenging in cases of a patient with a known history of malignancy. Moreover, in addition to liver metastases, other differential diagnoses on US

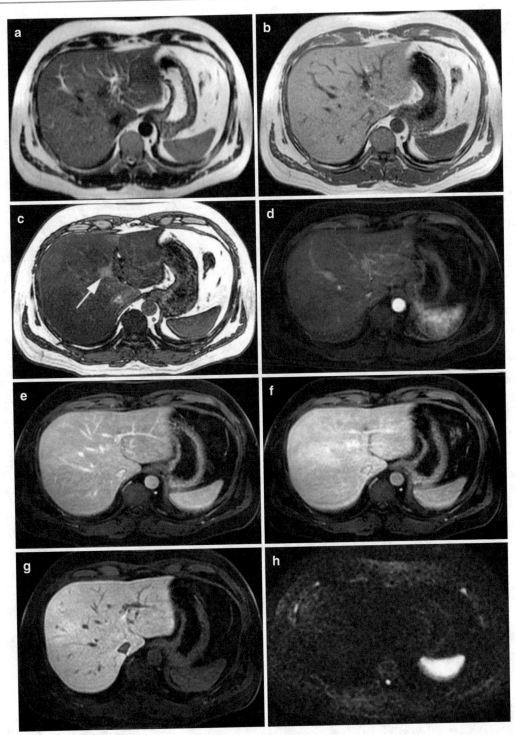

Fig. 23 Focal fat-sparing area on MRI. T2-weighted (**a**) and T1-weighted "in phase" (**b**) images demonstrating no focal lesions. T1-weighted "out-of-phase" (**c**) image shows a focal hyperintense area at the typical location in segment IV (arrow) on the background of a diffuse liver dropout of the signal. Dynamic study after contrast administration showing no alteration during the arterial (**d**), portal (**e**), delayed (**f**) and hepatobiliary (**g**) phases. Diffusion-weighted image (**h**) revealing no signal restrictions

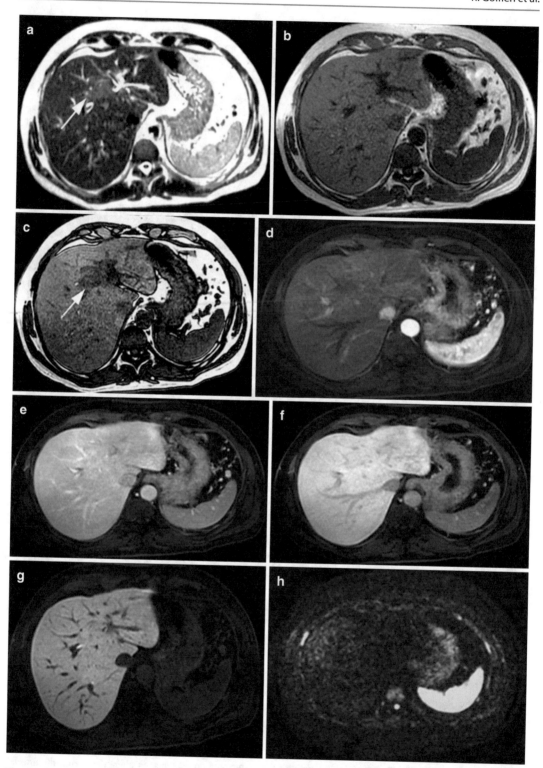

Fig. 24 Focal steatosis on MRI. T2-weighted image (**a**) depicts a focal hyperintense area in segment IV (arrow). T1-weighted images showing isointensity to the adjacent parenchyma on the "in-phase" image (**b**) and hypointensity of the focal area (arrow) on the "out-of-phase" image (**c**). Dynamic study after contrast administration does not show signal alteration during the arterial (**d**), portal (**e**) and delayed (**f**) phases, and isointensity to the adjacent parenchyma during the hepatobiliary phase (**g**). Diffusion-weighted image (**h**) confirms the absence of diffusion restriction in the area of the focal steatosis

and CT include lymphoma, sarcoidosis, abscesses, candidiasis, hemangiomatosis and biliary hamartomas. Magnetic resonance imaging is valuable for the correct differential diagnosis of fat deposition in oncological patients, due to the possibility of identifying microscopic fat within the lesions using T1-weighted images exploiting chemical shift artifacts. Moreover, the stability in size of these pseudolesions in the follow-up could indicate the exact diagnosis. In cirrhotic patients, multifocal fat deposition often corresponds to the fat degeneration within multiple RNs.

References

Alpern MB, Lawson TL, Foley WD et al (1986) Focal hepatic masses and fatty infiltration detected by enhanced dynamic CT. Radiology 158:45–49

Ames JT, Federle MP, Chopra K (2009) Distinguishing clinical and imaging features of nodular regenerative hyperplasia and large regenerative nodules of the liver. Clin Radiol 64:1190–1195

Angulo P (2002) Nonalcoholic fatty liver disease. N Engl J Med 346:1221–1231

Bhayana D, Kim TK, Jang HJ et al (2010) Hypervascular liver masses on contrast-enhanced ultrasound: the importance of washout. AJR Am J Roentgenol 194:977–983

Bookstein JJ, Cho KJ, Becker GB, Dail D (1982) Arterioportal communications: observations and hypotheses concerning transsinusoidal and transvasal types. Radiology 142:581–590

Boyce CJ, Pickhardt PJ, Kim DH et al (2010) Hepatic steatosis (fatty liver disease) in asymptomatic adults identified by unenhanced low-dose CT. AJR Am J Roentgenol 194:623–628

Brancatelli G, Federle MP, Blachar A, Grazioli L (2001) Hemangioma in the cirrhotic liver: diagnosis and natural history. Radiology 219:69–74

Brancatelli G, Federle MP, Grazioli L et al (2002a) Benign regenerative nodules in Budd Chiari syndrome and other vascular disorders of the liver: radiologic-pathologic and clinical correlations. Radiographics 22:847–862

Brancatelli G, Federle MP, Grazioli L et al (2002b) Large regenerative nodules in Budd-Chiari syndrome and other vascular disorders of the liver: CT and MR findings with clinico-pathologic correlation. AJR Am J Roentgenol 178:877–883

Brancatelli G, Baron RL, Peterson MS, Marsh W (2003) Helical CT screening for hepatocellular carcinoma in patients with cirrhosis: frequency and causes

of false-positive interpretation. Am J Roentengnol 180:1007–1014

Brancatelli G, Federle MP, Ambrosini R et al (2007) Cirrhosis: CT and MR imaging evaluation. Eur J Radiol 61:57–69

Brancatelli G, Baron RL, Federle MP et al (2009) Focal confluent fibrosis in cirrhotic liver: natural history studied with serial CT. AJR Am J Roentgenol 192:1341–1347

Brannigan M, Burns PN, Wilson SR (2004) Blood flow patterns in focal liver lesions at microbubble-enhanced US. Radiographics 24:921–935

Breen DJ, Rutherford EE, Stedman B et al (2004) Intrahepatic arterioportal shunting and anomalous venous drainage: understanding the CT features in the liver. Eur Radiol 14:2249–2260

Breitkopf K, Nagy LE, Beier JI et al (2009) Current experimental perspectives on the clinical progression of alcoholic liver disease. Alcohol Clin Exp Res 33:1647–1655

Brunt EM, Tiniakos DG (2002) Pathology of steatohepatitis. Best Pract Res Clin Gastroenterol 16:691–707

Cazals-Hatem D, Vilgrain V, Genin P et al (2003) Arterial and portal circulation and parenchymal changes in Budd-Chiari syndrome: a study in 17 explanted livers. Hepatology 37:510–509

Chen JH, Chai JW, Huang CL et al (1999a) Proximal arterioportal shunting associated with hepatocellular carcinoma: features revealed by dynamic helical CT. Am J Roentgenol 172:403–407

Chen WP, Chen JH, Hwang JI et al (1999b) Spectrum of transient hepatic attenuation differences in biphasic helical CT. Am J Roentgenol 172:419–424

Chen W, DelProposto Z, Wu D et al (2012) Improved Siderotic nodule detection in cirrhosis with susceptibility-weighted magnetic resonance imaging: a prospective study. PLoS One 7:e36454

Chen Y, Pan Y, Shen KR et al (2017) Contrast-enhanced multiple-phase imaging features of intrahepatic mass-forming cholangiocarcinoma and hepatocellular carcinoma with cirrhosis: a comparative study. Oncol Lett 14:4213–4219

Couinaud C (1988) The paraliliary venous system. Surg Radiol Anat 10:311–316

D'Amico G, Garcia-Tsao G, Pagliaro L (2006) Natural history and prognostic indicators of survival in cirrhosis: a systematic review of 118 studies. J Hepatol 44:217–231

De Sousa JM, Portmann B, Williams R (1991) Nodular regenerative hyperplasia of the liver and Budd-Chiari syndrome. Case report, review of the literature and reappraisal of pathogenesis. J Hepatol 12:28–35

Décarie PO, Lepanto L, Billiard JS et al (2011) Fatty liver deposition and sparing: a pictorial review. Insights Imaging 2:533–538

DeLeve LD, Shulman HM, McDonald GB (2002) Toxic injury to hepatic sinusoids: sinusoidal obstruction syndrome (veno-occlusive disease). Semin Liver Dis 22:27–42

Dioguardi Burgio M, Ronot M, Paulatto L et al (2016) Avoiding pitfalls in the interpretation of gadoxetic acid-enhanced magnetic resonance imaging. Semin Ultrasound CT MR 37:561–572

Doo KW, Lee CH, Choi JW et al (2009) "Pseudo washout" sign in high-flow hepatic hemangioma on gadoxetic acid contrast-enhanced MRI mimicking hypervascular tumor. AJR Am J Roentgenol 193:W490–W496

Duran R, Ronot M, Kerbaol A et al (2014) Hepatic hemangiomas: factors associated with T2 shine-through effect on diffusion-weighted MR sequences. Eur J Radiol 83:468–478

Duran R, Ronot M, Di Renzo S et al (2015) Is magnetic resonance imaging of hepatic hemangioma any different in liver fibrosis and cirrhosis compared to normal liver? Eur J Radiol 84:816–822

Elsayes KM, Shaaban AM (2015) Specialty imaging: pitfalls and classic signs of the abdomen and pelvis. Elsevier, Philadelphia, PA

Francisco FA, de Araújo AL, Oliveira Neto JA, Parente DB (2014) Hepatobiliary contrast agents: differential diagnosis of focal hepatic lesions, pitfalls and other indications. Radiol Bras 47:301–309

Galia M, Taibbi A, Marin D et al (2014) Focal lesions in cirrhotic liver: what else beyond hepatocellular carcinoma? Diagn Interv Radiol 20:222–228

Goodwin MD, Dobson JE, Sirlin CB et al (2011) Diagnostic challenges and pitfalls in MR imaging with hepatocyte-specific contrast agents. Radiographics 31:1547–1568

Gryspeerdt S, Van Hoe L, Marchal G, Baert AL (1997) Evaluation of hepatic perfusion disorders with double-phase spiral CT. Radiographics 17:337–348

Hamer OW, Aguirre DA, Casola G et al (2006) Fatty liver: imaging patterns and pitfalls. Radiographics 26:1637–1653

Hanna RF, Aguirre DA, Kased N et al (2008) Cirrhosis-associated hepatocellular nodules: correlation of histopathologic and MR imaging features. Radiographics 28:747–769

Hellekant CH (1976) Vascular complications following needle puncture of the liver. Acta Radiol 17:209–222

Hussain SM, Semelka RC, Mitchell DG (2002) MR imaging of hepatocellular carcinoma. Magn Reson Imaging Clin N Am 10:31–52

International Working Party (1995) Terminology of nodular hepatocellular lesions. Hepatology 22:983–993

Itai Y, Matsui O (1997) Blood flow and liver imaging. Radiology 202:306–314

Itai Y, Matsui O (1999) 'Nonportal' splanchnic venous supply to the liver: abnormal findings on CT, US and MRI. Eur Radiol 9:237–243

Itai Y, Saida Y (2002) Pitfalls in liver imaging. Eur Radiol 12:1162–1174

Itai Y, Murata S, Saida Y, Minami M (1994) Central zone and peripheral zone of the liver based on portal and hepatic arterial blood supply; imaging approach to deformity of cirrhotic liver. Jpn J Clin Radiol 39:1553–1559

Itai Y, Murata S, Kurosaki Y (1995) Straight border sign of the liver: spectrum of CT appearances and causes. Radiographics 15:1089–1102

Ito K, Mitchell DG, Gabata T et al (1999) Hepatocellular carcinoma: association with increased iron deposition in the cirrhotic liver at MR imaging. Radiology 212:235–224

Jang HJ, Kim TK, Lim HK et al (2003) Hepatic hemangioma: atypical appearances on CT, MR imaging, and sonography. AJR Am J Roentgenol 180:135–141

Jang HJ, Yu H, Kim TK (2009a) Contrast-enhanced ultrasound in the detection and characterization of liver tumors. Cancer Imaging 9:96–103

Jang HJ, Yu H, Kim TK (2009b) Imaging of focal liver lesions. Semin Roentgenol 44:266–282

Karhunen PJ (1986) Benign hepatic tumours and tumour like conditions in men. J Clin Pathol 39:183–188

Kemper J, Jung G, Poll LW et al (2002) CT and MRI findings of multifocal hepatic steatosis mimicking malignancy. Abdom Imaging 27:708–710

Khalili K, Lan FP, Hanbidge AE et al (2003) Hepatic subcapsular steatosis in response to intraperitoneal insulin delivery: CT findings and prevalence. AJR Am J Roentgenol 180:1601–1604

Kim TK, Jang HJ, Wilson SR (2006) Benign liver masses: imaging with microbubble contrast agents. Ultrasound Q 22:31–39

Kim TK, Lee E, Jang HJ (2015) Imaging findings of mimickers of hepatocellular carcinoma. Clin Mol Hepatol:326–343

Kim B, Byun JH, Kim HJ et al (2016) Enhancement patterns and pseudo-washout of hepatic haemangiomas on gadoxetate disodium-enhanced liver MRI. Eur Radiol 26:191–198

Kobayashi S, Gabata T, Matsui O (2010) Radiologic manifestation of hepatic pseudolesions and pseudotumors in the third inflow area. Imaging Med 2:519–528

Kondo F (2001) Benign nodular hepatocellular lesions caused by abnormal hepatic circulation: etiological analysis and introduction of a new concept. J Gastroenterol Hepatol 16:1319–1328

Krinsky GA, Lee VS, Nguyen MT et al (2000) Siderotic nodules at MR imaging: regenerative or dysplastic? J Comput Assist Tomogr 24:773–776

Krinsky GA, Lee VS, Nguyen MT et al (2001) Siderotic nodules in the cirrhotic liver at MR imaging with explant correlation: no increased frequency of dysplastic nodules and hepatocellular carcinoma. Radiology 218:47–53

Krinsky GA, Zivin SB, Thorner KM et al (2002) Low grade siderotic dysplastic nodules: determination of premalignant lesions on the basis of vasculature phenotype. Acad Radiol 9:336–341

Kroncke TJ, Taupitz M, Kivelitz D et al (2000) Multifocal nodular fatty infiltration of the liver mimicking metastatic disease on CT: imaging findings and diagnosis using MR imaging. Eur Radiol 10:1095–1100

Kudo M (2009) Multistep human hepatocarcinogenesis: correlation of imaging with pathology. J Gastroenterol 19:112–118

Lee SJ, Lim JH, Lee WJ et al (1997) Transient subsegmental hepatic parenchymal enhancement on dynamic CT: a sign of postbiopsy arterioportal shunt. J Comput Assist Tomogr 21:355–360

Makhlouf HR, Ishak KG (2002) Sclerosed hemangiomas and sclerosing cavernous hemangioma of the liver: a comparative clinicopathologic and immunohistochemical study with emphasis on the role of mast cells in their histogenesis. Liver 22:70–78

Marrero JA, Ahn J, Rajender Reddy K (2014) American College of Gastroenterology. ACG clinical guideline: the diagnosis and management of focal liver lesions. Am J Gastroenterol 109:1328–1347

Martin J, Puig J, Darnell A, Donoso L (2002) Magnetic resonance of focal liver lesions in hepatic cirrhosis and chronic hepatitis. Semin Ultrasound CT MR 23: 62–78

Mastropasqua M, Kanematsu M, Leonardou P et al (2004) Cavernous hemangiomas in patients with chronic liver disease: MR imaging findings. Magn Reson Imaging 22:15–18

Mathiesen UL, Franzen LE, Aselius H et al (2002) Increased liver echogenicity at ultrasound examination reflects degree of steatosis but not of fibrosis in asymptomatic patients with mild/moderate abnormalities of liver transaminases. Dig Liver Dis 34: 516–522

Mathieu D, Paret M, Mahfouz AE et al (1997) Hyperintense benign liver lesions on spin-echo T1-weighted MR images: pathologic correlations. Abdom Imaging 22:410–417

Mathieu D, Luciani A, Achab A et al (2001) Hepatic Pseudolesions. Gastroenterol Clin Biol 25:B158–B166

Matsui O, Kadoya M, Takahashi S et al (1995) Focal sparing of segment IV in fatty livers shown by sonography and CT: correlation with aberrant gastric venous drainage. AJR Am J Roentgenol 164:1137–1140

Mitchell DG, Rubin R, Siegelman ES et al (1991) Hepatocellular carcinoma within siderotic regenerative nodules: appearance as a nodule within a nodule on MR images. Radiology 178:101–103

Mittal S, El-Serag HB (2013) Epidemiology of hepatocellular carcinoma: consider the population. J Clin Gastroenterol 47.(suppl:S2–S6

Motosugi U, Ichikawa T, Sou H et al (2010) Distinguishing hypervascular pseudolesions of the liver from hypervascular hepatocellular carcinomas with gadoxetic acid-enhanced MR imaging. Radiology 256(1):151–158

Murata S, Itai Y, Asato M et al (1995) Effect of temporary occlusion of the hepatic vein on dual blood in the liver: evaluation with spiral CT. Radiology 197:351–356

Nicolau C, Brú C (2004) Focal liver lesions: evaluation with contrast-enhanced ultrasonography. Abdom Imaging 29:348–359

O'Malley ME, Takayama Y, Sherman M (2005) Outcome of small (10-20 mm) arterial phase-enhancing nodules seen on triphasic liver CT inpatients with cirrhosis or chronic liver disease. Am J Gastroenterol 100:1523–1528

Ohtomo K, Baron RL, Dodd GD 3rd et al (1993a) Confluent hepatic fibrosis in advanced cirrhosis: appearance at CT. Radiology 188:31–35

Ohtomo K, Baron RL, Dodd GD 3rd et al (1993b) Confluent hepatic fibrosis in advanced cirrhosis: evaluation with MR imaging. Radiology 189:871–874

Okuda K, Musha H, Nakajima Y et al (1978) Frequency of intrahepatic arteriovenous fistula as a sequela to percutaneous needle puncture of the liver. Gastroenterology 74:1204–1207

Park YN, Kim M-J (2011) Hepatocarcinogenesis: imaging-pathologic correlation. Abdom Imaging 36:232–243

Park YS, Lee CH, Kim BH et al (2013) Using Gd-EOB-DTPA-enhanced 3-T MRI for the differentiation of infiltrative hepatocellular carcinoma and focal confluent fibrosis in liver cirrhosis. Magn Reson Imaging 31:1137–1142

Prasad SR, Wang H, Rosas H et al (2005) Fat-containing lesions of the liver: radiologic-pathologic correlation. Radiographics 25:321–333

Renzulli M, Lucidi V, Moscni C et al (2011) Large regenerative nodules in a patient with Budd-Chiari syndrome after TIPS positioning while on the liver transplantation list diagnosed by Gd-EOB-DTPA MRI. Hepatobiliary Pancreat Dis Int 10:439–442

Ronot M, Dioguardi Burgio M, Purcell Y et al (2017) Focal lesions in cirrhosis: not always HCC. Eur J Radiol 93:157–168

Sadek AG, Mitchell DG, Siegelman ES et al (1995) Early hepatocellular carcinoma that develops within macroregenerative nodules: growth rate depicted at serial MR imaging. Radiology 195:753–756

Scheuer PJ, Lefkowitch JH (2000) Fatty liver and lesions in the alcoholic. In: Liver biopsy interpretation, 6th edn. Saunders, Philadelphia, PA, pp 111–129

Shimizu A, Ito K, Koike S et al (2003) Cirrhosis or chronic hepatitis: evaluation of small (<or=2-cm) early-enhancing hepatic lesions with serial contrast-enhanced dynamic MR imaging. Radiology 226:550–555

Siegelman ES, Chauhan A (2014) MR characterization of focal liver lesions. Magn Reson Imaging Clin N Am 22:295–313

Siegelman ES, Mitchell DG, Semelka RC (1996) Abdominal iron deposition: metabolism, MR findings, and clinical importance. Radiology 199:13–22

Sohn J, Siegelman E, Osiason A (2001) Unusual patterns of hepatic steatosis caused by the local effect of insulin revealed on chemical shift MR imaging. AJR Am J Roentgenol 176:471–474

Steiner PE (1959) Nodular regenerative hyperplasia of the liver. Am J Pathol 35:943–953

Stromeyer FW, Ishak KG (1981) Nodular transformation (nodular "regenerative" hyperplasia) of the liver. A clinicopathologic study of 30 cases. Hum Pathol 12:60–71

Sun HY, Lee JM, Shin CI et al (2010) Gadoxetic acid-enhanced magnetic resonance imaging for differentiating small hepatocellular carcinomas (< or =2 cm in diameter) from arterial enhancing pseudolesions: special emphasis on hepatobiliary phase imaging. Investig Radiol 45(2):96–103

Takayasu K, Muramatsu Y, Moriyama N et al (1994) Radiological study of idiopathic Budd-Chiari syndrome complicated by hepatocellular carcinoma. A report of four cases. Am J Gastroenterol 89:249–253

Tamada T, Ito K, Yamamoto A et al (2011) Hepatic hemangiomas: evaluation of enhancement patterns at dynamic MRI with gadoxetate disodium. AJR Am J Roentgenol 196:824–830

Tanaka M, Wanless IR (1998) Pathology of the liver in Budd-Chiari syndrome: portal vein thrombosis and the histogenesis of veno-centric cirrhosis, veno-portal cirrhosis, and large regenerative nodules. Hepatology 27:488–496

Terada T, Nakanuma Y (1989) Survey of iron-accumulative macroregenerative nodules in cirrhotic livers. Hepatology 10:851–854

Terada T, Kadoya M, Nakanuma Y, Matsui O (1990) Iron-accumulating adenomatous hyperplastic nodule with malignant foci in the cirrhotic liver histopathologic, quantitative iron, and magnetic resonance imaging in vitro studies. Cancer 65:1994–2000

Vilgrain V, Lewin M, Vons C et al (1999) Hepatic nodules in Budd-Chiari syndrome: imaging features. Radiology 210:443–450

Vilgrain V, Lagadec M, Ronot M (2016) Pitfalls in liver imaging. Radiology 278:34–51

Wachsberg RH, Bahramipour P, Sofocleous CT, Barone A (2002) Hepatofugal flow in the portal venous system:

pathophysiology, imaging findings, and diagnostic pitfalls. Radiographics 22:123–140

Wanless IR (1990) Micronodular transformation (nodular regenerative hyperplasia) of the liver: a report of 64 cases among 2,500 autopsies and a new classification of benign hepatocellular nodules. Hepatology 11:787–797

Wanless IR, Mawdsley C, Adams R (1985) On the pathogenesis of focal nodular hyperplasia of the liver. Hepatology 5:1194–1200

Wilson SR, Jang HJ, Kim TK et al (2008) Real-time temporal maximum-intensity-projection imaging of hepatic lesions with contrast-enhanced sonography. AJR Am J Roentgenol 190:691–695

Yoshimitsu K, Honda H, Kuroiwa T et al (1999) Pseudolesions of the liver possibly caused by focal rib compression: analysis based on hemodynamic change. AJR Am J Roentgenol 172:645–649

Yoshimitzu K, Honda H, Kuroiwa T et al (2001) Unusual hemodynamics and pseudolesions of the noncirrhotic liver at CT. Radiographics 21:S81–S96

Yu JS, Kim KW, Sung KB et al (1997) Small arterial-portal venous shunts: a cause of pseudolesions at hepatic imaging. Radiology 203:737–742

Yu JS, Kim KW, Yeong MG et al (2000) Non tumorous hepatic arterial-portal venous shunts: MR imaging findings. Radiology 217:750–756

Zhang J, Krinsky GA (2004) Iron-containing nodules of cirrhosis. NMR Biomed 17:459–464

Part III

Therapy of Hepatic Tumours and Post-treatment Changes in the Liver

Percutaneous Ablation of Liver Tumors

Arcangelo Merola, Silvia Brocco, and Emilio Quaia

Contents

Abstract

Primary and secondary liver tumors are very common. In developed countries, hepatocellular carcinoma (HCC) is the third cause of

cancer death with a poor survival rate in advanced cases. If a curative treatment can be applied at an early stage the overall survival is markedly improved.

Many patients (80–90%) cannot undergo radical surgery due to general health status, previous abdominal surgery, diffuse lesion with insufficient liver remnant after their complete removal, or anatomical unfavorable locations.

For these reasons, percutaneous treatments have become auspicious treatments for liver tumors due to minimal invasiveness, effectiveness, repeatability, and low costs.

A. Merola · S. Brocco · E. Quaia (✉)
Radiology Unit, Department of Medicine - DIMED,
University of Padova, Padova, Italy
e-mail: emilio.quaia@unipd.it

© Springer Nature Switzerland AG 2021
E. Quaia (ed.), *Imaging of the Liver and Intra-hepatic Biliary Tract*,
Medical Radiology Diagnostic Imaging, https://doi.org/10.1007/978-3-030-39021-1_12

Different modalities are accepted for percutaneous ablation procedures and can be divided into thermal and non-thermal ablation techniques.

Thermal techniques are monopolar and multipolar radiofrequency ablation (RFA), microwave ablation (MWA), laser ablation (LSA), cryoablation (CRA), and high-intensity focused ultrasound (HIFU). Non-thermal techniques are percutaneous ethanol injection (PEI) and irreversible electroporation. Combinations of the different techniques are possible.

These ablative techniques provide necrotization of tumor tissue in different ways, such as thermal coagulation, rapid freezing, or chemical cell dehydration.

The procedural planning is divided into three different phases (1) preprocedural planning, (2) intraprocedural targeting, monitoring, and modification, (3) postprocedural assessment.

Imaging techniques are of crucial importance in all these phases.

Complication after percutaneous techniques occurs in 3–7% of patients.

1   Introduction

In developed countries, hepatocellular carcinoma (HCC) is the third cause of cancer death with a poor survival rate in advanced cases (5 year overall survive 10–15%). If a curative treatment can be applied at an early stage the overall survival is markedly improved (De Angelis et al. 2014).

Secondary liver tumors are even more frequent than HCC.

Colorectal cancer is the second cause of cancer-related mortality. About 40–76% of patients with colorectal cancer develop liver metastases (Puijk et al. 2018; Liang et al. 2013; Van Tilborg et al. 2016) and, in general, liver metastases are identified in 50% of patients with gastrointestinal malignancies (Greenlee et al. 2001; Landis et al. 1999).

Liver transplant is considered the gold standard curative treatment for HCC but it is available for a small number of patients due to high costs and constant presence of organ shortage due to the small numbers of donors (Bruix and Sherman 2011).

In selected cases of HCC and secondary liver tumors, especially for metastases of colorectal origin, surgical resection significantly improves overall survival (Llovet et al. 1999; de Haas et al. 2010; de Haas et al. 2011; Gilliams et al. 2015).

However, many patients (about 80–90%) cannot undergo partial hepatectomy because they have a compromised health status or multiple previous abdominal surgical procedures due to diffuse metastatic liver involvement with insufficient liver remnant after their complete removal or even anatomically unfavorable metastasis location (Sotirchos et al. 2016; Van Tilborg et al. 2016).

For this reason, percutaneous treatments, thanks to their minimal invasiveness, effectiveness, and low costs, have become really favorable approaches to primary and secondary liver tumors. This happens especially for lesions <3 cm in diameter, in which local control after radiofrequency ablation is equivalent to resection in terms of therapeutic results. (Mulier et al. 2008).

Percutaneous ablation includes various techniques. These techniques improved in the last two decades, giving the possibility to treat a progressively increasing number of patients, with great efficacy in controlling liver disease (Breen and Lencioni 2015).

Different modalities are accepted for percutaneous ablation procedures and can be divided into thermal and non-thermal ablation techniques.

Thermal techniques are monopolar and multipolar radiofrequency ablation (RFA), microwave ablation (MWA), laser ablation (LSA), cryoablation (CRA), and high-intensity focused ultrasound (HIFU). Non-thermal techniques are percutaneous ethanol injection (PEI) and irreversible electroporation. The use of different combinations of these techniques is possible too.

These ablative techniques provide tumor tissue coagulative or colliquative necrosis in different ways, such as thermal coagulation, rapid freezing, or chemical cell dehydration

(Chinnaratha et al. 2016; Yang et al. 2015; Wang et al. 2015b; Orlacchio et al. 2014).

PEI was one of the first ablating techniques used for the treatment of HCC (Verslype et al. 2012). Radiofrequency ablation and microwave ablation have been used in the last two decades due to their minimal invasiveness, efficacy, the possibility of multiple repeated treatments, and low costs (Crocetti et al. 2010; Martin et al. 2010). The international guidelines for the treatment of HCC usually refer to these two methods (Bruix and Llovet 2009), but also other available techniques can achieve important effective therapeutic effects.

2 Indication and Percutaneous Ablation Techniques

Percutaneous ablation techniques are considered an alternative to surgery and in selected cases is considered curative.

To achieve this goal, the staging of primary and secondary liver tumors is fundamental. In the case of HCC in cirrhotic patients, the Barcelona Clinic Liver Cancer (BCLC) staging system should be used. This staging system identifies those patients with early HCC (stage 0 - tumor <2cm, Performance Status = 0, and Child-Pugh A - and A - single tumour of any size, or up to 3 tumours all <3 cm, Performance Status = 0, and Child-Pugh A or B) who may benefit from curative therapies, those at intermediate (stage B - multiple lesions, Performance Status = 0, and Child-Pugh A or B -) or advanced stage (stage C - tumor has spread into the blood vessels, lymph nodes or other body organs, Performance Status = 1 or 2, and Child-Pugh A or B -) who may benefit from palliative treatments and those patients with a very poor life expectancy (stage D - Performance Status = 3 or 4, and Child-Pugh C -) (Verslype et al. 2012).

To establish the possibilities of a percutaneous approach to be curative in the treatment of secondary liver tumors, a multidisciplinary evaluation is fundamental and must keep in mind the features and the extension of the original tumor and must consider the possibility of a combined multimodality approach (Tombesi et al. 2018).

2.1 Radiofrequency Ablation (RFA)

HCC can be treated by RFA in the case of very early (<2 cm) and early-stage disease (< 3 cm). Following BCLC criteria in these cases, RFA can be considered curative (Bruix et al. 2001) and complete response is obtained in >90% of cases with good long term outcomes (Livraghi et al. 2008). In nodules >2 cm RFA provides better control than PEI (Lencioni 2010).

RFA must consider the size and location of the tumor to be curative. The presence of a vessel larger than 3 mm in diameter creates the heath sink effect. Consequently, treatment with RFA of tumors located close to large vessels has a low ablation efficacy (Lu et al. 2003). At the same time, if the lesion is large, it can require multiple ablations because more applicators are needed, or sometimes their position is unfavorable to obtain a safe ablation margin. For this reason, RFA is preferentially indicated in lesions <3 cm in size or <5 cm in size when hook shape expandable electrode tines with a diameter of 3.5 cm at expansion are available (Chen et al. 2006). In the unfavorable event of a lesion >5 cm in size, the tumor control rate reported after RFA is quite low, ranging from 6 to 10% in different studies (Chen et al. 2006; Kudo 2004; Lencioni and Crocetti 2008).

It has been designed a mathematical model for the treatment of lesions with radiofrequency. Those tumors with diameters between 3 and 3.30 cm require at least four ablations. Tumors with diameters between 3.31 cm and 4.12 cm require at least six ablations. Tumors from 4.13 cm to 6.23 cm in size need at least 12 ablations (Khajanchee et al. 2004).

The HCC lesions treated with RFA in the same liver should not exceed the number of five and they must not be >5 cm in size.

Bile ducts can be damaged during the procedure and tumor seeding has been reported in case of percutaneous RFA in 0–12.5% (median 0.9%) of the cases depending on the studies (Stigliano et al. 2007).

In *liver metastases*, surgery is considered the treatment of choice with 5-years survival rates of 31–58%. It is feasible just in 10–15% of cases and patients must be carefully selected due to the frequent presence of multiple and multicentric lesions. Many of these patients usually undergo systemic chemotherapy treatments but the survival at 5 years is poor (de Haas et al. 2010; de Haas et al. 2011; Gilliams et al. 2015). For this reason, RFA is often proposed as an alternative to surgery. It owns a very low risk of complication, with a complete ablation at follow-up CT scan of 45% (Dodd et al. 2000). Among various studies, the 3 and 5 years survival rates range from 28 to 46% with a median survival of 30–40 months. In particular, Solbiati et al. showed a survival rate of 33% at 3 years with higher recurrence in patients with larger lesions (>3 cm in diameter) (Solbiati et al. 2001). Gilliam and Lees demonstrated a 28% and 25% survival rate at 3 and 5 years in patients treated with up to five liver metastases (Gilliam and Lees 2005), and Lee evidenced a survival rate at 3 and 5 years respectively of 53.3% and 42.6% in the treatment of solitary colorectal cancer metastases (Lee et al. 2008).

Hildebrand et al. (2006) demonstrated that the success of the procedure is also linked to the presence of a dedicated and experienced team in RFA.

A more recent position paper on the treatment of colorectal liver metastases by RFA showed a five-year survival after RFA of 31% (Gilliams et al. 2015).

RFA can be used even in resectable liver metastases in addition to surgical resection, in liver metastases with a partial response after chemotherapy and for recurrent liver metastases or metastatic lesions showing disease progression (Vogl et al. 2014a). The US monitoring is very helpful to determinate the radicality of the procedure. The transient hyperechoic zone within the target lesion and the surrounding normal tissue may be considered in the treatment management.

2.2 Microwave Ablation (MWA)

The main limit of MWA is the tumor size. If in the past it was confined to 2 cm, with recent advances in techniques this treatment can be extended to lesions up to 3 cm in diameter (Thamtorawat et al. 2016). Nowadays MWA can be considered a treatment of the first choice for lesions ≤3 cm in size. It is useful in particular if they are located near large bile ducts or larger blood vessels, with lower damage to these structures but also with a reduced heath sink effect that is instead important with RFA (Dong et al. 2003).

In *HCC* nodules the 3-year survival rate is 72.85% while 5-year survival rate is 56.70% in case of nodules ranging from 1.2 cm to 8 cm in size (mean 4.1 cm), with significantly shorter survival in patients with lesions >5 cm and better survival in patients with lesions <3 cm. (Dong et al. 2003).

In *liver metastases,* several studies demonstrated that the use of MWA allows a 3-year survival rate of 46–51% and a 5-year survival rate of 17_32% with a median survival time of 20–48 months (Liang et al. 2003; Tanaka et al. 2006; Ogata et al. 2008). The ability of MWA to achieve larger ablation areas than RFA with shorter application times to obtain safe free margins is fundamental in the treatment of liver metastases because they show a typical infiltrative growth and absence of well-defined margins (Tombesi et al. 2018). RFA and MWA do not differ in the local tumor progression at 2 years in HCC <4 cm (Violi et al. 2018).

2.3 Laser Ablation

Laser ablation (LSA) uses cannulation needles through which optical quartz fibers are inserted in the lesion to treat. These laser optical fibers deliver lights that are transformed in heath. This high energy laser radiation spread into liver parenchyma, leading to coagulative necrosis. The main advantage of laser ablation is the size of the needle that is very small (21 gauge) making this technique to be particularly suitable to treat high-risk locations.

LSA appears very flexible since it allows the treatment of lesions of different sizes depending on the number of optical fibers used. To treat nodules up to 1.5 cm one or two fibers are needed, three fibers are used to treat nodules from 1.5 cm to 2.5 cm while to treat nodules >2.5 cm four fibers are required. Fibers are positioned paying attention to correct spacing and using different geometrical distribution to achieve the maximum ablative effect (Francica et al. 2012a and 2012b; Di Costanzo et al. 2014).

The multiple fibers approach leads to the possibility to treat primary and secondary liver lesions up to 5 cm in diameter with good results. Di Costanzo et al. (2014) reported a complete ablation in 93.6% of nodules <3 cm and a complete ablation rate in 79.6% in nodules >3 cm.

LSA has recently shown results comparable to those of RFA and MWA (Francica et al. 2007; Pacella et al. 2005; di Costanzo et al. 2013). In patients with HCC and Child-Pugh A, liver cirrhosis nodules up to 5 cm in diameter treated with multiple fibers achieved a complete response rate ranging from 82 to 97%. Cumulative 3-year survival rates reached 73% (Di Costanzo et al. 2014; Pacella et al. 2009).

Eichler et al. (2012) showed that 98% of patients achieved complete necrosis with a safe margin 5 mm by using LSA. The survival rate at 3 and 5 years were respectively of 54% and 30% (Eichler et al. 2012). A complete response rate of 95.5% has also been reported in tumors with high-risk locations (Di Costanzo et al. 2013).

In presence of liver metastases, LSA is the percutaneous technique of choice if they are multiple, of different size and with a bi-lobar distribution, in case of a recurrence after surgery or if the patient has unresectable lesions or other major general contraindication to surgery. Usually, LSA is not performed if there is a concomitant extrahepatic disease (Tombesi et al. 2015; Sartori et al. 2017). Several studies considering liver metastases showed that 3-year survival is of 28–74% and 5-year survival is of 10–37% in lesions smaller than 5 cm (Vogl et al. 2004; Puls et al. 2009; Vogl et al. 2014b).

2.4 Percutaneous Ethanol Injection (PEI)

Percutaneous ethanol injection (PEI) is considered a well-tolerated and safe treatment with low costs. It is one of the more studied percutaneous techniques and one of the first to be applied for the treatment of liver tumors. Nowadays it has been replaced by RFA and is used just when RFA cannot be feasible, for example in entero-biliary reflux or when there is the adhesion of the tumor to the gastrointestinal tract (Omata et al. 2017). In many studies, PEI showed great safety. Mortality is very low ranging from 0 to 3.2% while morbidity ranges are 0–0.04%. In particular, Livraghi et al. (1995) described 1.7% of severe complications and a mortality of 0.1%, while Shiina et al. (2012) reported complications in 2.1% of cases with 0.09% of deaths. Di Stasi et al. (1997) had similar results with 3.2% of complications and 0.09% of mortality, while Ebara et al. (2005) reported no treatment-related deaths and 2.2% of complications. Sung et al. (2006) reported absence of complications in his case series.

The main complication reported were hemorrhages and tumor seeding. As a collateral effect of PEI, pain may be effectively treated by analgesics. Fever has been reported. More sessions are needed to obtain the necrosis of the tumor, ranging from 2 to 14 (Di Stasi et al. 1997).

Various factors are related to outcomes of PEI. Fundamental is the tumor size, the liver function measured with the Child-Pugh score, the levels of alfa-fetoprotein, the numbers of nodules, and the age of the patient. (Shiina et al. 2012)

A reasonable indication for PEI therapy is HCC < 3cm in greatest dimension (Ishii et al. 1996). Patients with a single nodule of HCC < 5 cm in size and Child-Pugh A showed the best outcome with survival rates of 47–79%, decreasing progressively in Child-Pugh B patients (29–63%) and Child-Pugh C patients (0–12%) at 3–5 years (Livraghi et al. 1995). Other studies reported a 5-year survival rate in patients undergoing PEI of 38–60% (Ebara et al. 2005, Sung et al. 2006, Shiina et al. 2012), while the local progression rates range from 6 to 31% and are mainly related to the tumoral size (Livraghi et al. 1995), Ishii et al. 1996, Di Stasi et al. 1997, Ebara et al. 2005, Sung et al. 2006, Shiina et al. 2012). In particular, a tumoral size >3 cm was associated with a higher rate of local recurrence within 2 years from treatment (Ishii et al. 1996).

2.5 Irreversible Electroporation (IRE)

IRE in a new percutaneous ablation technique. It is a nonthermal ablative method that delivers short electric pulses of high power and intensity between two electrodes located in the liver parenchyma. A high electromagnetic field is created that causes the formation of pores in the cellular membrane leading cells to apoptosis. The limits of the area that can be treated correspond to those in which a high electromagnetic field can be generated. For this reason, as a general rule two electrodes are needed to treat lesions up to 1 cm, three electrodes for lesions up to 2 cm, four electrodes for lesions between 2 and 3 cm and five to six electrodes for lesions between 3 and 5 cm in diameter (Narayanan et al. 2014; Scheffer et al. 2014).

Due to the use of electric pulses delivered synchronized to cardiac pulses IRE is contraindicated in patients with cardiac arrhythmia and pace-makers (Seror 2015). According to the absence of thermal energy, the risk of thermal injury to the skin and normal structures is low and there is no heat sink effect. Thus, this technique is particularly suitable for high-risk locations like biliary structures that usually preclude the application of thermal ablation techniques (Dollinger et al. 2015).

Ding et al. (2017) reported IRE treatment efficacy for HCC in 58 patients not treatable by thermal techniques. Complete ablation was observed in 92% of cases. The technique showed a good safety profile since IRE seems to lead less frequently than RFA to liver failure enabling the treatment of patients with worse liver function, for example, Child–Pugh class B patients (Bhutiani et al. 2016; Sutter et al. 2017). Sutter et al. (2017) studied other 58 patients with HCC lesions chosen for IRE because of difficulty in treating areas or compromised medical status. This study showed an ablation rate of 77.3% after one session, 89.3% after two sessions, and 92% after three sessions of IRE therapy. The progression-free survival at 6 months was 87% while at 12 months was 70% with 5% risk of complications after the procedure (Sutter et al. 2017).

2.6 Cryoablation

The first studies about cryoablation (CRA), carried out with first-generation equipment, reported a high incidence of adverse events. The most worrisome was cryo-shock. It developed after the ablation of large liver lesions producing multiorgan failure and consequent death. Furthermore, in several studies, CRA seemed to have less efficacy than RFA (Pearson et al. 1999; Tait et al. 2002; Adam et al. 2002; Huang et al. 2013). With latest advances in this technique, cryo-shock has not been reported anymore and various studies focalized on HCC treatment have been published (Mahnken et al. 2018). In 2015 a controlled multicenter study was published in which Child-Pugh A and B patients with HCC <4 cm were treated. CRA showed a lower local progression rate compared to RFA for HCC >3 cm (7.7% vs. 18.2%), with no difference in survival rate. Safety of CRA appeared similar to RFA (complication rate of 3.9% in CRA vs. 3.3% in RFA) (Wang et al. 2015b). There are no clear guidelines about liver metastasis treatment with CRA because of limited data that are difficult to compare due to association with different therapies. However, CRA showed an acceptable safety profile in tumors <4 cm in size with severe complications ranging from 5.8—8.7% in larger lesions (Littrup et al. 2016; Glazer et al. 2017). Results about local progression rates are quite different among studies, with a local progression rate of 11.1% after 1.8 years (Littrup et al. 2016) and of 25.4% at 2.5 years (Glazer et al. 2017) in colorectal liver metastases. CRA showed promising results for other types of primary tumors as breast and ovarian cancer (Zhang et al. 2014; Gao et al. 2015).

2.7 High Intensity Focused Ultrasound (HIFU)

HIFU ablation is one of the latest treatments introduced for the treatment of HCC and liver metastases. It consists of a totally extracorporeal non-invasive treatment modality that uses focused ultrasound energy causing coagulative necrosis of the target lesion. It does not need surgical incision because it is performed via intact skin (Cheung et al. 2013). It appears to be well tolerated in patients with advanced age and advances stages of liver cirrhosis. Often, HIFU is not considered curative but rather is considered as a bridge to liver transplant in patients with HCC (Cheung et al. 2013; Ng et al. 2011). In fact, HIFU is usually applied to those patients who cannot undergo surgical resection because of inadequate liver remnant due to advanced and decompensated cirrhosis or previous major hepatectomy (Cheung et al. 2012; Cheung et al. 2013) or in patients not suitable for RFA or PEI because the nodules to treat are too large or near major vessels (Zhu et al. 2009; Zhang et al. 2009).

HIFU has shown satisfying outcomes in various studies. In HCCs <3 cm in size, patients can achieve an ablation rate of 82.4% in one treatment session (Ng et al. 2011).

In other studies, tumor necrosis was achieved in 69.6% of lesions with a single HIFU session with complete necrosis after the second session and a survival rate at 5 year of 55.6% (Zhu et al. 2009). In a study by Zhang et al. (2009) half of the treated lesions were necrotic after the first session of HIFU treatment. In the second session, complete necrosis of all lesions was achieved with a 5-year survival rate of 31.8%. Fewer data are available for the treatment of liver metastases with HIFU and many studies conducted involved little groups of patients, showing a good safety profile. In liver metastases, HIFU is used when other percutaneous techniques are not indicated and particularly when lesions are located in difficult areas such as close to large blood vessels or bile ducts, near gallbladder, bowel, stomach, or heart (Orsi et al. 2010). In his study, Orsi et al. (2010) showed a complete response almost in all treated liver metastases after one HIFU session, as found by Park et al. (2009) assessing the use of HIFU in treatment of liver metastases from colon and stomach cancers in which the efficacy after the first treatment session was close to 100%. HIFU minor complications are represented by skin redness and burnt affecting all patients treated, or necrosis of rib or vertebrae located near the treated areas. The major complication reported were biliary obstructions, symptomatic pleural effusions, and fistulas and were reported in 5% of all patients treated (Jung et al. 2011).

3 Procedural Planning

The procedural planning is divided into three different phases (1) preprocedural planning, (2) intraprocedural targeting, monitoring, and modification, (3) postprocedural assessment.

Imaging techniques are of crucial importance in all of them.

3.1 Preprocedural Planning

Imaging techniques must be used to determine the target of interventional procedure, normal anatomy or anatomical variants, potential injury to close structures, presence of necrotic areas which should not be included in the treated liver region (Solomn and Silverman 2010), the procedure indication and the best approach to be employed. During this phase, even the duration and the number of the treatments should be assessed. Many imaging techniques are used in preprocedural planning:

US, CEUS. B-mode US is the most employed imaging technique because it is fast, feasible, iodine and radiation-free, is repeatable, allows real-time assessment, and presents low costs. The utility of US in detecting liver HCC has been studied by many groups (Lee et al. 2010; Chan et al. 2001; Dodd III et al. 1992; Bennett et al. 2002) and the results are quite heterogeneous. In fact, the detection rate is between 35 and 78.5% with a sensitivity of 38% and a specificity of 92% (Chan et al. 2001).

The detection of liver nodules could be a failure because of heterogeneous liver echotexture in patients with liver cirrhosis (owing to fibrosis, fatty infiltration, regeneration nodules, and parenchymal necrosis) and became more difficult when the lesion is near the diaphragm (Lee et al. 2010; Takayasu et al. 1990) because this portion of the liver is surrounded by the lung. The more the liver cirrhosis process is advanced the more difficult is to detect HCC (Lee et al. 2010).

US contrast agents could provide a contrast enhancement assessment of lesions to be treated without any risk related to iodine contrast agents and radiation. CEUS could be used to determine more accurately lesion size and margins, to detect small lesions not visible on the unenhanced US and to identify lesion necrosis (Chen et al. 2007).

CT, MRI. These are the imaging techniques more frequently used to detect target lesion and to evaluate anatomy, anatomical variants, the relationship between lesions and normal structures, and presence of lesion necrosis.

CT exposes the patient to ionizing radiation but is faster, more widespread, less expensive, more suitable for claustrophobic patients, and can be used for patients who cannot undergo to an MRI scan due to unsafe or unconditional devices.

3.2 Intraprocedural Targeting, Monitoring, and Modification

During real-time percutaneous procedures, the operator has to recognize the lesion and the adjacent normal anatomical landmarks previously identified during preprocedural planning. Lesion monitoring is the fundamental component of the intra-procedure time during which the operator has the possibility to assess target lesion morphologic changes during ablation treatment, the radicality of the procedure, and the safety of adjacent structures. When necessary, the operator has to recognize if the procedure is not feasible and the potential risk to compromise the adjacent anatomical structures and should modify the procedure strategy.

3.3 Real-Time Imaging Guiding Techniques and Associated Techniques

US, CEUS. Sometime the evaluation of target lesion could be insufficient because of the deep lesion localization (especially those lesions close to the diaphragm), small size, cirrhosis, and intervening intestinal gas (Lee et al. 2010). Intraprocedural injection of US contrast agents improves the real-time visualization of the target lesion, needle placement, and most importantly, the safe margins (Kim et al. 2015).

Probe placement below the costal margin increases difficulties due to interference of intra-pulmonary gas; artificial pleural effusion often provides better visibility for hepatic malignancies located near the diaphragm (Wang et al. 2015a).

CECT enables a 3D visualization of target lesion and of adjacent anatomical structures, and even of the needle, and ablation dome. CT-guided microwave ablation of tumors is associated with a high technical success rate, high rate of complete response, and low rate of complications (Asvadi et al. 2016) (Fig. 1).

MRI - guided liver tumor ablation is similar to real-time percutaneous thermal ablation (Crocetti et al. 2010; Solomn and Silverman 2010). This technique is used to monitoring local temperature (MR thermometry) during thermo-ablation and evaluate when the tumor is completely treated and the critical structure is not harmed (de Senneville et al. 2007). Different tissues have different thresholds for temperature - induced necrosis, and if the tissue temperature could be estimated the dying cell type could be predicted.

With MR thermometry tissue temperature change within 1 °C can be estimated (Quesson et al. 2000). By keeping temperature of 54 °C for more than 1 second we determine all cell necrosis (Sapareto and Dewey 1984). The temperature measurement by MR thermometry could represent a quantitative non-invasive method for procedure evaluation.

Even CT and US could be used to evaluate temperature changes (Fallone et al. 1982; Arthur et al. 2005) based on CT Hounsfield number change during thermal ablation treatment.

Fusion imaging refers to a partially transparent overlay of one imaging database over another. In interventional oncology many images coming from different techniques could be matched, for example, PET with CT or MRI;

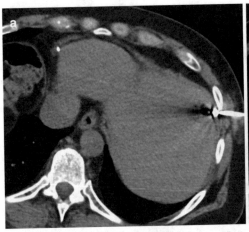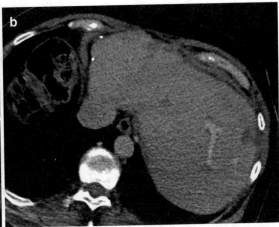

Fig. 1 HCC relapse in the second liver segment following right liver lobe resection treated by CT-guided radiofrequency ablation. (**a**) Lesion targeting based on CT guidance; (**b**) Contrast-enhanced CT, portal venous phase. Ablation assessment 1 week after treatment. Subcapsular ablation area with no evidence of residual disease

CT with US; fluoroscopy with conventional angiography, CT, or MRI. Fusion imaging leads to a more accurate 3D targeting and improves evaluation of little lesions (<5 mm in diameter) or undetectable lesions (Mauri et al. 2015; Ahn et al. 2017).

The optimal needle tracking is planned on 3D images that are transferred to the workstation. The needle is projected over 3D images in real-time (Rajagopal and Venkatesan 2016). Stereotactic ablation limits the number of needle adjustments and is useful in those lesions located in a difficult position as the hepatic dome.

During percutaneous ablation procedures, *High-Frequency Jet Ventilation* (HFJV) can be used. This ventilation technique is characterized by mechanical intra-tracheal ventilation due to a small catheter that reduces the respiratory movements and therefore the liver movements (Denys et al. 2014). HFJV produces a higher risk of barotraumatic pneumothorax. Another particular technique that can be used is *Transarterial catheter-assisted ablation*. This technique improves target detection on CT arterial portography (CTAP) or Hepatic arteriography (CTHA). During CTAP e CTHA a catheter is placed within superior mesenteric artery or hepatic artery, respectively, and contrast agent injection allows real-time contrast enhancement assessment. This technique improves lesion conspicuity, differentiation between scar and pathologic tissue, and treatment accuracy (Puijk et al. 2018, van Tilborg et al. 2014 and 2015).

3.4 Valuation of Technical Success

With both thermal and nonthermal percutaneous ablation techniques, technical success is achieved when energy is provided to the tissue and produces a spherical ablation zone.

Immediate contrast-enhanced post-procedural imaging could demonstrate the extension of percutaneous ablation that should contain tumor and a free-tumor 5 mm safety margins around the lesion (Ahmed et al. 2014).

US, CT, MR imaging, and intraprocedural contrast-enhanced imaging could be performed to evaluate the radicality of the ablation. After thermal ablation, US shows transient hyperechogenicity that disappears after several minutes. A well-delimited hypodense zone with hyperdense peripheral rim (transient peripheral hyperemia) can be seen on CECT (Crocetti et al. 2010).

On MRI, immediately after percutaneous ablation, the treated zone appears heterogeneously hyperintense on T1-w and homogeneously hyperintense on T2-w images (Solomon et al. 2010).

During CRA an echogenic mass with distal acoustic shadowing is visualized, corresponding to the ice ball (Mala et al. 2004). These ice balls could be visualized even by CT or MRI as non-enhancing areas on CECT and hypointense areas at T2-w and iso- to hyperintense areas at T1-w MR images (Silverman et al. 2005).

3.4.1 Postprocedural Assessment

For the imaging of post-procedural assessment and follow-up, we refer to the specific chapter (Imaging of Treated Liver Tumors and Assessment of Tumor Response to Cytostatic Therapy and Post-Treatment Changes in the Liver).

3.5 Complication

Complication after percutaneous techniques occur in 3–7% of patients (Jaskolka et al. 2005; Livraghi et al. 2003; Crocetti et al. 2010; Shibata et al. 2003) and include intraperitoneal bleeding, liver abscess, intestinal perforation, pneumothorax and hemothorax, bile duct stenosis and tumor seeding; the procedure mortality rate is on 0.1—0.5%.

The most common complications are hepatic abscesses, intraperitoneal bleeding, hepatic decompensation, and bile duct injury. The most common causes of death are sepsis, hepatic failure, colon perforation, and portal vein thrombosis. An uncommon late complication is tumor seeding along the needle track (1%).

Risk is related to size and location of the tumor. However there are also other components, for example, the abscess risk increases in patients after bilioenteric anastomoses or other manipulation as stent displacement or sphincterotomy (Shibata et al. 2003).

For the imaging assessment of complications after ablation, we refer to the specific chapter (Imaging of Treated Liver Tumors and Assessment of Tumor Response to Cytostatic Therapy and Post-Treatment Changes in the Liver).

References

Adam R, Hagopian EJ, Linhares M et al (2002) A comparison of percutaneous cryosurgery and percutaneous radiofrequency for unresectable hepatic malignancies. Arch Surg 37:1332–1339

Ahn SJ, Lee JM, Lee DH et al (2017) Real-time US-CT/MR fusion imaging for percutaneous radiofrequency ablation of hepatocellular carcinoma. J Hepatol 66:347–354

Ahmed M, Solbiati L, Brace CL et al (2014) Image-guided Tumor Ablation: Standardization of Terminology and Reporting Criteria—A 10-Year Update. Radiology 273(1):241–260

Arthur RM, Straube WL, Trobaugh JW, Moros EG (2005) Non-invasive estimation of hyperthermia temperatures with ultrasound. Int J Hyperth 21(6):589–600

Asvadi NH, Anvari A, Uppot RN (2016) CT-guided percutaneous microwave ablation of tumors in the hepatic dome: assessment of efficacy and safety. JckVIR 27:496–502

Bennett GL, Krinsky GA, Abitbol RJ, Kim SY et al (2002) Sonographic detection of hepatocellular carcinoma and dysplastic nodules in cirrhosis: correlation of pretransplantation sonography and liver explant pathology in 200 patients. AJR 179:75–80

Bhutiani N, Philips P, Scoggins CR et al (2016) Evaluation of tolerability and efficacy of irreversible electroporation (IRE) in treatment of child-Pugh B (7/8) hepatocellular carcinoma (HCC). HPB 18:593–599

Breen DJ, Lencioni R (2015) Image-guided ablation of primary liver and renal tumours. Nat Rev Clin Oncol 12:175–186

Bruix J, Llovet JM (2009) Major achievements in hepatocellular carcinoma. Lancet 373(9664):614–616

Bruix J, Sherman M American association for the study of liver diseases. (2011) management of hepatocellular carcinoma: an update. Hepatology 53(3):1020–1022

Bruix J, Sherman M, Llovet JM, EASL Panel of Experts on HCC et al (2001) Clinical management of hepatocellular carcinoma. Conclusions of the Barcelona-2000 EASL conference. European Association for the Study of the liver. J Hepaetol 35(3):421–430

Chan KK, Jae HL, Won JL (2001) Detection of hepatocellular carcinomas and dysplastic nodules in cirrhotic liver. J Ultrasound Med 20:99–104

Chen MH, Yang W, Yan K, Dai Y, Wu W, Fan ZH, Callstrom MR, Charboneau JW (2007) The role of contrast-enhanced ultrasound in planning treatment protocols for hepatocellular carcinoma before radio-frequency ablation. Clinical Radiology 62(8):752–760

Chen MS, Li JQ, Zheng Y et al (2006) A prospective randomized trial comparing percutaneous local ablative therapy and partial hepatectomy for small hepatocellular carcinoma. Ann Surg 243(3):321–328

Cheung TT, Chu FS, Jenkins CR et al (2012) Tolerance of high-intensity focused ultrasound ablation in patients with hepatocellular carcinoma. World J Surg 36:2420–2427

Cheung TT, Fan ST, Chan CS et al (2013) High-intensity focused ultrasound ablation: an effective bridging therapy for hepatocellular carcinoma patients. World J Gastroenterol 19(20):3083–3089

Chinnaratha MA, Chuang MA, Fraser RJ et al (2016) Percutaneous thermal ablation for primary hepatocellular carcinoma: a systematic review and meta-analysis. J Gastroenterol Hepatol 31:294–301

Crocetti L, de Baere T, Lencioni R (2010) Quality improvement guidelines for radiofrequency ablation of liver tumours. Cardiovasc Intervent Radiol 33:11e7

De Angelis R, Sant M, Coleman MP et al (2014) Cancer survival in Europe 1999–2007 by country and age: results of EUROCARE–5-a population-based study. Lancet Oncol 15:23–34

Denys A, Lachenal Y, Duran R, Chollet-Rivier M, Bize P (2014) Use of high-frequency jet ventilation for percutaneous tumor ablation. Cardiovasc Intervent Radiol 37:140–146

Di Costanzo GG, D'Adamo G, Tortrora R et al (2013) A novelneedle guide system to perform percutaneous laser ablation of liver tumors using the multi fiber technique. Acta Radiol 54(8):876–881

Di Costanzo GG, Francica G, Pacella CM (2014) Laserablation of small hepatocellular caricoma: state of the art and future perspectives. World J Hepatol 6(10):704–715

Di Stasi M, Buscarini L, Livraghi T et al (1997) Percutaneous ethanol injection in the treatment of hepatocellular carcinoma: a multicenter survey of evaluation practices and complication rates. Scand J Gastroenterol 32(11):1168–1173

Ding J, Zhou Y, Wang Y et al (2017) Percutaneous microwave ablation of exophytic tumours in hepatocellular carcinoma patients. Liver Int 37(9):1365–1372

Dodd GD, Soulen MC, Kane RA et al (2000) Minimally invasive treatment of malignant hepatic tumors: at the threshold of a major breakthrough. Radiographics 20(1):9–27

Dodd III GD, MIller WJ, Baron RL, Skolnick ML, Campbell WL (1992) Detection of Malignant Tumors in End-Stage Cirrhotic Livers : Efficacy of Sonography as a Screening Technique. Am J Roentgenol 159:727–733

Dollinger M, Beyer LP, Haimerl M et al (2015) Adverse effects of irreversible electroporation of malignant liver tumors under CT fluoroscopic guidance: a single-center experience. Diagn Interv Radiol 21:471–475

Dong B, Liang P, Yu X et al (2003) Percutaneous sonographically guided microwave coagulation therapy for hepatocellular carcinoma: results in 234 patients. Am J Roentgenol 180(6):1547–1555

Ebara M, Okabe S, Kita K et al (2005) Percutaneous ethanol injection for small hepatocellular carcinoma: terapeutic efficacy based on 20-year observation. J Hepatol 43(3):458–464

Eichler K, Zangos S, Gruber-Rouh T et al (2012) Magnetic resonance- guided laser-induced thermotherapy in patients with oligonodular hepatocellular carcinoma: long-term results over a 15-years period. J Clin Gastroenterol 46(9):796–801

Fallone BG, Moran PR, Podgorsak EB (1982) Noninvasive thermometry with a clinical x-ray CT scanner. Med Phys 9(5):715–721

Francica G, Iodice G, Delle Cave M et al (2007) Factors predicting complete necrosis rate after ultrasound-guided percutaneous laser thermoablation of small hepatocellular carcinoma tumors in cirrhotic patients: a multivariate analysis. Acta Radiol 48(5):514–519

Francica G, Petrolati A, Di Stasio E et al (2012a) Effectiveness, safety, and local progression after percutaneous laser ablation of hepatocellular carcinoma nodules up to 4 cm are not affected by tumor location. AJR Am J Roentgenol 199(6):1393–1401

Francica G, Petrolati A, Di Stasio E et al (2012b) Influence of ablative margin on local tumor progression and survival in patients with HCC ≤4 cm after laser ablation. Acta Radiol 53(4):384–400

Gao W, Guo Z, Zhang X et al (2015) Percutaneouscryoablationofovarian cancer metastasis to the liver: initial experience in 13 patients. Int J Gynecol Cancer 25:802–808

Gilliam AR, Lees WR (2005) Radiofrequency ablation of colorectal liver metastases. Abdom Imaging 30(4):419–426

Gilliams A, Goldberg N, Ahmed M et al (2015) Thermal ablation of colorectal liver metastases: a position paper by an international panel of ablation experts, the interventional oncology sans frontières meeting 2013. Eur Radiol 25(12):3438–3454

Glazer DI, Tatli S, Shyn PB et al (2017) Percutaneous Image-Guided Cryoablation of hepatic tumors: single-center experience with intermediate to long-term outcomes. Am J Roentgenol 209:1381–1389

Greenlee RT, Hill Harmon MB, Murray T et al (2001) Cancer statistics, 2001. CA Cancer J Clin 51(1):15–36

de Haas RJ, Wicherts DA, Salloum C et al (2010) Long-term outcomes after hepatic resection for colorectal metastases in young patients. Cancer 116(3): 647–658

de Haas RJ, Wicherts DA, Andreani P et al (2011) Impact of expanding criteria for resectability of colorectal metastases on short- and long-term outcomes after hepatic resection. Ann Surg 253(6):1069–1079

Hildebrand P, Leidbecke T, Kleemann M et al (2006) Influence of operator experience in radiofrequency ablation of malignant liver tumors on treatment outcome. Eur J Surg Oncol 32(4):430–434

Huang YZ, Zhou SC, Zhou H et al (2013) Radiofrequency ablation versus cryosurgery ablation for hepatocellular carcinoma: a meta-analysis. Hepato-Gastroenterology 60:1131–1135

Ishii H, Okada S, Nose H (1996) Local recurrence of hepatocellular carcinoma after percutaneous ethanol injection. Cancer 77(9):1792–1796

Jaskolka JD, Asch MR, Kachura JR et al (2005) Needle tract seeding after radio-frequency ablation of hepatic tumors. J Vasc Interv Radiol 16:485–491

Jung SE, Cho SH, Jang JH et al (2011) High-intensity focused ultrasound ablation in hepatic and pancreatic cancer: complications. Abdom Imaging 36: 185–195

Khajanchee YS, Streeter D, Swanstrom LL, Hansen PD (2004) A mathematical model for preoperative planning of radiofrequency ablation of hepatic tumors. Surg Endosc 18(4):696–701

Kim TK, Khalili K, Jang HJ (2015) Local ablation therapy with contrast-enhanced ultrasonography for hepatocellular carcinoma: a practical review. Ultrasonography 34:235–245

Kudo M (2004) Local ablation therapy for hepatocellular carcinoma: current status and future perspectives. J Gastroenterol 9(3):205–214

Landis SH, Murray T, Bolden S et al (1999) Cancer statistics, 1999. CA Cancer J Clin 49(1):8–31

Lee MW, Kim YJ, Park HS, Yu NC, Jung SI, Ko SY, Jeon HJ (2010) Targeted Sonography for Small Hepatocellular Carcinoma Discovered by CT or MRI: Factors Affecting Sonographic Detection. AJR American Journal of Roentgenology 194(5): W396–W400

Lee WS, Yun SH, Chun HK et al (2008) Clinical outcomes of hepatic resection and radiofrequency ablation in patients with solitary colorectal liver metastasis. J Clin Gastroenterol 42(8):945–949

Lencioni R (2010) Loco-regional treatment of hepatocellular carcinoma. Hepatologyvol 52:762–773

Lencioni R, Crocetti L (2008) Image-guided thermal ablation of hepatocellular carcinoma. Crit Rev Oncol Hematol 66(3):200–207

Liang P, Dong D, Yu X et al (2003) Prognostic factors for percutaneous microwave coagulation therapy of hepatic metastases. AJR Am J Roentgenol 181(5):1319–1325

Liang P, Yu J, MDet al L (2013) Practice guidelines for ultrasound-guided percutaneous microwave ablation for hepatic malignancy. World J Gastroenterol 19:8

Littrup PJ, Aoun HD, Adam B et al (2016) Percutaneouscryoablationofhepatic tumors: long-term experience of a large U. S. Series. Abdom Radiol 41:767–780

Livraghi T, Giorgio A, Marin G et al (1995) Hepatocellular carcinoma and cirrhosis in 746 patients: long-term results of percutaneous ethanol injection. Radiologyvol 197(1):101–108

Livraghi T, Solbiati L, Meloni MF, Gazelle GS, Halpern EF, Goldberg SN (2003) Treatment of focal liver tumors with percutaneous radio-frequency ablation: complications encountered in a multicenter study. Radiology 226:441–451

Livraghi T, Meloni F, Di Stasi M et al (2008) Sustained complete response and complications rates after radiofrequency ablation of very early hepatocellular carcinoma in cirrhosis: is resection still the treatment of choice? Hepatology 47:82–89

Llovet JM, Fuster J, Bruix J (1999) Intention-to-treat analysis of surgical treatment for early hepatocellular carcinoma: resection versus transplantation. Hepatology 30(6):1434–1440

Lu DS, Raman SS, Liamond P et al (2003) Influence of large peritumoral vessels on outcome of radiofrequency ablation of liver tumors. J Vasc Interv Radiol 14(10):1267–1274

Mahnken AH, König AM, Figiel JH (2018) Current technique and application of percutaneous Cryotherapy. Fortschr Röntgenstr 190:836–846

Mala T, Aurdal L, Frich L et al (2004) Liver tu-mor cryoablation: a commentary on the need of improved

procedural monitoring. Technol Cancer Res Treat 3(1):85–91

Martin RC, Scoggins CR, McMasters KM (2010) Safety and efficacy of microwave ablation of hepatic tumors: a prospective review of a 5-year experience. Ann Surg Oncol 17:171e8

Mauri G, Cova L, De Beni S, Ierace T, Tondolo T, Cerri A, Goldberg SN, Solbiati L (2015) Real-Time US-CT/MRI Image Fusion for Guidance of Thermal Ablation of Liver Tumors Undetectable with US: Results in 295 Cases. CardioVascular and Interventional Radiology 38(1):143–151

Mulier S, Ruers T, Jamart J et al (2008) Radiofrequency ablation versus resection for resectable colorectal liver metastases: time for a randomized trial? An update. Dig Surg 25(6):445–460

Narayanan G, Bhatia S, Echenique A et al (2014) Vessel patency post-irreversible electroporation. Cardiovasc Intervent Radiol 37(6):1523–1529

Ng KK, Poon RT, Chan SC et al (2011) High-intensity focused ultrasound for hepatocellular carcinoma a single-center experience. Ann Surg 253:981–987

Ogata Y, Uchida S, Hisaka T et al (2008) Intraoperative thermal ablation therapy for small colorectal metastases to the liver. Hepato-Gastroenterology 55(82–83):550–556

Omata M, Cheng AL, Kokudo N et al (2017) Asia–Pacific clinical practice guidelines on the management of hepatocellular carcinoma: a 2017 update. Hepatol Int 11(4):317–370

Orlacchio A, Bolacchi F, Chegai F et al (2014) Comparative evaluation of percutaneous laser and radiofrequency ablation in patients with HCC smaller than 4 cm. Radiol Med 119:298–308

Orsi F, Zhang L, Amone P et al (2010) High-intensity focused ultrasound ablation: effective and safe therapy for solid tumors in difficult locations. Am J Roentgenol 195:W245–W252

Pacella CM, Bizzarri G, Francica G et al (2005) Percutaneouslaser ablation in the treatment of hepatocellular carcinoma with small tumors: analysis of factors affecting the achievement of tumor necrosis. J Vasc Interv Radiol 16(11):1447–1457

Pacella CM, Francica G, Di Lascio FM et al (2009) Long-term outcome of cirrhotic patients with early hepatocellular carcinoma treated with ultrasound-guided percutaneous laser ablation: a retrospective analysis. J Clin Oncol 27(16):2615–2621

Park MY, Jung SE, Cho SH et al (2009) Preliminary experience using high intensity focused ultrasound for treating liver metastasis from colon and stomach cancer. Int J Hyperth 5(3):180–188

Pearson AS, Izzo F, Fleming RY et al (1999) Intraoperative radiofrequency ablation or cryoablation for hepatic malignancies. Am J Surg 178:592–599

Puijk RS, Ruarus AH, Scheffer HJ et al (2018) Percutaneus liver tumor ablation: image guidance, end point assessment, and quality control. Can Assoc Radiol J 69:51–62

Puls R, Langner S, Rosenberg C et al. (2009) Laser ablation of liver metastases from colorectal

Quesson B, de Zwart JA, Moonen CT (2000) Magnetic resonance temperature imaging for guidance of thermotherapy. J Magn Reson Imaging 12(4):525–533

Rajagopal M, Venkatesan AM (2016) Image fusion and navigation platforms for percutaneous image-guided interventions. Abdom Radiol (NY) 41:620–628

Sapareto SA, Dewey WC (1984) Thermal dose determination in cancer therapy. Int J Radiat Oncol Biol Phys 10(6):787–800

Sartori S, Di Vece F, Ermili F et al (2017) Laser ablation of liver tumors: an ancillary technique, or an alternative technique to radiofrequency and microwave? World J Radiol 9(3):91–96

Scheffer HJ, Melenhorst MC, van Tilborg AA et al. (2014) Percutaneous irreversible electroporation of a large centrally located hepatocellular adenoma in a woman with a pregnancy wish. Cardiovasc Intervent Radiol 2014

de Senneville BD, Mougenot C, Quesson B, Dragonu I, Grenier N, Moonen CT (2007) MR thermometry for monitoring tumor ablation. Eur Radiol 17(9):2401–2410

Seror O (2015) Ablative therapies: advantages and disadvantages of radiofrequency, cryotherapy, microwave and electroporation methods, or how to choose the right method for an individual patient? Diagn Interv Imag 96:617–624

Shibata T, Yamamoto Y, Yamamoto N et al (2003) Cholangitis and liver abscess after percutaneous ablation therapy for liver tumors: incidence and risk factors. J Vasc Interv Radiol 14:1535–1542

Shiina S, Tateishi R, Imamura M et al (2012) Percutaneous ethanol injection for hepatocellular carcinoma: 20-years outcome and prognostic factors. Liver Int 32(9):1434–1442

Silverman SG, Tuncali K, Morrison PR (2005) MR imaging-guided percutaneous tumor ablation. Acad Radiol 12(9):1100–1109

Solbiati L, Ierace T, Tonolini M et al (2001) Radiofrequency thermal ablation of hepatic metastases. Eur J Ultrasound 13(2):149–158

Solomn SB, Silverman SG (2010) Imaging in interventional oncology. Radiology 257(Number 3):624–640

Sotirchos VS, Petrovic LM, Gonen M et al (2016) Colorectal cancer liver metastases: biopsy of the ablation zone and margins can be used to predict oncologic outcome. Radiology 280:949e59

Stigliano R, Marelli L, Yu D et al (2007) Seeding following percutaneous diagnostic and therapeutic approaches for hepatocellular carcinoma. What is the risk and the outcome? Seeding risk for percutaneous approach of HCC. Cancer Treat Revvol 33:437–447

Sung YM, Choi D, Lim HK et al (2006) Long-term results of percutaneous ethanol injection for the treatment of hepatocellular carcinoma in Korea. Korean J Radiol 7(3):187–192

Sutter O, Calvo J, N'Kontchou G et al (2017) Safety and efficacy of irreversible electroporation for the treatment of hepatocellular carcinoma not amenable to thermal ablation techniques: a retrospective single-center case series. Radiology 161413

Tait IS, Yong SM, Cuschieri SA (2002) Laparoscopic in situ ablation of liver cancer with cryotherapy and radiofrequency ablation. Br J Surg 89: 1613–1619

Takayasu K, Moriyama N, Makuuchi M et al (1990) The diagnosis of small hepatocellular carcinoma: efficacy of various imaging procedures in 100 patients. AJR 155:49–54

Tanaka K, Shimada H, Nagano Y et al (2006) Outcome after hepatic resection versus combined resection and microwave ablation for multiple bilobar colorectal metastases to the liver. Surgery 139(2):263–273

Thamtorawat S, Hicks RM, Yu J et al (2016) Preliminary outcome of microwave ablation of hepatocellular carcinoma: breaking the 3-cm barrier? J Vasc Interv Radiol 27(5):623–630

Tombesi P, Di Vece F, Sartori S (2015) Radiofrequency, microwave, and laser ablation of liver tumors: time to move toward a tailored ablation technique? Hepatom Res 1:52–57

Tombesi P, Di Vece F, Bianchi L et al (2018) Thermal ablation of liver Tumours: how the scenario has changed in the last decade. EMJ Hepatol 6(1):88–94

Van Tilborg AA, Scheffer HJ, de Jong MC et al (2016) MWA versus RFA for perivascular and peribiliary CRLM: a retrospective patient- and lesion- based analysis of two historical cohorts. Cardiovasc Intervent Radiol 39:14e38e46

van Tilborg AA, Scheffer HJ, van der Meijs BB, van Werkum MH, Melenhorst MC, van den Tol PM, Meijerink MR (2015) Transcatheter CT Hepatic Arteriography–Guided Percutaneous Ablation to Treat Ablation Site Recurrences of Colorectal Liver Metastases: The Incomplete Ring Sign. J Vasc Interv Radiol 26(4):583–587

van Tilborg AA, Scheffer HJ, Nielsen K, van Waesberghe JH, Comans EF, van Kuijk C, van den Tol PM, Meijerink MR (2014) Transcatheter CT Arterial Portography and CT Hepatic Arteriography for Liver Tumor Visualization during Percutaneous Ablation. J Vasc Interv Radiol 25(7):1101–1111

Verslype C, Rosmorduc O, Rougier P, on behalf of the ESMO Guidelines Working Group (2012) Hepatocellular carcinoma: ESMO–ESDO clinical practice guidelines for diagnosis, treatment and follow-up. Ann Oncol 23(Supplement 7):vii41–vii48

Violi NV, Duran R, Guiu B, Cercueil JP, Aubé C, Digklia A, Pache I, Deltenre P, Knebel JF, Denys A (2018) Efficacy of microwave ablation versus radiofrequency ablation for the treatment of hepatocellular carcinoma in patients with chronic liver disease: a randomised controlled phase 2 trial. Lancet Gastroenterol Hepatol 3(5):317–325

Vogl TJ, Straub R, Zangos S et al (2004) MR-guided laser- induced thermotherapy (LITT) of liver tumours: experimental and clinical data. Int J Hyperth 20(7):713–724

Vogl TJ, Farshid P, Naguib NN et al (2014a) Thermal ablation of liver metastases from colorectal cancer: radiofrequency, microwave and laser ablation therapies. Radiol Med 119(7):451–461

Vogl TJ, Dommermuth A, Heinle B et al (2014b) Colorectal cancer liver metastases: long-term survival and progression-free survival after thermal ablation using magnetic resonance-guided laser-induced interstitial thermotherapy in 594 patients: analysis of prognostic factors. Investig Radiol 49(1):48–56

Wang G, Sun Y, Cong L, Jing X, Yu J (2015a) Artificial pleural effusion in percutaneous microwave ablation of hepatic tumors near the diaphragm under the guidance of ultrasound. Int J Clin Exp Med 8: 16765–16771

Wang C, Wang H, Yang W et al (2015b) Multicenter randomized controlled trial of percutaneous cryoablation versus radiofrequency ablation in hepatocellular carcinoma. Hepatology 61:1579–1590

Yang B, Zan RY, Wang SY et al (2015) Radiofrequency ablation versus percutaneous ethanol injection for hepatocellular carcinoma: a meta-analysis of randomized controlled trials. World J Surg Oncol 13:96

Zhang L, Rao F, Setzen R (2009) High-intensity focused ultrasound (HIFU): effective and safe therapy for hepatocellular carcinoma adjacent to major hepatic veins. Eur Radiol 19(2):437–445

Zhang W, Yu H, Guo Z et al (2014) Percutaneouscryoablationofliivermetastases from breast cancer: initial experience in 17 patients. Clin Radiol 69: 231–238

Zhu H, Zhou K, Zhang L et al (2009) High intensity focused ultrasound (HIFU) therapy for local treatment of hepatocellular carcinoma: role of partial rib resection. Eur J Radiol 72(1):160–166

Transarterial Chemoembolisation and Combined Therapy

Alberta Cappelli, Giuliano Peta, and Rita Golfieri

Contents

Abstract

In Hepatocellular carcinoma (HCC), transarterial chemoembolisation (TACE) is the most widely used loco-regional treatment not only in the intermediate stage, but often also in early or advanced disease ("treatment stage migration"), but is the least standardised, both in terms of indications and techniques. The rationale for the efficacy of transarterial therapies is that the vascularisation of HCC is, for the most part, dependent on the hepatic artery.

A. Cappelli · G. Peta · R. Golfieri (✉)
Radiology Unit, Department of Experimental, Diagnostic and Speciality Medicine, Sant'Orsola Hospital, University of Bologna, Bologna, Italy
e-mail: rita.golfieri@unibo.it

Conventional TACE (cTACE) consists of the intra-arterial administration of a chemotherapeutic drug emulsified with Lipiodol followed by embolisation of the tumour-feeding vessels with an embolic agent (most commonly gel foam particles).

Drug-eluting bead-TACE (DEB-TACE) is progressively challenging cTACE; DEB-TACE is supposed to maximise the concentration of a cytotoxic drug at the tumour level, with a slower release of the drug into the tumour and minimal systemic exposure. Beads, along with their embolic properties, segregate the chemotherapeutic agent and release it over a one-week period. At present, data from the literature do not confirm the superiority of DEB-TACE over cTACE in terms of patient survival, tumour response and

© Springer Nature Switzerland AG 2021
E. Quaia (ed.), *Imaging of the Liver and Intra-hepatic Biliary Tract*,
Medical Radiology Diagnostic Imaging, https://doi.org/10.1007/978-3-030-39021-1_13

safety, and the choice is therefore left to the operator. Several cytotoxic drugs are administered in both conventional and DEB-TACE. The most widely used is doxorubicin, with no evidence of its superiority over other chemotherapeutics.

Transarterial embolisation (TAE) consists of the embolisation of tumour-feeding arteries with embolic agents without adding any chemotherapeutic drugs. To date, the relative effectiveness of TACE over TAE has not been established in randomised trials.

Combined treatment (radiofrequency ablation (RFA) plus TACE) is safe and effective for the treatment of unresectable patients with early/intermediate HCC exceeding 3 cm in size.

Hepatic arterial infusion chemotherapy (HAIC) is frequently adopted for the treatment of locally advanced HCC in Japan, based on reports of high response rates and favourable long-term outcomes. Firm evidence of the superiority of one over the other has not yet been established. In the future, a demonstration of the survival advantage of HAIC over systemic therapies and the recognition of HAIC as one of the standard treatments for patients with advanced HCC are expected.

In intrahepatic cholangiocarcinoma (ICC), hepatic arterial therapy (HAT) seems to be a promising strategy for improving outcomes in patients with unresectable ICC. The best outcomes in terms of response and OS are reported by HAIC even it is associated with increased toxicity. Targeted treatment strategy based on patient-disease characteristics is a goal for future research.

In liver metastases, liver-directed therapies have become common due to the increased complexity of hepatic surgery. Intra-arterial treatment options include TACE, TAE, HAIC and ablative techniques, such as microwave irradiation (MWI) or RF ablation. The evidence supports their use to provide salvage options when first-line treatment has failed. Although these treatments have been applied without high-level clinical evidence, they have allowed tailoring the clinical approach to the individual based on disease status and clinical condition.

In patients with well-differentiated unresectable hypervascular neuroendocrine tumour (NET) liver metastases, TAE, TACE and selective transarterial radioembolisation (TARE) are the preferred choices among other treatment modalities. Transarterial embolisation and TACE generally achieve average symptomatic, biological and radiological responses of 75%, 56% and 50%, respectively with a progression-free survival of 12–18 months, with acceptable tolerance.

1 Intra-Arterial Treatments of IICC

1.1 Transarterial Chemoembolisation (TACE): Basic Principles

Transarterial chemoembolisation (TACE) is the most diffuse treatment for unresectable hepatocellular carcinoma (HCC) and is the recommended first-line therapy for patients with the intermediate-stage disease (Barcelona Clinic Liver Cancer [BCLC] B) (EASL 2018).

Transarterial chemoembolisation treatment aims to induce tumour necrosis, thanks to the predominant arterial vascularisation of HCC; moreover, TACE combines the efficacy of the chemotherapy injected locally with the embolic effect of the particles. On the one hand, the embolisation induces ischemia and prevents washout of the injected chemotherapeutic agents from the tumour; on the other hand, the blood supply to the surrounding liver is still maintained by blood flow from the portal vein, minimising damage to the liver. Moreover, chemotherapeutic agents, thanks to ischemic damage, remain in the tumour for a long period at a higher concentration. In addition, the high tumour concentration of chemotherapeutic agents results in lower systemic drug levels and, therefore, in less toxicity. These combined effects are reported to be synergistic in obtaining high anti-tumour effects with a high objective response rate. However, it is mandatory to preserve the surrounding cirrhotic liver parenchyma. As a consequence, the selection of the most appropriate treatment option for HCC patients depends not only on tumour burden but also on liver function and the general performance status (PS) of the patient.

Data from the literature showed that the prognosis of HCC patients is mainly related to three factors: tumour burden (lesion number and size, the presence of vascular invasion, and extrahepatic spread), liver function (the presence of cancer-related symptoms) and, finally, treatment accomplished (i.e., resection, liver transplantation, ablation, TACE, systemic therapy, or best supportive care).

In Western countries, the most commonly used staging system for establishing prognosis and determining the choice of treatment for HCC is the BCLC system, originally proposed in 1999 (LLovet et al. 1999) and subsequently updated (Forner et al. 2010; Forner et al. 2012; Forner et al. 2018). It consists of five stages: very early,

early, intermediate, advanced and terminal, according to the variables related to tumour burden, liver function (Child-Pugh class), clinical status and cancer-related symptoms (Eastern Cooperative Group Performance Status [ECOG PS]) (Table 1). The BCLC staging system has also been endorsed for HCC management by the guidelines of the American Association for the Study of Liver Diseases (AASLD), the American Gastroenterology Association (AGA), the European Association for the Study of Liver (EASL) and the European Organization for Research and Treatment of Cancer (EORTC) (Bruix and Sherman 2011; Marrero et al. 2018; EASL 2018). Moreover, the BCLC staging system is the only staging system that assigns treatment strategies based on specific prognostic subclasses.

Other guidelines also include tumour resectability and are based on the modified Union of International Cancer Control staging system and the Child-Pugh class of liver function. The more recent and detailed Asia-Pacific guidelines

Table 1 Barcelona clinic liver cancer (BCLC) staging system and treatment strategy (modified from Forner et al. 2018)

ECOG PS Eastern Cooperative Oncology Group Performance Status

Table 2 Treatment algorithm for hepatocellular carcinoma (modified from Omata et al. 2017)

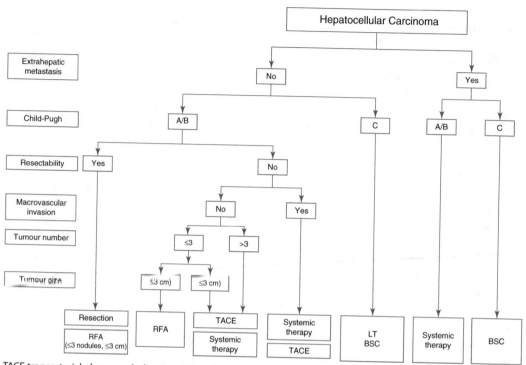

TACE transarterial chemoembolisation, *RFA* radiofrequency ablation, *LT* liver transplantation, *BSC* best supportive care

(Table 2) (Omata et al. 2017) are evidence-based and consider six parameters: extrahepatic diffusion, Child-Pugh classes, resectability, macrovascular invasion, tumour number and tumour size.

According to the European Association for the Study of the Liver (EASL) guidelines (EASL 2018) and the AASLD guidelines (Marrero et al. 2018), TACE is the current standard of care for intermediate-stage disease (BCLC stage B) which includes unresectable patients with multinodular HCCs without vascular invasion or extrahepatic spread and with well-preserved liver function who cannot benefit from curative treatment; they are defined as Child-Pugh (CP) ≤ B7 stage with preserved performance status (PS = 0–1).

Absolute and relative contraindications to TACE are reported in Table 3.

A precise anatomical evaluation is essential for performing TACE; thus, accurate pretreatment imaging (Computed Tomography (CT) or Magnetic Resonance (MR) examina-

Table 3 Absolute and relative contraindications to TACE (modified from Facciorusso et al. 2015)

Absolute
• Child-Pugh ≥ B8
• Massive replacement of both lobes
• Technical impossibility to hepatic artery catheterization
• Impaired portal blood flow
Relative
• Tumor size ≥ 10 cm
• Varices at high risk of bleeding
• Bile duct occlusion
• Severe cardiopulmonary comorbidities
• Kidney failure

tions) should be achieved preliminary to TACE treatment in order to detect all the feeding arteries of the tumour including any possible extrahepatic arteries which may supply the tumour (Covey et al. 2002), since HCC can have multiple feeding arteries which can originate from different trunks and may develop more

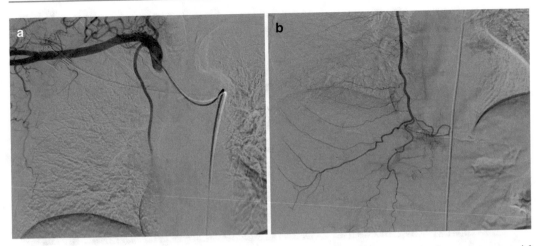

Fig. 1 Angiographic study showing selective catheterisation of the axillary artery (**a**) and subsequent transarterial chemoembolisation performed via the right internal mammary artery (**b**)

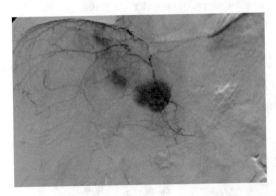

Fig. 2 Angiographic study showing the adrenal artery as the main feeding nodule vessel

frequently after the first treatment (Chung et al. 2006) (Figs. 1, 2 and 3).

Kim et al. (2005) described 2104 extrahepatic collateral vessels in 1622 TACE sessions performed on 860 patients; TACE procedures were performed via 1556 extrahepatic collateral vessels (74%) in 732 patients (1281 sessions).

More recently introduced cone-beam computed tomographic angiography (CBCTA) can help in identifying the collateral vessels and provide a detailed map of every feeding vessel to the target lesions, also useful in catheter guidance during the procedure. It has been shown to improve the technical success of TACE which may lead to a better outcome of the treatment (Fig. 4) (Angle et al. 2013, Miyayama et al. 2011, Yao et al. 2018).

Furthermore, it is well established that the use of selective/superselective TACE more often results in better outcomes and fewer adverse events (AEs). A selective/superselective procedure achieves better antitumoural effects and reduces both the dose of the drugs and the number of TACE sessions needed to achieve extensive tumour necrosis (Ji et al. 2008, Matsui et al. 1994, Miyayama et al. 2007, Park et al. 2007, Golfieri et al. 2011).

1.1.1 Conventional TACE (cTACE)

Conventional TACE was developed in the early 1980s in Japan and broadly adopted worldwide after two randomised control trials (RCTs) (Llovet et al. 2002, Lo et al. 2002) and a meta-analysis demonstrated he superiority of Lipiodol TACE to best supportive care. Conventional TACE has been established as the standard treatment for intermediate-stage HCC without portal vein invasion and consists of the intra-arterial injection of doxorubicin (LLovet et al. 2002) or cisplatinum (Lo et al. 2002) mixed with Lipiodol, followed by the administration of an embolic agent.

1.1.1.1 cTACE Protocol

Preliminary triple-phase cross-sectional imaging should be carried out before the procedure to identify major anatomic variants in the hepatic arterial anatomy and, during the TACE procedure, dedicated mesenteric and celiac

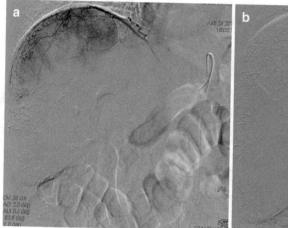
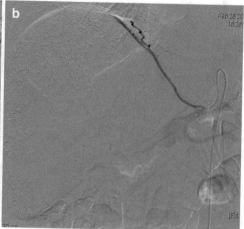

Fig. 3 (**a**) Superselective transarterial chemoembolisation into the right inferior phrenic artery contributing to the perfusion of a nodule of the dome of the liver. (**b**) Angiographic study performed after chemotherapy mix ture injection, showing complete stasis of the arterial flow through the vessels feeding the nodule, maintaining the flow into the proximal trunk of the phrenic artery

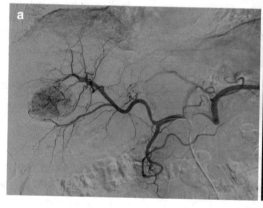
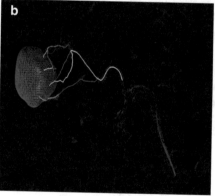

Fig. 4 (**a**) Angiographic study showing selective catheterisation of the right hepatic artery (the left hepatic artery originates from the left gastric artery (black arrow). (**b**) Cone-beam computed tomographic angiography (CBCTA) reconstruction using EmboGuide software (Philips®) showing the nodule feeding vessels, useful in guiding the catheterisation preliminary to performing the transarterial chemoembolisation

angiography is required to detect subtle arterial anatomic variants; maximal effort should be made to identify possible branches to the extrahepatic structures and possible extrahepatic collaterals supplying the liver tumour (i.e., the inferior phrenic artery, internal mammary artery, adrenal artery, and intercostal artery).

Chemotherapeutic Agents. Conventional TACE with Lipiodol involves the intra-arterial injection of a cytotoxic drug, such as anthracyclines (doxorubicin, epirubicin), mitomycin C, cisplatin, idarubicin alone, or a combination of doxorubicin and cisplatin emulsified in the oily radio-opaque agent Lipiodol (Lipiodol® Ultra-Fluid, Guerbet Laboratories, Roissy, France) (Fig. 5). At the end of the intra-arterial infusion of the drug/Lipiodol emulsion, an embolic agent, such as a gelatin sponge (Gelita® Medical)

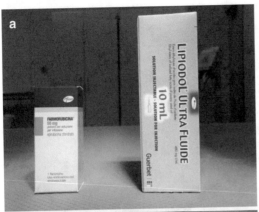

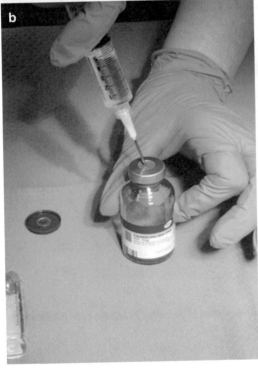

Fig. 5 cTACE protocol and therapeutic agents. (**a**) Farmorubicin® and Lipiodol® packages. (**b**) Image showing the emulsion of the chemotherapeutic agent with Lipiodol®

(Fig. 6), polyvinyl alcohol particles (PVAs), or microspheres are injected in order to induce complete stasis. Both the chemotherapeutic mixture and the embolising agent are delivered as close to the tumour as possible, with the catheter tip placed superselectively in order to penetrate not only into the HCC but also into the drainage area, including daughter nodules or microsatellites.

Regarding the ideal dose of chemotherapeutic agents, data from the literature reported a usual dose of 10–70 mg for doxorubicin and 10–120 mg for cisplatin per session (Marelli et al. 2007, Bruix et al. 2004). The criteria to determine the optimal doses are not standardised: some authors refer to patient body surface area (BSA), weight, tumour burden or bilirubin level, and some used a fixed dose. In the literature, there are a few RCTs that have failed to show significant differences in survival between the use of different drugs (doxorubicin, cisplatin or epirubicin), and different doses (Kasugai et al. 1989, Kawai et al. 1997, Watanabe et al. 1994). Marelli et al. (2007) have not demonstrated the superiority of any single chemotherapeutic agent over other drugs or for mono-drug chemotherapy versus combination chemotherapy.

Lipiodol (Lipiodol® Ultra-Fluid, Guerbet Laboratories, Roissy, France) is an iodinated ethyl ester of poppy seed oil, first used as an oily contrast medium in lymphangiographic studies. Its use dates back to 1974 (Doyon et al. 1974) and in the early 1980s (Nakakuma et al. 1983), with the spread of cTACE, Lipiodol was introduced as a drug carrier. Lipiodol is a microvessel embolic agent, a carrier of chemotherapeutic agents into the tumour (Kan et al. 1997, Raoul et al. 1992) and it retains them inside the tumour for a long time (Kan et al. 1994a, b) enhancing the antitumour effects, thanks to the filling into the portal veins.

In the normal liver parenchyma, Lipiodol accumulates in the portal venules using arterio-portal shunts; it is gradually released into the systemic circulation via the hepatic sinusoids or undergoes phagocytosis by Kupffer cells (Kan et al. 1993, Kan et al. 1994a, b). On the contrary, in HCC and hypervascular liver metastases, Lipiodol has the property of preferential accumulation and longer retention than in the normal liver. The rationale lies in the fact that HCC is hyper-vascularised and thus determines a "siphoning effect" which is enhanced by the absence of Kupffer cells inside the tumour tissues, resulting in the embolic effects on smaller vessels (Ohishi et al. 1985). Another fundamental role of Lipiodol is its capacity to carry

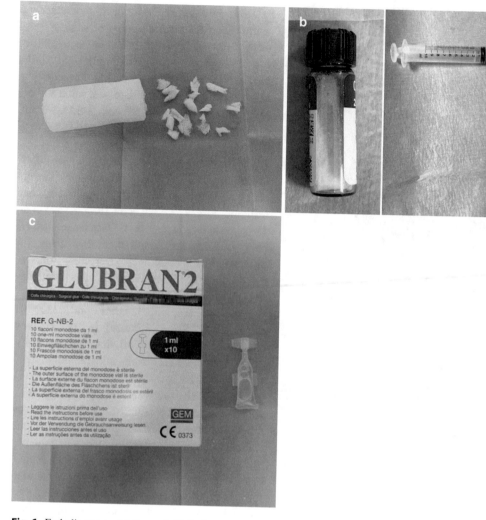

Fig. 6 Embolic agents. (**a**) Spongel (Gelita® Medical). (**b**) Polyvinyl alcohol particles (PVAs). (**c**) Glue (Glubran®)

chemotherapeutic agents into the tumour. When the emulsion is injected, the drug is slowly released from the Lipiodol and remains in high concentration within the tumour for a prolonged period. When injected into the hepatic artery, Lipiodol selectively remains in the tumour nodules for several weeks to over a year.

Furthermore, Lipiodol circulates beyond the tumour-feeding arteries into the distal portal branches because of arterioportal communication through the peribiliary capillary plexus and the drainage route from the tumour itself (Kan et al. 1994a, b, Terayama et al. 2001). Lipiodol also exerts a temporary embolic effect both on the hepatic artery and the portal branches (de Baere et al. 1998, Kan et al. 1994a, b).

Another major advantage of Lipiodol TACE is the ability to control the delivery of the treatment by continuous visualisation of the therapeutic agents due to the radio-opacity of Lipiodol. The Lipiodol drug emulsion is actively monitored until the tumour vascular bed is saturated, and stasis is obtained in the very peripheral branches. Opacification of the small peripheral portal branches around the tumour with Lipiodol is a common finding and has been demonstrated as a predictive factor for tumour response to treatment associated with a lower rate of local recurrence (Miyayama et al. 2007), complete necrosis (Miyayama et al. 2007), including necrosis of the liver parenchyma around the lesion and its satellite nodules, and achieving safety margins in a manner similar to radiofrequency ablation (Miyayama et al. 2009). Local tumour recurrence was significantly lower when a greater degree of portal vein visualisation with Lipiodol was demonstrated during TACE (Fig. 7) (Miyayama et al. 2007). The deposition of Lipiodol in the portal veins around a tumour has been reported to have stronger antitumour effects than embolisation without Lipiodol.

Moreover, intratumoural retention of Lipiodol, as detected on postprocedure CT scan, is useful in detecting the response to the treatment and in predicting overall survival (OS) (Fig. 8). (Kim et al. 2012; Kim et al. 2009).

Although Marelli L et al. (2007) reported that the use of Lipiodol in TACE has been challenged, nowadays robust evidence confirms the efficacy of the use of Lipiodol, and it is still widely adopted in TACE protocol.

Embolic agents. Embolisation can be performed using either permanent or temporary embolic agents. Different embolic agents have been reported in the literature; the most commonly used include gelatin sponges (Gelita® Medical), PVA particles and microspheres. Steel coils, autologous blood clots and degradable starch microspheres have also been reported. Of these, PVA, microspheres and steel coils are permanent embolic agents while the others embolise temporarily. No consensus is available on which is the most appropriate embolic agent; as a general rule, the optimal embolic agent is that which can embolise the peripheral portions of the hepatic artery as much as possible in order to stop the hepatic arterial flow and prevent the development of collateral feeding arteries to the tumour. A gelatin sponge is the most widely used embolic agent; it can be prepared in various forms (particles, pledgets or fragments), and its

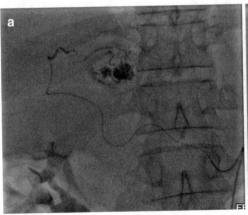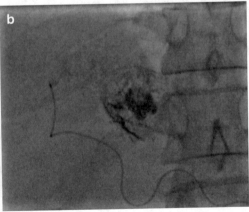

Fig. 7 Angiogram showing the superselective catheterisation of a large hepatocellular carcinoma (HCC) and the injection of the chemotherapeutic mixture (**a**); (**b**) the injection was stopped when the deposition of Lipiodol® into the portal vein around the tumour was reported

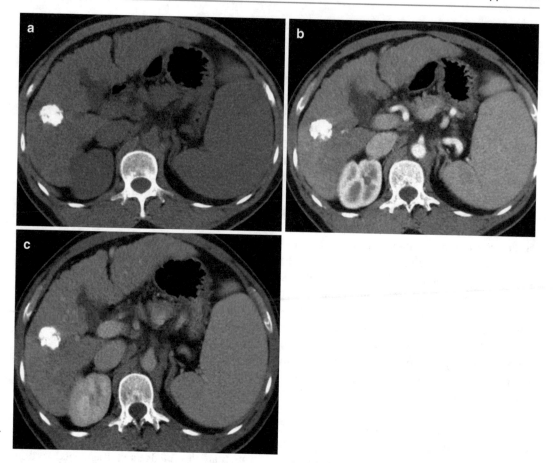

Fig. 8 A computed tomography (CT) scan performed 1 month after cTACE of a nodule located in the V segment. The pre-contrast CT scan shows a compact Lipiodol® uptake (**a**) The arterial phase (**b**) The venous phase (**c**) Showing no viable residual tumour, indicating a complete response to treatment

major advantage is that it induces temporary occlusion and allows revascularisation within 2 weeks, enabling a sequential treatment (Coldwell 1994). An experimental study on animals (Kan, 1993) has demonstrated that hepatic artery embolisation with a gelatin sponge alone does not cause any damage to the liver.

1.1.1.2 cTACE: Therapeutic Efficacy/ Clinical Results

Chemotherapeutic agent injection and embolisation induce tumour necrosis which is evaluated by the pathological identification of the necrosis of the target nodules by a reduction in the viable tumour burden identified on contrast-enhanced CT scans and by a decrease in tumour marker serum levels (Ji et al. 2008).

However, the therapeutic efficacy of TACE in inducing tumour necrosis does not necessarily mean longer survival rates for HCC patients. Death from tumour progression is reported in almost 70–80% of patients treated with TACE, due to the recurrence of HCC or HCC nodules de novo.

Until 2002, small RCTs failed to show a survival advantage of TACE/transarterial embolisation (TAE) versus inactive treatment; the use of TACE remained controversial in patients not suitable for curative therapies (Bruix et al. 1998, GETCH 1995, Lin et al. 1988, Pelletier et al. 1990, Pelletier et al. 1998).

In 2002, two RCTs (Llovet et al. 2002, Lo et al. 2002) demonstrated the superiority of cTACE over best supportive care (BSC) for intermediate-stage HCC. Llovet et al. (2002) showed significantly longer mean survival after cTACE (28.6 months) as compared to BSC (17.9 months; $p = 0.009$), and Lo et al. (2002), confirmed that cTACE has a benefit over BSC in terms of survival rate (57% vs. 32% at 1 year; 31% vs. 11% at 2 years; 26% vs. 3% at 3 years, respectively, $p = 0.002$).

These RCTs were followed by the publication of a cumulative meta-analysis by Camma et al. (2002) and a systematic review of randomised trials (LLovet et al. 2003) showing that TACE significantly reduced the overall 2-year mortality rate as compared to conservative treatments (odds ratios [ORs]: 0.53 and 0.54; 95% confidence intervals: 0.32–0.89 and 0.33–0.89; $p = 0.015$ and 0.017, respectively). According to the EASL-EORTC Clinical Practice Guidelines, in 2012 (EASL-EORTC 2012, EASL 2018), cTACE became the gold standard treatment for intermediate-stage HCC with the highest grade of recommendation (1A).

Of all the possible therapies for HCC, TACE is the least standardised, widely varying as to the chemotherapeutic agents injected, treatment devices used and therapeutic schedule (Facciorusso et al. 2018, Lencioni et al. 2016a, b). This poor standardisation is outlined in some Society guidelines, such as those from the Chinese National Health and Family Planning Commission, which recommend performing individualised chemoembolisation protocols (Zhou et al. 2018).

Since then, cTACE has been reported in many publications, performed using different methods of preparation and administration; in 2016, a worldwide expert panel published consensus technical recommendations in order to encourage cTACE standardisation as reported in Table 4 (de Baere et al. 2016a, b).

1.1.1.3 Complications of cTACE

Transarterial chemoembolisation can cause complications that arise from underlying causative

Table 4 Summary of the technical recommendations from experts on how to perform reproducible cTACE (modified from Raoul et al. 2019)

Item	Recommendations for reproducible cTACE
Patient selection	Pay particular attention to underlying liver disease and Performance Status (PS)
Pre-procedure imaging	Perform multiphasic computed tomography (CT) or dynamic contrast-enhanced-magnetic resonance imaging (MRI) of the liver before treatment allocation
Patient preparation	Discuss systematic antiemetic treatment, intravenous hydration, and pain killer use as well as antibiotic prophylaxis according to the risk of liver abscess
Per-procedure imaging	Use cone beam (CB)-CT for tumor visualization, targeting, and assessment of treatment completion
Chemotherapy	Use doxorubicin 50–75 mg/m² body surface area or cisplatin 50–100 mg/m²
Lipiodol emulsion	To improve tumour deposit prepare water-in-oil emulsion (aqueous chemotherapy droplets in internal phase and Lipiodol in continuous external phase). The water-in-oil emulsion is obtained by mixing one volume of drug solution with two to three volumes of Lipiodol by pushing the drug syringe into the syringe containing Lipiodol
Embolizing agent	Gelatin sponge is commonly used. Alternatively, the size of calibrated microspheres should be 100–300 μm in order to ensure distal occlusion with preservation of feeding segmental arteries
Selectivity	Super selective cTACE, using microcatheter when treating a single tumour or low number of tumours
Endpoint	Lipiodol opacification of the small arterioportal sinusoids should be used as a predictive factor for tumor response, tumor necrosis, and local recurrence
Response evaluation	Assess tumour viability using the mRECIST criteria
cTACE regimen	Perform at least two cTACE procedures 2–8 weeks apart before stopping due to a lack of response

PS performance status, *CT* computed tomography, *MRI* magnetic resonance imaging, *(CB)-CT* cone-beam computed tomography, *cTACE* conventional transarterial chemoembolisation, *mRECIST* Modified Response Evaluation Criteria In Solid Tumours factors or an application of erroneous techniques. Major factors that induce complications include compromised liver function, main portal vein obstruction, biliary tract obstruction, a previous history of bile duct surgery, Lipiodol overdose, hepatic artery occlusion due to repeated TACE and nonselective TACE (Chung et al. 1996, Golfieri et al. 2011). The most common complication of TACE is postembolisation syndrome occurring in 60–80% of the patients after the procedure. It consists of transient abdominal pain, fever and elevation of the level of hepatic transaminases (Wigmore et al. 2003). It is uncertain if postembolisation syndrome reflects damage to the normal liver parenchyma or tumour necrosis; it is mostly self-limiting within 3–4 days; however, a prolonged hospital stay may be required to monitor the patient and control pain

The most serious complication is a hepatic failure which is related to TACE-induced ischemic damage to the non-target liver tissue and portal vein obstruction. A high dose of anticancer drugs and Lipiodol, a high basal level of bilirubin, prolonged prothrombin time and advanced Child-Pugh class have been identified as risk factors (Chan et al. 2002). Although the definition of TACE-induced hepatic failure is different in each study, its incidence varied widely from 0–49%, with a median incidence of 8% (Marelli et al. 2007).

Other TACE-related complications occur in less than 10% of cases and include ischemic cholecystitis (mainly due to inadvertent injection of the Lipiodol mixture or embolisation of the cystic artery), hepatic abscesses and biliary strictures (Bruix et al. 2004); however, the majority of cases are asymptomatic and rarely require percutaneous drainage or a cholecystectomy. Liver abscess is a rare complication reported in 0.2% of a series of 6255 TACE procedures (Song et al. 2001), more frequently occurring in patients who had undergone previous intervention in the biliary system which is prone to ascending biliary infection. The prophylactic use of antibiotics should be considered in these patients. Another possible complication, even though rare (0.5–2% incidence), is biloma (Kim et al. 2001; Wang et al. 2005). Upper gastrointestinal complica-

tions, such as gastritis, ulceration and bleeding, can occur after TACE due to the reflux of the embolic agents into the gastric arteries and the presence of anatomic variants (e.g., an accessory left gastric artery arising from the left hepatic artery). Upper gastrointestinal bleeding occurred in 3% (median) of the patients (range, 0–22%) in 23 trials which involved 2593 patients (Marelli et al. 2007). It is very important to recognise any of the anatomic variants and to prevent the reflux of a drug into the gastrointestinal organs.

1.1.2 Drug-Eluting Bead (DEB)-TACE

Although conventional Lipiodol-based TACE is the most popular TACE technique, the introduction of an embolic drug-eluting bead (DEB) has provided an attractive alternative to conventional regimens.

Drug-eluting bead microspheres are composed of a hydrophilic, ionic polymer that can bind anthracyclines via an ion-exchange mechanism, and they were developed to have the ability to sequester the chemotherapeutic agent and release it over time (a one-week period).

Transarterial chemoembolisation with drug-eluting beads (DEB-TACE), using calibrated microspheres preloaded with doxorubicin, has shown more sustained drug release in a slow and controlled manner with concomitant permanent embolisation, thus obtaining low circulating drug levels. With this technique, the pharmacokinetic profile is substantially improved, the side effects are reduced with lower systemic drug exposure due to the minimum passage of doxorubicin in the systemic circulation and significantly reduced liver toxicity as compared with cTACE. DEB-TACE also provides levels of consistency and repeatability not available with cTACE, offering the opportunity of implementing a standardised approach to HCC treatment.

1.1.2.1 DEB-TACE Protocol

Bead size. Commercialised DEBs are composed of various hydrophilic ionic polymers that bind to anthracycline drugs via an anion exchange mechanism. Up to 37.5 mg of doxorubicin per mL of microspheres can be loaded in from 30 min to 2 h. The beads are available in several diameters

Table 5 Drug-eluting beads (DEBs) present on the market and different available bead sizes

Type	After loading with Doxo	Size ranges smaller size	◄·····················►		Size ranges larger size
Tandem ™ (Boston Scientific-Celonova, Marlborough, Massachusetts)	Size reduction of 5–9%	40 ± 10 μm	75 ± 15 μm	100 ± 25 μm	
LifePearl ™ (Terumo European Interventional Systems, Leuven, Belgium)	Size reduction of 20–25%	100 ± 25 μm	200 ± 50 μm	400 ± 50 μm	
DC Bead ™ (BTG, Farnham, United Kingdom)	Size reduction of 20%	70–150 μm (DC Bead™)	100–300 μm	300–500 μm	500–700 μm
HepaSphere ™ (Merit Medical, South Jordan,Utah).	Expand up to 4 times	30–60 μm dry 120–240 μm expanded	50–100 μm dry 200–400 μm expanded	100–150 μm dry 400–600 μm expanded	150–200 μm dry 600–1000 μm expanded

Table 6 Change in the diameters of unloaded and Doxorubicin-loaded Microspheres (from de Baere et al. 2016)

Microsphere type	Diameter (μm)	
	Unloaded	Doxorubicin-loaded
DC Bead™	173 ± 53	138 ± 46
LifePearl™	199 ± 24	151 ± 18
Tandem™	98 ± 15	89 ± 15
HepaSphere™	NA	165 ± 28

ranging from 40 to 900 μm (Table 5) and they change in diameter after the drug is loaded (Table 6) (Lewis et al. 2006).

The choice of the best bead size depends on precise calibration, a high drug-loading capacity which means deeper penetration into the tumour vessels and increased spatial density (to avoid clumping in larger vessels upstream of the tumour). Moreover, ideal beads should also be able to cover the perinodular drainage area. There are differences in drug loading and release related to the type and the size of the microspheres as in vitro analysis has demonstrated (Lewis et al. 2006, deBaere et al.2016a, b)

1.1.2.2 DEB-TACE: Therapeutic Efficacy/Clinical Evidences

There are currently no definitive recommendations on which DEBs should be preferred since there is a lack of RCTs that compare the different DEB devices and only retrospective single centre studies are, for the most part, available.

The smaller commercialised DC Bead M1® (70–150 μm) (BTG) has been evaluated in recent studies (Malagari et al. 2012; Spreafico et al. 2015) which showed an objective response rate (ORR) ranging from 77 to 93%.

HepaSphere® microspheres (Merit Medical) are another type of commercialised superabsorbent microspheres (30–60 μm) which expand in diameter according to the suspension protocol: 166–242 μm in diameter in saline and 145–213 μm in a doxorubicin solution (Liu et al. 2012). In 2014, Malagari et al. (2014) evaluated the outcome of 45 patients treated with HepaSphere® (30–60 μm) and reported an ORR of 68.9% with no serious adverse events.

In 2018, the MIRACLE I pilot study showed that Embozene TANDEM® 75 μm microsphere (Boston Scientific) loaded doxorubicin provided good local tumour control (95%) in a small cohort of patients with the unilobar disease (Richter et al. 2018)

Aliberti et al. suggested that TACE with LifePearl® microspheres (Terumo) loaded with doxorubicin was efficient and safe for the treatment of unresectable primary liver cancer (Aliberti et al. 2016)

In the first phase II trial of DEB-TACE, Varela et al. demonstrated that the DEB-TACE group (DC Beads® 500–700 μm (BTG)) had a lower plasma doxorubicin Cmax and Area Under the Curve (AUC) for up to 7 days as compared to the cTACE group (Varela 2007)

In 2012, two retrospective studies comparing DEB-TACE using 100–300 μm to 300–500 μm microspheres in select BCLC-A or -B patients (Burrel et al. 2012; Malagari et al. 2012) showed that the median OSs in the two groups was 43.8 months and 48 months, respectively. Although no studies have compared the efficacy of different sizes of DC-Bead®, the 100–300 μm beads became the most frequently used microspheres.

1.1.3 Patient Selection and Repetition Protocols

The ability to predict prognosis after the first or repeated TACE for HCC is mandatory to maximise treatment outcomes. Therefore, over time, different risk stratification scores have been developed to identify patients who may or may not benefit from the first treatment and/or from TACE repetition.

Two scores were developed to improve patient selection for the first TACE treatment: the Selection for Transarterial chemoembolisation treatment (STATE) score (Hucke et al. 2014), which includes serum albumin level, tumour load, and C-reactive protein (CRP) level, and the Hepatoma arterial-embolisation prognostic (HAP) score (Kadalayil et al. 2013), which is based on four parameters (albumin, bilirubin, alfa-fetoprotein (AFP) and tumour size).

Two score systems were developed to select patients for TACE repetition: the Assessment for Retreatment with TACE (ART) score (Siegart et al. 2013) and the ABCR (α-fetoprotein, Barcelona Clinic Liver Cancer, Child-Pugh, and Response) score (Adhoute et al. 2015).

The ART score includes a serum aspartate aminotransferase (AST) increase >25% after the first TACE, an increase in the Child-Pugh score of 1, 2 or more points after the first TACE, and the absence of radiological tumour response. The START strategy combines the STATE and the ART score and aims to indicate patient selection both for the first treatment and for retreatment.

The ABCR score includes an AFP level ≥ 200 ng/mL at baseline, the BCLC stage at baseline, an increase in the Child-Pugh score of

≥2 points from baseline after the first TACE session, and radiologic response after the first TACE session (Kloeckner et al. 2017).

A study published in 2016, (Cappelli et al. 2016) suggested that an individual prognostication tool is feasible, based on easily available pre-TACE parameters, such as the number of tumours, serum albumin, total bilirubin, alpha-fetoprotein and maximum tumour size. For this reason, a web-based calculator (optimised for smartphones) was developed and published online at http://www.liver-cancer.eu/mhap3.html. This enables physicians to calculate survival during their daily routine, an outpatient examination or even directly at the patient's bedside.

None of the scoring systems have been validated prospectively, and their ability to prognosticate in other Eastern and Western cohorts has been variable. Larger multicentre series are necessary.

Considering a median dose of 50–75 mg/m² of doxorubicin for a single TACE procedure and a maximum cumulative dose of 450 mg/m² to prevent cardiotoxicity, 6–9 TACE treatments are allowed in a single patient.

However, according to European guidelines (EASL 2018), TACE should not be repeated when substantial.

necrosis is not achieved after two rounds of treatment or when follow-up treatment fails to induce.

marked necrosis at sites that have progressed after the initial tumour response. The guidelines also set the limit of cumulative doxorubicin which should be administered at 450 mg/m². However, the maximum number of TACE procedures to be performed on each patient should be decided on by a multidisciplinary tumour board, according to the lobar/bilobar tumour distribution, the response in the lesion/s treated and individual tolerance to the treatment. To date, tumour burden, BCLC stage at baseline, Child-Pugh score and radiologic response are considered to be the most predictive factors for TACE retreatment decision-making.

In summary, TACE should not be repeated when complete necrosis is not achieved after

TACE treatments or when there is progression or liver function impairment, worsening of performance status, portal vein tumour thrombosis or extrahepatic metastases (Facciorusso et al. 2015, Terzi et al. 2012, Terzi et al. 2014). Transarterial chemoembolisation can be repeated continuously in the case of a suspicious viable tumour seen in follow-up imaging. No real consensus exists regarding the frequency of TACE and the interval between two TACE treatments. Experts in the field propose on-demand repetition with longer intervals between treatments rather than a regular predefined schedule (Raoul et al. 2011, Bolondi et al. 2012)

A treatment algorithm for patients undergoing TACE proposed by Bolondi et al. for the Italian Association for the Study of the Liver (Bolondi et al. 2013) recommends that TACE *should not be repeated (untreatable progression)* when:

- substantial necrosis is not accomplished after two initial sessions
- follow-up treatment fails to induce marked necrosis at sites which have progressed after an initial response
- major progression (substantial liver involvement, vascular invasion, or extrahepatic spread) occurs after an initial response; retreatment is unsafe due to deterioration of the liver function

The corresponding reported algorithm proposed is reported in (Table 7) (Position paper AISF. 2013).

Table 7 Treatment algorithm for patients undergoing transarterial chemoembolisation (modified from Position paper of the Italian Association for the Study of the Liver (AISF): the multidisciplinary clinical approach to hepatocellular carcinoma 2013)

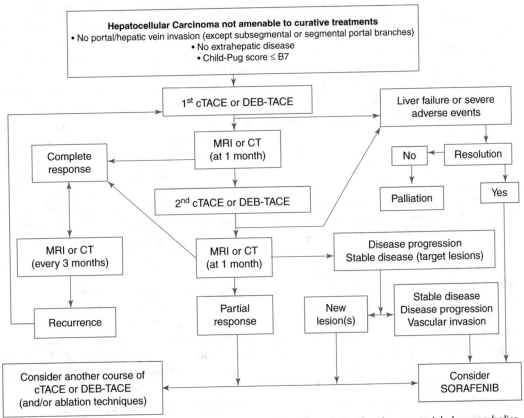

cTACE conventional transarterial chemoembolisation, *DEB-TACE* drug-eluting bead transarterial chemoembolisation, *MRI* magnetic resonance imaging, *CT* computed tomography

1.1.4 Choosing Between cTACE and DEB-TACE: Tumour Response and Survival

Several trials have compared cTACE and DEB-TACE in terms of both efficacy and safety. Nowadays, the best choice between cTACE and DEB-TACE follows the evidence coming from two well-conducted RCTs.

The first was the PRECISION V multicentre RCT phase II trial (Lammer et al. 2010), showing that DEB-TACE performed with DC Bead® 300–500 μm followed by DC Bead® 500–700 μm, is not superior over cTACE for tumour response at 6 months after the procedure ($p = 0.11$), which was the primary endpoint of the trial.

The second phase III RCT of Golfieri et al. (2014) for the PRECISION ITALIA STUDY GROUP enrolled 177 patients (89 in the DEB-TACE group and 88 in the cTACE group). The results showed no difference in tumour response and in median time-to-progression (9 months in both arms). The 1- and 2-year survival rates were similar: 86.2% and 56.8% after DEB-TACE, respectively, and 83.5% and 55.4%. after cTACE, respectively ($p = 0.949$).

Although the heterogeneity in patient selection makes it difficult to draw definitive conclusions regarding the best treatment, the meta-analysis of Facciorusso et al. (2016) which included 1449 patients, confirmed the non-superiority of DEB-TACE over cTACE in terms of tumour response and survival.

According to the Italian Association of Medical Oncology (AIOM) (AIOM 2018), due to the lack of convincing evidence in favour of DEB-TACE over cTACE in terms of survival, the choice depends on the single centre or operator experience. In Italy, according to a recent survey, DEB-TACE was performed more frequently than cTACE (52% vs. 32%) (Bargellini et al. 2014). According to the position of the Italian Association for the Study of the Liver (AISF): the multidisciplinary clinical approach to hepatocellular carcinoma 2018), DEB-TACE may be preferred to cTACE in Child-Pugh B or ECOG PS 1 patients (Grade of recommendations 2b-B).

The current European guidelines do not endorse one technique over the other, due to the lack of sufficient evidence, and leave the choice to the operator (EASL Guidelines 2018).

1.1.4.1 CTACE and DEB-TACE: Choice of Drug

An additional debatable point is the choice of the chemotherapeutic drug to use. In fact, there is no univocal agreement on the optimal chemotherapy to use in TACE, and no cytotoxic agent has definitively been proven to be superior to the others (Marelli et al. 2007). Despite being the most frequently used, there is no evidence that doxorubicin is the most appropriate chemotherapeutic agent for TACE in HCC. The rationale for its use is quite limited, and no rigorous preclinical data have ever supported its preferential use with respect to other cytotoxic agents. Randomised control trials, focusing on other outcomes and a meta-analysis have demonstrated that doxorubicin administered in the setting of DEB-TACE is as effective as when administered emulsified with Lipiodol (Lammer et al. 2010, Golfieri et al. 2014). Moreover, regarding safety, no substantial differences were observed. The two RCTs which compared Doxorubicin to epirubicin in cTACE for HCC did not show any difference in terms of efficacy (Watanabe et al. 1994, Kawai et al. 1997).

In DEB-TACE, with respect to specific techniques, in vitro studies have demonstrated that the microspheres can be loaded with several different drugs (Jordan et al. 2010, Lee et al. 2010); epirubicin is one of them and the data available have shown that DEB- TACE with epirubicin is effective and safe (Sattler et al. 2018). In DEB-TACE, the pharmacokinetics of the drug in patients treated with epirubicin-loaded microspheres is similar to that of doxorubicin (Sottaniet al. 2012).

1.1.4.2 Choosing Between cTACE and DEB-TACE: Safety

Both DEB-TACE and cTACE may be responsible for the typical postembolisation syndrome. Data from the literature (Lammer et al. 2010, Golfieri et al. 2014, Facciorusso et al. 2018) have failed to find any difference between DEB-TACE and cTACE in terms of safety. In the PRECISION V study, there was no significant difference in serious adverse events ($p = 0.86$) in DEB-TACE and cTACE within 30 days of the procedure (20.4% and 19.4% after DEB-TACE and cTACE, respectively) (Lammer et al. 2010). In the PRECISION ITALIA STUDY GROUP trial, post-procedural pain was less frequent in the DEB-TACE arm (Golfieri et al. 2014). Similarly, a recent meta-analysis pooled 9 studies and included 1026 patients reported to have a severe AE rate with no statistical difference between the cTACE and the DEB-TACE groups (OR 0.85, 0.60–1.20, $p = 0.36$) (Facciorusso et al. 2018). Interestingly, regarding the cirrhotic HCC group, other studies have reported at least one liver/biliary injury in 30.4% of the DEB-TACE procedures versus 4.2% of the cTACE procedures ($p < 0.001$) (Guiu et al. 2012)

Recently, a retrospective study compared TACE-related hepatic toxicities 3 months after cTACE and DEB-TACE in 151 patients and reported a significantly higher incidence of biloma in the DEB-TACE group than in the cTACE group ($p < 0.001$) (Monier et al. 2017).

Regarding the incidence and predictors of hepatic arterial damage after DEB-TACE versus cTACE treatment, some authors have proven that the incidence was significantly higher after DEB-TACE when analysed per branch (OR 6.36; $p < 0.001$) and per patient (OR 3.15; $p = 0.005$), and the doxorubicin dose results was a possible risk factor (Lee et al. 2017).

1.1.4.3 Choosing Between cTACE and DEB-TACE: Cost

The use of DEB-TACE in HCC patients led to a significantly lower rate of rehospitalisation for the management of TACE-related toxicities with a better economic profile (Vadot et al. 2015).

An Italian group (Cucchetti et al. 2016) presented a cost-effective analysis comparing cTACE and DEB-TACE which included 1860 patients performed from the healthcare-provider point of view following a Markov simulation model from the first TACE until death. They showed that the direct incremental cost of DEB-TACE was not particularly high and would be amortised by the shorter hospital stay, the better quality of life and the mild survival improvement obtained. Because of a longer ($p = 0.001$) in-hospital stay after cTACE, due to more frequent postembolisation syndrome, the global cost was not significantly lower for cTACE as compared to DEB-TACE. The authors concluded that DEB-TACE was cost-effective as compared to the conventional procedure.

1.1.5 Assessment of Tumour Response

Conventional criteria based on tumour diameter shrinkage (Response Evaluation Criteria In Solid Tumour [RECIST] criteria) (Lencioni et al. 2010) were poor predictors of survival of HCC patients undergoing intra-arterial therapies and locoregional treatments (Ronot et al. 2014)

Therefore, modified RECIST (mRECIST) criteria were introduced in 2010; they take into account the residual viable tumour after TACE, detected at multiphasic CT and MRI as enhancing areas in the late arterial phase and washout in the portal/delayed phases. (Lencioni et al. 2010).

After DEB-TACE, tumour response can be assessed using either dynamic CT or MRI whereas, after cTACE, MRI is preferred over CT where the dense Lipiodol deposition can obscure a residual hypervascular tumour and underestimate its extent.

The completeness of Lipiodol deposition is also considered to be a helpful tool in evaluating the response rate after treatment for patients with large HCC lesions (Forner et al. 2009, Takayasu et al. 2000, Chen et al. 2016a, b). In particular, complete Lipiodol tumour deposition is considered to indicate tumour necrosis; a partial deposition suggests that a residual viable tumour is present, and the patient can be scheduled for TACE repetition.

1.1.6 The Real-World Indications for TACE

According to the BCLC staging system, TACE should only be indicated as the first-line treatment for patients with intermediate-stage HCC; nevertheless, TACE is widely used not only in intermediate HCCs but also outside this specific scenario. In clinical routine practice, approximately 40% of TACE procedures are performed on either BCLC A or, although more rarely, on BCLC C patients (Bargellini et al. 2014). The heterogeneous practices among interventional radiologists have been outlined in two surveys in terms of indications, techniques and also in the assessment of tumour response (Bargellini et al. 2014; Fohlen et al. 2018).

Have recently proposed an updated treatment algorithm to treat HCC patients of any stage based on the new evidence from the literature, which is additionally detailed for any stage, thus justifying the "treatment stage migration" strategy (i.e., "a therapeutic choice by which a treatment theoretically recommended for a different stage is selected as the best 1st line treatment option") (Table 8).

An updated algorithm decision tree for TACE in managing early, intermediate and advanced stage HCC can be the following.

- *Early stage (Stage A)*

Patients with BCLC early stage disease who cannot benefit from the recommended option (surgery and/or percutaneous ablation) can benefit from TACE treatment, according to the literature and also mentioned in the most recent EASL guidelines as "stage migration strategy" (Burrel et al. 2012, EASL 2018; Terzi et al. 2012, Bargellini et al. 2012, Golfieri et al. 2011).

In some series, more than 40% of cases with solitary nodules, the majority with early-stage disease, were treated with TACE (Terzi et al. 2012, Takayasu et al. 2012). Furthermore, the role of TACE as neoadjuvant therapy prior to liver transplantation (LT) is widely accepted, either as a bridge between treatments in patients on the waiting list or to downstage the tumour. In this setting, cTACE has been shown to reduce HCC recurrence after LT and to improve a post-transplant OS when the waiting list period is longer than 6–12 months (Pompili et al. 2013). Drug-eluting bead TACE has not been widely evaluated as bridging therapy, and the current evidence is not as strong as for cTACE.

- *Intermediate Stage (BCLC B)*

Table 8 A proposal of an algorithm decision tree for transarterial chemoembolisation in the management of the different stages of HCC (modified from Raoul et al. 2019)

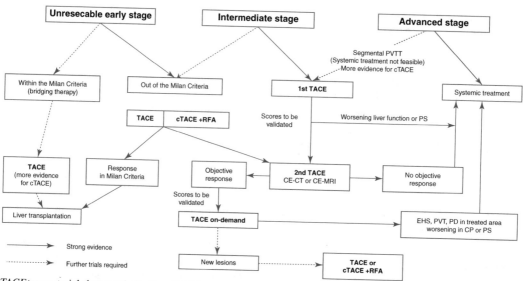

TACE transarterial chemoembolisation, *HCC* hepatocellular carcinoma, *Seg PVTT* segmental portal vein tumour thrombosis, *RFA* radio-frequency ablation, *CECT* contrast-enhanced computed tomography, *CE-MRI* contrast-enhanced magnetic resonance imaging, *CP* Child-Pugh, *cTACE* conventional transarterial chemoembolisation, *EHS* extrahepatic spread, *PD* progressive disease, *PS* performance status, *PVT* portal vein tumour thrombosis

The Barcelona Clinic Liver Cancer (BCLC) intermediate and advanced stages (BCLC B and C) of HCC both include heterogeneous populations. Patients classified as BCLC stage B present with different tumour burdens, and, as is known, the recommended treatment is TACE.

For BCLB stage B, in 2012, a panel of experts (Bolondi et al. 2012) proposed a subclassification which identified four substages (B1–B4) of intermediate HCC, incorporating the new concept of joint consideration of the tumour burden according to the "beyond Milan" and the "within up-to-7" criteria together with the Child-Pugh score and PS (Table 9). The authors advised TACE as the first/alternative options for different substages of BCLC B patients due to their rather limited tumour bulk and substantially preserved hepatic function. Following this paper, in 2014, Ha et al. (2014) validated the model by examining 466 BCLC B patients undergoing TACE. They developed a modified subclassification in which B3 and B4 subclasses were merged as BIII while BI and BII corresponded to B1 and B2 of the Bolondi model. Median survival significantly differed among the three subclasses (41.0 vs. 22.1 vs. 16.6 months, respectively, $p \leq 0.001$), confirming it to be an effective tool for stratifying the BCLC B stage group. The most recent evaluation of the prognostic capability of the subclassification of Bolondi et al. (2012) was carried out by Kim et al. (2017) on 821 patients treated with TACE. The B1, B2 and B3 subclasses showed significantly different survival rates between the contiguous stages with a median survival of 51.5, 26, and 14.8 months, respectively ($p < 0.001$ for each comparison with the contiguous stratum until B3). The authors suggested a reclassification, adopting the so-called "up-to-11" criteria, instead of the "up-to-7-2 criteria. According to the new proposal, median survival progressively decreased from B1 (44.8 months) to B2 (21.5 months) and B3 (11.3 months), with a significant difference between the contiguous stages ($p < 0.001$ for the comparison of each stage with the subsequent one).

An additional BCLC B subclassification has been developed by Kudo et al. (2015) who has proposed the "Kinki criteria" which incorporate the idea of classifying patients by Child-Pugh scores (up to 7 and 8–9) and the "beyond Milan" and the "up-to-7" criteria from the Bolondi et al. classification. The Kinki staging system relies on three substages (Table 10). The authors include the combined therapies (TACE and ablation) in the potential treatment options in order to extend the ablation area if the tumour size was close to 5 cm. Moreover, in patients with several nodules, superselective conventional TACE (cTACE) could be considered in order to carefully treat the tumours one by one with curative intent. When

Table 9 A proposal for a subclassification of the intermediate stage of hepatocellular carcinoma (modified from Bolondi L et al. 2012)

Intermediate substage	B1	B2	B3	B4	Quasi C
Child-Pugh score	5–7	5–6	7	8–9[a]	A
Beyond Milan criteria and within the up-to-7 criteria	in	out	out	any	any
ECOG performance status (tumour-related)	0	0	0	0–1	0
Portal vein tumour thrombosis	no	no	no	no	yes (segmental)
1st option	TACE	TACE or TARE	research trial	LT[b]	or subsegmental) sorafenib
Alternative	LT TACE + ablation	sorafenib	TACE sorafenib		TACE or TARE
Median survival time, months	41.0	22.1	14.1	17.2	

TACE transarterial chemoembolisation, *LT* liver transplantation, *TARE* transarterial radioembolisation, *ECOG* Eastern Cooperative Group Performance Status
[a]With severe/refractory ascites and/or jaundice
[b]Only if "up-to-7 IN" and PS 0

Table 10 Subclassification and treatment strategy of intermediate-stage HCC according to the Kinki criteria (modified from Kudo et al. 2015)

BCLC substage	B1	B2	B3	
Child-Pugh score	5–7	5–7	8–9	
Beyond Milan and	IN	OUT	ANY	
Within up-to-7			IN	OUT
Substage			B3 A	B3 B
Concept of treatment strategy	curative intent	non-curative, palliative	curative intent if within up-to-7	palliative, no treatment
Treatment option	resection ablation superselective cTACE	DEB-TACE[a] HAIC[b] sorafenib[c]	transplantation ablation superselective cTACE	HAIC selective DEB-TACE
Alternative	DEB-TACE (large, Child-Pugh score 7) B-TACE[d]	cTACE	DEB-TACE B-TACE, HAIC	BSC

HAIC hepatic arterial infusion chemotherapy, *TACE* transarterial chemoembolisation, *DEB-TACE* drug-eluting bead transarterial chemoembolisation, *cTACE* conventional transarterial chemoembolisation, *BSC* best supportive care
[a]DEB-TACE is recommended for very large tumours >6 cm
[b]HAIC (hepatic arterial infusion chemotherapy) is recommended for multiple tumours >6 cm
[c]Sorafenib is recommended for patients having liver function with a Child-Pugh score of 5 and 6
[d]B-TACE (balloon-occluded TACE) is recommended when there are fewer tumours

superselective catheterisation was not applicable, TACE with drug-eluting beads (DEB-TACE) or balloon-occluded TACE (Irie et al. 2013) could be alternative options. Other proposals of subclassification of the BCLB stage were widely described in the review of Golfieri et al. (2019). The authors concluded that movements to subdivide the BCLC intermediate stage were underway due to the marked diversity of patients included in this stage. Before being endorsed by guidelines and followed in clinical practice, substaging systems must be externally validated in terms of prognostic ability and suitability to indicate the most appropriate therapy for each patient.

- *Advanced stage (BCLC C)*

Similar to the intermediate stage, heterogeneity of tumour burden and liver function can be found among patients classified as advanced stage HCC (BCLC stage C), which includes a wide variety of patients with one or more adverse predictors, such as symptomatic tumours causing a decline in PS (ECOG PS 1 or 2), macrovascular invasion (MVI) regardless of its location (hepatic veins [HV] or portal trunks)

and extension, and/or extrahepatic spread, such as lymph node involvement or distant metastases, in patients with a wide range of residual liver function, defined by Child-Pugh class A or B (Guglielmi et al. 2008). The Western guidelines (EASL 2018) recommend systemic therapy as a unique treatment option for patients with advanced HCC and preserved liver function (Child-Pugh class A). (Forner et al. 2012, Forner et al. 2018, EASL 2018, Cheng et al. 2009). As a consequence, several proposals of subclassification for both these stages have been suggested in recent years, differentiating the more appropriate treatment for each substage.

Unlike Western guidelines, the Hong Kong Liver Cancer (HKLC) staging system and the Japanese guidelines consider TACE, resection, hepatic intra-arterial chemotherapy (HAIC) and molecular-targeted agents as possible treatment alternatives in advanced-stage patients, depending on the patient's clinical condition and tumour extension (Omata et al. 2017, Yau et al. 2014).

However, in the advanced stage, no tumoural portal vein thrombosis (PVT) can be considered prognostically equivalent since they have a different disease course according to the involvement of the peripheral, segmental, lobar or main trunk portal veins (Park et al. 2008), and the extent of the PVT should be assessed and staged differently. In 2010, Shi et al. (2010) classified PVT into four categories for surgical purposes: (1) tumour thrombi involving only sectoral or segmental portal branches, (2) involvement of the right/left portal vein, (3) involvement of the main portal trunk and (4) involvement of the main portal trunk up to the superior mesenteric vein. The same authors reported differences in survival based on the portal vein invasion patterns cited. This result was in line with a previous study by Park et al. (2018) who, in a series of 904 HCC patients, showed that both the presence and the extent of the PVT (no portal vein invasion, first and second branch invasion, and main portal vein invasion) were independent predictors of survival.

Considering the different clinical outcomes based on the extent of PVT in the proposed subclassification of intermediate-stage HCC, Bolondi et al. (2012) introduced a substage beyond B4, called "quasi C," which represents a sort of overlap between the intermediate and the advanced stages (Table 9). This stage includes Child-Pugh class A, PS 0 patients with peripheral (subsegmental or segmental) PVT for whom TACE or TARE could also be considered as alternative treatment options to sorafenib.

Have recently published a detailed review highlighting the need for a subclassification due to the marked diversity of patients included in the BCLC stages.

The authors concluded that subclassifications are urgently needed for achieving better prognostic performance, for proposing an updated guide for proper intervention, and for benchmarking the results of the different interventional options.

1.2 Transarterial Embolisation (TAE)

Transarterial embolisation (TAE) consists of the occlusion of the feeding arteries to the tumour using embolic agents without adding any chemotherapeutic drug. To date, the relative effectiveness of TACE over TAE has not been established in randomised trials.

The 2002 RCT from Llovet, which represented the milestone of the superiority of TAE/TACE over BSC (Llovet et al. 2002), did not demonstrate any difference in median OS after TAE and TACE, but a significant survival benefit was observed with respect to BSC only in TACE arm. However, TAE was performed by the injection of a suboptimal agent, such as gelatin sponge fragments, very large particles only temporarily occluding the tumour-feeding vessels (Tsochatzis et al. 2012). A meta-analysis published in 2007, including three RCTs comparing TAE and TACE, showed no difference in mortality (Marelli et al. 2007), although they consisted of trials using this suboptimal agent.

Many of the clinical studies evaluating the effectiveness of TAE and/or TACE in the treatment of HCC patients are confounded by the use of a wide range of treatment strategies, including the type of embolic agents, type of drug, type of emulsifying agent and number of treatment sessions.

Ideally, embolisation should be carried out with the smallest and permanently occluding particles to ensure more selective occlusion of the small feeding tumour arteries and fewer side effects. In 2006, drug-eluting beads (DEBs) were introduced, specifically designed to slowly release chemotherapy, thus reducing the plasmatic peak of doxorubicin-caused drug-related side effects, and maintaining the same therapeutic efficacy as cTACE (Varela et al. 2007, Golfieri et al. 2014, Poon et al. 2007), with a favourable cost-effectiveness profile (Cucchetti et al. 2016).

Two additional RCTs regarding DEB-TACE and TAE with beads have been carried out, and neither showed any differences in survival (Malagari et al. 2010, Meyer et al. 2013).

A recent RCT (Brown et al. 2016) compared DEB-TACE and TAE, and reported no difference in response, progression-free survival (PFS) or OS (OS 19.6 vs. 20.8 months after TAE and DEB-TACE, respectively). However, they used particles of 100–300 microns first, increasing bead diameter if stasis was not achieved, up to 700–900 m; thus, the final treatment was attained with particles similar to those of gel foam (Sergio et al. 2008). The latest retrospective study (Massarweh et al. 2016) analysed the outcome of TACE and TAE in 405 patients with propensity score adjustments and found no differences in median OS (20.1 vs. 23 months). This study was limited by the small number of patients treated with TAE and by variability in the agent used over the 8-year study period. Osuga et al. (2008) reported a median OS of 30 months after TAE and radiologically stable disease in the vast majority (81%) of patients. A limitation of this study was the lack of a TACE control group. However, when compared to outcomes for TACE from a population-level cohort of contemporary patients treated in the same setting, the results after TAE compared favourably. The results from the studies cited raise the question: why do we continue to add doxorubicin to embolisation? No survival benefit was observed between TACE and TAE while the latter has a lower cost and avoids the side effects of chemotherapy (Tsochatzis et al. 2010, Tsochatzis et al. 2013)

According to the most recent AISF position paper *(Digestive and liver disease 2018),* even though TACE is the most frequently used transarterial treatment for HCC, there is not yet any convincing evidence in favour of TACE over TAE in terms of patient survival.

1.3 Combined Treatments

1.3.1 Combining TACE and Local Ablation

Hepatic resection (HR) and LT are curative therapies for HCC; when they are not possible, percutaneous ablation using radiofrequency (RFA) or microwave (MWA) is considered a suitable alternative (Cho et al. 2009, Chen et al. 2006).

It is well known that RFA is only indicated for early-stage HCC patients with fewer than three tumours, due to the local range of the treatment action, and with tumours less than 3-cm in size, due to a complete response rate of less than 50% in larger lesions, which is clearly poor for a treatment intended to cure the tumour. However, it is well known that percutaneous ablation suffers from the dimensional limit of approximately 3 cm: below this size, the complete response is 70–80% whereas, above this size, complete pathologic necrosis falls to very low percentages (approximately 30%) (Takaki et al. 2007, Serra et al. 2019).

Based on literature data (Iezzi et al. 2014, Takuma et al. 2013), the combined treatment seems to be safe and effective for the treatment of unresectable patients with early/intermediate HCC; furthermore, this approach provides better results than RFA and TACE alone in the treatment of large HCCs exceeding 3 cm in size. It can also extend the indication for RFA to previously contraindicated "complex cases", with an increased risk of thermal ablation-related complications due to tumour location, or to "complex patients" with high bleeding risk.

The ischemia and cytotoxicity associated with TACE can increase the thermal damage induced with RF/MWI ablation. The combination of TACE-RFA may reduce local tumour progression because of the synergistic effects of the two treatments. When using the combination of RFA (thermal damage) and TACE (ischemic and/or cytotoxic injury) rather than one of these treatments alone, it is possible to obtain complete tumour necrosis of HCCs larger than 3 cm, as has also been confirmed by other authors (Cheng et al. 2008, Peng et al. 2013).

However, the term "combined treatment" is not clearly defined and is often misinterpreted: TACE and then RFA (to enhance the thermal damage), RFA and then TACE (to enhance the cytotoxic injury).

When TACE is performed before RFA (the most common option), obtaining feeding vessel occlusion, the heat-sink effect can be reduced and the RFA treatment area extended, thus increasing the "safety margin" with the coagulation of the satellite nodules. Transarterial chemoembolisation can reduce the cooling effect of the hepatic blood flow by decreasing hepatic arterial flow and increasing the necrotising effect of RFA therapy at the tumour level. Furthermore, the oedematous change in the tumour tissue induced by ischemia and inflammation after TACE is expected to enlarge the area of tumour necrosis during RFA treatment, thereby increasing the ablation safety margin and reducing local recurrence.

On the contrary, when RF/MW ablation is performed followed by TACE, the aim is to obtain a sustained anticancer effect from the sublethal heating created in the large area surrounding the heating zone. A higher concentration of the drug in the residual vital tissue is expected, together with less cellular resistance to cytotoxic damage from the drug with the best drug release due to hyperaemia. In this area, a number of phenomena are present, including increased blood flow, increased vascular permeability and effects on multiple cell targets. Transarterial chemoembolisation performed after RFA could increase its therapeutic effect, acting on the large zones of sublethal heating obtained during RFA application in the tissues surrounding the electrode.

An experimental trial on animal models comparing four different sequences of combinations and different beads size for TACE demonstrated that bland TAE before RFA is more effective than post-ablation TACE, reaching larger necrotic areas. The use of very small 40-μm microspheres enhances the efficacy of RFA more than the use of larger particles (Tanaka et al. 2013).

In 2010, Morimoto et al. (2010) compared RFA combined with TACE to RFA alone in 37 patients with solitary HCCs (diameter, 3.1–5.0 cm at their the greatest dimension) divided into two groups: the TACE-RFA group, in which the patients received TACE followed by RFA on the same day, and the RFA group, in which the patients received only RFA. The rates of local tumour progression at the end of the third year in the RFA and TACE-RFA groups were 39% and 6%, respectively ($P = 0.012$). The 3-year survival rates of the patients in the RFA and TACE-RFA groups were 80% and 93%, respectively ($P = 0.369$).

In 2012, an RCT (Peng et al. 2012) involving patients with a single nodule up to 5 cm in diameter demonstrated the superiority of combined treatment (first cTACE and then RFA) over RFA alone, reporting 1-, 3-, and 5- year overall survival rates of 94%, 69%, and 46%, respectively,

for combined treatment and 82%, 47%, and 36%, respectively, for RFA alone ($p = 0.037$). One year later, the same authors published (Peng et al. 2013) the results of an RCT in patients with single HCC lesions less than 7 cm or with a maximum of three nodules each less than 3 cm, showing significantly better overall survival and recurrence-free survival in patients treated with cTACE + RFA than in patients treated with RFA alone ($p = 0.009$, respectively).

In the proposal of the subclassification by Kudo et al. ("Kinki criteria"), combined therapies (TACE and ablation) are included as potential treatment options in order to extend the ablation area if the tumour size is close to 5 cm. (Kudo et al. 2015).

Two meta-analyses, one from Lu (Lu et al. 2013) including seven RCTs and another from Wang (Wang et al. 2016) including 21 studies with 3073 patients showed that RFA plus TACE significantly improved the survival rates of patients with HCC at 1 and 3 years more than RFA alone. Unfortunately, in the first meta-analysis (Lu et al. 2013), there were issues of sample size (studies ranging from 19 to 69 patients), tumour size (ranging from 1.7 to 6.7 cm), and trials inadequately powered for outcome evaluation. A more recent meta-analysis included small RCTs from Asia which were significantly underpowered to evaluate survival or response rates (Chen et al. 2016a, b). Therefore, at this time, the combination of RFA with TACE may be considered a good alternative option in patients not suitable for HR, even though to date, no trial has been adequately powered and no trial has compared cTACE alone versus cTACE + RFA. This topic requires additional clinical trials.

In summary, for 3–5 cm HCCs, a combination of intra-arterial therapy and percutaneous ablation seems to provide benefits in OS and recurrence-free survival (RFS); data are lacking for 5–7 cm HCCs to support the role of single or combined therapy over other treatment options.

1.3.2 Combining TACE and Systemic Therapy

The rationale for the combination of TACE plus anti-angiogenic drugs is to control tumour progression and improve the survival of HCC patients; the acute hypoxia induced by TACE, leading to an upregulation of the vascular endothelial growth factor (VEGF), which might promote tumour local recurrence, can be controlled by systemic therapy with tyrosine kinase inhibitors which inhibit both revascularisation and tumour proliferation.

Two phase II/phase III RCTs and the SPACE trial (Lencioni et al. 2016a, b, Meyer et al. 2017) compared the combination of TACE+ sorafenib to TACE alone. Two other RCTs compared TACE to a combination of TACE+ brivanib in the BRISK-TA study (Kudo et al. 2014;) and to orantinib in the ORIENTAL study (Kudo et al. 2018a, b).

All four trials failed to demonstrate any clinical benefit from combined therapy as has recently been summarised (Kudo et al. 2017).

1.4   Hepatic Arterial Infusion Chemotherapy (HAIC)

Hepatic arterial infusion chemotherapy has often been selected as a therapeutic option for advanced HCC with intrahepatic metastases or portal vein thrombosis which is not eligible for hepatic resection, tumour ablation or embolisation. Of the various regimens, HAIC, consisting of 5-fluorouracil (5-FU) in combination with either low-doses of cisplatin (CDDP) or interferon-alpha has been reported to improve the response rates for advanced HCC.

In a small retrospective series, Moriguchi et al. (2017) reported significantly longer survival in patients with tumour thrombus involving the main trunk and the first branches of the portal vein (types III and IV of the Shi classification) treated with HAIC as compared to sorafenib, suggesting that HAIC should be the first-line therapy in these patients, followed by sorafenib in case of no response.

Hepatic arterial infusion chemotherapy could also represent a safe treatment option in selected Child-Pugh class B patients who are contraindicated to sorafenib (Saeki et al. 2018, Ikeda et al. 2016).

Ikeda et al. (2016) prospectively evaluated 108 patients in a multicentre phase II trial in chemonaïve patients with advanced HCC having Child-Pugh scores of 5–7. The patients were randomised to receive sorafenib alone ($n = 42$) or sorafenib combined with HAIC with cisplatin ($n = 66$). The combination HAIC plus sorafenib yielded favourable OS when compared with sorafenib alone (median survival of 10.6 vs. 8.7 months, respectively). However, the median TTP and the response rate were similar, that is, 2.8 months and 7.3% in the sorafenib arm and 3.1 months and 21.7% in the combination arm, respectively.

In a retrospective analysis involving 179 Child-Pugh class B patients treated with HAIC, Terashima et al. (2016) reported an improvement in liver function in patients with Child Pugh scores of 7 and 8 who responded to HAIC, with a median OS of 12.1 and 11.9 months, respectively. On the contrary, no advantages were demonstrated for patients with a Child-Pugh score of 9. A more recent phase III trial (SILIUS) tested the combination of sorafenib with continuous HAIC with cisplatin and fluorouracil, via an implanted catheter system, against sorafenib alone in patients with advanced, unresectable HCC (Kudo et al. 2018a, b).

The results of all these studies failed to demonstrate a significant improvement of OS with the addition of HAIC to sorafenib and there are no currently established criteria used for the selection of advanced HCC patients to receive either sorafenib or HAIC.

As HAIC requires the use of an implanted port-catheter system, maintaining the patency of the hepatic arteries is a critical factor for intrahepatic drug distribution and the efficacy of HAIC.

However, the long-term outcome or the survival benefit remains unclear with HAIC, and it may be significantly affected by liver function and cirrhosis. None of the above-mentioned regimens have been proven to be the ideal standard for HAIC, and prospective multi-centre clinical studies with a standardised protocol are needed in the future. For these reasons, HAIC is not recommended as the standard of care in major guidelines, even in the updated versions (EASL 2018), except for Japanese guidelines (Omata et al. 2017).

2 Intra-Arterial Treatment of Intrahepatic Cholangiocarcinoma (ICC)

Intrahepatic cholangiocarcinoma (ICC) is the second most common primary liver malignancy after HCC and accounts for 10–20% of all primary liver cancers (Shaib et al. 2004, Bridgewater et al. 2014). Surgical intervention is possible in approximately 54–70% of patients at the time of diagnosis; the prognosis for these patients is poor with a reported median survival of 3 to 8 months. Traditionally, systemic chemotherapy has a poor response; therefore, the role of intra-arterial therapy is increasingly being investigated for these patients.

Table 11 shows the overall median survival across the intra-arterial strategies. The median

Table 11 Summary of the main studies of intra-arterial therapies, and outcomes and response for Unresectable Intrahepatic Cholangiocarcinoma (ICC) (modified from Boehm et al. 2015)

Author (year)	Study design	Sample	Treatment regimen	EHD %	RECIST response (CR + PR)	Median survival (months)	Toxicities[a]
HAIC							
Tanaka et al. (2002)	PC	11	5-FU, Doxorubicin, MMC, Cisplatin	36.4	7	26[b]	NR
Jarnagin et al. (2009)	PC	26	FUDR	0	14	31	6
Inaba et al. (2011)	PC	25	Gemcitabine	36	3	11.3	12
Burger et al. (2005)	PC	17	Cisplatin + MMC + Doxorubicin	29.4	NR	23[c]	1
TACE							
Herber et al. (2007)	RS	15	MMC	0	1	16.3	2
Gusani et al. (2008)	RS	42	Gemcitabine, Cisplatin Oxaliplatin	45.2	0	9.1	7
Shitara et al. (2008)	RS	20	MMC	85	10	14.1	7
Andrasina et al. (2010)	PC	17	5-FU + Cisplatin	0	NR	25.2[c]	0
Park et al. (2011)	RS	72	Cisplatin	54.2	15	12.2[c,d]	36
Kiefer et al. (2011)	PC	62	Cisplatin + MMC + Doxorubicin	30.6	5	15	5
Kuhlman et al. (2012)	PC	10	MMC	40	1	5.7	3
Halappa et al. (2012)	RS	29	Cisplatin + MMC + Doxorubicin	NR	NR	16[c,d]	NR
Vogl et al. (2012)	RS	115	MMC, Gemcitabine, Cisplatin	0	10	13	0
Scheuermann et al. (2013)	RS	32	MMC	0	NR	11	NR
DEB-TACE							
Aliberti et al. (2008)	PC	11	Doxorubicin DEB-Tace	NR	10	13	1
Kuhlman et al. (2012)	PC	26	Irinotecan DEB-Tace	42.3	1	11.7	11

ICC intrahepatic cholangiocarcinoma, *HAIC* hepatic arterial infusion chemotherapy, *TACE* transarterial chemoembolisation, *DEB-TACE* drug-eluting bead transarterial chemoembolisation, *EHD* extrahepatic disease, *CR* complete response to therapy, *PR* partial response to therapy, *PC* prospective cohort study, *RC* retrospective study, *NR* not reported, *5-FU* 5-fluorouracil, *MMC* mitomycin C, *FUDR* floxuridine

[a]National Cancer Institute (NCI)/World Health Organization (WHO) Grade III/IV Toxicities

[b]Represents mean survival as median survival was not reported in the group

[c]Survival calculated from the date of diagnosis

[d]Treatment-naive group (therefore, date of diagnosis was assumed to be the date of initiation of hepatic arterial therapy (HAT) for the purpose of analysis) and c: World Health Organisation Tumour Response Criteria

overall survival was 14.5 months (95% CI: 12.5–16.4), suggesting a beneficial effect when compared to traditional systemic chemotherapy regimens (5–8 months) (Khan SA 2005). The median time to tumour response evaluation was 3 (range 1–6) months after HAIC.

Table 12 reports the results of the response rates (complete or partial) stratified according to treatment strategy (HAIC group (56.9%, 95% CI: 41.0–72.8) vs. TACE (17.3%, 6.8–27.8)) and DEB-TACE. Overall, partial or complete response was observed in 28.5% (95% CI: 18.0–39.1, n 390) of the evaluable subjects. The rate of stable disease was highest in the DEB-TACE group (61.5%; 95% CI: 42.8–80.2) versus TACE (46.9%; 35.5–58.4) versus HAIC (42.2%; 17.1–67.2).

The rate of grade III/IV complications was highest for HAIC (0.35, 95% CI: 0.22–0.48) versus TACE (0.26, 0.21) versus DEB-TACE (0.32, 0.17–0.48) (Boehm et al. 2015).

The hepatic toxicity was highest for HAIC (0.75, 95% CI: 0.65–0.86) versus TACE (0.09, 0.06–0.12) versus DEB-TACE (0.08, 0.0–0.17). Therefore, HAT seems to be a promising strategy for improving outcomes for patients with unresectable ICC. The best outcomes in terms of response and OS are reported by HAIC even if they are associated with increased toxicity. Targeted treatment strategy based on patient-disease characteristics is a goal for future research.

3 Intra-Arterial Treatment of Liver Metastases

Liver-directed therapies to treat metastatic tumours of the liver have become common due to the increased complexity of hepatic surgery. Intra-arterial treatment options include TACE, TAE, HAIC and ablative techniques, such as MWI or RF ablation. Evidence supports their use in providing salvage options when first-line treatment has failed.

3.1 Colorectal Liver Metastases (CLRM)

Colorectal cancer is the third most common cancer in terms of incidence and is the second leading cause of death both in Europe and worldwide, with an estimated 881,000 deaths in 2018. (Bray et al. 2018, Ferlay et al. 2015).

This is one of the main reasons why colorectal liver metastases (CRLMs) have been those most thoroughly evaluated. The standard for treatment is surgical resection with curative intent combined with systemic chemotherapy (NCCN 2018), but only approximately 25% of patients are amenable to standard resection at diagnosis (Engstrand et al. 2018). Moreover, up to 80% of patients develop liver recurrence up to 10 years post-surgery, the majority within the first 2 years (Misiakos et al. 2011).

Thus, a multidisciplinary approach to treat patients with unresectable disease or potentially resectable disease has been developed to treat recurrences and prolong these patients' survival.

Different interventional radiology procedures are considered as either alternative to surgery or ancillary treatment methods in the management of CLRM patients. The most widely used treatment methods include percutaneous ablation

Table 12 Results of a meta-analysis regarding median OS and tumour response using the Recist Criteria, stratified according to treatment strategy for unresectable intrahepatic cholangiocarcinoma (ICC) (modified from Boehm et al. 2015)

	TACE (95% CI)	HAIC (95% CI)	DEB-TACE (95% CI)
Cumulative median OS (months)	12.4(10.9–13.9)	22.8(9.8–35.8)	12.3 (11.0–13.5)
RECIST tumor response Complete/partial response	17.3 (6.8–27.8)	56.9 (41.0–72.8)	—
Stable disease	46.9(35.5–58.4)	42.2 (17.1–67.2)	61.5 (42.8–80.2)

HAIC hepatic arterial infusion chemotherapy, *TACE* transarterial chemoembolisation, *DEB-TACE* drug-eluting bead transarterial chemoembolisation, *OS* Overall survival, *RECIST* Response evaluation criteria in solid tumours (radiofrequency, microwave), TACE and selective internal radiation therapy (TARE).

Nowadays, the intra-arterial treatment options for CRLM include cTACE, DEB-TACE, transarterial radioembolisation (TARE) and HAIC. These therapies are generally indicated for patients with the oligometastatic disease who are not suitable for surgery or other curative locoregional therapies, and without any response, disease progression or toxicity/contraindication to systemic chemotherapy.

3.1.1 Intra-Arterial Treatments (TACE, DEB-TACE)

The safety and efficacy of both cTACE and DEB-TACE have been studied extensively; highlights from the literature are summarised in Table 13. Nowadays intra-arterial chemotherapy regimens, also including HAIC and TARE, are considered a good therapeutic approach for patients with colorectal cancer and liver-limited disease in whom the available chemotherapeutic options had failed (Wasan et al. 2017, Kemeny et al. 2006, Levi et al. 2016)

- *cTACE.* In 1998, Tellez et al. (1998) analysed the outcome of TACE in 30 patients with CRLMs who had failed standard-of-care chemotherapy, showing a median OS of 8.6 months. The authors concluded that cTACE is a feasible treatment for patients with CRLMs in a salvage setting.

Other authors (Albert et al. 2011) have reported the results of TACE with cisplatin, doxorubicin, mitomycin C and a lipiodol mixture followed by PVA particles in an analogous population (245 treatments in 121 patients), showing a median TTP in the liver treated of 5 months and a median survival of 33 months from initial diagnosis and 9 months from TACE procedure. As expected, OS was significantly better when TACE was performed after first- or second-line systemic therapy than after various lines of chemotherapy.

Later, Vogl et al. (2007) reported the results of a wide population (463 patients) treated with cTACE including mitomycin C alone, mitomycin C with gemcitabine or mitomycin C with irinotecan followed by microsphere embolisation. The authors concluded that the 1-year survival rate after cTACE was 62% and 2-year survival was 28% without significant differences between cTACE regimens.

- *DEB-TACE.* Since 2006, several groups have investigated the safety and efficacy of irinotecan-loaded DEBs (DEBIRI) for the treatment of CRLMs in patients who had failed systemic chemotherapy. Martin et al. (2009) reported that DEBIRI is safe and well tolerated in patients with non-responsive CRLMs with an OS of 19 months and a PFS of 11 months. In 2011, the results of a phase II study of DEBIRI in 82 patients with CRLMs

Table 13 Summary of the leading papers on cTACE/DEB-TACE for the treatment of colorectal liver metastases (modified from Tsitskari et al. 2019)

Study	Study details	Median OS (months)
Vogl et al. (2009)	TACE, mitomycin C alone or with gemcitabine vs. irinotecan Prospective cohort, 463 patients	14
Albert et al. (2011)	TACE, cisplatin, doxorubicin, mitomycin C Retrospective cohort, 121 patients	9
Martin et al. (2011)	DEB-TACE (DEBIRI), irinotecan Prospective cohort, 55 patient	19
Florentini et al. (2012)	DEB-TACE (DEBIRI), irinotecan Randomized controlled trial, 74 patients, DEBIRI vs FOLFIRI	15
Narayanan et al. (2013)	DEB-TACE (DEBIRI) Retrospective cohort, 28 patients	13.3
Iezzi et al. (2015)	DEB-TACE (DEBIRI), irinotecan+Capecitabine Prospective phase II Trial, 20 patients	7.3

TACE transarterial chemoembolisation, *DEB-TACE* drug-eluting beads transarterial chemoembolisation, *DEBIRI* irinotecan-loaded DEB, *OS* Overall survival, *FOLFIRI* folinic acid–fluorouracil–irinotecan who had failed at least two lines of chemotherapy, showed a median OS of 25 months with a PFS of 8 months (Aliberti et al. 2011).

The best-developed evidence for DEB-TACE in the setting of CRLMs derives from two randomised controlled trials. The first compared DEBIRI versus systemic chemotherapy with FOLFIRI (folinic acid, fluorouracil and irinotecan) in patients with unresectable CRLMs not responsive to second- or third-line therapy (Fiorentini et al. 2012), showing a prolonged median overall survival (22 vs. 15 months, $p = 0.031$) in the DEBIRI arm. The second trial compared modified FOLFOX (fluorouracil and oxaliplatin) with bevacizumab with and without DEBIRI. The study showed no difference in OS (Martin et al. 2015). As DEB-TACE is well tolerated, it represents a good treatment option, particularly to downsize tumours.

According to this evidence, local ablation and locoregional therapies have been included in the armamentarium of the updated European Society for Medical Oncology (ESMO) guidelines for the treatment of CRLMs as potential treatment options. These guidelines recommend ablation alone or in combination with surgical resection either initially, or possibly after systemic therapy in patients with oligometastatic disease in order to achieve long-term disease control. In patients with the more advanced liver-limited disease, TACE and TARE are recommended once other chemotherapeutic options have failed.

3.1.2 Hepatic Artery Infusion Chemotherapy (HAIC)

The use of HAIC for metastatic liver lesions dates back to at least the 1960s, reported as a possible treatment option for unresectable CRLMs as a salvage treatment, as adjuvant therapy following hepatic resection or to downstage patients for surgery (Sullivan et al. 1964); it was considered a valid alternative treatment option. In a large RCT comparing HAIC versus systemic chemotherapy (135 patients with unresectable CRLMs), HAIC showed an improved OS and response rate (Kemeny et al. 2006). More recently, Levi et al. (2016) conducted a phase II

trial (OPTILIV) demonstrating that HAIC is able to convert almost 30% of patients to resectability by using HAIC with 5-fluorouracil, oxaliplatin and irinotecan, and this rate is almost double that of systemic chemotherapy which typically converts only 15% of patients.

In a prospective phase II trial, some authors have recently demonstrated that chemo-naive patients had high response rates and a 5-year OS of 51% while patients converted to resection after HAIC had a 5-year survival of 63% (Pak et al. 2018). As a salvage therapy, HAIC still appears to offer a survival advantage over modern systemic chemotherapy alone; even for patients refractory to standard systemic chemotherapy, HAIC offers a response rate of 33% (Dhir et al. 2017, Cercek et al. 2016).

Currently, in the era of modern biologic agents, these trials seem out of date; nevertheless, they demonstrate a continued survival benefit on propensity score-matched comparison of HAIC versus systemic chemotherapy alone (Groot et al. 2017). In this scenario, even though HAIC appears obsolete, there still appears to be an advantage if performed at experienced centres in the setting of a multidisciplinary team decision. Additional multicentre trials are warranted to determine the appropriate role and timing of HAIC in the setting of unresectable CRLMs.

Although these treatment options have been applied without high-level clinical evidence, they have allowed tailoring the clinical approach to the individual based on disease status and clinical condition. Additional comparative or randomised studies are required to better define the role and sequence of these therapies used in combination with surgery and standard systemic therapy.

3.2 Hypervascular Neuroendocrine (NET) Liver Metastases

The management of patients with well-differentiated non-resectable neuroendocrine tumour (NET) liver metastases, is challenging. Transarterial embolisation, TACE and selective TARE ae preferred to other treatment modalities. Transarterial embolisation and TACE generally achieve average symptomatic, biological and radiological responses of 75%, 56% and 50%, respectively, with progression-free survival of 12–18 months and acceptable tolerance. Although not clearly demonstrated, TACE may be more effective than TAE in pancreatic NETs, but not in small-intestine NET. Transarterial radioembolisation has been developed more recently and may achieve similar results, with improved tolerance, but with decreased cost-effectiveness, although no prospective comparison has been published to date. There are currently no strong arguments for choosing between TAE, TACE and TARE, and they have not been compared to other treatment modalities. The evaluation of their efficacy has, for the most part, relied on criteria based on size variations, which does not take into account tumour viability and metabolism, and thus may not be relevant. These techniques may be especially effective when performed as first-line therapy in patients with non-major liver involvement (<75%) and with hypervascular metastases. Finally, studies exploring their combination with systemic therapies are ongoing (de Mestier et al. 2017). However, the utilisation of intra-arterial therapy is based on a low level of evidence, due to the lack of prospective data, the absence of comparative studies and considerable heterogeneity between local practices. The quality and strength of the reports available do not allow any modality to be determined as superior in terms of imaging response, symptomatic response or impact on survival. Transarterial radioembolisation may have advantages over TAE and TACE since it causes fewer side effects and requires fewer treatments. Based on the current European Neuroendocrine Tumour Society (ENETS) Consensus Guidelines, TARE can be substituted for TAE or TACE in patients with either liver-only disease or those with limited extrahepatic metastases (Kennedy et al. 2015).

References

Adhoute X, Penaranda G, Naude S et al (2015) Retreatment with TACE: the ABCR SCORE, an aid to the decision-making process. J Hepatol 62:855–862

Albert M, Kiefer MV, Sun W et al (2011) Chemoembolization of colorectal liver metastases

with cisplatin, doxorubicin, mitomycin C, ethiodol, and polyvinyl alcohol. Cancer 117:343–352

Aliberti C, Carandina R, Sarti D et al (2016) Hepatic arterial infusion of polyethylene glycol drug-eluting beads for primary and meta- static liver cancer therapy. Anticancer Res 36:3515–3521

Angle JF (2013) Cone-beam CT: vascular applications. Tech Vasc Interv Radiol 16:144–149

de Baere T, Denys A, Briquet R et al (1998) Modification of arterial and portal hemodynamic after injection of iodized oil in the hepatic artery: experimental study. J Vasc Interv Radiol 9:305–330

de Baere T, Arai Y, Lencioni R et al (2016a) Treatment of liver tumors with lipiodol TACE: technical recommendations from experts. Cardiovasc Interv Radiol 39:334–343

de Baere T, Plotkin S, Yu R et al (2016b) An in vitro evaluation of four types of drug-eluting microspheres loaded with doxorubicin. J Vasc Interv Radiol 27:1425–1431

Bargellini I, Sacco R, Bozzi E et al (2012) Transarterial chemoembolization in very early and early-stage hepatocellular carcinoma pa- tients excluded from curative treatment: a prospective cohort study. Eur J Radiol 81:1173–1178

Bargellini I, Florio F, Golfieri R et al (2014) Trends in utilization of transarterial treatments for hepatocellular carcinoma: results of a survey by the Italian Society of Interventional Radiology. Cardiovasc Intervent Radiol 37:438–444

Boehm LM, Jayakrishnan TT, Miura JT et al (2015) Comparative effectiveness of hepatic artery based therapies for unresectable intrahepatic cholangiocarcinoma. J Surg Oncol 111:213–220

Bolondi L, Burroughs A, Dufour JF et al (2012) Heterogeneity of patients with intermediate (BCLC B) hepatocellular carcinoma: proposal for a subclassification to facilitate treatment decisions. Semin Liver Dis 32:348–359

Bolondi L, Cillo U, Colombo M et al (2013) Position paper of the Italian Association for the Study of the liver (AISF): the multidisciplinary clinical approach to hepatocellular carcinoma. Dig Liver Dis 45(9):712–723

Bray F, Ferlay J, Soerjomataram I, Siegel RL et al (2018) Global cancer statistics 2018: GLOBOCAN estimates of incidence and mortality worldwide for 36 cancers in 185 countries. CA Cancer J Clin 68:394–424

Bridgewater J, Galle PR, Khan SA et al (2014) Guidelines for the diagnosis and management of intrahepatic cholangiocarcinoma. J Hepatol 60:1268–1289

Brown KT, Do RK, Gonen M et al (2016) Randomized trial of hepatic artery embolization for hepatocellular carcinoma using doxorubicin-eluting microspheres compared with embolization with microspheres alone. J Clin Oncol 34:2046–2053

Bruix J, Sala M (2004) Llovet JMChemoembolization for hepatocellular carcinoma. Gastroenterology 127:S179–S188

Bruix J, Sherman M (2011) Management of hepatocellular carcinoma: an update. American Association for the Study of Liver Diseases. Hepatology 53:1020–1022

Bruix J, Llovet JM, Castells A et al (1998) Transarterial embolization versus symptomatic treatment in patients with advanced hepatocellular carcinoma: results of a randomized, controlled trial in a single institution. Hepatology 27:1578–1583

Burrel M, Reig M, Forner A et al (2012) Survival of patients with hepatocellular carcinoma treated by transarterial chemoembolisation (TACE) using drug eluting beads. Implications for clinical practice and trial design. J Hepatol 56:1330–1335

Camma C, Schepis F, Orlando A et al (2002) Transarterial chemoembolization for unresectable hepatocellular carcinoma: meta-analysis of randomized controlled trials. Radiology 224:47–54

Cappelli A, Cucchetti A, Cabibbo G et al (2016) Refining prognosis after trans-arterial chemo-embolization for hepatocellular carcinoma. Liver Int 3:729–736

Cercek A, Boucher TM, Gluskin JS et al (2016) Response rates of hepatic arterial infusion pump therapy in patients with metastatic colorectal cancer liver metastases refractory to all standard chemotherapies. J Surg Oncol 114:655–663

Chan AO, Yuen MF, Hui CK et al (2002) A prospective study regarding the complications of transcatheter intraarterial Lipiodol chemoembolization in patients with hepatocellular carcinoma. Cancer 94:1747–1752

Chen MS, Li JQ, Zheng Y et al (2006) A prospective randomized trial comparing percutaneous local ablative therapy and partial he- patectomy for small hepatocellular carcinoma. Ann Surg 243:321–328

Chen CS, Li FK, Guo CY et al (2016a) Tumor vascularity and Lipiodol deposition as early radiological markers for predicting risk of disease progression in patients with unresectable hepatocellular carcinoma after transarterial chemoembolization. Oncotarget 7:7241–7252

Chen QW, Ying HF, Gao S et al (2016b) Radiofrequency ablation plus chemoembolization versus radiofrequency ablation alone for hepatocellular carcinoma: a systematic review and meta-analysis. Clin Res Hepatol Gastroenterol 40:309–314

Cheng BQ, Jia CQ, Liu CT et al (2008) Chemoembolization combined with radiofrequency ablation for patients with hepatocellular carcinoma larger than 3 cm: a randomized controlled trial. JAMA 299:1669–1677

Cheng AL, Kang YK, Chen Z et al (2009) Efficacy and safety of sorafenib in patients in the Asia- Pacific region with advanced hepatocellular carcinoma: a phase III randomised, double-blind, placebo- controlled trial. Lancet Oncol 10:25–34

Cho YK, Kim JK, Kim MY et al (2009) Systematic review of randomized trials for hepatocellular carcinoma treated with percutaneous ablation therapies. Hepatology 49:453–459

Chung JW, Park JH, Han JK et al (1996) Hepatic tumors: predisposing factors for complications of transcatheter oily chemoembolization. Radiology 198:33–40

Chung JW, Kim HC, Yoon JH et al (2006) Transcatheter arterial chemoembolization of hepatocellular carcinoma: prevalence and causative factors of extrahepatic collateral arteries in 479 patients. Korean J Radiol 7:257–266

Coldwell DM, Stokes KR, Yakes WF (1994) Embolotherapy: agents, clinical applications, and techniques. Radiographics 14:623–643

Covey AM, Brody LA, Maluccio MA (2002) Variant hepatic arterial anatomy revisited: digital subtraction angiography performed in 600 patients. Radiology 224:542–547

Cucchetti A, Trevisani F, Cappelli A et al (2016) Cost-effectiveness of doxorubicin-eluting beads versus conventional trans-arterial chemo-embolization for hepatocellular carcinoma. Dig Liver Dis 48:798–805

Dhir M, Jones HL, Shuai Y et al (2017) Hepatic arterial infusion in combination with modern systemic chemotherapy is associated with improved survival compared with modern systemic chemotherapy in patients with isolated unresectable colorectal liver metastases. Ann Surg Oncol 24:150–158

Doyon D, Mouzon A, Jourde AM et al (1974) Hepatic, arterial embolization in patients with malignant liver tumours (author's transl). Ann Radiol 17:593–603

Engstrand J, Nilsson H, Stromberg C et al (2018) Colorectal cancer liver metastases - a population-based study on incidence, management and survival. BMC Canc 18:78

European Association for the Study of the Liver (2018) EASL clinical practice guidelines: management of hepatocellular carcinoma. J Hepatol 69:182–236

European Association For The Study Of The Liver; European Organisation For Research And Treatment Of Cancer (2012) EASL-EORTC clinical practice guidelines: management of hepatocellular carcinoma. J Hepatol 56:908–943

Facciorusso A (2018) Drug-eluting beads transarterial chemoembolization for hepatocellular carcinoma: current state of the art. World J Gastroenterol 24:161–169

Facciorusso A, Bhoori S, Sposito C et al (2015) Repeated transarterial chemoembolization: an overfitting effort? J Hepatol 62:1440–1442

Facciorusso A, Di Maso M, Muscatiello N et al (2016) Drug-eluting beads versus conventional chemoembolization for the treatment of unresectable hepatocellular carcinoma: a meta-analysis. Dig Liver Dis 48:571–577

Ferlay J, Soerjomataram I, Dikshit R et al (2015) Cancer incidence and mortality worldwide: sources, methods and major patterns in GLOBOCAN 2012. Int J Cancer 136:359–386

Fiorentini G, Aliberti C, Tilli M et al (2012) Intra-arterial infusion of irinotecan-loaded drug-eluting beads (DEBIRI) versus intravenous therapy (FOLFIRI) for hepatic metastases from colorectal cancer: final results of a phase II study. Anticancer Res 32:1387–1395

Fohlen A, Tasu JP, Kobeiter H et al (2018) Transarterial chemoembolization (TACE) in the management of hepatocellular carcinoma: results of a French national survey on current practices. Diagn Interv Imaging 99:527–535

Forner A, Ayuso C, Varela M et al (2009) Evaluation of tumor response after locoregional therapies in hepatocellular carcinoma: are response evaluation criteria in solid tumors reliable? Cancer 115:616–623

Forner A, Reig ME, de Lope CR et al (2010) Current strategy for staging and treatment: the BCLC update and future prospects. Semin Liver Dis 30:61–74

Forner A, Llovet JM, Bruix J (2012) Hepatocellular carcinoma. Lancet 379:1245–1255

Forner A, Reig M, Bruix J (2018) Hepatocellular carcinoma. Lancet 391:1301–1314

Golfieri R, Cappelli A, Cucchetti A et al (2011) Efficacy of selective transarterial chemoembolization in inducing tumor necrosis in small (<5 cm) hepatocellular carcinomas. Hepatology 53:1580–1589

Golfieri R, Giampalma E, Renzulli M et al (2014) Randomised controlled trial of doxorubicin-eluting beads vs conventional chemoembolisation for hepatocellular carcinoma. Br J Cancer 111:255–264

Groot Koerkamp B, Sadot E, Kemeny NE et al (2017) Perioperative hepatic arterial infusion pump chemotherapy is associated with longer survival after resection of colorectal liver metastases. J Clin Oncol 71:834–839

Groupe d'Etude et de Traitement du Carcinome Hépatocellulaire (1995) A comparison of lipiodol chemoembolization and conservative treatment for unresectable hepatocellular carcinoma. N Engl J Med 332:1256–1261

Guglielmi A, Ruzzenente A, Pachera S et al (2008) Comparison of seven staging systems in cirrhotic patients with hepatocellular carcinoma in a cohort of patients who underwent radiofrequency ablation with complete response. Am J Gastroenterol 103:597–604

Guiu B, Deschamps F, Aho S et al (2012) Liver/biliary injuries following chemoembolisation of endocrine tumours and hepatocellular carcinoma: Lipiodol vs. drug-eluting beads. J Hepatol 56:609–617

Ha Y, Shim JH, Kim SO et al (2014) Clinical appraisal of the recently proposed Barcelona clinic liver Cancer stage B subclassification by survival analysis. J Gastroenterol Hepatol 29:787–799

Hucke F, Pinter M, Graziadei I et al (2014) How to STATE suitability and START transarterial chemoembolization in patients with inter- mediate stage hepatocellular carcinoma. J Hepatol 61:1287–1296

Iezzi R, Pompili M, Gasbarrini A et al (2014) Sequential or combined treatment? That is the question. Radiology 272:612–613

Iezzi R, Marsico VA, Guerra A, et al (2015) Trans-Arterial Chemoembolization with Irinotecan-Loaded Drug-Eluting Beads (DEBIRI) and Capecitabine in Refractory Liver Prevalent Colorectal Metastases: A Phase II Single-Center Study. Cardiovasc Intervent Radiol 38(6):1523–1531

Ikeda M, Shimizu S, Sato T (2016) Sorafenib plus hepatic arterial infusion chemotherapy with cisplatin versus sorafenib for advanced hepatocellular carcinoma: randomized phase II trial. Ann Oncol 27:2090–2096

Irie T, Kuramochi M, Takahashi N et al (2013) Dense accumulation of lipiodol emulsion in hepatocellular carcinoma nodule during selective balloon-occluded transarterial chemoembolisation: measurement of balloon-occluded arterial stump pressure. Cardiovasc Intervent Radiol 36:706–713

Ji SK, Cho YK, Ahn YS et al (2008) Multivariate analysis of the predictors of survival for patients with hepatocellular carcinoma undergoing transarterial chemoembolization: focusing on superselective chemoembolization. Korean J Radiol 9: 534–540

Jordan O, Denys A, De Baere T et al (2010) Comparative study of chemoembolization loadable beads: in vitro drug release and physical properties of DC bead and hepasphere loaded with doxorubicin and irinotecan. J Vasc Interv Radiol 21:1084–1090

Kadalayil L, Benini R, Pallan L et al (2013) A simple prog- nostic scoring system for patients receiving transarterial embolisation for hepa-tocellular cancer. Ann Oncol 24:2565–2570

Kan Z, Sato M, Ivancev K et al (1993) Distribution and effect of iodized poppyseed oil in the liver after hepatic artery embolization: experimental study in several animal species. Radiology 186:861–866

Kan Z, Ivancev K, Lunderquist A et al (1994a) Peribiliary plexa– important pathways for shunting of iodized oil and silicon rubber solution from the hepatic artery to the portal vein. An experimental study in rat. Invest Radiol 29:671–676

Kan Z, McCuskey PA, Wright KC et al (1994b) Role of Kupffer cells in iodized oil embolization. Investig Radiol 29:990–993

Kan Z, Wright K, Wallace S et al (1997) Ethiodized oil emulsions in hepatic microcirculation: in vivo microscopy in animal models. Acad Radiol 4: 275–282

Kasugai H, Kojima J, Tatsuta M et al (1989) Treatment of hepatocellular carcinoma by transcatheter arterial embolization combined with intraarterial infusion of a mixture of cisplatin and ethiodized oil. Gastroenterology 97:965–997

Kawai S, Tani M, Okamura J et al (1997) Prospective and randomized trial of Lipiodol-transcatheter arterial chemoembolization for treatment of hepatocellular carcinoma: a comparison of epirubicin and doxorubicin (second cooperative study). The cooperative study Group for Liver Cancer Treatment of Japan. Semin Oncol 24:S6–38-S6-45

Kemeny NE, Niedzwiecki D, Hollis DR et al (2006) Hepatic arterial infusion versus systemic therapy for hepatic metastases from colorectal cancer: a randomized trial of efficacy, quality of life, and molecular markers (CALGB 9481). J Clin Oncol 24:1395e1403

Kennedy A, Bester L, Salem R et al (2015) NET-Liver-Metastases Consensus Conference. Role of hepatic intra-arterial therapies in metastatic neuroendocrine tumours (NET): guidelines from the NET-liver-metastases consensus conference. HPB (Oxford) 17:29–37

Khan SA, Thomas HC, Davidson BR et al (2005) Cholangiocarcinoma. Lancet 366:1303–1314

Kim HK, Chung YH, Song BC et al (2001) Ischemic bile duct injury as a serious complication after transarterial chemoembolization in patients with hepatocellular carcinoma. J Clin Gastroenterol 32:423–427

Kim HC, Chung JW, Lee W (2005) Recognizing extrahepatic collateral vessels that supply hepatocellular carcinoma to avoid complications of transcatheter arterial chemoembolization. Radiographics 25:S25–S39

Kim SJ, Choi MS, Kang JY et al (2009) Prediction of complete necrosis of hepatocellular carcinoma treated with transarterial che-moembolization prior to liver transplantation. Gut Liver 3:285–291

Kim DY, Ryu HJ, Choi JY et al (2012) Radiological response predicts survival following transarterial chemoembolisation in patients with un-resectable hepatocellular carcinoma. Aliment Pharmacol Ther 35:1343–1350

Kim JH, Shim JH, Lee HC et al (2017) New intermediate-stage subclassification for patients with hepatocellular carcinoma treated with transarterial chemoembolization. Liver Int 37:1861–1868

Kloeckner R, Pitton MB, Dueber C et al (2017) Validation of clinical scoring systems ART and ABCR after Transarterial chemoembolization of hepatocellular carcinoma. J Vasc Interven Radiol 28:94–102

Kudo M, Arizumi T (2017) Transarterial chemoembolization in combination with a molecular targeted agent: lessons learned from negative trials (post-TACE, BRISK-TA, SPACE, ORIENTAL, and TACE-2). Oncology 93:127–134

Kudo M, Han G, Finn RS et al (2014) Brivanib as adjuvant therapy to transarterial chemoembolization in patients with hepatocellular carcinoma: a randomized phase III trial. Hepatology 60:1697–1707

Kudo M, Arizumi T, Ueshima K et al (2015) Subclassification of BCLC B stage hepatocel- lular carcinoma and treatment strategies: proposal of modified Bolondi's subclassification (Kinki criteria). Dig Dis 33:751–758

Kudo M, Cheng A-L, Park J-W (2018a) Orantinib versus placebo combined with transcatheter arterial chemoembolization in patients with unresectable hepatocellular carcinoma (ORIENTAL): a randomised, double-blind, placebo-controlled, multicentre, phase 3 study. Lancet Gastroenterol Hepatol 3:37–46

Kudo M, Ueshima K, Yokosuka O (2018b) SILIUS study group: Sorafenib plus low-dose cisplatin and fluorouracil hepatic arterial infusion chemotherapy versus sorafenib alone in patients with advanced hepatocellular carcinoma (SILIUS): a randomised, open label, phase 3 trial. Lancet. Gastroenterol Hepatol 3:424–432

Lammer J, Malagari K, Vogl T et al (2010) Prospective randomized study of doxorubicin-eluting-bead embolization in the treatment of hepatocellular carcinoma: results of the PRECISION V study. Cardiovasc Intervent Radiol 33:41–52

Lee K-H, Liapi EA, Cornell C et al (2010) Doxorubicin-loaded QuadraSphere microspheres: plasma pharmacokinetics and intratumoral drug concentration in an animal model of liver cancer. Cardiovasc Intervent Radiol 33:576–582

Lee S, Kim KM, Lee SJ et al (2017) Hepatic arterial damage after transarterial chemoembolization for the treatment of hepatocellular carcinoma: comparison of drug-eluting bead and conventional chemoembolization in a retrospective controlled study. Acta Radiol 58:131–139

Lencioni R, Llovet JM (2010) Modified RECIST (mRECIST) assessment for hepatocellular carcinoma. Sem Liver Dis 30:52–60

Lencioni R, de Baere T, Soulen MC et al (2016a) Lipiodol transarterial chemoembolization for hepatocellular carcinoma: a systematic review of efficacy and safety data. Hepatology 64(1):106–116

Lencioni R, Llovet JM, Han G et al (2016b) Sorafenib or placebo plus TACE with doxorubicin-eluting beads for intermediate stage HCC: the SPACE trial. J Hepatol 64:1090–1090

Levi FA, Boige V, Hebbar M et al (2016) Conversion to resection of liver metastases from colorectal cancer with hepatic artery infusion of combined chemotherapy and systemic cetuximab in multicenter trial OPTILIV. Ann Oncol 27:267–274

Lewis AL, Gonzalez MV, Lloyd AW et al (2006) DC bead: in vitro characterization of a drug-delivery device for transarterial chemoemboliza- tion. J Vasc Interv Radiol 17:335–342

Lin DY, Liaw YF, Lee TY et al (1988) Hepatic arterial embolization in patients with unresectable hepatocellular carcinoma—a randomized controlled trial. Gastroenterology 94:453–456

Linee guida AIOM, Edizione 2018. https://www.aiom.it/linee-guida-aiom-2018-epatocarcinoma

Liu DM, Kos S, Buczkowski A et al (2012) Optimization of doxorubicin loading for superabsorbent polymer microspheres: in vitro analysis. Cardiovasc Interv Radiol 35:391–398

Llovet JM, Bruix J (2003) Systematic review of randomized trials for unresectable hepatocellular carcinoma: chemoembolization improves survival. Hepatology 37:429–442

Llovet JM, Bru C, Bruix J (1999) Prognosis of hepatocellular carcinoma: the BCLC staging classification. Semin Liver Dis 19:329–338

Llovet JM, Real MI, Montana X (2002) Arterial embolisation or chemoembolisation versus symptomatic treatment in patients with unresectable hepatocellular carcinoma: a randomised controlled trial. Lancet 359:1734–1739

Lo CM, Ngan H, Tso WK (2002) Randomized controlled trial of transarterial lipiodol chemoembolization for unresectable hepatocellular carcinoma. Hepatology 35:1164–1171

Lu Z, Wen F, Guo Q et al (2013) Radiofrequency ablation plus chemoembolization versus radiofrequency ablation alone for hepatocellular carcinoma: a meta-analysis of randomized-controlled trials. Eur J Gastroenterol Hepatol 25:187–194

Malagari K, Pomoni M, Kelekis A et al (2010) Prospective randomized comparison of chemoembolization with doxorubicin-eluting beads and bland embolization with BeadBlock for hepatocellular carcinoma. Cardiovasc Intervent Radiol 33:541–551

Malagari K, Pomoni M, Moschouris H et al (2012) Chemoembolization with doxorubicin-eluting beads for unresectable hepatocellular carcinoma: five-year survival analysis. Cardiovasc Interv Radiol 35:1119–1128

Malagari K, Pomoni M, Moschouris H et al (2014) Chemoembolization of hepatocellular carcinoma with HepaSphere 30–60 μm. Safety and efficacy study. Cardiovasc Interv Radiol 37:165–175

Marelli L, Stigliano R, Triantos C et al (2007) Transarterial therapy for hepatocellular carcinoma: which technique is more effective? A systematic review of cohort and randomized studies. Cardiovasc Intervent Radiol 30:6–25

Marrero JA, Kulik LM, Sirlin CB et al (2018) Diagnosis, Staging, and Management of Hepatocellular Carcinoma: 2018 Practice Guidance by the American Association for the Study of Liver Diseases. Hepatology 68:723–750

Martin RC, Robbins K, Tomalty D et al (2009) Transarterial chemoembolisation (TACE) using irinotecan-loaded beads for the treatment of unresectable metastases to the liver in patients with colorectal cancer: an interim report. World J Surg Oncol 7:80

Martin RC, Scoggins CR, Schreeder M et al (2015) Randomized controlled trial of irinotecan drug-eluting beads with simultaneous FOLFOX and bevacizumab for patients with unresectable colorectal liver-limited metastasis. Cancer 121:3649–3658

Massarweh NN, Davila JA, El-Serag HB et al (2016) Transarterial bland versus chemoembolization for hepatocellular carcinoma: rethinking a gold standard. J Surg Res 200:552–559

Matsui O, Kadoya M, Yoshikawa J et al (1994) Subsegmental transcatheter arterial embolization for small hepatocellular carcinomas: local therapeutic effect and 5-year survival rate. Cancer Chemother Pharmacol 33:S84–S88

de Mestier L, Zappa M, Hentic O et al (2017) Liver transarterial embolizations in metastatic neuroendocrine tumours. Rev Endocr Metab Disord 18:459–471

Meyer T, Kirkwood A, Roughton M et al (2013) A randomised phase II/III trial of 3-weekly cisplatin-based sequential transarterial chemoembolisation vs embolisation alone for hepatocellular carcinoma. Br J Cancer 108(2):1252–1259

Meyer T, Fox R, Ma YT et al (2017) Sorafenib in combination with transarterial chemoembolisation in patients with unresectable he- patocellular carcinoma (TACE 2): a randomised placebo-controlled, double-blind, phase 3 trial. Lancet Gastroenterol Hepatol 2:565–575

Misiakos EP, Karidis NP, Kouraklis G et al (2011) Current treatment for colorectal liver metastases. World J Gastroenterol 17:4067–4075

Miyayama S, Matsui O, Yamashiro M et al (2007) Ultraselective transcatheter arterial chemoembolization with a 2-f tip microcatheter for small hepatocellular carcinomas: relationship between local tumor recurrence and visualization of the portal vein with iodized oil. J Vasc Interv Radiol 18:365–376

Miyayama S, Mitsui T, Zen Y et al (2009) Histopathological findings after ultraselective transcatheter arterial chemoembolization for hepatocellular carcinoma. Hepatol Res 39:374–381

Miyayama S, Yamashiro M, Hattori Y et al (2011) Efficacy of cone-beam computed tomography during transcatheter arterial chemoembolization for hepatocellular carcinoma. Jpn J Radiol 29:371–377

Monier A, Guiu B, Duran R et al (2017) Liver and biliary damages following transarterial chemoembolization of hepatocellular carcinoma: comparison between drug-eluting beads and lipiodol emulsion. Eur Radiol 27:1431–1439

Moriguchi M, Aramaki T, Nishiofuku H (2017) Sorafenib versus hepatic arterial infusion chemotherapy as initial treatment for hepatocellular carcinoma with advanced portal vein tumor thrombosis. Liver Cancer 6:275–286

Morimoto M, Numata K, Kondou M et al (2010) Midterm outcomes in patients with intermediate-sized hepatocellular carcinoma: a randomized controlled trial for determining the efficacy of radiofrequency ablation combined with transcatheter arterial chemoembolization. Cancer 116:5452–5460

Nakakuma K, Tashiro S, Hiraoka T et al (1983) Studies on anticancer treatment with an oily anticancer drug injected into the ligated feeding hepatic artery for liver cancer. Cancer 52:2193–2200

Narayanan G, Barbery K, Suthar R et al (2013) Transarterial chemoembolization using DEBIRI for treatment of hepatic metastases from colorectal cancer. Anticancer Res 33(5):2077–2083

Ohishi H, Uchida H, Yoshimura H et al (1985) Hepatocellular carcinoma detected by iodized oil. Use of anticancer agents. Radiology 154:25–29

Omata M, Cheng AL, Kokudo N (2017) Asia-Pacific clinical practice guidelines on the management of hepatocellular carcinoma: a 2017 update. Hepatol Int 11:317–370

Osuga K, Hori S, Hiraishi K et al (2008) Bland embolization of hepatocellular carcinoma using superabsorbent polymer microspheres. Cardiovasc Intervent Radiol 31:1108

Pak LM, Kemeny NE, Capanu M et al (2018) Prospective phase II trial of combination hepatic artery infusion and systemic chemotherapy for unresectable colorectal liver metastases: long term results and curative potential. J Surg Oncol 117:634–643

Park SH, Cho YK, Ahn YS et al (2007) Local recurrence of hepatocellular carcinoma after segmental transarterial chemoembolization: risk estimates based on multiple prognostic factors. Korean J Radiol 8:111–119

Park KW, Park JW, Choi JI et al (2008) Survival analysis of 904 patients with hepatocellular carcinoma in a hepatitis B virus-endemic area. J Gastroenterol Hepatol 23:467–473

Pelletier G, Roche A, Ink O et al (1990) A randomized trial of hepatic arterial chemoembolization in patients with unresectable hepatocellular carcinoma. J Hepatol 11:181–184

Pelletier G, Ducreux M, Gay F et al (1998) Treatment of unresectable hepatocellular carcinoma with Lipiodol chemoembolization: a multicenter randomized trial. Groupe CHC. J Hepatol 29:129–134

Peng ZW, Zhang YJ, Liang HH et al (2012) Recurrent hepatocellular carcinoma treated with sequential transcatheter arterial chemoembolization and RF ablation versus RF ablation alone: a prospective randomized trial. Radiology 262:689–700

Peng ZW, Zhang YJ, Chen MS et al (2013) Radiofrequency ablation with or without transcatheter arterial chemoembolization in the treatment of hepatocellular carcinoma: a prospective randomized trial. J Clin Oncol 31:426–432

Pompili M, Francica G, Ponziani FR et al (2013) Bridging and downstaging treatments for hepatocellular carcinoma in patients on the waiting list for liver transplantation. World J Gastroenterol 19:7515–7530

Poon RT, Tso WK, Pang RW et al (2007) A phase I/II trial of chemoembolization for hepatocellular carcinoma using a novel intra-arterial drug-eluting bead. Clin Gastroenterol Hepatol 5:1100–1108

Raoul JL, Heresbach D, Bretagne JF et al (1992) Chemoembolization of hepatocellular carcinomas. A study of the biodistribution and pharmacokinetics of doxorubicin. Cancer 70:585–590

Raoul JL, Sangro B, Forner A (2011) Evolving strategies for the management of intermediate-stage hepatocellular carcinoma: available evidence and expert opinion on the use of transarterial chemoembolization. Cancer Treat Rev 37(3):212–220

Richter G, Radeleff B, Stroszczynski C et al (2018) Safety and feasibility of chemoembolization with doxorubicin-loaded small cali- brated microspheres in patients with hepatocellular carcinoma: results of the MIRACLE I prospective multicenter study. Cardiovasc Intervent Radiol 41:587–593

Ronot M, Bouattour M, Wassermann J et al (2014) Alternative response criteria (Choi, European association for the study of the liver, and modified Response Evaluation Criteria in Solid Tumors [RECIST]) versus RECIST 1.1 in patients with advanced hepatocellular carcinoma treated with sorafenib. Oncologist 19:394–402

Saeki I, Yamasaki T, Maeda M, Hisanaga T, Iwamoto T, Matsumoto T, Hidaka I, Ishikawa T, Takami T, Sakaida I (2018) Evaluation of the "assessment for continuous treatment with hepatic arterial infusion chemotherapy" scoring system in patients with advanced hepatocellular carcinoma. Hepatol Res 48:E87–E97

Sattler T, Bredt C, Surwald S et al (2018) Efficacy and safety of drug eluting bead TACE with microspheres <150 mum for the treatment of hepatocellular carcinoma. Anticancer Res 38:1025–1032

Sergio A, Cristofori C, Cardin R et al (2008) Transcatheter arterial chemoembolization (TACE) in hepatocellular carcinoma (HCC): the role of angiogenesis and invasiveness. Am J Gastroenterol 103:914–921

Serra C, Cucchetti A, Felicani C et al (2019) Assessment of radiofrequency ablation efficacy for hepatocellular carcinoma by histology and pretransplant radiology. Liver Transpl 25:88–97

Shaib Y, El-Serag HB (2004) The epidemiology of cholangiocarcinoma. Semin Liver Dis 24:115–125

Shi J, Lai EC, Li N et al (2010) Surgical treatment of hepatocellular carcinoma with portal vein tumour thrombus. Ann Surg Oncol 17:2073–2080

Song SY, Chung JW, Han JK et al (2001) Liver abscess after transcatheter oily chemoembolization for hepatic tumors: incidence, predisposing factors, and clinical outcome. J Vasc Interv Radiol 12:313–320

Sottani C, Poggi G, Quaretti P et al (2012) Serum pharmacokinetics in patients treated with transarterial chemoembolization (TACE) using two types of epirubicin-loaded microspheres. Anticancer Res 32:1769–1774

Spreafico C, Cascella T, Facciorusso A et al (2015) Transarterial chemoembolization for hepatocellular carcinoma with a new generation of beads: clinical-radiological outcomes and safety profile. Cardiovasc Interv Radiol 38:129–134

Sullivan RD, Norcross JW, Watkins E et al (1964) Chemotherapy of metastatic liver cancer by prolonged hepatic-artery infusion. N Engl J Med 270:321–327

Takaki H, Yamakado K, Nakatsuka A et al (2007) Radiofrequency ablation combined with chemoembolization for the treatment of hepatocellular carcinomas 5 cm or smaller: risk factors for local tumour progression. J Vasc Interv Radiol 18(7):856–861

Takayasu K, Arii S, Matsuo N et al (2000) Comparison of CT findings with resected specimens after chemoembolization with iodized oil for hepatocellular carcinoma. AJR Am J Roentgenol 175:699–704

Takayasu K, Arii S, Kudo M et al (2012) Superselective transarterial chemoembolization for hepatocellular carcinoma. Validation of treatment algorithm proposed by Japanese guidelines. J Hepatol 56:886–892

Takuma Y, Takabatake H, Morimoto Y et al (2013) Comparison of combined transcatheter arterial chemoembolization and radiofrequency ablation with surgical resection by using propensity score matching in patients with hepatocellular carcinoma within Milan criteria. Radiology 269:927–937

Tanaka T, Isfort P, Braunschweig T et al (2013) Superselective particle embolization enhances efficacy of radiofrequency ablation: effects of particle size and sequence of action. Cardiovasc Intervent Radiol 36:773–782

Tellez C, Benson AB 3rd, Lyster MT et al (1998) Phase II trial of chemoembolization for the treatment of metastatic colorectal carcinoma to the liver and review of the literature. Cancer 82:1250–1259

Terashima T, Yamashita T, Arai K (2016) Response to chemotherapy improves hepatic reserve for patients with hepatocellular carcinoma and child-Pugh B cirrhosis. Cancer Sci 107:1263–1269

Terayama N, Matsui O, Gabata T et al (2001) Accumulation of iodized oil within the nonneoplastic liver adjacent to hepatocellular carcinoma via the drainage routes of the tumour after transcatheter arterial embolization. Cardiovasc Intervent Radiol 24:383–387

Terzi E, Golfieri R, Piscaglia F et al (2012) Response rate and clinical outcome of HCC after first and repeated cTACE performed "on demand". J Hepatol 57:1258–1267

Terzi E, Terenzi L, Venerandi L et al (2014) The ART score is not effective to select patients for transarterial chemoembolization re- treatment in an Italian series. Dig Dis 32:711–716

Tsochatzis E, Meyer T, Marelli L et al (2010) Which transarterial therapy is best for hepatocellular carcinoma? – the evidence to date. J Hepatol 53:588

Tsochatzis EA, Meyer T, Burroughs AK et al (2012) Hepatocellular carcinoma. N Engl J Med 366:92–93

Tsochatzis E, Meyer T, O'Beirne J et al (2013) Transarterial chemoembolisation is not superior to embolisation alone: the recent European Association for the Study of the liver (EASL) - European Organisation for Research and Treatment of Cancer (EORTC) guidelines. Eur J Cancer 49:1509–1510

Vadot L, Boulin M, Guiu B et al (2015) Clinical and economic impact of drug eluting beads in transarterial chemoembolization for hepatocellular carcinoma. J Clin Pharm Ther 40:83–90

Varela M, Real MI, Burrel M et al (2007) Chemoembolization of hepatocellular carcinoma with drug eluting beads: efficacy and doxorubicin pharmacokinetics. J Hepatol 46:474–481

Vogl TJ, Zangos S, Eichler K et al (2007) Colorectal liver metastases: regional chemotherapy via transarterial chemoembolization (TACE) and hepatic chemoperfusion: an update. Eur Radiol 17:1025–1034

Wang MQ, Shao RH, Ye HY et al (2005) Investigation of bile duct injury after transcatheter arterial chemoembolization. Zhonghua Zhong Liu Za Zhi 27:609–612

Wang Y, Deng T, Zeng L et al (2016) Efficacy and safety of radiofrequency ablation and transcatheter arterial chemoembolization for treatment of hepatocellular carcinoma: a meta-analysis. Hepatol Res 46:58–71

Wasan HS, Gibbs P, Sharma NK et al (2017) First-line selective internal radiotherapy plus chemotherapy versus chemotherapy alone in patients with liver metastases from colorectal cancer (FOXFIRE, SIRFLOX, FOXFIRE-global). Lancet Oncol 18:1159e1171

Watanabe S, Nishioka M, Ohta Y et al (1994) Prospective and randomized controlled study of chemoembolization therapy in patients with advanced hepatocellular carcinoma. Cooperative study Group for Liver Cancer Treatment in Shikoku area. Cancer Chemother Pharmacol 33:S93–S96

Wigmore SJ, Redhead DN, Thomson BN et al (2003) Postchemoembolisation syndrome—tumour necrosis or hepatocyte injury? Br J Cancer 89:1423–1427

Yao X, Yan D, Jiang X et al (2018) Dual-phase conebeam CT-based navigation imaging significantly enhances tumor detectability and aids Superselective Transarterial hemoembolization of liver Cancer. Acad Radiol 25:1031–1037

Yau T, Tang VYF, Yao T et al (2014) Development of Hong Kong liver cancer staging system with treatment stratification for patients with hepatocellular carcinoma. Gastroenterology 146:1691–1700

Zhou J, Sun H, Cong W et al (2018) Guidelines for diagnosis and treatment of primary liver Cancer in China (2017 edition). Liver Cancer 7:235–260

Transarterial 90Yttrium Radioembolisation

Cristina Mosconi and Rita Golfieri

Contents

C. Mosconi · R. Golfieri (✉)
Radiology Unit, Department of Experimental, Diagnostic and Speciality Medicine, Sant'Orsola Hospital, University of Bologna, Bologna, Italy
e-mail: rita.golfieri@unibo.it

Abstract

The term transarterial radioembolisation includes those procedures in which intra-arterially injected radioactive microspheres are used for internal radiation purposes. This procedure aims to selectively target radiation to liver tumours and to limit the dose involving the normal liver parenchyma. The yttrium-90 microspheres

© Springer Nature Switzerland AG 2021
E. Quaia (ed.), *Imaging of the Liver and Intra-hepatic Biliary Tract*,
Medical Radiology Diagnostic Imaging, https://doi.org/10.1007/978-3-030-39021-1_14

delivered through the hepatic artery are implanted into liver tumours in a ratio ranging from 3:1 to 20:1 as compared to a normal liver. A work-up, involving computed tomography scanning, contrast-enhanced magnetic resonance imaging and hepatic angiography, is essential for assessing the appropriateness of yttrium-90 treatment for each patient. A simulation of the procedure, carried out with technetium-99 m-labelled macroaggregated albumin particles, which approximate the size of microspheres, is used to identify the shunting of microparticles to the lungs or the gastrointestinal tract, thus helping in patient selection.

Excellent periprocedural care, discharge planning and follow-up are essential for assessing treatment response and ensuring that the short-term side effects of radioembolisation are adequately managed.

The purpose of this chapter is to summarise the relevant recent results regarding technical aspect, dosimetric advances, adverse events, safety and efficacy of radioembolisation in the treatment of hepatocellular carcinoma, intrahepatic cholangiocarcinoma and liver metastasis.

1 Introduction

Transarterial radioembolisation (TARE) is a form of brachytherapy in which intra-arterially injected yttrium-90 (^{90}Y)-loaded microspheres serve as a source for internal radiation. It produces average disease control rates exceeding 80%; it is usually very well tolerated and, for these reasons, it is a consolidated therapy for hepatocellular carcinoma (HCC), intrahepatic cholangiocarcinoma (ICC) and secondary liver disease (Sangro et al. 2012).

Currently the main application of TARE is for the treatment of HCC. In Western countries, the most commonly used staging system for establishing prognosis and determining the choice of treatment for HCC is the Barcelona Clinic Liver Cancer (BCLC) system (Forner et al. 2018);

moreover, it has been reported that, in tertiary referral centres, deviations from BCLC therapeutic recommendations occur in up to 50% of patients and this is especially true in stages B and C. In particular, in intermediate HCC (BCLC-B stage), it has been shown that transarterial chemoembolisation (TACE) which is recommended has a lower efficacy in large (>5 cm) and in multinodular tumours (Kim et al. 2012; Golfieri et al. 2013) while, in the advanced stage, sorafenib and the more recent lenvatinib are recommended; they are associated with important side effects and often dose reduction or suspension must be used (Llovet et al. 2008; Cheng et al. 2009). This scenario has led to new therapies for the best management of intermediate/advanced-stage HCC and, in this setting, the data available have shown that TARE could be an effective therapeutic option.

Transarterial radioembolisation also seems to be promising as a locoregional treatment in intrahepatic cholangiocarcinoma (ICC) which is a relatively rare and rapidly fatal malignancy; without early intervention and surgical resection, the prognosis for patients with ICC remains unequivocally dismal (Bridgewater et al. 2014; Yang et al. 2012). Although therapeutic options for unresectable disease are limited (Roayaie et al. 1998), various palliative options have been tested. Given the relative radiosensitivity of the normal liver parenchyma, external beam radiation has historically played a limited role in the treatment of liver malignancies. Traditional systemic chemotherapies have been relatively useless in treating patients with advanced disease, and locoregional therapies, such as radiofrequency ablation (RFA) and TACE, have also been used with varying degrees of success (Valle et al. 2010; Kim et al. 2011; Boehm et al. 2015). Given the relative radiation sensitivity of ICCs, preliminary studies involving TARE treatment have reported good results regarding safety and efficacy (Ibrahim et al. 2008; Saxena et al. 2010a, b; Hoffmann et al. 2012; Mouli et al. 2013; Rafi et al. 2013).

Transarterial radioembolisation is also widely used in the treatment of liver metastasis, particularly from colorectal cancer (CRC). In this setting, the liver is often the dominant site of metastatic disease (being the most relevant clinical problem) (Schindl et al. 2002). Five-year overall survival (OS) for patients with metastatic CRC is approximately 13% (National Cancer Institute 2016), and resection results in five-year survival rates of 30–40% (Adam et al. 2009); however, fewer than 25% of patients are suitable for resection at diagnosis (Delaunoit et al. 2005). Chemotherapy alone or combined with biological agents can also result in significant tumour downstaging, allowing for subsequent resection of liver metastases. For patients with liver-isolated or dominant CRC metastases unfit for potentially curative resection, in addition to systemic chemotherapy, TARE (Benson et al. 2013; Maawy et al. 2016) can be an option. Recently, TARE has been used for the treatment of metastases from other tumours including neuroendocrine tumours, gastric cancer, pancreatic cancer, breast cancer and lung cancer. After careful pretreatment assessments and proper patient selection, TARE has been shown to have tolerable toxicity with good results regarding response and survival.

2   Technical Aspects

TARE is defined as the intra-arterial delivery of micron-sized embolic particles loaded with a radioisotope in order to carry high focal doses of radiation selectively to liver tumours while sparing the normal liver parenchyma. This is achieved by the deposition of microspheres carrying a high-energy radiation source (yttrium-90 (^{90}Y), 0.97 MeV), a β-emitter, into the tumour capillary bed so that a tumouricidal dose of radiation (100–1000+ Gy) is absorbed for a short time over a limited area (mean tissue penetration 2.5 mm, maximum 11 mm). ^{90}Y decays to stable zirconium-90 with an average half-life of 2.67 days (64.2 h) (Kennedy et al. 2012).

The preferential release of ^{90}Y to liver tumours is based on anatomic and pathologic factors which are typical of solid liver and hepatic tumours; the liver parenchyma derives approximately all ($\geq$75%) of its blood from the portal vein whereas liver cancers (both metastatic and primary tumours as small as 0.5 mm in diameter) derive 80–100% of their blood supply from the hepatic artery (Ackerman et al. 1970). In addition, the neovascularisation of the plexus surrounding the tumour leads to increased microvascular density in liver lesions as compared to the normal liver parenchyma. These characteristics cause the ^{90}Y microspheres, released into the hepatic artery, to preferentially pile up in the periphery of tumours in at least a ratio ranging from 3:1 to 20:1 as compared to the normal liver (Kennedy et al. 2007). The size of the microspheres is essential for obtaining an optimal implantation within the network of tumour vessels to be efficacious (Kennedy et al. 2007). Therefore, it is necessary that the particles used for radioembolisation are small enough (~20 to 40 mm) to allow optimal access into the nodules and deposition within the tumour plexus, but also large enough to avoid the passage of the microspheres through the capillary bed into the venous circulation, thus escaping the liver. Any particles situated within the afferent tumour vessels, but distant more than 3 mm from the tumour, do not have a direct antitumour effect and can destroy the feeding arteries.

The principles and mode of action of radioembolisation are fundamentally different from conventional embolisation or TACE. For the latter to be effective, the feeding vessels are filled with chemotherapeutic agents and are then embolised to maximise exposure to those agents and to promote ischemic necrosis. Instead, to be effective, TARE needs optimal perfusion and blood flow maintenance to allow the generation of free radicals by means of ionisation of the water molecules near the DNA of the tumour cells. In the presence of normal oxygen tension, permanent DNA damage is caused to one or both DNA strands, and apoptosis is initiated or reproductive death is eventually achieved (Kennedy et al. 2012). Maximal cytoreduction by radiation requires not only normal oxygen tension in the target cells but also sufficient microsphere coverage of the tumour nodule in order to avoid gaps in cumulative radiation due to crossfire—"cold spots"—or a low total dose of radiation in the tumour (Kennedy et al. 2012).

There are two types of devices on the market:

- ^{90}Y resin microspheres (Sir-Spheres® 2017; Sirtex Medical Europe GmbH, Bonn, Germany)
- ^{90}Y glass microspheres (TheraSphere; MDS Nordion, Ottawa, Canada)

In both resin and glass microspheres, the primary mechanism of action is a localised radio-therapeutic effect (brachytherapy) rather than microvascular embolisation and tumour ischemia (Bilbao et al. 2009; Mackie et al. 2011). The adsorbed radiation dose depends on the microsphere distribution within the tumour, mainly resulting from the arterial hepatic hemo-dynamic and tumour vascularization. In TARE, dosimetry planning, the administration and delivery of the radiation, modification of the dose on the basis of tumour and hepatic volume and the knowledge required regarding radiation effects on tissue make this therapy a brachyther-apy procedure as well.

3   TARE Procedure

3.1   Patient Selection for Radioembolisation

All patients undergo a multidisciplinary clinical evaluation which includes history, physical examination, and a laboratory profile of liver function. In addition, detailed radiologic imaging is needed, showing unequivocal and measurable computed tomography (CT) or magnetic reso-nance imaging (MRI) evidence of hepatic lesions which cannot be surgically resected or ablated with curative intent (Coldwell et al. 2011). The best candidates for radioembolisation are patients with unresectable liver-only or liver-dominant tumours (Kennedy et al. 2007). Generally, patients are not excluded from treatment based on prior therapy or age. A multidisciplinary team consisting of professionals from interventional radiology, hepatology, medical, surgical and radi-ation oncology and nuclear medicine is involved in selecting suitable patients for radioembolisa-tion. Patients are selected according to the fol-lowing criteria:

- Inclusion criteria: (1) diagnosis of a hepatic lesion; (2) unresectable tumour; (3) an Eastern Cooperative Oncology Group (ECOG) perfor-mance status of (0, 1) or (2, 4) adequate hae-matology, including an absolute neutrophil count >1.5 3109/L, a platelet count >50 3109/L, renal function with creatinine level < 2.0 mg/dL, adequate liver function with bilirubin <2.0 mg/dL and (5) the possi-bility of undergoing angiography and selec-tive visceral catheterisation
- Exclusion criteria: (1) flow to the gastroin-testinal tract not correctable by coil embolisation on visceral angiography, (2) estimated radia-tion doses to the lungs exceeding 30 Gy in a single administration and (3) significant extra-hepatic disease representing an imminent life-threatening outcome

The important indications of adequate liver tolerance include the absence of ascites, normal synthetic liver function (albumin >3 g/dL) and total bilirubin of less than 2.0 mg/dL (<34 μmol/L).

A limited number of patients are unsuitable for treatment due to either vascular variants or the extent of lung shunting (Coldwell et al. 2011). These criteria are established at the work-up pro-cedure performed by the interventional radiolo-gists before treatment, thereby preventing inappropriate treatment of the patient. Excessive shunting to the gastrointestinal tract can some-times be corrected by the interventional radiolo-gist. It is very important to isolate the liver arterial tree from the gastric and small bowel arteries and to exclude patients with arteriovenous fistulae in tumours which allow more than 20% of the microspheres to pass through the liver capillary bed to the lungs. Even if the contraindications have been defined, the benefits of radioembolisa-tion in patients with relative exclusion parameter(s) need to be judged on a case-by-case basis to assess whether they represent an inap-propriate risk (Coldwell et al. 2011).

3.2   Pretreatment Evaluation

Yttrium-90 radioembolisation is a two-stage process involving an extensive work-up procedure for assessing the appropriateness of the patient for treatment and for preparing the treatment procedure itself. All patients undergo the following procedures approximately 1–3 weeks before the first planned treatment.

- Pretreatment cross-sectional imaging is essential for treatment planning and post-treatment response assessment; during the work-up, three-phase contrast computed tomography and/or gadolinium-enhanced magnetic resonance of the liver should be carried out for the

assessment of tumour and non-tumour volume (necessary for dosimetry), portal vein patency or not and the extent of extrahepatic disease (Fig. 1a–c).

- *Pretreatment Angiography:* All patients evaluated for TARE must undergo pretreatment angiography due to the high propensity of arterial variants and hepatic tumours to exhibit arteriovenous shunting (Memon et al. 2011). This permits planning the treatment according to each patient's individual anatomy and helps to avoid any inadvertent spread of the microspheres to non-target organs; this can be mitigated by prophylactic embolisation of the aberrant vessels to non-hepatic targets (Memon et al. 2011). Celiac trunk and/or

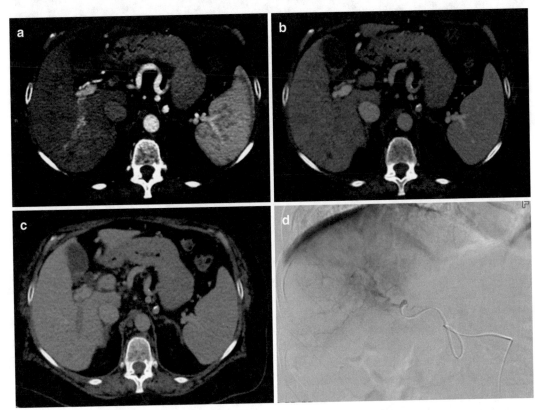

Fig. 1 Pretreatment CT showing infiltrative HCC in the *VI-VII segments* with associated tumour thrombosis of the corresponding portal branches, as visualised in the arterial (**a**), portal (**b**) and delayed phases (**c**). The pretreatment angiogram performed with a selective catheterisation of the hepatic artery for the *VI-VII segments* confirms the hypervascularization of the venous thrombus (**d**). The pretreatment 99mTc-MAA SPECT images showed the cor-

responding uptake of MAA in the region of interest (tumour thrombus) (**e**). The CT performed 3 months after treatment showed both a significant decrease in the enhancement of the portal venous thrombus and a reduction in the enlargement of the portal branch as a sign of response, as visualised in the arterial (**f**), portal (**g**) and delayed phases (**h**)

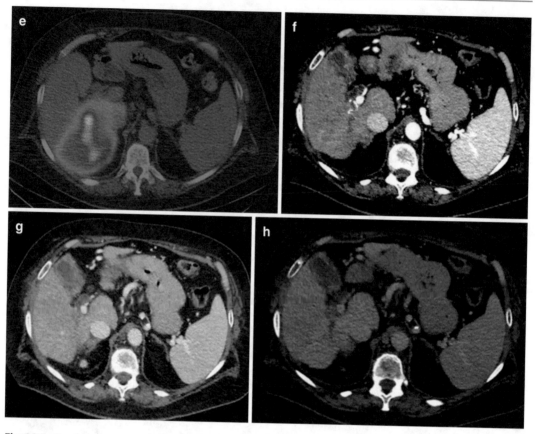

Fig. 14.1 (continued)

superior mesenteric angiograms, using a 4-F or 5-F catheter, give the interventional radiologist an opportunity to study the hepatic vascular anatomy. Subsequently, the tumour feeding arteries are cannulated using a highly flexible coaxial microcatheter passed through the 4-F or 5-F catheter previously placed in the artery itself. The tip of the microcatheter is placed into the hepatic arterial branch afferent to the segment or lobe where the tumour is located. In the case of superselective transarterial treatment, the tip of the catheter is advanced further into the subsegmental branches feeding the tumour (Fig. 1d).

- In some cases, prophylactic embolisation of the gastroduodenal artery and right gastric artery is recommended as a safe and efficacious mode of minimising the risks of hepatoenteric flow since this can lead to the inadvertent deposition of the microspheres into the gastrointestinal tract causing severe ulcers which are highly symp-

tomatic and difficult to manage (Cosin et al. 2007). Other vessels which need to be investigated and potentially embolised are the falciform, inferior oesophageal, left inferior phrenic, accessory left gastric, supraduodenal and retroduodenal arteries.

- Diagnostic angiography is essential to ensure that the blood supply to the tumour(s) has been adequately identified since incomplete identification of the blood supply to the tumour may lead to incomplete targeting and treatment. This facilitates accurate calculation of the target volumes because the artery or arteries into which the microspheres are injected define the volume of liver tissue exposed to radiation.

- *Pulmonary shunting and technetium-99 m-labelled macroaggregated albumin (99mTc-MAA) scan*: In some primary liver cancers (especially in HCC), one of the angiographic features is direct arteriovenous shunting, bypassing the capillary bed to the liver; the shunting of ^{90}Y microspheres to the lungs therefore becomes worrisome because this could result in radiation pneumonitis (Memon et al. 2011). Since the size of the 99mTc macroaggregated albumin (MAA) particle is similar to ^{90}Y, the distribution of the two will be identical; this concept is utilised in assessing splanchnic and pulmonary shunting (Fig. 1e). It is important to correlate the findings of angiography to those of the 99mTc-MAA scan as the proximity of some portions of the gastrointestinal tract to the liver may confuse the findings of nuclear medicine scans. The lung shunt fraction (LSF) is used to calculate the dose delivered to the lungs, and appropriate adjustment for this parameter minimizes the risk of radiation pneumonitis. If the LSF is deemed to be high, an appropriate reduction is made in the overall dose administered.

3.3 ^{90}Y Radioembolisation Procedure

The tumour is approached under fluoroscopic guidance; the first part of the procedure is similar to pretreatment angiography after which the activity vial is injected into the vessel feeding the tumour. Tumour distribution guides the selectivity of the treatment to one or more lobes/segments as required. The device for administering the ^{90}Y is designed to minimise radiation exposure of the personnel involved in the procedure. A physicist is present throughout the procedure to ensure that proper protocols are followed in order to minimise accidental radiation exposure. In some hospitals, a Bremsstrahlung (gamma) scan or positron emission tomography (PET)-CT is performed to evaluate ^{90}Y distribution immediately after treatment.

4 Dosimetry and ^{90}Y Microsphere Activity Selection

Personalised treatment planning is desirable for TARE and can be carried out using 99mTc-MAA SPECT images and volumes obtained

from CT scans. The image fusion of the CT and the single-photon emission computerised tomography (SPECT) images can help in delineating the volumes involved in the treatment. An important limitation of TARE is the dose to the normal liver because an excessive dose to the normal parenchyma could induce radiation hepatitis and liver failure. The spatial distribution of the microspheres is crucial and may be very different for the two types of spheres. When using resin microspheres, the dose absorbed by the normal liver should be kept lower than 40 Gy to minimise the risk of liver failure, especially in patients having compromised liver function (Sangro et al. 2008). Although personalised dosimetry would be the best approach to TARE, it has not been standardised and is often not achievable. For these reasons, the majority of TARE treatments are performed calculating the injected activity based on empiric formulas suggested by the manufacturers instead of following scrupulous dosimetric formalism. In the following paragraphs, the standard methods for activity assessment are briefly described for both glass and resin microspheres.

4.1 Glass Microspheres

The activity determination for glass microspheres, proposed by the manufacturer (TheraSphere Yttrium-90 Glass Microspheres Users Manual, BTG), is based on a nominal target dose (80–150 Gy) to the treated mass (M), which can be measured by CT images. This approach assumes a uniform distribution of the microspheres throughout the treated volume, including the tumour and the normal parenchyma:

$$A(GBq)_{glass} = \frac{D(Gy) \times M(kg)}{50}$$

The dose arriving to the lung should be kept to less than 30 Gy for a single injection and less than 50 Gy as a cumulative dose for multiple injections (Leung et al. 1995). Using the above formula, the dose delivered to the tumour is not known; however, going on the assumption that tumours have a higher vascularity as compared to the normal parenchyma, it is reasonable to predict that the prescribed dose be at least that which is absorbed by the tumour in order to prevent liver fibrosis.

4.2 Resin Microspheres

Two methods have been proposed by SIRTEX to determine the activity of ^{90}Y to be injected: the empiric method and the body surface area (BSA) method (Sirtex Medical Limited 2007).

The empiric method suggests a standard amount of activity based on tumour involvement only, considering three varying degrees of tumour involvement:

Tumour ≤25% of the total mass of the liver by CT scan = 2 GBq whole-liver delivery.

Tumour ≥25% but ≤50% of the liver mass by CT scan = 2.5 GBq whole-liver delivery.

Tumour ≥50% of the liver mass by CT scan = 3 GBq for whole-liver delivery.

It is important to point out that this method is not recommended by the scientific community (Kennedy et al. 2007).

The *BSA (body surface area) method* is a variant of the empiric method which calculates the injected activity, taking into account the patient's BSA and the fraction of liver volume involved by the tumour:

$$A(GBq) = (BSA - 0.2) + \frac{V_{tumor}}{V_{tumor} + V_{normal\ liver}}$$

where BSA (m²) = 0.20247 × height(m)0.725 × weight(kg)0.425.

The BSA formula is considered safe for patients with compromised liver function or for particularly small patients. A reduction of the amount of activity up to 20% is recommended for lung shunts greater than 15%.

4.3 Dosimetric Approach

The empiric methods suggested by both manufacturers do not represent a real dosimetric approach to the treatment because the distribu-

tion of the ^{90}Y microspheres and the uptake ratio between the tumour and the normal parenchyma are never considered, thus preventing any accurate dosimetric evaluation.

A dosimetric approach based on Medical Internal Radiation Dosimetry (MIRD) formalism was proposed by SIRTEX as a "partition model" and has been formalised with MIRD equations by Gulec and colleagues (Gulec et al. 2006). The MIRD formalism is based on the determination of the fraction of activity (fractional uptake) which is trapped by the tumour, normal liver and lungs, and by the masses of each compartment which are calculated using CT images. The fractional uptake, representing the fraction of activity reaching each compartment, is measured by 99mTc-MAA SPECT images, calculating the tumour to liver ratio (TLR) and the lung shunt fraction. Because the dose to the normal parenchyma is the most important limiting factor, the administered activity can be calculated as the activity delivering the selected nominal dose to the liver, as follows:

$$A(GBq)_{injected} = \frac{D(Gy)_{liver} \times M(kg)_{liver}}{50}$$

where:

$A(GBq)$ is the ^{90}Y injected activity.

$D(Gy)$ is the nominal dose to the liver.

$M(kg)$ is the liver mass.

50 is a constant which depends on the physical characteristics of ^{90}Y.

Once the fraction of activity reaching each compartment/tissue is measured, the corresponding absorbed dose is evaluated using the following formula:

$$D(Gy)_{tissue} = \frac{50 \times A(GBq)_{tissue}}{M(kg)_{tissue}}$$

The 99mTc-MAA particles are considered a surrogate of the microspheres, and their distribution inside tissues is representative of the microsphere distribution. It is very important to point out that, using 99mTc-MAA SPECT images, it is possible to carry out provisional dosimetry before the ^{90}Y infusion, although it presents several limitations. In particular, the major limitations of this approach are the different sizes and specific gravities of 99mTc-MAA and the ^{90}Y microspheres, the different volumes and velocities of injection, the reproducibility of the exact site of injection and the haemodynamic conditions inside the tumour which can be considerably different between the 99mTc-MAA and the ^{90}Y treatments. Furthermore, the MIRD approach assumes the uniform distribution of the microspheres and measures average doses while, especially in tumour masses, the dose is strongly dependent on heterogeneous vessel density.

However, despite the limitations listed above, the higher mean dose absorbed by the tumour masses, calculated with 99mTc-MAA SPECT images, was predictive of a better tumour response in patients affected by HCC for both resin (Strigari et al. 2010) and glass microsphere (Chiesa et al. 2011) treatments. Furthermore, the intrinsic differences between the two types of microspheres and, in particular, their different numbers and specific activities are responsible for the different distribution of the microspheres inside the tissues, more uniform for resin than for glass microspheres. Consequently, the published data regarding dosimetry have reported higher values of the tumour dose response for glass microspheres than for resin microspheres (Garin et al. 2010).

4.4 Post-Treatment Assessment and Follow-Up

Clinical, laboratory and radiologic follow-up is very important for evaluating response to treatment and identifying any toxicity. A regular laboratory follow-up includes the hepatic panel and tumour markers. Cross-sectional imaging is carried out 1 month after treatment and every 3 months thereafter in order to assess the response to treatment or the progression of the disease.

To provide post-treatment care, the follow-up involves an office visit and interval and physical examination, laboratory tests and imaging.

Follow-up Care: Within 4 weeks after radioembolisation, patients should schedule a follow-up office visit with their treating physician. At that time, the physician will conduct a review of

systems, carry out a physical examination and program laboratory tests.

Recommended Laboratory Tests: The following laboratory tests are recommended: complete blood count, basic metabolic panel, liver function tests, coagulation panel (prothrombin time (PT)/ activated partial thromboplastin time (APTT)/ international normalized ratio (INR)) and tests for the presence of tumour markers.

Recommended Imaging: Imaging studies play an essential role in assessing the response to radioembolisation (Fig. 1f–h). The following scans are recommended: CT scanning scheduled for 4 weeks post-treatment and then every 3 months for the first year (note: there is usually only a modest response in liver tumours at 4 weeks); however, extrahepatic and new hepatic disease can be detected. Imaging after TARE is required to monitor the tumour response but it is not always easy to interpret. Imaging usually shows a change in both the appearance of the tumour and the surrounding liver. Since the effect of the radiation may not be evident until 30 days after treatment, imaging at 1 month after the procedure is usually not representative of the tumour response. However, a common early feature is the appearance of rim enhancement surrounding the lesion; this is an early sign of a fibrotic capsule, and it is fundamental that it not be erroneously considered to be a residual tumour (Riaz et al. 2009a, b). Instead, in a period ranging from 8 to 12 weeks after TARE, there is noticeable tumour shrinkage and the parenchyma also becomes atrophic as a consequence of hepatic fibrosis and capsular retraction of the treated area; atrophy of the treated area induces compensatory hypertrophy of the contralateral lobe especially after lobar procedures (rather than after a segmental or subsegmental approach). Another common feature is the appearance of transient perfusion abnormalities in the treated area which should be differentiated from residual or recurrent tumours. Furthermore, transient hypoattenuating perivascular oedema near the hepatic and portal veins can also be observed on imaging.

Computed tomography is capable of identifying changes in the size of the lesions and alterations in vascularity and enhancement; the appearance of new intra- or extrahepatic lesions are well defined with this technique but may limit the capability of documenting tumour necrosis.

Magnetic resonance imaging, especially using diffusion-weighted imaging (DW-MRI) and gadolinium-ethoxybenzyl-diethylenetriamine/pentaacetic acid imaging (Gd-EOB-DTPA-MRI), identifies necrosis and cell death earlier (6–8 weeks post-procedure in some cases) and better than CT (Schelhorn et al. 2015).

5 Side Effects and Complications

Complications after TARE can be classified into the following groups: post-radioembolisation syndrome (PRS), hepatic dysfunction, biliary sequelae, portal hypertension, radiation pneumonitis, gastrointestinal (GI) ulceration, vascular injury, lymphopenia and a miscellaneous category (Riaz et al. 2009a, b). The current reports in the literature use the Common Toxicity Criteria for Adverse Events 3.0.

PRS: The incidence of PRS in the literature ranges from 20 to 55% (Riaz et al. 2009a, b). Post-radioembolisation syndrome consists of the following clinical symptoms: fatigue, nausea, vomiting, anorexia, fever, abdominal discomfort and cachexia. The duration of PRS has not been studied; however, hospitalization is usually not required. Post-radioembolisation syndrome is less severe than the post-treatment syndromes observed after other embolic therapies in which fatigue and constitutional symptoms predominate (Coldwell et al. 2011). Mild abdominal pain may be experienced after radioembolisation (Riaz et al. 2009a, b). Patients can take steroids and antiemetic agents to reduce the incidence of PRS. A 2-week follow-up after radioembolisation is recommended to investigate the clinical evidence of the PRS. Symptomatic management may be required.

Hepatic Dysfunction: The incidence of radiation-induced liver disease (RILD) after ^{90}Y administration ranges from 0 to 4% (Sangro et al. 2008). Radiation-induced liver disease results from the exposure of the normal liver parenchyma to high doses of radiation. Clinical correlation is essential; in fact, this may lead to biochemical aberrations with minimal clinical manifestations. Follow-up laboratory evaluation is routinely recommended at 1 month after treatment and, if RILD is clinically manifest, supportive management is recommended. The diagnosis of RILD can be confirmed by a biopsy of the normal parenchyma. It is seen most often in patients with pre-existing liver function abnormalities; therefore, patients with baseline bilirubin levels of more than 2 mg/dL are generally not considered ideal candidates. Whole-liver radioembolisation in a single session is not recommended. Sangro et al. (2008) studied liver disease induced by the radioembolisation of liver tumours in 45 patients who underwent treatment for primary or secondary liver tumours, and they showed that the incidence of RILD was associated with increasing age, whole-liver treatment and increased baseline bilirubin levels.

Biliary Sequelae: The incidence of biliary sequelae after TARE is less than 10% . It results from radiation-induced injury to the biliary structures or the microembolic effect of the therapy. The majority of biliary complications are not manifested clinically; clinical correlation with imaging findings is recommended. Abscesses may need antibiotics and sometimes drainage. Radiation cholecystitis requiring surgical intervention is present in less than 1% of cases. Radiation cholecystitis may be prevented by identifying the cystic artery and injecting microspheres distal to its origin. It is possible to consider embolisation of the cystic artery if the blood flow into it is significant and radioembolisation distal to its origin is not feasible. Patients with a history of systemic polychemotherapy may also be at high risk of developing biliary complications.

Portal Hypertension: The clinically significant occurrence of portal hypertension is low (Jakobs et al. 2008). Radiation leads to fibrosis which causes shrinkage of the liver parenchyma. This can radiologically appear with signs of portal hypertension even if clinically relevant manifestations (reduced platelet counts (<100,000/dL) or variceal bleeding) are rarely seen. It is recom-

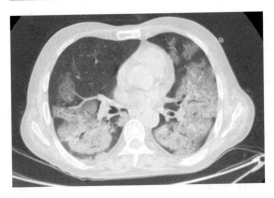

Fig. 2 Lung CT: batwing appearance of radiation pneumonitis

mended to routinely check for radiological and clinical evidence of portal hypertension as this is not an acute process (Gaba et al. 2009).

Radiation Pneumonitis: The incidence of radiation pneumonitis is less than 1% if standard dosimetry models are used (Wright et al. 2012). Radiation pneumonitis manifests as a restrictive ventilatory dysfunction. On chest CT, it has a batwing appearance (Fig. 2); management is medical with steroids. Other complications, such as atelectasis and pulmonary effusion, are rarely observed. A 99mTc-MAA scan is essential for calculating the LSF. A high LSF translates into a high percentage of activity (and, hence, the dose) being delivered to the lungs. Lung doses less than 30 Gy per treatment and less than 50q Gy cumulatively are recommended.

GI Complications: If proper percutaneous techniques are used, the incidence of GI ulceration is well below 5%. The cause of this complication is the ectopic distribution of radioembolic microspheres into the lining of the GI tract. Severe epigastric pain after treatment should be managed aggressively; endoscopy may be required to confirm the diagnosis. Cases refractory to proton pump inhibitors may require surgical management. As opposed to a normal ulcer which develops at the mucosal surface, ^{90}Y-induced ulcers originate from the serosal surface. This may theoretically decrease the ability of the ulcer to heal and complicate the surgical field from scars/adhesions should surgery be required. For these reasons, pretreatment angiography is essential for identifying the vessels

which may supply the GI tract; in fact, prophylactic embolisation of the gastroduodenal artery (GDA) is recommended if a high number of microspheres are to be delivered. Moreover, if the right gastric artery originates from the proper hepatic artery, it would be better to embolise it. A left hepatic angiogram is carried out to identify the left gastric, inferior oesophageal and right gastric arteries. Prolonged and delayed angiography of the left hepatic artery is recommended; opacification of the coronary vein confirms gastric or oesophageal flow. A right hepatic angiogram is required to identify the supraduodenal and retroportal arteries.

A 99mTc-MAA scan may show splanchnic flow but must be correlated to angiographic findings (Hamami et al. 2009). Prophylactic gastric acid suppressive agents are recommended after therapy. As stated earlier, the degree of pretreatment prophylactic embolisation should be determined based on the treating physician's experience, vessel size, planned treatment location and the radioembolic device being considered. However, gastrointestinal toxicities can be avoided by using meticulous techniques.

Vascular Injury: Radioembolisation is an invasive procedure. The incidence of vascular injury is very low (<1%) and is, for the most part, seen in patients previously exposed to systemic chemotherapy; this could cause increased fragility of the artery wall leading to susceptibility to injury (spasm, dissection). They are therefore related to the technique and/or previous chemotherapy rather than to the dose of microspheres.

6 TARE in HCC: Treatment Outcomes and Survival

Hepatocellular carcinoma represents approximately 90% of primary liver cancers and constitutes a major health problem worldwide (Akinyemiju et al. 2017). The most commonly used staging system for establishing prognosis and determining the choice of treatment for HCC management is the BCLC system endorsed by the guidelines for HCC management of the

American Association for the Study of Liver Diseases (AASLD), the American Gastroenterology Association (AGA) and the European Association for the Study of Liver (EASL) (EASL guidelines 2018). It consists of five stages: very early, early, intermediate, advanced and terminal, according to variables related to tumour burden, liver function (Child-Pugh class), clinical status and cancer-related symptoms (Eastern Cooperative Group Performance Status (ECOG PS)) (Forner et al. 2018).

When diagnosed at an early stage of the disease, HCC may benefit from potentially curative treatments, such as liver resection, liver transplantation or local ablation, while, despite the effectiveness of the treatment in early and very early stages, the majority of patients are diagnosed or progress to an intermediate or advanced stage, in which treatment options are limited and the prognosis is poor (EASL guidelines 2018; Golfieri et al. 2019). In fact, even if TACE is recommended for patients with intermediate-stage HCC according to a systematic review by Llovet and Bruix (2003) which reported an increased survival rate in patients treated with TACE, its low efficacy has however been demonstrated in large (>5 cm) and in multinodular tumours (Kim et al. 2012; Sangro et al. 2011; Golfieri et al. 2011, 2013) and confirmed by a multicentric Japanese study (Takayasu et al. 2012). This study showed a significant decrease in 3-year survival after superselective TACE for lesions larger than 5 cm and for multiple lesions (four or more) and an inverse correlation between survival and tumour size and number.

In the advanced stage, the recommended treatment is sorafenib, a receptor tyrosine kinase inhibitor, according to two large randomised trials (Llovet et al. 2008; Cheng et al. 2009) that reported a benefit in terms of survival rate in advanced HCC with distant metastasis and/or vascular invasion; moreover, the latest BCLC update has acknowledged the positive results of recent randomised trials, introducing lenvatinib, which has not been proven to be inferior to sorafenib, as in first-line therapy and regorafenib, which has been shown to improve survival as compared to a placebo in selected patients progressing after sorafenib as second-line therapy (EASL guidelines 2018; Golfieri et al. 2019). However, the tolerability of sorafenib and the other chemotherapies were revealed to be suboptimal, especially when sorafenib was down-dosed in more than half of the patients and interrupted in 45% of patients due to severe adverse events (AEs) or liver function deterioration (Iavarone et al. 2011).

Therefore, this scenario has led to new therapies for the best management of intermediate/advanced-stage HCC and, in this setting, available data have shown that TARE could be an effective therapeutic option. Additional studies regarding the safety and efficacy of TARE have led to its adoption across BCLC stages, with treatment goals ranging from complete tumour control to symptom palliation. Clinical practice guidelines, however, do not recommend TARE in clinical practice. In particular, in the recent EASL guidelines, TARE is not recommended in BCLC B and C patients due to its failure to demonstrate a survival benefit when compared to sorafenib (EASL guidelines 2018) in two recent random controlled trials (RCTs) (Vilgrain et al. 2017; Chow et al. 2018). However, in the same RCTS, TARE has demonstrated durable local control and a good safety profile, and ongoing trials are seeking to elucidate its optimal patient population.

6.1 Clinical Results of TARE in HCC Treatment

The role of TARE in HCC was first explored in the setting of portal vein thrombosis (PVT). It is estimated that approximately one in three HCC patients will develop PVT (Okuda et al. 1985) and, historically, TACE in patients with PVT was relatively contraindicated out of concern for iatrogenically induced acute liver failure unless superselective or segmental embolisation could be achieved. In 2004, Salem and colleagues reported on the safety of ^{90}Y glass microspheres in unresectable HCC patients with PVT (Salem et al. 2004). In a cohort of 15 patients with PVT of one or both first order segmental portal vein branches who underwent TARE, the treatment was well tolerated with grade 1–2 bilirubin toxicity noted in only five patients, and it was attributed to intrahepatic disease progression rather than treatment effect. No patient experienced liver failure and, for the first time, TARE was confirmed to be safe in HCC patients with PVT. Furthermore, it was found that due to the minimally embolic nature of ^{90}Y glass microspheres, this treatment did not preclude future intra-arterial treatments, such as TACE (Salem et al. 2004). In 2008, a similar two-centre phase 2 study investigated the safety and efficacy of TARE in 108 unresectable HCC patients with and without PVT of the branch or the main portal vein (Kulik et al. 2008), building upon previous results in this patient population. No cases of radiation-induced gastritis or pneumonitis were reported, and post-treatment elevations of bilirubin and the development of ascites were higher in the group with main PVT. Importantly, there was no increased risk of hepatic failure or encephalopathy between patients with main PVT versus those with branch or no PVT. Moreover, there were no significant treatment-related complications or treatment-related deaths. With respect to efficacy, partial responses (PRs) were noted in 42.2% of patients using the World Health Organization (WHO) criteria and in 70% of patients using the EASL criteria.

In 2013, treatment sequencing of HCC patients with PVT was further elucidated. In a cohort of 63 patients treated with TARE who experienced disease progression, investigators noted that 64% of the patients were deemed ineligible for systemic treatment or clinical trials due to a worsened Child-Pugh status (Child-Pugh B or C) at the time of progression (Memon et al. 2013). In addition, survival was significantly shorter when comparing Child-Pugh A versus B groups (13.8 vs. 6.5 months). These findings led investigators to conclude that an adjuvant approach to sequencing in which systemic treatment is administered after TARE but before disease progression/declines in liver function may be beneficial in this patient population.

With the safety profile of TARE better understood and its efficacy coming to light, several studies began to examine long-term treatment outcomes across stages. In the first long-term outcome analysis for 291 HCC patients treated with TARE using glass microspheres, Salem et al. measured response rate, time to progression (TTP), and survival across stages (Salem et al. 2010). The investigators noted objective response rates (ORR) of 42 and 57% based on the WHO and the EASL criteria, respectively. Time to progression for the entire patient cohort was 7.9 months and varied by Child-Pugh stage as did survival outcomes. Patients with Child-Pugh A disease survived significantly longer than those with Child-Pugh B disease (17.2 vs. 7.7 months). Moreover, patients with Child-Pugh B disease and PVT had the worst outcomes with a median OS of 5.6 months. This study was the first to demonstrate the varying TTPs and outcomes by Child-Pugh status.

Moreover, even if PVT is not a contraindication for radioembolisation, the prognosis is, however, closely correlated to the PVT extension; in fact, Kulik et al. (2008) reported, using glass microspheres, an OS of 4.4 months in patients with main PVT, of 9.9 in patients with branch PVT and of 15.4 months in patients without PVT. Similar results were obtained with the resin microspheres (OS of 9.7 in patients with main PVT, 10.7 in patients with branch PVT and 15.3 in patients with patent PVT) (Sangro et al. 2012). In 2013, Mazzaferro and colleagues conducted the first phase 2 study examining efficacy and long-term outcomes of ^{90}Y radioembolisation in BCLC intermediate and advanced HCC (Mazzaferro et al. 2013). In 52 patients with a median follow-up time of 36 months, they observed that OS was correlated to Child-Pugh status and, in particular, to the presence and the extension of PVT; in fact, they reported that patients with Child-Pugh A and branch PVT have OS similar to patients with Child-Pugh A without PVT (17 months vs. 18 months). Another European series of 104 patients showed a median OS which differed significantly between patients with segmental and lobar/main PVT ($p = 0.031$); moreover, OS was 17 months in both those with patent vessels and those with segmental PVT (Golfieri et al. 2015a, b). More recently, Spreafico et al. (2018) proposed a prognostic score (validated by other groups (Mosconi et al. 2018)) for survival in patients with HCC and PVT undergoing TARE where the only variables independently correlated with OS were bilirubin, extension of PVT and tumour burden. Three prognostic categories were identified: favourable prognosis (0 points), intermediate prognosis (2–3 points) and dismal prognosis (>3 points) and the median OS in the three categories was 32.2 months, 14.9 months and 7.8 months, respectively ($p < 0.0001$), confirming the relevant role of liver function and the presence/extension of PVT.

More recently, a retrospective analysis by Gordon et al. sought to elucidate baseline patient characteristics and prognostic factors in unresectable HCC patients called "super survivors," those remaining alive >3 years after ^{90}Y treatment (Gordon et al. 2018). Sixty-seven "super survivors" were identified. Upon further analysis, the common variable among these patients was an imaging response after treatment. Moreover, the Child-Pugh score and main PVT stratified median OS and segmental versus lobar PVT, ^{90}Y was associated with improved OS.

6.2 Comparisons to TACE and Sorafenib

In recent years, there have been several studies comparing the efficacy of ^{90}Y radioembolisation to TACE and systemic therapies in the settings of definitive treatment and in downstaging as a bridge to transplantation.

6.2.1 TARE vs. TACE

The first paper regarding this topic was published in 2011 by Salem et al. (2011); they reported that patients with HCC treated with TACE or TARE had similar survival times (20.5 months vs. 17.4 months, respectively, $P = 0.232$); however, TARE resulted in longer time-to-progression (13.3 months vs. 8.4 months, respectively, $P = 0.046$) and less toxicity than TACE. In patients with intermediate-stage disease, survival was similar between the groups which received

TACE (17.5 months) and TARE (17.2 months, $P = 0.42$). Other retrospective studies obtained similar results; in fact, Lance et al. did not report any significant differences in survival when comparing 38 patients treated with TARE and 35 treated with TACE (median 8.0 months vs. 10.3 months, respectively, $p = 0.33$) (Lance et al. 2011) in line with other papers (Moreno-Luna et al. 2013; El Fouly et al. 2015).

In 2016, a systematic review and meta-analysis of 5 studies and 553 patients with unresectable HCC who underwent TACE or TARE was carried out (Lobo et al. 2016). The analysis showed no significant survival differences between the groups for up to 4 years. Furthermore, partial and complete response (CR) rates were similar as were the complication profiles between the two treatments, although it was noted that patients receiving TACE had increased post-treatment pain (Lobo et al. 2016). However, in 2016, the results of the PREMIERE trial, a landmark phase 2 study comparing the TTP for 45 BCLC A and B patients randomized to TACE or TARE, were released (Salem et al. 2016). The investigators discovered a significantly longer median TTP for patients receiving ^{90}Y radioembolisation when compared to TACE (26 months vs. 6.8 months), although no differences in survival were noted "suggesting local control is insufficient for survival improvement in cirrhotic patients with competing risks of death" (Salem et al. 2016). It should be noted that the trial was closed early due to slow accrual.

A meta-analysis of Facciorusso et al. (2016) confirmed these data; in fact, analysing a total of ten studies, of which two were randomised controlled trials, the survival rate assessed at 1 year showed absolute similarity between the two treatment groups (odds ratio (OR) = 1.01; 95% confidence level (CI), 0.78–1.31; $P = 0.93$) but the longer the period after the treatment, OS tended to significantly increase with increase in time after the treatment, thus indicating better long-term outcomes in patients who underwent TARE (2-year SR (OR = 1.43, 1.08–1.89, $P = 0.01$), 3-year SR (OR = 1.48, 1.03–2.13, $P = 0.04$)). A recent meta-analysis (Casadei Gardini et al.

2018) considering only randomised studies in order to provide the highest possible level of evidence reported that overall survival and progression-free survival at 1 year were similar between the two treatment groups; the authors only demonstrated a higher proportion of patients undergoing transplantation in the TARE group (30% vs. 20.8%), even if it was not statistically significant. Despite the lack of survival benefits, the increased TTP reported in some studies for patients treated with TARE could decrease transplant list dropout, making TARE an attractive alternative to transplant-eligible HCC patients when compared to TACE. In the setting of downstaging for transplant eligibility, a comparative analysis of TACE versus TARE demonstrated the superior performance of TARE in downstaging HCC patients from United Network for Organ Sharing (UNOS) T3–T2 (Lewandowski et al. 2009). In this study of 86 patients, partial response rates were significantly higher in the ^{90}Y patients, and downstaging was achieved in more TARE patients when compared to TACE patients (58% vs. 31%). By more efficiently downstaging patients from T3 to T2 and thus placing them within the confines of the Milan criteria, ^{90}Y radioembolisation may more quickly allow for a UNOS priority status upgrade and quicker access to donor organs.

However, significant data regarding comparison between TARE and TACE are lacking due to the well-known heterogeneity of the BCLC-B stage, which includes different tumour characteristics in terms of tumour number and size. For this reason, Bolondi et al. (2013) proposed a subclassification of the intermediate stage; they identified the B2 group, which included patients with Child-Pugh class A status exceeding the up-to-7 criterion as good candidates for TARE, and some subsequent studies seem to confirm these data (Cappelli et al. 2019).

6.2.2 TARE vs. Sorafenib

The relative efficacy of TARE versus sorafenib for advanced HCC patients was evaluated in the Strengthening and Stretching for Rheumatoid Arthritis of the Hand (SARAH) trial (Vilgrain et al. 2017). This was a phase III, randomised,

controlled, open-label, multicentre trial which included 459 locally advanced HCC patients (BCLC C) or those previously treated with two unsuccessful rounds of TACE. Patients were randomised to sorafenib or TARE using resin microspheres; the primary endpoint was OS, with secondary endpoints including PFS, TTP, response rate, adverse events and quality of life (QOL). The median OS was not significantly different between the two treatment arms, with patients surviving 8.0 months in the TARE group and 9.9 months in the sorafenib group. The median PFS was similar between the two groups in both the intention-to-treat (ITT) population and in the per-protocol population. The ORR was significantly higher in the TARE intention to treat population. Furthermore, higher rates of treatment-related adverse events including fatigue, haematologic abnormalities, diarrhoea, abdominal pain and dermatologic reactions were noted in the sorafenib group.

More recently, a randomised, phase III, open-label, multicentre trial comparing sorafenib to TARE using resin microspheres in 360 patients with locally advanced HCC patients with and without vascular invasion was conducted (selective internal radiation therapy versus sorafenib (SIRveNIB)) (Chow et al. 2018). The primary endpoint was OS and the secondary endpoint was PFS, tumour response rate, toxicity and QOL. Median OS was not statistically different between the two groups (8.8 vs. 10.0 months in the TARE and sorafenib groups, respectively), although patients treated with TARE were noted to have higher tumour response rates and twofold fewer adverse events. These results were similar to the SARAH study (Vilgrain et al. 2017); both studies were negative and demonstrated no survival benefits for TARE when compared to sorafenib. However, as reported in some recent papers (Sposito and Mazzaferro 2018), these results must be interpreted with caution and there are many questionable points to think about. First of all, as stated elsewhere, failure of rejecting the null hypothesis in a superiority trial should be distinguished from the concept used in a non-inferiority trial, in which a non-inferiority margin is set a priori and generally larger sample sizes are needed (Llovet and Finn 2018). Consequently, neither the results of the SIRveNIB trial nor the results of the SARAH trial could have been instrumental in claiming for an equivalency between TARE and sorafenib. Thus, how should the results of these two recent RCTs be interpreted in the light of previously published studies and clinical experience which showed a promising efficacy of TARE even if at a lower level of evidence? Should TARE be abandoned as a treatment for HCC or should it be pursued in some specific subsets of patients? To answer these questions, the difficulties and potential biases undermining trials which compare an interventional procedure to a drug should be carefully analysed.

The second relevant point is that radioembolisation is a sophisticated technical procedure which requires great skill and multidisciplinary management involving a medical and non-medical team after a considerable learning curve. The expertise in managing this treatment might have been highly heterogeneous in both the SIRveNIB trial (which was conducted at 11 centres of which only 5 had facilities to perform TARE) and the SARAH trial (which was conducted at 25 centres). The majority of the cohort studies reporting promising results of TARE were carried out on series from single centres which were highly experienced (Rognoni et al. 2016); the relatively poor results of TARE in both RCTs might be partially explained by the diluting effect of the multicentricity of the design, with some contributing centres having little experience of administering TARE. Moreover, considering that TARE is a form of radiotherapy, dosimetric considerations should have been better elucidated. In the two RCTs, the planned activity and ^{90}Y treatment dose were based on body surface area; no endpoints regarding tumour-absorbed dose and liver-absorbed dose were planned while a clear tumour dose-response relationship with glass microspheres had already been demonstrated in several studies (Chiesa et al. 2011). Finally, as already explained, the appropriate population in which a benefit of TARE over sorafenib could be shown still needs to be defined. Local treatment, such as TARE, and surgical resection have been demonstrated to be particularly effective in those patients with PVT limited to primary or secondary order branches of the portal vein and less or noneffective in patients with occlusion of the main portal trunk (Rognoni et al. 2016; Spreafico et al. 2018; Kokudo et al. 2016). In both the SIRveNIB and the SARAH trials, subgroup analyses did not demonstrate a significant survival benefit in patients with PVT undergoing TARE. Apart from being underpowered by definition, subgroup analyses in both studies were not designed to target survival differences according to PVT extension. In conclusion, the SIRveNIB and the SARAH trials failed to prove the superiority of TARE over sorafenib in patients with advanced HCC. However, these trials were pivotal since they were the first RCTs confirming the safety and efficacy of TARE in patients with locally advanced HCC. Both studies suggested that TARE might be better tolerated than sorafenib in those patients, and these results were in line with what is felt by the majority of clinicians dealing with TARE. A clear superiority of TARE with respect to sorafenib in inducing tumour response was confirmed; the reasons why this result did not translate into a benefit in OS or in PFS should probably be researched with a better and more restrictive patient selection for the procedure. In particular, until new trials are designed, it would be more correct that the results of large cohort studies demonstrating that radioembolisation provides a significant survival benefit in patients with HCC and PVT (Rognoni et al. 2016) not be disregarded because of the present two negative RCTs which included a broader spectrum of intermediate and advanced HCC patients.

6.3 TARE in ICC: Treatment Outcomes and Survival

Intrahepatic cholangiocarcinoma is the second most common primary liver cancer after HCC (Bridgewater et al. 2014]. Although relatively rare, its incidence is increasing worldwide, accounting for up to 15% of primary liver cancers with an age-adjusted rate of about 2.1 per 100,000 people/year in western countries (Yang et al. 2012). The only potential curative treatment is surgical treatment; however, only 30–40% of ICCs are diagnosed at a stage which meets the criteria for curative resection (Bridgewater et al. 2014). Furthermore, curative-intent surgery is mainly limited by the high recurrence rate of this cancer; however, it can increase median overall survival from 27 to 36 months. If untreated, unresectable ICCs have a median survival of less than 8 months (Roayaie et al. 1998; Chou et al. 1997) which can be increased to approximately 12 months with systemic chemotherapy (gemcitabine and cisplatin) (Valle et al. 2010).

For these reasons, locoregional therapies, such as RFA or transarterial therapies, including hepatic artery infusion (HAI) and TACE, have been employed. However, given the relative radiation sensitivity of ICC (Chou et al. 2007), TARE could be promising as a locoregional treatment for this tumour (Fig. 3). Preliminary analyses of safety and efficacy have been reported in some small studies (Ibrahim et al. 2008; Rafi et al. 2013), with median survival ranging from 9 to 22 months.

6.3.1 Clinical Results of TARE in ICC Treatment

For patients with ICC, some data exists regarding the utility and efficacy of TARE in patients with unresectable ICC. The first study of Ibrahim et al. (2008) reported the results of TARE in 24 patients with histologically proven ICC; they showed (follow-up available for 22 patients), according to the WHO Criteria, a partial response in 6 patients (27%), stable disease in 15 patients (68%) and disease progression in 1 patient (5%) and, according to the EASL Criteria, a complete response in 2 patients (9%) and a partial response in 17 patients (77%). The median OS was 14.9 months from the time of the first treatment. Median survival was significantly prolonged in patients with ECOG performance status 0 as compared to those with status 1 and 2 (31.8 months vs. 6.1 months and 1 month, respectively, $P < 0.0001$) and in patients without PVT (31.8 months vs. 5.7 months, $P = 0.0003$); the median survival of patients with peripheral ver-

sus infiltrative tumours was 31.8 months and 5.7 months, respectively ($P = 0.0005$).

A second and more recent study of the same group (Mouli et al. 2013) confirmed these initial results. In evaluating the response based on the WHO criteria, disease control was evident in 98% of patients, and, based on the EASL Criteria, 73% of patients exhibited greater than 50% necrosis on follow-up imaging. Survival varied according to the presence of multifocal (5.7 months vs. 14.6 months), infiltrative (6.1 months vs. 15.6 months) or bilobar disease (10.9 months vs. 11.7 months).

In a series of 33 patients, Hoffmann et al. (Hoffmann et al. 2012) reported a median OS of 22 months from the time of the first treatment and disease control (partial response or stable disease (SD)) in 85% of patients, all evaluated according to the Response Evaluation Criteria in Solid Tumours (RECIST) Criteria. The median TTP was 9.8 months. Survival and TTP were significantly prolonged in patients with ECOG 0 vs. ECOG 1 or 2 (median OS (29.4, 10 and 5.1 months, respectively), TTP (17.5, 6.9 and 2.4 months, respectively)), in those with a tumour burden ≤25% (OS, 26.7 vs. 6 months; TTP, 17.5 vs. 2.3 months) or in those with tumour response (partial response or stable disease vs. progressive disease (PD); OS (35.5, 17.7 vs. 5.7 months, respectively), TTP (31.9, 9.8 vs. 2.5 months, respectively)).

Saxena et al. (2010a, b) demonstrated disease control in 74% of patients according to the RECIST Criteria and a median OS of 9.3 months in a study of 25 patients; survival was significantly correlated to two factors, peripheral tumour type (vs. infiltrative, $P = 0.004$) and an ECOG performance status of 0 (vs. 1 and 2, $P < 0.001$). Furthermore, in a series of 19 patients, Rafi et al. (Rafi et al. 2013) showed a median survival of 345 ± 128 days from the time of the first TARE but the median survival was not correlated with the ECOG performance status or the presence of extrahepatic metastases.

Camacho et al. (2014) reported a median OS of 16.3 months (95% CI, 7.2–25.4 months). Using the mRECIST and the EASL Criteria applied to the delayed phases of dynamic

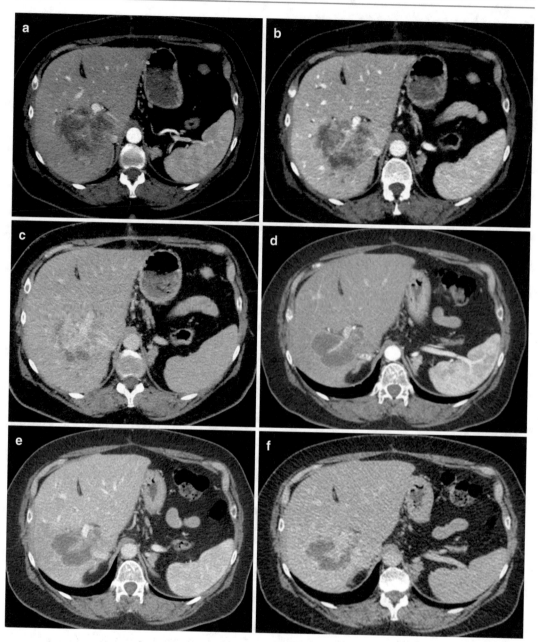

Fig. 3 A pretreatment CT showed a large, hypervascular, biopsy-proven cholangiocarcinoma in the right lobe as visualised in the arterial (**a**), portal (**b**) and delayed phases (**c**). The CT performed after 3 months (**d**–**f**) demonstrates marked lesions shrinkage with almost complete necrosis

contrast-enhanced cross-sectional imaging, the target ORRs (CR and PR) were 56.2% for mRE-CIST, 50% for EASL and only 6.2% for RECIST. The overall ORRs were 0% for RECIST and 37.5% for mRECIST. They found significant differences in survival between mRE-CIST and EASL versus RECIST when categoris-ing patients into responders and nonresponders ($P < 0.001$).

Al-Adra et al. (2015) carried out a comprehensive review of the current studies and clinical outcomes of unresectable ICCs treated with TARE, identifying 12 studies with relevant data. Based on a pooled analysis, they found partial responses in

28% and stable disease in 54% of patients at 3 months, and the overall weighted median survival was 15.5 months. However, the authors pointed out the heterogeneity of the study populations included in the pooled OS; in fact, all the studies reported survival after the initiation of TARE but, in some cases, the patients had undergone systemic chemotherapy prior to or during the treatment. Therefore, the overall pooled survival may have underestimated the effects of TARE if some patients had already undergone previous therapies.

Recently, Edeline et al. (2015) and Mosconi et al. (2016) showed that TARE combined with chemotherapy seemed to be a promising strategy as a first-line treatment for unresectable intrahepatic cholangiocarcinoma; Edeline observed a median progression-free survival after TARE of 10.3 months; a longer PFS was observed when chemotherapy was given concomitantly with TARE than when it was given before TARE, with a respective median of 20.0 versus 8.8 months ($P = 0.001$) (median OS was not reached). Mosconi et al. showed a median OS of 17.9 months (14.3–21.4 months, 95% CI) with significantly better median survival in the treatment-naive patients as compared with previously treated patients (52 vs. 16 months, $p = 0.009$).

Moreover, Cucchetti et al. (2017) recently carried out a meta-regression study, obtaining two very relevant results: first, naïve ICCs treated with TARE have a 2-year survival of 50.4% while ICCs treated after failure/recurrence of a previous treatment have a 2-year survival of 23.6%, with a statistically significant difference; second, they found a significant correlation between the 1-year survival rates reported in the literature and the number of infiltrative ICCs included in each study, with a median pooled survival of the infiltrative type estimated to be 8.2 months, considerably lower than that estimated for peripheral ICC of 19.3 months.

6.4 TARE in in Metastatic CRC (mCRC): Treatment Outcomes and Survival

Colorectal cancer is the third leading cause of cancer death in both the United States and Europe (Grothey et al. 2004; Jemal et al. 2002). The liver is often the dominant site of metastatic disease, thus being the most significant clinical problem (Zacharias et al. 2015), with approximately 50% of those diagnosed developing metastases, either synchronous or metachronous, within 2 years after diagnosis of the primary tumour (Schindl et al. 2002). The 5-year OS for patients with metastatic CRC is approximately 13% (National Cancer Institute 2016). Resection has a five-year survival rate of 30–40% in the treatment of colorectal liver metastases (Adam et al. 2004), but fewer than 25% of patients are suitable for resection at diagnosis (Delaunoit et al. 2005). Chemotherapy alone or combined with biological agents can also result in significant tumour downstaging, allowing for the subsequent resection of liver metastases. For these patients, a five-year survival of 33% can be achieved. A proportion of patients with initially unresectable liver disease become suitable for resection following systemic chemotherapy (12.5–40%) (Adam et al. 2009; Alberts et al. 2005). Although liver resection can achieve long-term survival, the majority of patients have extrahepatic disease or are unresectable due to tumour size and number, location, or an inadequate residual liver. For patients with unresectable disease, five-year survival remains just over 10% and, hence, exploration of treatments targeted for liver-only or liver-dominant disease is potentially important (Townsend et al. 2016).

There are several non-surgical treatment options in addition to systemic chemotherapy for patients with liver-isolated or liver-dominant CRC metastases who are not candidates for potentially curative resection. However, there has been growing interest and utilisation of other hepatic arterial therapies, in particular TARE (Benson et al. 2013; Maawy et al. 2016) which has been shown to have tolerable toxicity with good results regarding response and survival. The relevant studies in this setting are summarised below, with particular attention paid to randomised controlled trial evidence of the use of TARE in the management of advanced CRC as a first-line therapy and as a salvage treatment.

6.4.1 Clinical Results of TARE in mCRC Patients

6.4.1.1 First-Line Therapy

SIR-Spheres® has been approved in the USA, based upon results from a single controlled trial in which 74 patients with liver-isolated CRC metastases were randomly assigned to hepatic artery infusion with fluorodeoxyuridine (FUDR) alone or in conjunction with the single intrahepatic artery administration of TARE (Gray et al. 2001). Although, in this trial, patients were not excluded from participation if they had received prior systemic chemotherapy for metastatic disease, only five patients in each arm had received this therapy. In addition, accrual did not reach the planned target of 90 patients and it was perhaps underpowered as a result. Combined HAI-FUDR/TARE therapy was associated with a significantly better objective complete response rate (44 vs. 18%) and median time to progression (16 vs. 10 months), with similar toxicity grades of 3 and 4 when compared to HAI-FUDR alone. Although the 1-, 2-, 3- and 5-year overall survival rates for patients receiving TARE (72, 39, 17 and 4%, respectively) did not differ significantly from those of patients in the control arm (68, 29, 7 and 0%, respectively), Cox regression analysis suggested a survival benefit for patients who lived longer than 15 months. A reasonable conclusion from this trial was that TARE was active in the setting of HAI-FUDR-based therapy.

Following this study, other studies have analysed the role of TARE in this setting, showing a high response rate (>80%), with a prolonged mean survival (30 months) (Van Hazel et al. 2004; Tie et al. 2010). The results of the SIRFLOX clinical trial and the combined analysis of three multicentre, randomised, phase III trials (FOXFIRE, SIRFLOX and FOXFIRE-Global) (Wasan et al. 2017) have recently been published. SIRFLOX was a randomised, multicentre trial designed to assess the efficacy and safety of the addition of TARE to mFOLFOX6-based chemotherapy with or without bevacizumab in patients with previously untreated metastatic CRC. Chemotherapy-naïve patients with liver metastases plus or minus limited extra-hepatic metastases were randomly assigned to receive either modified FOLFOX (mFOLFOX6)—control group—or mFOLFOX6 plus TARE plus or minus bevacizumab. The primary endpoint was PFS at any site as assessed by an independent centralised radiology review blinded-to-study arm. The authors randomised 530 patients, assigned to each treatment (control, 263; TARE, 267). Median PFS at any site was 10.2 vs. 10.7 months in the control group versus the TARE group ($P = 43$) while median PFS in the liver by competing risk analysis was 12.6 in the control group vs. 20.5 months in the TARE group ($P = 0.002$). The ORRs at any site were similar (68.1% in the control group vs. 76.4% in the TARE group; $P = 0.113$) while the ORR in the liver was improved with the addition of TARE (68.8% in the control group vs. 78.7% in the TARE group; $P = 0.042$). The authors concluded that the addition of TARE to FOLFOX-based first-line chemotherapy in patients with liver-dominant or liver-only CRC metastases did not improve PFS at any site but significantly delayed disease progression in the liver while waiting for the results regarding survival published in the combined analysis of three multicentre, randomised, phase 3 trials (FOXFIRE, SIRFLOX and FOXFIRE-Global). The results were published in September 2017; FOXFIRE, SIRFLOX and FOXFIRE-Global (Wasan et al. 2017) were randomized phase III trials carried out in hospitals and specialist liver centres in 14 countries worldwide (Australia, Belgium, France, Germany, Israel, Italy, New Zealand, Portugal, South Korea, Singapore, Spain, Taiwan, the UK and the USA). Chemotherapy-naïve patients with mCRC WHO performance status (0 or 1) with liver metastases not suitable for curative resection or ablation were randomly assigned (1:1) to either oxaliplatin-based chemotherapy (FOLFOX: leucovorin, fluorouracil and oxaliplatin) or FOLFOX plus single TARE treatment concurrent with cycle 1 or cycle 2 of chemotherapy. The primary endpoint was OS (with 2 years of follow-up), using a two-stage meta-analysis of pooled individual patient data.

Five hundred and forty-nine patients were randomly assigned to FOLFOX alone and 554 patients were assigned FOLFOX plus TARE; the median survival time in the FOLFOX plus TARE group was 22.6 months (95% CI, 21.0–24.5) versus 23.3 months (95% CI, 21.8–24.7) in the FOLFOX-alone group, without statistically significant differences ($p = 0.61$). Therefore, this analysis showed that the significant improvement in liver disease control assessed by competing risk analyses did not correspond to a benefit in OS. This result is completely different from the result of the European Organization for Research and Treatment of Cancer (EORTC) Chemotherapy + Local Ablation versus Chemotherapy (CLOCC) study (Ruers et al. 2017) which showed that a significant effect of TARE ablation with or without surgery on progression-free survival translated into a highly significant overall survival benefit in patients; however, in this study, patients did not have a primary tumour in situ or extrahepatic metastases at trial entry. On the contrary, in the FOXFIRE, SIRFLOX and FOXFIRE-Global studies, half of the study population had a primary tumour in situ and approximately a third had extrahepatic metastases; therefore, the absence of benefit of adding TARE to FOLFOX on PFS and OS in the combined study could be partly explained by the high proportion of patients who developed first progression at an extrahepatic site, independently of whether the metastases were liver-only at baseline or whether there were extrahepatic metastases or primary tumours in situ at baseline. However, the demonstrated absence of an OS benefit suggested that the early use of TARE in combination with first-line oxaliplatin-based chemotherapy cannot be recommended in unselected patients with mCRC.

6.4.2 TARE as a Single Treatment in mCRC Chemotherapy-Refractory Patients

Multiple retrospective studies have reported outcomes when TARE was used as a salvage therapy in chemotherapy-refractory patients, showing significantly extended PFS, TTP and OS in patients with unresectable liver-only or liver-dominant CRC metastases who had failed standard-of-care systemic chemotherapy. The most significant comparative and non-comparative studies carried out in this group of patients (Golfieri et al. 2015a, b; Sofocleous et al. 2015) obtained good results regarding OS which ranged from 8 to 13 months. In particular, Bester et al. reported the results of a retrospective study which evaluated the safety to the liver and the survival of patients with chemotherapy-refractory mCRC who were treated with resin microsphere TARE (n D224) as compared with patients who underwent standard/supportive care (Bester et al. 2012). The median OS after TARE was 11.9 months as compared to 6.3 months for the standard care cohort. Moreover, the study by Seidensticker et al. (2012) evaluated OS after TARE with resin microspheres vs. best supportive care (BSC) in patients with chemotherapy-refractory liver-dominant mCRC. Twenty-nine patients who received TARE were retrospectively matched with a contemporary cohort of 500 patients who received BSC, with prolonged survival in the TARE group (median, 8.3 vs. 3.5 months; $p < 0.001$). In a phase II multicentre clinical trial, Cosimelli et al. (2010) reported an ORR of 24% using RECIST. The median TTP was 3.7 months and the median OS was 12.6 months. A systematic review by Saxena et al. (n = 979) reported a median time to intrahepatic progression of 9 months (range 6–16) and a median overall survival of 12 months (range 8.3–36). After treatment, the average reported value of patients with a complete radiological response, partial response and stable disease was 0% (range 0–6%), 31% (range 0–73%) and 40.5% (range 17–76%), respectively (Saxena et al. 2014). The number of previous lines of chemotherapy (≥ 3), poor radiological response to treatment, extrahepatic disease and extensive liver disease ($\geq 25\%$) were the factors most commonly associated with poorer overall survival.

Therefore, the median OS of patients who failed third-line therapy ranged from 4 to 6 months; therapy with TARE may improve survival outcomes. The utility of concomitant chemotherapy requires additional exploration.

6.5 TARE in Non-colorectal Cancer Liver Metastases: Treatment Outcomes and Survival

6.5.1 Clinical Results of TARE in Non-colorectal Cancer Liver Metastasis Treatment

Neuroendocrine liver metastases (NELMs) appear as an ideal target for this treatment modality due to their hypervascularity, well-preserved liver function and good general condition in the majority of patients despite their advanced tumour stage. Additional favourability may be found in the substantial potential for TARE in the symptomatic relief of patients with carcinoid syndrome from hormonally active NELMs. There are some studies regarding the use of TARE in this setting. Moreover, a recent meta-analysis by Frilling et al. (2019) demonstrated evidence of the clinical effectiveness and safety of TARE for neuroendocrine liver metastases. They reported a cumulative ORR of 51% and a disease control rate of 88% with median overall survival of 32 months. However, neuroendocrine cancer is a complex disease; therefore, the possibility of intra- and extrahepatic disease recurrence predicates a mandate for systemic adjuvant treatment after TARE. Saxena et al. (2010a, b) identified five factors indicative for improved survival in 48 patients with NELMs: complete/partial response, low hepatic tumour burden, well-differentiated tumours, female gender and absence of extrahepatic disease. Female gender, well-differentiated tumours and the absence of extrahepatic disease were associated with complete/partial response. Inversely, higher tumour grade and tumour burden were reported to negatively impact hepatic progression-free survival and overall survival after embolisation therapy of patients treated for NELMs (TARE in 64 cases) (Chen et al. 2017). In another study, ECOG performance score 0, a tumour burden of 25%, albumin <3.5 g/dL and bilirubin <1.2 mg/dL were positive prognostic factors of survival on univariate analysis while, on multivariate analysis, only ECOG performance score 0 and bilirubin <1.2 mg/dL were prognosticators of a favourable outcome (Memon et al. 2012). High

lung shunt (>10%), total serum bilirubin >1.2 mg and lack of pretreatment with octreotide were identified on multivariate analysis as factors predicting poor survival in another study (Ludwig et al. 2016). A novel approach with promising outcomes was taken in a phase 1b study in 13 patients, analysing three dose levels of everolimus (2.5, 5 and 10 mg/day), pasireotide (600 mg twice daily) and SIR-Spheres (administered on days 9 and 37). The authors hypothesised that everolimus and pasireotide, both shown to be effective in a palliative setting in neuroendocrine tumours (NETs), may potentiate TARE radiosensitisation and inhibit rebound angiogenesis. The median progression-free survival was 19 months and overall survival was 46 months. No major toxicity or clinical side effects occurred (Kim et al. 2018). In the first published randomised phase II trial run at the University of Gothenburg, Sweden, radioembolisation with ^{90}Y-labelled microspheres was compared with transarterial embolisation (TAE) in 11 patients with NELMs of the small intestine (Elf et al. 2018). The primary endpoint was response to treatment according to RECIST 1.1 assessed by diffusion-weighted magnetic resonance imaging at 3 months post-treatment. At 3 months, all metastases in both treatment arms had decreased in size; however, the decrease was significantly larger in patients treated with TAE ($n = 5$). The in-hospital stay was significantly longer in the TAE group (4 days) when compared to the TARE cohort (2 days). At 6 months, no difference in RECIST 1.1 response was seen between the TARE and the TAE groups, indicating a delay in imaging response following TARE. A similar experience has been reported by Fidelman et al. (2016) who documented time to maximal response after TARE on imaging at a median of 2.8 months (1.0–21.9) in patients treated for colorectal liver metastases (n-21) and at a median of 1.1 months (0.7–4.5) in patients treated for cholangiocarcinoma ($n = 7$) as compared to 11.0 months (5.0–29.6) for those treated for NELMs ($n = 11$). At the same time, the ORR, the disease control rate (DCR), median PFS and median OS were more favourable in patients with NELMs than in those with colorectal liver metastases or cholangiocarcinoma. These studies demonstrated evidence of the safety and efficacy of TARE in this setting which should be assessed by local and national clinical commissioning groups. Additional randomised controlled trials with not only standard endpoints but also quality of life assessment and economic aspects are urgently needed to highlight and explain the differences between radioembolisation and other palliative treatment options for patients with unresectable neuroendocrine liver metastases. A combination of clinical and translational research goals should be set to identify those patients who might benefit from TARE as a first-line treatment and those with a predictably poor response to treatment.

Breast cancer liver metastases (BRCLMs): Breast cancer is the most commonly diagnosed cancer in women, expected to account for 29% of all new cancers diagnosed among women (Siegel et al. 2014). Breast cancer confined to the primary site has a promising prognosis, with estimated 5-year survival rates exceeding 99% (Siegel et al. 2014). The outlook significantly worsens for the estimated 20–30% of patients who develop distant metastatic disease, with 5-year survival rates as low as 16–25% (Purushotham et al. 2014) and median survival in patients with unresectable, chemoresistant BRCLMs ranges from 3 and 10 months. Even if solitary liver metastases are rare in the setting of breast cancer (<5%), of the studies on TARE regarding nonconventional liver metastases, breast cancer is the most studied; the first study investigating survival of BRCLM patients undergoing TARE was by Bangash et al. (2007) who assessed 27 patients with progressing liver metastases being treated with polychemotherapy. Of the 23 patients, 39.1% showed either complete or partial response according to the WHO criteria; median survival for the 21 patients with a tumour burden <25% and 6 patients with a tumour burden >25% were 9.4 and 2.0 months, respectively. The authors concluded that although the tumour response with TARE was encouraging, the influence on survival remained unclear. A larger study in 2007 by Coldwell et al. (2007) included a total of 44 women with unresectable chemorefractory

BRCLMs; 47% of the 36 patients had a partial response according to the RECIST criteria and 95% of all 44 patients showed a response on PET scan. Based on an expected median survival of patients with advanced breast cancer responding to standard chemotherapy of 14 months, the authors predicted the patients would demonstrate an increase in overall survival. However, at 14 months, 86% of patients were still alive. Patients nonresponsive to CT or PET had a median survival of 3.6 months. In 2013, the largest study to date reported the use of TARE in 77 unresectable chemorefractory BRCLM patients. Response rates were consistent with prior studies having a partial response rate of 56% according to the RECIST criteria. Median survival was 11.5 months; in patients with ECOG 0, with <25% of tumour burden and no extrahepatic disease, median survival was promising at 14.3 months (Cianni et al. 2013).

Metastatic Melanoma: Melanoma is a particularly lethal form of skin cancer, accounting for 75% of skin cancer-related deaths; the most common types of melanoma are cutaneous (over 90%) and ocular (around 5%) (Markovic et al. 2007; Bakalian et al. 2008). Ocular (uveal) melanomas have a tendency to metastasise to the liver (95% of ocular metastatic disease) whereas liver metastasis occurs in just 15%–20% of metastatic cutaneous melanomas. As a first-line treatment, standard chemotherapy has traditionally been ineffective in metastatic patients; liver-directed therapy is a preferred approach to reduce the tumour burden and prolong overall survival. Four studies have been using TARE regarding melanoma liver metastases; in 2011, Gonsalves et al. (2011) studied a larger cohort consisting of 32 patients with hepatic metastasis of uveal melanoma. Median OS was 10.0 months but only 6% had treatment response according to the RECIST criteria. The low response rate was attributed to the inclusion of salvage patients with bulky, treatment-resistant progressive lesions and a high tumour burden (seven patients had >25% hepatic tumour burden). Given the hypervascular and aggressive nature of melanoma liver metastases, locoregional treatment with TARE appears to be a reasonable approach at reducing disease progression. Median overall survival ranges from 7.6 to 10.1 months, substantially improved over the expected less than 3 months reported decades ago.

Metastatic pancreatic cancer carries a notoriously dismal prognosis (Ghaneh et al. 2002). Systemic chemotherapy, the current mainstay of treatment, has poor median overall survival (Cunningham et al. 2009). A paucity of clinical data exists regarding TARE for liver metastases of pancreatic cancer patients; the first small study in 2010 by Cao et al. (2010) included seven pancreatic adenocarcinoma patients with liver metastases. Two patients died prior to the initial follow-up and two (40%) of the remaining five patients exhibited partial response according to the RECIST criteria. Average median survival was not provided, but the authors reported that one patient survived nearly 15 months after TARE therapy. A second, slightly larger, study in 2014 by Michl et al. (2014) on 19 chemorefractory pancreatic patients with metastatic liver disease reported an encouraging median overall survival of 9.0 months. Five patients died and one patient was lost to the study due to disease progression prior to the initial follow-up. Of the 13 patients at initial follow-up, 64.3% exhibited partial response according to the RECIST criteria; nine patients received adjuvant chemotherapy after surgery. The authors also found a correlation with serum markers CA 19–9 and C-reactive protein (CRP) and shorter overall survival.

Metastatic renal cell carcinoma (RCC): Renal cell carcinoma is currently responsible for 2–3% of malignancies in the USA; approximately 33–50% of patients with RCC eventually develop metastatic disease (Aloia et al. 2006). Metastatic disease to the liver affects 20–40% of patients, and the overwhelming majority (over 96%) are accompanied by widespread disease (McKay et al. 2014). Patients with hepatic involvement have a reported median overall survival of 7.4 months (Ballarin et al. 2011). The pilot study for TARE of chemorefractory renal cell carcinoma liver metastases was carried out by Abdelmaksoud et al. in 2012 (Abdelmaksoud et al. 2012). Median overall survival for six patients was 12 months. Of the five patients who made it to the initial follow-up, three (60%) had a complete response and one (20%) had a partial response according to the RECIST criteria. In the treatment of liver metastasis from renal cell carcinoma, TARE is limited by the rarity of liver-dominant metastases and the known resistance to radiation.

References

Abdelmaksoud MH, Louie JD, Hwang GL et al (2012) Yttrium-90 radioembolization of renal cell carcinoma metastatic to the liver. J Vasc Interv Radiol 23:323–330

Ackerman NB, Lien WM, Kondi ES et al (1970) The blood supply of experimental liver metastases. I. The distribution of hepatic artery and portal vein blood to "small" and "large" tumors. Surgery 66: 1067 1072

Adam R, Delvart V, Pascal G et al (2004) Rescue surgery for unresectable colorectal liver metastases downstaged by chemotherapy: a model to predict long-term survival. Ann Surgery 240:644–658

Adam R, Wicherts DA, de Haas RJ et al (2009) Patients with initially unresectable colorectal liver metastases: is there a possibility of cure? J Clin Oncol 27:1829–1835

Akinyemiju T, Abera S, Ahmed M et al (2017) The burden of primary liver cancer and underlying Etiologies from 1990 to 2015 at the Global, Regional, and National Level: Results From the Global Burden of Disease Study 2015. JAMA Oncol 3:1683–1691

Al-Adra DP, Gill RS, Axford SJ et al (2015) Treatment of unresectable intrahepatic cholangiocarcinoma with yttrium-90 radioembolization: a systematic review and pooled analysis. Eur J Surg Oncol 41:120–127

Alberts SR, Horvath WL, Sternfeld WC et al (2005) Oxaliplatin, fluouracil and leucovorin for patients with unresectable liver only metastases from colorectal cancer: a North Central Cancer Treatment Group phase II study. J Clin Oncol 23:2943–2949

Aloia TA, Adam R, Azoulay D et al (2006) Outcome following hepatic resection of metastatic renal tumors: the Paul Brousse Hospital experience. HPB (Oxford) 8:100–105

Bakalian S, Marshall JC, Logan P et al (2008) Molecular pathways mediating liver metastasis in patients with uveal melanoma. Clin Cancer Res 14:951–956

Ballarin R, Spaggiari M, Cautero N et al (2011) Pancreatic metastases from renal cell carcinoma: the state of the art. World J Gastroenterol 17:4747–4756

Bangash AK, Atassi B, Kaklamani V et al (2007) 90Y radioembolization of metastatic breast cancer to the liver: toxicity, imaging response, survival. J Vasc Interv Radiol 18:621–628

Benson AB 3rd, Geschwind JF, Mulcahy MF et al (2013) Radioembolisation for liver metastases: results from a prospective 151 patients multi-institutional phase II study. Eur J Cancer 49:3122–3130

Bester L, Meteling B, Pocock N et al (2012) Radioembolization versus standard care of hepatic metastases: comparative retrospective cohort study of survival outcomes and adverse events in salvage patients. J Vasc Interv Radiol 23:96–105

Bilbao JI, de Martino A, de Luis E et al (2009) Biocompatibility, inflammatory response, and recannalization characteristics of nonradioactive resin microspheres: histological findings. Cardiovasc Intervent Radiol 32:727–736

Boehm LM, Jayakrishnan TT, Miura JT et al (2015) Comparative effectiveness of hepatic artery based therapies for unresectable intrahepatic cholangiocarcinoma. J Surg Oncol 11:213–220

Bolondi L, Burroughs A, Dufour J-F et al (2013) Heterogeneity of patients with intermediate (BCLC B) hepatocellular carcinoma: proposal for a subclassification to facilitate treatment decisions. Semin Liver Dis 32:348–359

Bridgewater J, Galle PR, Khan SA et al (2014) Guidelines for the diagnosis and management of intrahepatic cholangiocarcinoma. J Hepatol 60:1268–1289

Camacho JC, Kokabi N, Xing M et al (2014) Evaluation Criteria in Solid Tumors and European Association for the Study of the liver criteria using delayed-phase imaging at an early time point predict survival in patients with unresectable intrahepatic cholangiocarcinoma following yttrium-90 radioembolization. J Vasc Interv Radiol 25:256–265

Cao C, Yan TD, Morris DL et al (2010) Radioembolization with yttrium-90 microspheres for pancreatic cancer liver metastases: results from a pilot study. Tumori 96:955–958

Cappelli A, Sangro P, Mosconi C et al (2019) Transarterial radioembolization in patients with hepatocellular carcinoma of intermediate B2 substage. Eur J Nucl Med Mol Imaging 46:661–668

Casadei Gardini A, Tamburini E, Iñarrairaegui M et al (2018) Radioembolization versus chemoembolization for unresectable hepatocellular carcinoma: a meta-analysis of randomized trials. Onco Targets Ther 11:7315–7321

Chen JX, Rose S, White SB et al (2017) Embolotherapy for neuroendocrine tumor liver metastases: prognostic factors for hepatic progression-free survival and overall survival. Cardiovasc Interv Radiol 40:69–80

Cheng AL, Kang YK, Chen Z et al (2009) Efficacy and safety of sorafenib in patients in the Asia-Pacific region with advanced hepatocellular carcinoma: a phase III randomised, double-blind, placebo-controlled trial. Lancet Oncol 10:25–34

Chiesa C, Maccauro M, Romito R et al (2011) Need, feasibility and convenience of dosimetric treatment planning in liver selective internal radiation therapy with (90)Y microspheres: the experience of the National Tumor Institute of Milan. Q J Nucl Med Mol Imaging 55:168–197

Chou FF, Sheen-Chen SM, Chen YS et al (1997) Surgical treatment of cholangiocarcinoma. Hepato-Gastroenterology 44:760–765

Chou FF, Nathan H, Pawlik TM, Wolfgang CL et al (2007) Trends in survival after surgery for cholangiocarcinoma: a 30-year population-based SEER Database analysis. J Gastrointest Surg 11:1488–1496

Chow PKH, Gandhi M, Tan SB et al (2018) SIRveNIB: selective internal radiation therapy versus sorafenib in Asia-Pacific patients with hepatocellular carcinoma. J Clin Oncol 36:1913–1921

Cianni R, Pelle G, Notarianni E et al (2013) Radioembolisation with (90)Y-labelled resin microspheres in the treatment of liver metastasis from breast cancer. Eur Radiol 23:182–189

Coldwell DM, Kennedy AS, Nutting CW (2007) Use of yttrium-90 microspheres in the treatment of unresectable hepatic metastases from breast cancer. Int J Radiat Oncol Biol Phys 69:800–804

Coldwell D, Sangro B, Wasan H et al (2011) General selection criteria of patients for radioembolization of liver tumors: an international working group report. Am J Clin Oncol 34:337–341

Cosimelli M, Golfieri R, Cagol PP et al (2010) Multicenter phase II clinical trial of yttrium-90 resin microspheres alone in unresectable, chemotherapy refractory colorectal liver metastases. Br J Cancer 103:324–331

Cosin O, Bilbao JI, Alvarez S et al (2007) Right gastric artery embolization prior to treatment with yttrium-90 microspheres. Cardiovasc Intervent Radiol 30:98–103

Cucchetti A, Cappelli A, Mosconi C et al (2017) Improving patient selection for selective internal radiation therapy of intra-hepatic cholangiocarcinoma: a meta-regression study. Liver Int 37:1056–1064

Cunningham D, Chau I, Stocken DD et al (2009) Phase III randomized comparison of gemcitabine versus gemcitabine plus capecitabine in patients with advanced pancreatic cancer. J Clin Oncol 27:5513–5518

Delaunoit T, Alberts SR, Sargent DJ et al (2005) Chemotherapy permits resection of metastatic colorectal cancer: experience from Intergroup N9741. Ann Oncol 16:425–429

Edeline J, Du FL, Rayar M et al (2015) Glass microspheres 90Y selective internal radiation therapy and chemotherapy as first-line treatment of intrahepatic cholangiocarcinoma. Clin Nucl Med 40:851–855

El Fouly A, Ertle J, El Dorry A et al (2015) In intermediate stage hepatocellular carcinoma: radioembolization with yttrium 90 or chemoembolization? Liver Int 35:627–635

Elf A-K, Andersson M, Henrikson O et al (2018) Radioembolization versus bland embolization for hepatic metastases from small intestinal neuroendocrine tumors: short-term results of a randomized clinical trial. World J Surg 42:506–513

European Association for the Study of the Liver (2018) EASL clinical practice guidelines: management of hepatocellular carcinoma. J Hepatol 69:182–236

Facciorusso A, Serviddio G, Muscatiello N (2016) Transarterial radioembolization vs chemoembolization for hepatocarcinoma patients: a systematic review and meta-analysis. World J Hepatol 8:770–778

Fidelman N, Kerlan RK, Hawkins RA et al (2016) Radioembolization with 90Y glass microspheres for the treatment of unresectable metastatic liver disease from chemotherapy- refractory gastrointestinal cancers: final report of a prospective pilot study. J Gastrointest Oncol 7:860–874

Forner A, Reig M, Bruix J (2018) Hepatocellular carcinoma. Lancet 391:1301–1314

Frilling A, Clift AK, Braat AJAT et al (2019) Radioembolisation with 90Y microspheres for neuroendocrine liver metastases: an institutional case series, systematic review and meta-analysis. HPB (Oxford) 21(7):773–783. https://doi.org/10.1016/j.hpb.2018.12.014

Gaba RC, Lewandowski RJ, Kulik LM et al (2009) Radiation lobectomy: preliminary findings of hepatic volumetric response to lobar yttrium-90 radioembolization. Ann Surg Oncol 16:1587–1596

Garin E, Rolland Y, Boucher L et al (2010) First experience of hepatic radioembolization using microspheres labelled with yttrium-90 (TheraSphere): practical aspects concerning its implementation. Eur J Nucl Med Mol Imaging 37:453–461

Ghaneh P, Kawesha A, Evans JD et al (2002) Molecular prognostic markers in pancreatic cancer. J Hepato-Biliary-Pancreat Surg 9:1–11

Golfieri R, Cappelli A, Cucchetti A et al (2011) Efficacy of selective transarterial chemoembolization in inducing tumor necrosis in small (<5 cm) hepatocellular carcinomas. Hepatology 53:1580–1589

Golfieri R, Renzulli M, Mosconi C et al (2013) Hepatocellular carcinoma responding to superselective transarterial chemoembolization: an issue of nodule dimension? J Vasc Interv Radiol 24:509–517

Golfieri R, Mosconi C, Cappelli A et al (2015a) Efficacy of radioembolization according to tumor morphology and portal vein thrombosis in intermediate-advanced hepatocellular carcinoma. Future Oncol 11:3133–3142

Golfieri R, Mosconi C, Giampalma E et al (2015b) Selective transarterial radioembolization of unresectable liverdominant colorectal cancer refractory to chemotherapy. Radiol Med 120:767–776

Golfieri R, Bargellini I, Spreafico C et al (2019) Patients with Barcelona clinic liver cancer Stages B and C hepatocellular carcinoma: time for a subclassification. Liver Cancer 8:78–91

Gonsalves CF, Eschelman DJ, Sullivan KL et al (2011) Radioembolization as salvage therapy for hepatic metastasis of uveal melanoma: a single-institution experience. AJR Am J Roentgenol 196:468–473

Gordon AC, Gabr A, Riaz A et al (2018) Radioembolization super survivors: extended survival in non-operative hepatocellular carcinoma. Cardiovasc Interv Radiol 41:1557–1565

Gray B, Van Hazel G, Hope M et al (2001) Randomised trial of SIR-spheres plus chemotherapy vs. chemo-

therapy alone for treating patients with liver metastases from primary large bowel cancer. Ann Oncol 12:1711–1720

Grothey A, Sargent D, Goldberg RM et al (2004) Survival of patients with advanced colorectal cancer improves with the availability of fluorouracilleucovorin, irinotecan and oxaliplatin in the course of treatment. J Clin Oncol 22:1209–1214

Gulec SA, Mesoloras G, Stabin M (2006) Dosimetric techniques in 90Y-microsphere therapy of liver cancer: the MIRD equations for dose calculations. J Nucl Med 47:1209–1211

Hamami ME, Poeppel TD, Muller S et al (2009) SPECT/CT with 99mTC-MAA in radioembolization with 90y microspheres in patients with hepatocellular cancer. J Nucl Med 50:688–692

Hoffmann RT, Paprottka PM, Schön A et al (2012) Transarterial hepatic yttrium-90 radioembolization in patients with unresectable intrahepatic cholangiocarcinoma: factors associated with prolonged survival. Cardiovasc Intervent Radiol 35:105–116

Iavarone M, Cabibbo G, Piscaglia F et al (2011) Field-practice study of sorafenib therapy for hepatocellular carcinoma: a prospective multicenter study in Italy. Hepatology 54:2055–2063

Ibrahim SM, Mulcahy MF, Lewandowski RJ et al (2008) Treatment of unresectable cholangiocarcinoma using yttrium-90 microspheres: results from a pilot study. Cancer 113:2119–2128

Jakobs TF, Saleem S, Atassi B et al (2008) Fibrosis, portal hypertension, and hepatic volume changes induced by intraarterial radiotherapy with (90)Yttrium microspheres. Dig Dis Sci 53:2556–2563

Jemal A, Thomas A, Murray T et al (2002) Cancer statistics, 2002. CA Cancer J Clin 52:23–47

Kennedy A, Nag S, Salem R et al (2007) Recommendations for radioembolization of hepatic malignancies using yttrium-90 microsphere brachytherapy: a consensus panel report from the Radioembolization Brachytherapy Oncology Consortium (REBOC). Int J Radiat Oncol Biol Phys 68:13–23

Kennedy A, Coldwell D, Sangro B et al (2012) Radioembolization for the treatment of liver tumors general principles. Am J Clin Oncol 35:91–99

Kim JH, Won HJ, Shin YM et al (2011) Radiofrequency ablation for the treatment of primary intrahepatic cholangiocarcinoma. AJR Am J Roentgenol 196:W205–W209

Kim DY, Ryu HJ, Choi JY et al (2012) Radiological response predicts survival following transarterial chemoembolisation in patients with unresectable hepatocellular carcinoma. Aliment Pharmacol Ther 35:1343–1350

Kim HS, Shaib WL, Zhang C et al (2018) Phase 1b study of pasireotide, everolimus, and selective internal radioembolization therapy for unresectable neuroendocrine tumors with hepatic metastases. Cancer 124:1992–2000

Kokudo T, Hasegawa K, Matsuyama Y et al (2016) Survival benefit of liver resection for hepatocellular carcinoma associated with portal vein invasion. J Hepatol 65:938–943

Kulik LM, Carr BI, Mulcahy MF et al (2008) Safety and efficacy of 90Y radiotherapy for hepatocellular carcinoma with and without portal vein thrombosis. Hepatology 47:71–81

Lance C, McLennan G, Obuchowski N et al (2011) Comparative analysis of the safety and efficacy of transcatheter arterial chemoembolization and yttrium-90 radioembolization in patients with unresectable hepatocellular carcinoma. J Vasc Interv Radiol 22:1697–1705

Leung TW, Lau WY, Ho SK et al (1995) Radiation pneumonitis after selective internal radiation treatment with intraarterial 90yttrium-microspheres for inoperable hepatic tumors. Int J Radiat Oncol Biol Phys 33:919–924

Lewandowski RJ, Kulik LM, Riaz A et al (2009) A comparative analysis of transarterial downstaging for hepatocellular carcinoma: chemoembolization versus radioembolization. Am J Transplant 9:1920–1928

Llovet JM, Bruix J (2003) Systematic review of randomized trials for unresectable hepatocellular carcinoma: chemoembolization improves survival. Hepatology 37:429–442

Llovet JM, Finn RS (2018) Negative phase 3 study of (90)Y microspheres versus sorafenib in HCC. Lancet Oncol 19:e69

Llovet JM, Ricci S, Mazzaferro V et al (2008) Sorafenib in advanced hepatocellular carcinoma. N Engl J Med 359:378–390

Lobo L, Yakoub D, Picado O et al (2016) Unresectable hepatocellular carcinoma: radioembolization versus chemoembolization: a systematic review and meta-analysis. Cardiovasc Interv Radiol 39:1580–1588

Ludwig JM, Ambinder EM, Ghodadra A et al (2016) Lung shunt fraction prior to yttrium-90 radioembolization predicts survival in patients with neuroendocrine liver metastases: single- center prospective analysis. Cardiovasc Interv Radiol 39:1007–1014

Maawy AA, Rose SC, Clary B (2016) Use of yttrium-90 radioembolization for management of colorectal liver metastases. Curr Colorectal Cancer Rep 12:226–231

Mackie S, de Silva S, Aslan P et al (2011) Super selective radio embolization of the porcine kidney with 90yttrium resin microspheres: a feasibility, safety and dose ranging study. J Urol 185:285–290

Markovic SN, Erickson LA, Rao RD et al (2007) Malignant melanoma in the 21st century, part 1: epidemiology, risk factors, screening, prevention, and diagnosis. Mayo Clin Proc 82:364–380

Mazzaferro V, Sposito C, Bhoori S et al (2013) Yttrium-90 radioembolization for intermediate-advanced hepatocellular carcinoma: a phase 2 study. Hepatology 57:1826–1837

McKay RR, Kroeger N, Xie W et al (2014) Impact of bone and liver metastases on patients with renal cell carcinoma treated with targeted therapy. Eur Urol 65:577–584

Memon K, Lewandowski RJ, Kulik L et al (2011) Radioembolization for primary and metastatic liver cancer. Semin Radiat Oncol 21:294–302

Memon K, Lewandowski RJ, Mulcahy MF et al (2012) Radioembolization for neuroendocrine liver metastases: safety, imaging, and long-term outcomes. Int J Radiat Oncol 83:887–894

Memon K, Kulik L, Lewandowski RJ et al (2013) Radioembolization for hepatocellular carcinoma with portal vein thrombosis: impact of liver function on systemic treatment options at disease progression. J Hepatol 58:73–80

Michl M, Haug AR, Jakobs TF et al (2014) Radioembolization with yttrium-90 microspheres (SIRT) in pancreatic cancer patients with liver metastases: efficacy, safety and prognostic factors. Oncology 86:24–32

Moreno-Luna LE, Yang JD, Sanchez W et al (2013) Efficacy and safety of transarterial radioembolization versus chemoembolization in patients with hepatocellular carcinoma. Cardiovasc Intervent Radiol 36:714–723

Mosconi C, Gramenzi A, Ascanio S et al (2016) Yttrium-90 radioembolization for unresectable/recurrent intrahepatic cholangiocarcinoma: a survival, efficacy and safety study. Br J Cancer 115:297–302

Mosconi C, Cucchetti A, Pettinato C et al (2018) Validation of response to yttrium-90 radioembolization for hepatocellular carcinoma with portal vein invasion. J Hepatol 69:259–260

Mouli S, Memon K, Baker T et al (2013) Yttrium-90 radioembolization for intrahepatic cholangiocarcinoma: safety, response, and survival analysis. J Vasc Interv Radiol 24:1227–1234

National Cancer Institute. Surveillance, Epidemiology, and End Results Program. Cancer Statistics. National Cancer Institute. Surveillance, Epidemiology, and End Results Program (updated 2016). Available from: http://seer.cancer.gov/statfacts/html/colorect.html

Okuda K, Ohnishi K, Kimura K et al (1985) Incidence of portal vein thrombosis in liver cirrhosis. An angiographic study in 708 patients. Gastroenterology 89:279–286

Purushotham A, Shamil E, Cariati M et al (2014) Age at diagnosis and distant metastasis in breast cancer—a surprising inverse relationship. Eur J Cancer 50:1697–1705

Rafi S, Piduru SM, El-Rayes B et al (2013) Yttrium-90 radioembolization for unresectable standard-chemorefractory intrahepatic cholangiocarcinoma: survival, efficacy, and safety study. Cardiovasc Intervent Radiol 36:440–448

Riaz A, Kulik L, Lewandowski RJ et al (2009a) Radiologic–pathologic correlation of hepatocellular carcinoma treated with internal radiation using yttrium–90 microspheres. Hepatology 49:1185–1193

Riaz A, Lewandowski RJ, Kulik LM et al (2009b) Complications following radioembolization with yttrium-90 microspheres: a comprehensive literature review. J Vasc Interv Radiol 20:1121–1130

Roayaie S, Guarrera JV, Ye MQ et al (1998) Aggressive surgical treatment of intrahepatic cholangiocarcinoma: predictors of outcomes. J Am Coll Surg 187:365–372

Rognoni C, Ciani O, Sommariva S et al (2016) Transarterial radioembolization in intermediate-advanced hepatocellular carcinoma: systematic review and meta-analyses. Oncotarget 7:72343–72355

Ruers T, Van Coevorden F, Punt CJ et al (2017) Local treatment of Unresectable colorectal liver metastases: results of randomized phase II trial. J Natl Cancer Inst 109(9):djx015. https://doi.org/10.1093/jnci/djx015

Salem R, Lewandowski R, Roberts C et al (2004) A. use of yttrium-90 glass microspheres (TheraSphere) for the treatment of unresectable hepatocellular carcinoma in patients with portal vein thrombosis. J Vasc Interv Radiol 15:335–345

Salem R, Lewandowski RJ, Mulcahy MF et al (2010) Radioembolization for hepatocellular carcinoma using yttrium-90 microspheres: a comprehensive report of long-term outcomes. Gastroenterology 138:52–64

Salem R, Lewandowski RJ, Kulik L et al (2011) Radioembolization results in longer time-to-progression and reduced toxicity compared with chemoembolization in patients with hepatocellular carcinoma. Gastroenterology 140:497–507

Salem R, Gordon AC, Mouli S et al (2016) Y90 radioembolization significantly prolongs time to progression compared with chemoembolization in patients with hepatocellular carcinoma. Gastroenterology 151:1155–1163

Sangro B, Gil-Alzugaray B, Rodriguez J et al (2008) Liver disease induced by radioembolization of liver tumors: description and possible risk factors. Cancer 112:1538–1546

Sangro B, Carpanese L, Cianni R et al (2011) Network on radioembolization with yttrium-90 resin microspheres (ENRY). Survival after yttrium-90 resin microsphere radioembolization of hepatocellular carcinoma across Barcelona clinic liver cancer stages: a European evaluation. Hepatology 54:868–878

Sangro B, Iñarrairaegui M, Bilbao JI (2012) Radioembolization for hepatocellular carcinoma. J Hepatol 56:464–473. http://www.ncbi.nlm.nih.gov/pubmed/21816126

Saxena A, Bester L, Chua TC et al (2010a) Yttrium-90 radiotherapy for unresectable intrahepatic cholangiocarcinoma: a preliminary assessment of this novel treatment option. Ann Surg Oncol 17:484–491

Saxena A, Chua TC, Bester L et al (2010b) Factors predicting response and survival after yttrium-90 radioembolization of unresectable neuroendocrine tumor liver metastases. Ann Surg 251:910–916

Saxena A, Bester L, Shan L et al (2014) A systematic review on the safety and efficacy of yttrium-90 radioembolization for unresectable, chemorefractory colorectal cancer liver metastases. J Cancer Res Clin Oncol 140:537–547

Schelhorn J, Best J, Reinboldt MP et al (2015) Does diffusion-weighted imaging improve therapy response evaluation in patients with hepatocellular carcinoma after radioembolization? Comparison of MRI using Gd-EOB-DTPA with and without DWI. J Magn Reson Imaging 42:818–827

Schindl M, Gruenberger T, Längle F (2002) Current strategies in the treatment of colorectal cancer liver metastases: aspects of surgical treatment. Eu Surg 34:332–336

Seidensticker R, Denecke T, Kraus P et al (2012) Matched-pair comparison of radioembolization plus best supportive care versus best supportive care alone for chemotherapy refractory liver-dominant colorectal metastases. Cardiovasc Intervent Radiol 35:1066–1073

Siegel R, Ma J, Zou Z et al (2014) Cancer statistics, 2014. CA Cancer J Clin 64:9–29

Sirtex Medical Limited. Sirtex medical training manual, training program physicians and institutions. Australia. Available at: http://www.sirtex.com/usa/_data/page/549/TRN-US-0320for20US1.pdf. Accessed October 16, 2007

Sotocleous CT, Violari EG, Sotirchos VS et al (2015) Radioembolization as a salvage therapy for heavily pretreated patients with colorectal cancer liver metastases: factors that affect outcomes. Clin Colorectal Cancer 14:296–305

Sposito C, Mazzaferro V (2018) The SIRveNIB and SARAH trials, radioembolization vs. sorafenib in advanced HCC patients: reasons for a failure, and perspectives for the future. HepatoBiliary Surg Nutr 7:487–489

Spreafico C, Sposito C, Vaiani M et al (2018) Development of a prognostic score to predict response to yttrium-90 radioembolization for hepatocellular carcinoma with portal vein invasion. J Hepatol 68:724–732

Strigari L, Sciuto R, Rea S et al (2010) Efficacy and toxicity related to treatment of hepatocellular carcinoma with 90Y-SIR spheres: radiobiologic considerations. J Nucl Med 51:1377–1385

Takayasu K, Arii S, Kudo M et al (2012) Superselective transarterial chemoembolization for hepatocellular carcinoma: validation of treatment algorithm proposed by Japanese guidelines. J Hepatol 56:886–892

Tie J, Yip D, Dowling R et al (2010) Radioembolization and systemic chemotherapy in patients with hepatic metastases from primary colorectal cancer. Ann Oncol 21:Abs.698

Townsend AR, Chong LC, Karapetis C et al (2016) Selective internal radiation therapy for liver metastases from colorectal cancer. Cancer Treat Rev 50:148–154

Valle J, Wasan H, Palmer DH et al (2010) ABC-02 Trial Investigators. Cisplatin plus gemcitabine vs. gemcitabine for biliary tract cancer. N Engl J Med 362:1273–1281

Van Hazel G, Blackwell A, Anderson J et al (2004) Randomised phase 2 trial of SIR-spheres plus fluorouracil/leucovorin chemotherapy versus fluorouracil/leucovorin chemotherapy alone in advanced colorectal cancer. J Surg Oncol 88:78–85

Vilgrain V, Pereira H, Assenat E et al (2017) Efficacy and safety of selective internal radiotherapy with yttrium-90 resin microspheres compared with Sorafenib in Locally Advanced and Inoperable Hepatocellular Carcinoma (SARAH): an open-label randomised controlled Phase 3 Trial. Lancet Oncol 18:1624–1636

Wasan HS, Gibbs P, Sharma NK et al (2017) First-line selective internal radiotherapy plus chemotherapy versus chemotherapy alone in patients with liver metastases from colorectal cancer (FOXFIRE, SIRFLOX, and FOXFIRE-Global): a combined analysis of three multicentre, randomised, phase 3 trials. Lancet Oncol 18:1159–1171

Wright CL, Werner JD, Tran JM et al (2012) Radiation pneumonitis following yttrium90 radioembolization: case report and literature review. J Vasc Interv Radiol 23:669–674

Yang JD, Kim B, Sanderson SO et al (2012) Biliary tract cancers in Olmsted County, Minnesota, 1976–2008. Am J Gastroenterol 107:1256–1262

Zacharias AJ, Jayakrishnan TT, Rajeev R et al (2015) Comparative effectiveness of hepatic artery based therapies for unresectable colorectal liver metastases: a meta-analysis. PLoS One 10:e0139940

Imaging of Treated Liver Tumors and Assessment of Tumor Response to Cytostatic Therapy and Post-Treatment Changes in the Liver

Silvia Brocco, Anna Sara Fraia, Anna Florio, and Emilio Quaia

Contents

Abstract

Liver represents a common site of metastatic spread of epithelial cancers, especially from the gastrointestinal tract, breast and lung, and a focus of primary hepatic tumors, including hepatocellular carcinoma (HCC), cholangiocarcinoma, and rare tumors such as angiosarcoma or hemangioendothelioma. Nowadays, the treatment of primary or metastatic liver lesions may count on a variety of therapeutic alternatives to surgery, such as new anticancer drugs and interventional-radiological procedures for tumor ablation. Imaging assessment remains the milestone to evaluate the tumor response to any kind of therapy, but these new locoregional treatments can lead to change in imaging that makes very challenging to identify residual or recurrent disease.

1 Choice of Tumor Treatment and Response Evaluation Criteria

A wide range of percutaneous ablation techniques is available to treat both primary liver tumors and hepatic metastases. The choice of the most suitable therapeutic procedure for each

S. Brocco · A. S. Fraia · A. Florio · E. Quaia (✉)
Radiology Unit, Department of Medicine - DIMED, University of Padova, Padova, Italy
e-mail: emilio.quaia@unipd.it

© Springer Nature Switzerland AG 2021
E. Quaia (ed.), *Imaging of the Liver and Intra-hepatic Biliary Tract*,
Medical Radiology Diagnostic Imaging, https://doi.org/10.1007/978-3-030-39021-1_15

patient often considers not only the features of the tumor but also the performance status of the patient and the liver function.

Percutaneous ablation of liver metastases is applied to patients who cannot undergo surgical resection and is much more effective for lesions smaller than 3 cm, in particular, if they are solitary lesions. In this case, outcomes can be compared with surgical resection (Kim et al. 2011).

Hepatocellular carcinoma (HCC) has an even more complex therapeutic approach. According to EASL guidelines on the treatment of HCC, patients are stratified in several stages following BCLC classification. This classification povides a prognostic indication and is focused to guide the treatment for each stage. The different stages include the features of the tumor, the number of HCC nodules and their size, their intra- and extrahepatic vascular spread and presence of vascular invasion, the liver function that is assessed by Child-Pugh score and the presence of general symptoms related to a neoplastic disease affecting the patient's performance status (Fig. 1a) (Galle et al. 2018).

A correct evaluation of therapy efficacy and consequently of post-therapeutic changes in tumor viability and vascularization is mandatory to guide the correct management of the patients (Memon et al. 2011). Usually, in clinical practice, the criteria used to determine tumor response to therapy are based on the size of treated nodules. These imaging criteria (WHO criteria, RECIST 1.0, and RECIST 1.1) are applicable le to describe tumor response to cytotoxic chemotherapies (Lencioni and Llovet 2010).

Instead, locoregional therapies, creating areas of necrosis and hemorrhage, may confer stability to tumor size or even a size increase after therapy. This peculiar feature limits the role of criteria based only on the size of the tumor to assess therapy response (Atassi et al. 2008; Horger et al. 2009). Thus, in liver treated with percutaneous techniques, it is fundamental to use other characteristics of the treated lesion together with the standard measurement guidelines based on size (Forner et al. 2009). This is true also for molecular targeted systemic therapies. These therapies affect tumor angiogenesis or cell signaling leading to apoptosis and cell death that can vary the morphology of the tumor but not its size.

For this reason, quantitative and functional criteria that are specific for tumor type and therapy have been developed. In 2000 and 2010 respectively EASL criteria, and a modified RECIST (mRECIST) system for liver tumors treated with locoregional therapies were proposed (Lencioni and Llovet 2010). EASL criteria consider not the size of the whole treated lesion but only the residual viable tissue that is represented by the tissue that enhances during the arterial phase in a treated HCC. This system gives a bidimensional measurement of the viable tumor considering the two longest diameters of the enhancing area.

mRECIST system gives unidimensional measurement considering the longest diameter of the enhancing part of HCC (Lencioni and Llovet 2010). In both systems, the viable tissue of a treated HCC is assessed in the arterial phase on CECT or CEMRI and must be measured avoiding necrotic areas.

According to mRECIST for HCC complete response (CR) corresponds to the disappearance of any intratumoral arterial enhancement in all target lesions; partial response (PR) corresponds to at least a 30% decrease in the sum of diameters of viable (contrast enhancement in the arterial phase) target lesions, taking as reference the baseline sum of the diameters of target lesions; progressive disease (PD) corresponds to increase of at least 20% in the sum of the diameters of viable (enhancing) target lesions, taking as reference the smallest sum of the diameters of viable (enhancing) target lesions recorded since the treatment started, or newly detected hepatic nodule(s) with longest diameter ≥1 cm and typical vascular pattern of HCC on dynamic imaging (hypervascularization in the arterial phase with washout in the portal venous or late venous phase) or liver lesions >1 cm that do not show a typical vascular pattern but with evidence of at least 1-cm-interval growth in subsequent scans; stable disease (SD) corresponds to any cases that do not qualify for either partial response or progressive disease (Lencioni and Llovet 2010) (Fig. 1b).

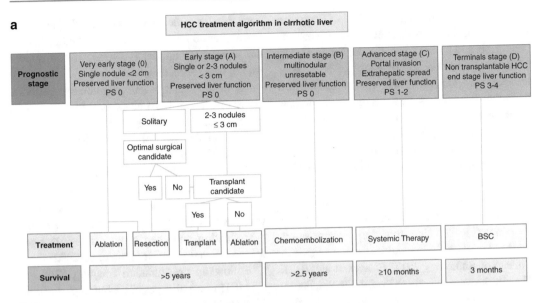

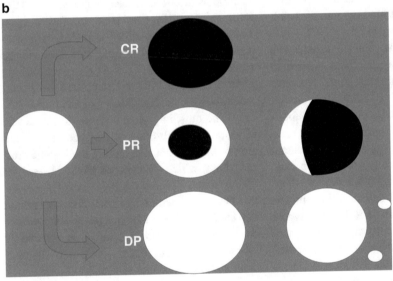

Fig. 1 (**a**) Diagram shows the modified BCLC staging system for hepatocellular carcinoma and the various treatment options related to its stages. Preserved liver function refers to patients with Child-Pugh A and without ascites. Optimal surgical candidate is a patient with expected perioperative mortality less than 3% and mortality less than 20% estimated on the basis of the presence of a compensated Child-Pugh class A cirrhosis with MELD score less than 10, the grade of portal hypertension and functional remaining liver parenchyma after surgery and the possibility to perform a mini-invasive surgical approach. Systemic therapy includes sorafenib as the first-line treatment and regorafenib as a second-line treatment, used when progression under sorafenib is detected. Other non-first-line possibilities include lenvatinib, cabozantinib, nivolumab. (From Galle et al. 2018, EASL Clinical Practice Guidelines: Management of hepatocellular carcinoma). (**b**) Diagram showing the modified RECIST (mRECIST criteria). Complete response (CR): disappearance of any intratumoral arterial enhancement in all target lesions; partial response (PR): at least a 30% decrease in the sum of diameters of viable (contrast enhancement in the arterial phase) target lesions, taking as reference the baseline sum of the diameters of target lesions; progressive disease (PD): increase of at least 20% in the sum of the diameters of viable (enhancing) target lesions, taking as reference the smallest sum of the diameters of viable (enhancing) target lesions recorded since the treatment started, or newly detected hepatic nodule(s) with longest diameter ≥ 1 cm and typical vascular pattern of HCC on dynamic imaging (hypervascularization in the arterial phase with washout in the portal venous or late venous phase) or liver lesions >1 cm that do not show a typical vascular pattern but with evidence of at least 1-cm-interval growth in subsequent scans; stable disease (SD): any cases that do not qualify for either partial response or progressive disease

Another classification, RECICL (Response Evaluation Criteria in Cancer of the Liver) has been proposed by the Liver Cancer Study Group of Japan to evaluate the response of HCC after locoregional therapies and molecular-targeted therapies. It considers the areas of tumor necrosis incorporating the ablation margins, suggests a correct timing for evaluation for every treatment strategy, and includes evaluation of tumor markers to assess the prognosis (Kudo et al. 2010).

Similarly to the modified Response Evaluation Criteria in Solid Tumors (mRECIST), the Liver Imaging Reporting and Data System Treatment Response (LR-TR) algorithm clarify tumor status at the level of individual lesions (American College of Radiology 2017; Elsayes et al. 2017). These lesions are categorized as LR-TR Nonviable, Equivocal, or Viable according to their imaging features. The LR-TR algorithm presents high predictive value for the viability of treated HCC. HCC nodule(s) may be assessed as viable—lesions with nodular, mass-like, or irregular thick enhancing viable tissue showing arterial phase hyperenhancement, portal venous or later phase washout, and/or enhancement similar to that before embolization—or nonviable—no intra lesional enhancement or treatment-specific expected enhancement pattern. However, LR-TR algorithm shows clear limitations since a substantial proportion of embolized lesions could not be definitively characterized and fall into the LR-TR equivocal category—lesions with indeterminate enhancement and which do not meet criteria for being probably or definitely viable (Shropshire et al. 2019) or those lesions which were incompletely necrotic at the histopathologic examination.

2 Imaging Post Percutaneous Ablation Therapies

Percutaneous ablation therapies induce in the treated liver parenchyma a region of coagulative necrosis that is called the ablation zone. This area must be at least 5–10 mm larger than the original tumor size, thus allowing the ablation of small satellite nodules and reducing the risk of tumor progression or relapse. The shape of the ablated zone can vary depending on the choice of the thermal or non thermal ablation technique and on the number of applicators used. It can appear round, oval, or rectangular.

In the peri-ablative and post-ablative period, a series of changes must be expected in the treated zone. These changes must be known to perform a correct evaluation of the tumor treatment response (Lee et al. 2016).

In the immediate post-ablation time, around the ablation area appears a zone of hyperemia because tissue injury evokes an inflammatory reaction that is evident in the first 3–6 months post-ablation and then progressively decreases during the first year (Dromain et al. 2002).

Follow up post-ablation imaging (CECT or CEMRI) is usually performed at 1, 3, 6, 9, and 12 months after the procedure (Lee et al. 2016; Kudo et al. 2010) considered the follow-up at 3 months the most suitable for the response evaluation when treatment does not need to be repeated.

CECT and CEMRI represent the most useful modalities for the assessment of treatment efficacy. The most important criterion to assess this efficacy is the absence of enhancement in the area of induced necrosis during the hepatic arterial phase, which corresponds to the absence of viable tumor. Some authors described a correlation between the size of the non-enhancing region depicted on CT and MR images and the size of coagulative necrosis measured at histologic examination within a range of 2 mm (Solbiati et al. 1997; Goldberg et al. 2000).

2.1 CT Findings

Immediately after the procedure, on unenhanced CT the ablated zone appears heterogeneously hypodense. This heterogenicity is due to hyperdense material representing hemorrhagic and fresh coagulative necrosis and carbonization products, whose presence is normally in small amount (Fig. 2). Over time the treated area becomes uniformly hypodense (Lee et al. 2016).

The inflammatory reaction and the presence of granulation tissue appear as a uniform, peripheral enhancement in the arterial phase and measure usually less than 1 mm.

In the immediate post-ablation period, this peripheral enhancement may sometimes be thicker and irregular. However, it must always be less than 5 mm and its persistence on portal venous phase imaging is fundamental. Its thick-

ness must also decrease and disappear with time (Goldberg et al. 2000; Livraghi et al. 1997). Yaghmai et al. described this rim in 89% of cases at 1 month, 56% at 1–3 months, and 22% at 3–6 months (Yaghmai et al. 2011) (Figs. 3 and 4).

These features can create confusion because of the overlap with disease progression repre-

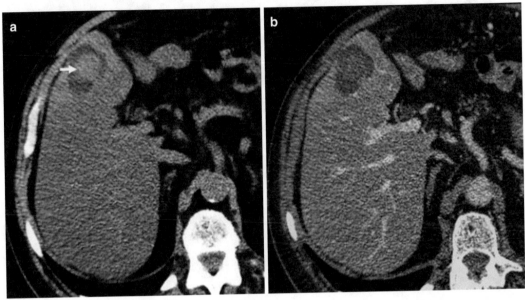

Fig. 2 60 years old man with cirrhosis (**a, b**). Immediately after the procedure, on unenhanced CT (**a**) the ablated zone appears heterogeneously hypodense and centrally hyperdense. This heterogenicity is due to hyperdense material representing hemorrhagic and fresh coagulative necrosis and carbonization products. Over time (**b**) the treated area becomes uniformly hypodense

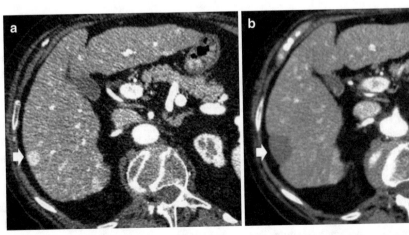

Fig. 3 62 years old man with cirrhosis. Complete response after thermal ablation in a patient with HCC. (**a, b**) CT scan on arterial phase before thermal ablation (**a**) and 30 days after microwave ablation (**b**). Hypodense treated area is evident (white arrow). These findings are consistent with complete response according to mRECIST criteria

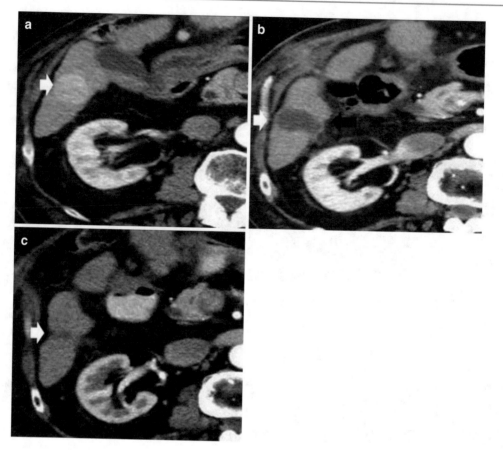

Fig. 4 55 years old man with cirrhosis. Complete response after thermal ablation in a patient with HCC. (**a**) CT scan on arterial phase before thermal ablation (**a**), 30 days and 6 months (**c**) after microwave thermal abla-tion (**b**). Hypodense treated area is evident (white arrow) with progressive shrinkage 6 months after treatment. These findings are consistent with complete response according to mRECIST criteria

sented by residual unablated tumor or local tumor progression.

These two disease progression patterns must be distinguished because they have different treatments. Residual unablated tumor is a tumor not treated during the ablating session that remains along the ablation margins. Local tumor progression is represented by tumor arising from the periphery of an ablation zone in an area previously without viable tissue (Ahmed et al. 2014).

Residual unablated tumor usually is treated with a new ablation, while in local tumor progres-sion other alternative therapies should be considered.

Unablated tumor or tumor progression mani-fest as a thick peripheral enhancement usually >5 mm, nodular and eccentric enhancing on arte-rial phase with or without wash-out on the portal or delayed phase (Figs. 5, 6, 7, and 8). The timing of visualization of these two different types of tumoral persistence is different (Smith and Gillams 2008; Brennan and Ahmed 2013). The first follow-up scan can show the residual unab-lated tumor that is always present at this time. Sometimes it cannot be recognized due to paren-chymal changes peripheral to the ablation area and can be seen only observing retrospectively the follow-up scans. In particular, thick nodular enhancement that persists in time indicates unab-lated tumor.

Local tumor progression has similar features but is evidenced later in the follow-up, along the ablation margin and in a zone that previously

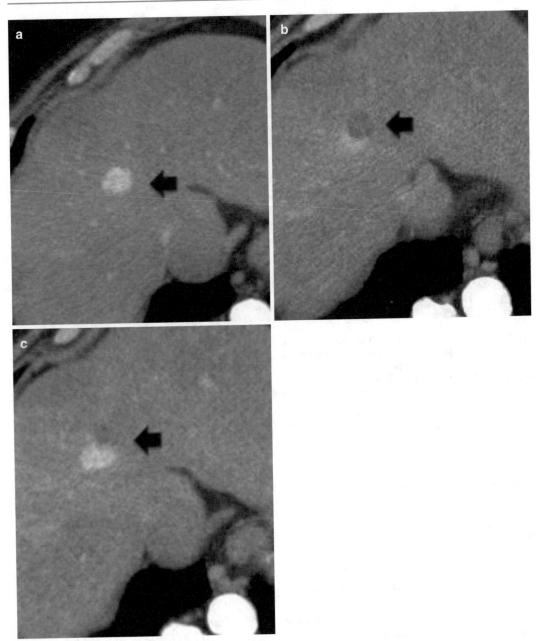

Fig. 5 (**a–c**) 70 years old man with cirrhosis and small HCC. Disease progression after thermal ablation. (**a**) CT scan on hepatic arterial phase before thermal ablation (**a**), 30 days (**b**) and 6 months (**c**) after microwave thermal ablation (**b**). Peripheral enhancing residual tumor is evident 30 days after treatment (**b**) with progressive increase in the enhancing tumor diameter as long as at 6 months disease progression is clearly evident (**c**)

demonstrated an absence of viable tissue (Lee et al. 2016). Specific attention must be paid to those ablated zones located near a blood vessel that is larger than 3 mm in diameter. It is common to visualize residual disease in this area due to an incomplete ablation linked to the phenomenon resulting from a "heat sink" effect (Lu et al. 2003). Tumoral seeding along the needle track is rare (Fig. 7). In a large metanalysis, it occurs only in 0.2% of cases (Mulier et al. 2002).

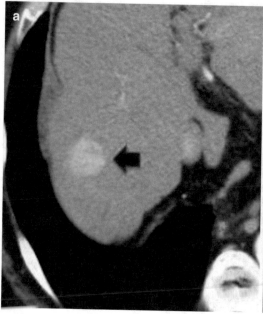
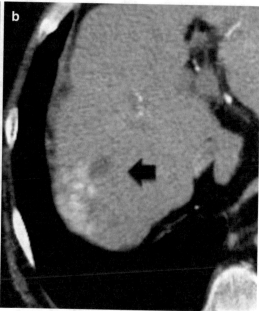
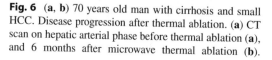

Fig. 6 (**a, b**) 70 years old man with cirrhosis and small HCC. Disease progression after thermal ablation. (**a**) CT scan on hepatic arterial phase before thermal ablation (**a**), and 6 months after microwave thermal ablation (**b**).

Multiple enhancing nodules (arrow) are evident peripherally to the ablation region in keeping with disease progression

After percutaneous ablation, the foci of air within the ablation zone can be seen in the peri-ablative period and up to 1 month after treatment or even later but their extension must be decreased (Lee et al. 2016).

2.2 MRI Findings

Contrast-enhanced magnetic resonance imaging (CE-MRI) together with CE-CT is a gold standard method to study patients after percutaneous ablation treatments. Arterial is the fundamental phase to assess the outcome of ablation therapies both at CE-CT and CE-MRI imaging.

Extracellular contrast agents are preferred to hepatocyte-specific contrast agents in MR imaging follow up after ablation of HCC. Hepatobiliary specific agents are taken up only by normal hepatocytes. In the detection of liver malignancies, both metastatic and primary HCCs will appear hypointense relative to background parenchymal uptake during the hepatobiliary phase. In this setting, MRI with hepatobiliary specific agents show a higher ability to detect new lesions (Ahn et al. 2010; Lee et al. 2015). However after percutaneous ablation treatments, the arterial phase is less intense after hepato-specific contrast agent injection due to the early uptake of the contrast agents in the hepatocytes that produce a rapid enhancement of the liver parenchyma and contemporary early reduction of vessel enhancement. This phenomenon makes the residual arterial phase enhancement in the treated lesion more difficult to detect (Vogl et al. 1996; Goodwin et al. 2011).

The features of the treated areas change over time due to the degradation of blood products. In the first 1 to 3 months after the procedure, at unenhanced MRI the ablation zone appears heterogeneously hyperintense in T1-w sequences and hypointense in T2-w sequences. The T1 hyperintensity depends on the presence of hemorrhage and coagulative necrosis expected after the treatment. Even with MR imaging, small foci of air may be seen in this period. They must be distinguished from the superinfection of the ablated zone if in conjunction with the presence

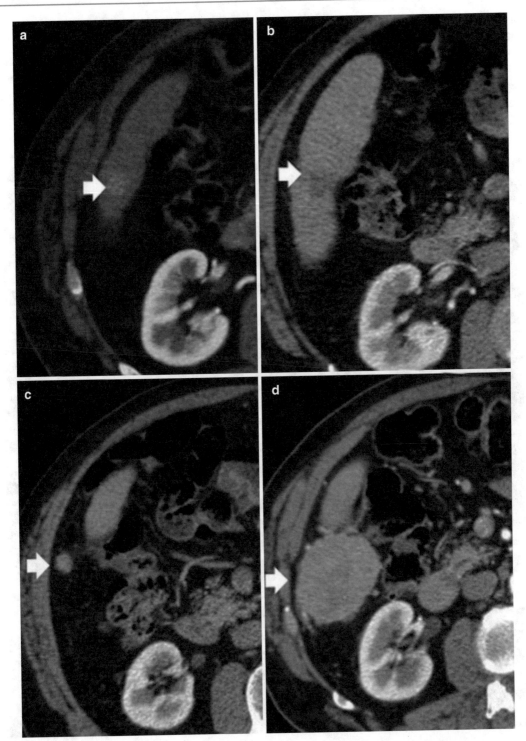

Fig. 7 (**a–d**) 68 years old man with cirrhosis and small HCC. Disease progression after thermal ablation. (**a**) CT scan on arterial phase before ablation showing one small arterially enhancing HCC nodule (arrow); (**b**) apparent complete response 30 days after thermal ablation; (**c**) evidence of one small extrahepatic nodule (arrow) adjacent to the treated liver area, along the needle track, 3 months after thermal ablation; (**d**) the same nodule presents a clear increase in dimension 6 months after thermal ablation in keeping with disease progression due to tumoral seeding along needle track after thermal ablation

of air, other systemic symptoms and signs are present including abdominal pain, fever, and leukocytosis (Lee et al. 2016).

The presence of a uniform hypointensity together with the absence of residual arterial enhancement at contrast-enhanced MRI sequences at 2–3 months within the ablated zone indicates the efficacy of the treatment.

Peripheral enhancement surrounding the zone of ablation due to inflammatory changes is evident in the arterial phase and persist in later phases, as in CT imaging (Dromain et al. 2002).

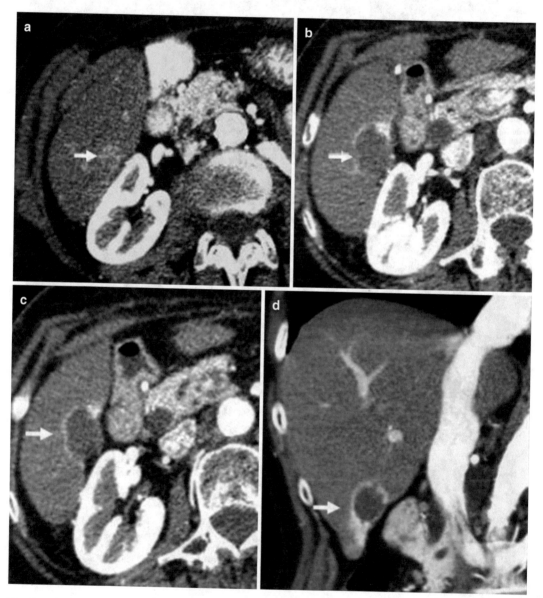

Fig. 8 (a–e) 70 years old man with cirrhosis and small HCC. Complete response after thermal ablation simulating disease progression on the transverse plane. (a) CT scan on arterial phase before thermal ablation treatment showing one enhancing nodule on the sixth liver segment; (b, c) CT scan on arterial phase 30 days after thermal showing peripheral enhancement simulating disease persistence. (d, e) Coronal reformats show that peripheral enhancement presents a wedge shape with a capsular base and is related to transient hepatic attenuation differences (THAD)

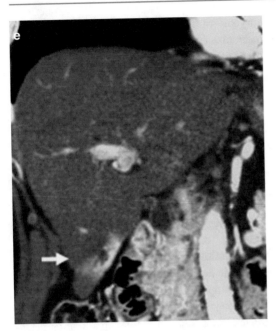

Fig. 8 (continued)

At 3 months follow-up, the ablated zone starts to decrease in size. A peripheral enhancement surrounding the zone of ablation can still be present on contrast-enhanced MRI sequences, but it must be thin and uniform. Sometimes persistence of small foci of T1 hyperintensity and heterogeneous T2 signal in the ablated zone can be seen (Lee et al. 2016). Hyperintense intra tumoral areas on T1-w MRI sequences may be due to hemorrhage or even presence of arterial enhancement in residual tumor. Subtraction T1-w MR images can distinguish the two cases.

On late follow-up in a period between 6 and 12 months after the ablation procedure, in pre-contrast sequences, the ablation zone appears iso-hypointense in T1-w and hypointense in T2-w MRI sequences due to thermal injury derived dehydration. At this time high hyperintensity on T2-w MRI sequences can indicate an evolution in liquefactive necrosis or biloma formation. Moderate T2 hyperintensity, less intense than fluid signal, can represent residual tumor. The ablation zone may contract in size with time due to the formation of scar tissue (Dromain et al. 2002). The thin and peripheral arterial enhancement surrounding the zone of ablation, sometimes persisting in later phases, should disappear at 12 months follow up with a concomitant decrease in the size of the area of ablation (Lee et al. 2016).

2.3 CEUS

Necrotic and remaining viable tumor tissue after treatment may have a similar appearance at US due to their similar echogenicity. The use of an ultrasound microbubble contrast agent that can clearly depict tumor vascularity provides the opportunity of a real-time imaging technique that plays an important role in the management of patients treated by ablation for malignant tumors (Wilson and Burns 2010).

CEUS highly depends on the investigator's experience and is not a panoramic technique. It does not allow a complete view of the entire parenchyma of the liver and some lesions, because of their location or due to the habitus of the patients, are very difficult to visualize. CEUS owns some important advantages: it does not use ionizing radiation, it has a low allergic potential, and offers the possibility to repeat the examination with additional contrast doses without any risk of acute kindey injury and a reduced risk of allergic reactions (Chung and Kim 2015).

According to EFSUMB guidelines in patients treated with ablation therapies CEUS is recommended in the setting of a periprocedural evaluation performed immediately or within 24 h after ablation or in follow-up when there is a contraindication to CE-CT and CE-MRI or when CE-CT or CE-MRI are inconclusive.

US is often used as a guide to target ablation therapy. During the ablation procedure, US shows a transient hyperechoic zone due to the high intensity of energy delivered to the liver parenchyma producing cavitation and vapors (Cha et al. 2000; Raman et al. 2000)

After this, CEUS shows areas of residual tumor that can be immediately re-treated. This reduces the incidence of local tumor progression and spares a second treatment session in 30% of patients (Meloni et al. 2012; Mauri et al. 2014). Thus, CEUS shows high sensitivity and specificity in the evaluation of the treatment effect immediately or within 24 h after ablation (Meloni et al. 2001; Vilana et al. 2006; Salvaggio et al. 2010). A complete response to ablation therapy is achieved if there is no enhancement within or at the periphery of the tumor. Residual unablated tumor shows focal enhancement with the same imaging characteristics of the original tumor (Wilson and Burns 2010).

CEUS cannot be used after PEI because the hyperechogenicity of the chemical agents and the gas bubbles created by the injection mask the microbubbles of the contrast agents (Cha et al. 2000; Raman et al. 2000). As it happens in CE-CT and CE-MRI, CEUS after ablation shows peripheral arterial enhancement surrounding the ablation zone due to reactive hyperemia: the differentiation between this peripheral reactive halo and residual unablated tumor can be difficult. Usually, uniform thickness of the hyperenhancing halo without wash-out in the late phase suggests reactive hyperemia, while residual tumor appears irregular, and the hypervascular components have the typical wash-out of the original tumor during the late phase. The fact that peripheral reactive halo can mask small microscopic foci of residual disease must be considered.

CEUS can also visualize active peritoneal hemorrhage, hepatic infarction, and hematomas allowing early detection of such complications (Mauri et al. 2014). In long-term follow-up, CEUS is used if CE-CT and CE-MRI, the gold standard techniques for their high diagnostic accuracy and panoramic view, are inconclusive or contraindicated (Ahmed et al. 2014). In the follow-up of ablated metastases, CEUS permits a complete examination of the liver during the prolonged late phase (Filice et al. 2011) with a high accuracy that is similar to CE-CT and CE-MRI (Cantisani et al. 2010; Larsen et al. 2007; Dietrich et al. 2006).

2.4 Complications

Complication after percutaneous procedures regards blood vessel, biliary tree, or superinfection of the treated zone.

Vascular complications include hemorrhage, arteriovenous fistula, hepatic arterial pseudoan-

eurysm, portal vein thrombosis, and hepatic infarction (Sainani et al. 2013). The most common vascular complications are parenchymal and intraperitoneal hemorrhage caused by direct mechanical injury to blood vessels. This risk is lower with heat-based ablation modalities than with cryoablation because of vessel cauterization induced by RF ablation and MWA. A small amount of parenchymal hemorrhage (hyperdense on CT or hyperintense on MRI) is normal. Hyperdensity in the peritoneum or during the arterial phase are signs of ongoing hemorrhage. Hemorrhage into the biliary tree manifests as the presence of blood into gallbladder lumen. Cholecystitis is a complication of obstruction of the cystic duct by blood clots.

Arterioportal fistulas may be created when a lesion near large hepatic arteries or portal veins is treated. Arterioportal fistulas manifest as perfusional abnormality in liver parenchyma with an early filling of portal veins during the arterial phase (Lee et al. 2016).

Biliary complications are represented by bilomas and biliary strictures. Biliary strictures, caused by damage to large bile ducts, usually become evident 6–12 months after ablation, when progressive enlargement of bile ducts can be seen on serial imaging. Bilomas due to biliary duct injury usually do not require any treatment because they resolve spontaneously in a few months. They require drainage if they become symptomatic or infected (Kim et al. 2004).

Hepatic abscess formation is described in 0.2–3% cases. The main risk factors are diabetes and bilioenteric anastomoses after RFA and MWA (Shankar et al. 2003; Choi et al. 2005). Their imaging features are similar to a hepatic abscess. The presence of air can be normal in the treated zone up to 2–3 weeks after treatment but it must decrease over time.

3 Imaging Post TACE

Transarterial chemoembolization (TACE) is a locoregional therapy of hepatic tumors consists of intraarterial administration of a viscous emulsion, made by a chemotherapeutic drug such as doxorubicin or cisplatin mixed with iodized oil, followed by embolization of the tumor-feeding blood vessels with embolic agents. It is based on the intense tumor neo-angiogenesis activity and its goal is to induce acute ischemic damage and a strong cytotoxic effect, enhanced by ischemia (Lencioni 2010).

It should be distinguished from transarterial embolization (TAE) without administration of the chemotherapeutic agent, or intra-arterial chemotherapy, where no embolization is performed.

The main indication for TACE is multinodular HCC without vascular invasion or extrahepatic spread, whose position or size do not allow other percutaneous treatment, in patients with relatively preserved liver function and absence of cancer-related symptoms; this condition is classified as intermediate stage according to Barcelona Clinic Liver Cancer staging system. Other indications are the treatment of selective metastatic disease, most commonly colorectal cancer, and in intra hepatic cholangiocarcinoma, or even in HCC as a bridge to a liver transplant.

Moreover, TACE is the most used palliative treatment for unresectable HCC (Maleux et al. 2009). For inoperable patients, the available treatment options are intraarterial chemoembolization, radiofrequency ablation, hepatic arterial infusion chemotherapy, sorafenib, and best supportive care. In actual practice, the choice among these therapies is not standardized (Achenbach et al. 2002) and determined by the clinical condition (Yim et al. 2015). According to some authors, TACE may significantly improve the survival of patients with unresectable liver tumors compared with supportive treatment (Llovet et al. 2002).

TACE is commonly performed in two ways: the conventional TACE (cTACE) uses an oily radiopaque material mixed with chemotherapeutic drugs followed by embolic particles (Pesapane et al. 2017); the second method, drug-eluting bead TACE (DEB-TACE), uses particles that slowly release the chemotherapeutic agent (Brown et al. 2016). Both techniques involve cannulation of the arteries feeding the tumor with a catheter or microcatheter, stopping the blood supply to the tumor.

The two procedures are characterized also by different radiological features during follow-up imaging. Lipiodol is visible in the treated area for months after cTACE, while the contrast used during DEB-TACE typically washes out after a few hours (Brennan and Ahmed 2013; Golowa et al. 2012). Compared to cTACE, the absence of iodized oil in DEB-TACE does not mask the arterial enhancement on contrast-enhanced CT or MR imaging and it makes it easier the assessment of residual viable tumor tissue.

In the first 24 hours following cTACE, the patients typically undergo unenhanced CT to define the lipiodol distribution within and around the target tumor, considering that only complete coverage of the treated area is associated to a greater degree of necrosis and an adequate response (Adam and Miller 2015). If the lipiodol does not stain the tumor, the patient may repeat a second TACE. The presence of areas of reduced uptake within the tumor may refer to pre-existing necrosis, or a tumor portion supplies by alternative branches. In this case, the untreated tumor feeding arteries should be sought and more than one TACE should be considered to achieve the maximal response (Riaz et al. 2011).

Contrast-enhanced Computer Tomography (CE-CT) and Magnetic Resonance imaging (CE-MRI) are the most common modalities to evaluate the therapeutic response in patients after TACE.

In comparison to CE-CT and contrast-enhanced ultrasound (CEUS), CE-MRI results to be the most sensitive and specific modality to define residual tumor following TACE treatment (Kubota et al. 2001).

Particularly, CE-MRI superiority compared to CE-CT to detect HCC relapse or persistance after TACE treatment is due to a better contrast delineation between the tumor and the underlying liver in the different sequences available, with or without contrast agent administration (Rostambeigi et al. 2016).

However, in comparison to CE-MRI CE-CT has been associated with reduced cost, requires less patient cooperation, and doesn't suffer the presence of a large volume of ascites (Westwood et al. 2013). CEUS is rarely used in patients treated by TACE and has not performed as well as either CE-CT or CE-MRI (Kubota et al. 2001).

Timing for post-treatment imaging follow-up is at 1 month, 3 months, and then every 3–6 months. Alternative follow-up schedules have been suggested by different author's institutions, but not generally accepted (Boas et al. 2015).

At the initial post-TACE examination, the HCC usually presents the same size as the pre-existing tumor. To evaluate the response after treatment, a method derived from modified RECIST (mRECIST) was developed. As described earlier, these criteria are based on tumor vascularity, which is represented by enhancement on arterial phase imaging (Choi et al. 2018) (Figs. 9 and 10).

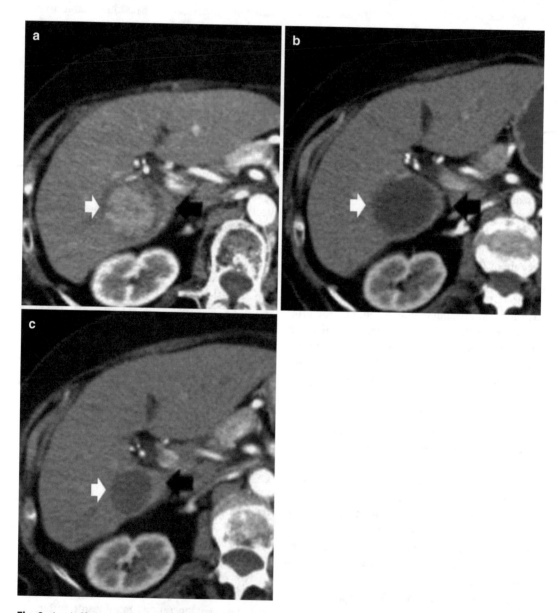

Fig. 9 (a–c) 62 years old man with cirrhosis. Complete response after trans arterial chemoembolization in a patient with HCC. (a–c) CT scan on arterial phase before thermal ablation (a) and 30 days (b) and 3 months (c) after microwave ablation. Hypodense treated area is evident (white arrow) which shows progressive reduction in diameter. These findings are consistent with complete response according to mRECIST criteria

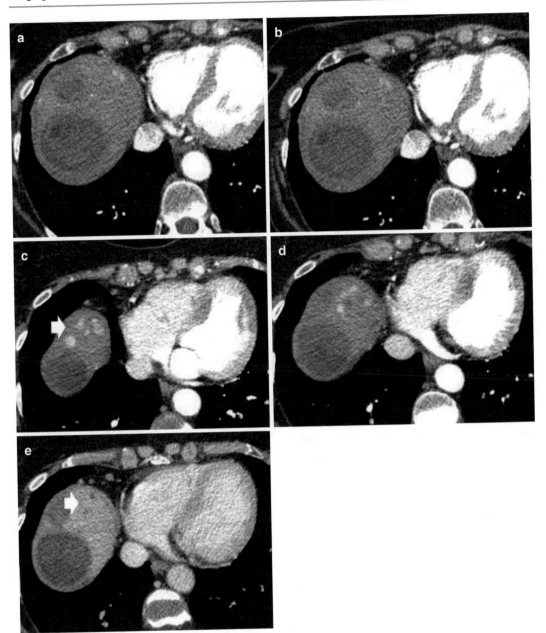

Fig. 10 (**a–e**) 70 years old man with cirrhosis and small HCC. Disease progression after TACE. (**a, b**) CT scan on arterial phase 30 days after TACE showing no evidence of residual enhancing tumor. (**c–e**) Six months after TACE. Multiple enhancing nodules (arrow) are evident peripherally to the treated region (**c, d**), with evidence of contrast washout on portal venous phase (**e**) in keeping with disease progression

On contrast-enhanced CT imaging, the tumor that retains iodized oil is considered necrotic, while tumoral tissue that shows enhancement represents a viable tumor. Beam hardening artifacts led to lipiodol deposition may obscure the enhancement of the arterial phase, reducing the sensitivity of CT. Recent advances in dual-energy CT may increase the sensitivity of contrast-enhanced CT following cTACE, but this technology is not readily available for clinical use (Altenbernd et al. 2011). The signal intensity of MRI is not influenced by the lipiodol, and it is considered superior in evaluating residual viable tumor after cTACE. Necrotic tumor shows variable signal intensity on non-enhanced T1-w images and T2-w images and a lack of enhancement after gadolinium administration (Riaz et al. 2011). Hyperintense foci may represent hemorrhage or residual tumor. Particularly, residual tumoral tissue is seen as a demarcated nodular area, usually >5 mm, that presents arterial enhancement and subsequent washout on portal venous phase images (Park et al. 2013). It is common to see a thin rim <5 mm around the treated lesion after TACE, which shows persistent enhancement, without washout on the portal phase (Brennan and Ahmed 2013). This finding should not be confused with recurrences, which are most commonly localized at the edge of the treatment area. The absence of washout is crucial to differentiate recurrences or residual tumor from pseudolesions, such as arteroportal shunts. More recently, diffusion-weighted imaging (DWI) is used to assess the persistence of tumor tissue after TACE, which results in an increase in the apparent diffusion coefficient values in areas of the tumor that undergo necrosis and signal restriction on DWI in tumoral persistance or recurrence (Sahin et al. 2012).

4 Imaging Post Systemic Therapy

Greater knowledge of cancer genomics for the study of genetic mutations involved in carcinogenesis has allowed the development of therapies that interact with specific molecular targets. Immunotherapies represent a new class of drugs that have significantly changed treatment strategies in advanced tumors. This type of systemic therapy goes to act on well-defined molecular targets, which interfere with tumor neoangiogenesis or cellular signaling (Braschi-Amirfarzan et al. 2017). The aim of immunotherapy is different from conventional cytotoxic therapies whose goal is to determine cell death; with immunotherapy, instead, the immune system is stimulated to activate and increase an inflammatory response against the neoplasm. This translates into a change in the

morphology of the tumor and not in its size as is used with cytotoxic chemotherapeutics that directly kill tumor cells (Karp and Falchook 2014). Immunotherapies improve the antitumor response of the immune system and increase its activity to achieve a more effective antitumor response. Based on the mode of action, the immunotherapies can have an active or passive mechanism: active immunotherapies, such as vaccines, recombinant cytokines, preformed monoclonal antibodies, and immunomodulatory antibodies stimulate humoral or cell-mediated immunity against tumoral cell (Mellman et al. 2011); passive immunotherapies, such as preformed monoclonal antibodies, inhibit the growth of tumor cells by blocking their receptors and signaling proteins, and consequently cause the death of cancer cells by signaling the tumor cells to be removed from the immune system (Schuster et al. 2006). These several immunotherapies, such as tumor antigen therapy, immune checkpoint inhibitors, and adoptive cell transfer (ACT) immunotherapy are currently being studied in HCC (Li et al. 2017).

For HCC conventional cytotoxic chemotherapy with capecitabine, oxaliplatin, cisplatin, fluoropyrimidine (5-FU or capecitabine), doxorubicin demonstrated limited efficacy on long-term (Brandi et al. 2013); hormonal agents, such as tamoxifen or octreotide, have failed to show an objective treatment response in placebo-controlled randomized trials, or when added to existing chemotherapeutic options (Becker et al. 2007; Chow et al. 2002). Generally, the response and success of traditional cytotoxic chemotherapy are given by the decrease in tumor size and the absence of new lesions. Response to treatment after immune-modulatory therapy may be associated with an initial delay in response to treatment, such as a slow decrease in the size of the tumor or even as the appearance of new lesions and tumor size increase followed by stable disease, or even partial or complete response (tumor pseudoprogression) (Kwak et al. 2015). It is also important to remember that immunotherapy activates immune system against cancer, which can also lead to unwanted activation of autoimmunity, with a consequent wide range of toxic effects (Chiou and Burotto 2015).

A great number of organs and tissues can be involved in immune-related adverse events (irAE): skin and mucosae, bowels, lung, liver, pancreas, endocrine glands (thyroid, hypophysis, adrenal glands), kidney, eyes, central nervous system, blood, muscles, and bones (Michot et al. 2016). The most common adverse events related to the activation of the immune system are dermatological, including vitiligo, rash and erythema, hand-foot skin reaction, arterial hypertension, fatigue, and diarrhea (Bruix et al. 2017); other reactions that may occur during follow-up are colitis, pneumatosis intestinalis, pneumonia, thyroiditis, hepatitis, pancreatitis, hypophysitis, and arthritis (Wang et al. 2017). These autoimmune toxic effects must be readily recognized and treated to avoid more serious complications.

As tumors respond differently to treatment with immunotherapy compared to traditional cytotoxic therapies, a consensus guideline - immune-related Response Evaluation Criteria in Solid Tumors (iRECIST) - was developed by the RECIST working group in cancer immunotherapy trials (Seymour et al. 2017). This is a guideline that describes a standard approach to a solid tumor, measurements and definitions for objective change in tumor size for use in clinical trials and to facilitate the ongoing collection of clinical trial data but not for the routine clinical use. iRECIST was published for the first time in 2017 and was based on RECIST 1.1 (Response Evaluation Criteria in Solid Tumors Responses) assigned using a prefix of "i" (i.e., immune) (Somarouthu et al. 2018). According to these criteria some parameters are considered: sum of target lesion maximum diameters (measurable lesions are >10 mm in diameter and lymph node lesion >15 mm in diameter), maximum 2 target lesions per organ, and maximum 5 target lesions in total. New tumoral lesions (maximum 2 for organ, 5 in total) are recorded and followed-up separately (Seymour et al. 2017) (Table 1).

But these criteria have not been yet validated in clinical practice because the dimensional criterion is not sufficient to quantify the change within the tumor determined by immunotherapy whichmodifies the neoangiogenesis or activates the immune response, and may result in a dimensional increase of the lesion itself or in the appearance of new lesions on imaging (pseudoprogression). The real novelty introduced by the iRECIST criteria, compared to the RECIST 1.1 criteria is the iUPD category (Table 1) and the

Table 1 iRECIST criteria 2017

iCR (complete response)—disappearance of all lesions—
Total remission of all the lesions (target and nontarget), lack of new lesion, and any lymph node should be less than 10 mm in short axis diameter. Imaging needs to be confirmed by another consecutive study in the next 4 weeks after the first one.
iSD (stable disease)—neither CR nor PD is met—
Change of the total tumor burden is reduced by less than 30% when compared with baseline or increase less than 20% when compared with baseline.
iPD (progressive disease)
≥ 20% increase in the nadir of the sum of target lesions with a minimum of 5 mm—at least 4 weeks after, and up to 8 weeks
iUPD (unconfirmed progressive disease)
Increase in the total tumor burden of at least 20% compared to nadir (minimum 5 mm) or progression of the non-target lesion. Further confirmation after 4 weeks is needed.
iCPD (confirmed progressive disease)
In order to confirm the progression, it must be an increase of target of non-target lesions. Increase in the sum of new target lesion >5 mm in the next assessment after the examination where progression was previously observed.
iPR (partial response)— ≥30% decrease from baseline—
Decrease of at least 30% in the total tumor burden compared to baseline. Non-unequivocal progression of non-target lesion and lack of new lesion. The study needs to be confirmed by another consecutive study in the next 4 weeks after the first one.

simultaneous evaluation of the patient's clinical status (Seymour et al. 2017).

According to the guidelines for the clinical practice of the 2018 EASL (European Association for the Study of the Liver) for the management of HCC (Galle et al. 2018) patients with advanced HCC (BCLC stage C) (Fig. 1), with cancer-related symptoms (symptomatic tumors, ECOG 1–2), macrovascular invasion (either segmental or portal invasion) or extrahepatic spread (lymph node involvement or metastases) have a poor prognosis, with expected median survival times of 6–8 months, or 25% at 1 year (Cabibbo et al. 2010).

For these patients, the therapeutic scenario has changed since 2007, thanks to sorafenib and immunotherapy. Around 20 molecular targeted therapies have been approved during recent years for patients with breast, colorectal, non-small cell lung, renal cancer, and HCC, among other malignancies (Llovet and Bruix 2008).

Sorafenib is an oral multikinase inhibitor that can interfere with tumor angiogenesis and growth, which usually does not lead to apparent tumor shrinkage and may alter tumor morphology blocking several molecular pathways that are important in tumor angiogenesis and progression, including serine-threonine kinases (c-RAF and BRAF), tyrosine kinases related to vascular endothelial growth factor receptor 2 and 3 (VEGFR-2 and VEGFR-3), and platelet-derived growth factor receptor (PDGFR) (Wilhelm et al. 2004). Among these pathways, VEGF is the main molecule that drives tumor angiogenesis (Jayson et al. 2016), Sorafenib destroys tumor blood vessels and facilitates vascular normalization (Heath and Bicknell 2009). Sorafenib is established as the standard systemic therapy for patients with well-preserved liver function (Child-Pugh A class) and with advanced HCC stage (BCLC C) or those HCCs at intermediate stage (BCLC B) showing disease progression after loco-regional therapies. The data reported in the trial SHARP phase III, showed that Sorafenib improved survival compared with placebo (Llovet et al. 2008). The results of the SHARP trial were confirmed also in the Asia-Pacific phase III trial (Cheng et al. 2009). In first-line systemic therapy also lenvatinib has been shown to be non-inferior to Sorafenib. Among second-line therapies, Regorafenib an oral multi-kinase inhibitor that blocks the activity of protein kinases involved in angiogenesis, oncogenesis, and the tumor micro-environment should be mentioned (Wilhelm et al. 2011). Cabozantinib is a MET (receptor tyrosine kinase for the hepatocyte growth factor), VEGFR2, and RET inhibitor, approved in patients with advanced HCC in second- or third-line treatment (Abou-Alfa et al. 2018).

4.1 Imaging Findings

The goal of monitoring the response to this new therapeutic agents by imaging should be to evaluate the reduction of tumoral vascularization and induced necrosis and internal tumoral hemorrhage as indicators of treatment response. Internal tumoral hemorrhage may thus be observed during immunotherapy treatment due to ischemia. Decreased tumor cellularity is another pathological finding seen during immunotherapy treatment.

On CE-CT, the contrast enhancement degree of HCC on the arterial phase may decrease during sorafenib therapy without necessarily affecting tumor size (Kim et al. 2011) and reflects the degree of neoangiogenesis. However, the assessment of tumoral contrast enhancement depends on the CE-CT scan protocol, the contrast agent injection protocol, and the patient's cardiovascular circle status at the time of scanning. During treatment with sorafenib, it is important to measure tumor density on both unenhanced and CE-CT images and to evaluate the change of tumoral vascularization caused by the therapy. It should be remembered that tumor attenuation on unenhanced CT may even increase due to hemorrhage (Figs. 11 and 12). Perfusion CT and its perfusion parameters such as peak enhancement, time to peak, transition time may allow more accurate quantification of tumor perfusion (Maksimovic et al. 2010; Sahani et al. 2007).

On MRI tumoral T1 and T2 signal varies according to the presence of hemorrhage and necrosis. CE-MRI can also show the reduction of tumor perfusion (Horger et al. 2009). The signal changes on T1-w and T2-w sequences, reflect the morphological changes in the tumor and can be observed as early as 2–4 weeks in therapy, which corresponds to the timing of the first post-therapy MRI scan. In the early acute phase (<1 week from therapy), the transformation of intracellular deoxyglobin into methaemoglobin leads to high signal intensity on T1-w sequences and low signal intensity on T2-w MRI sequences, while in the subacute phase (first weeks in therapy), presence of extracellular methemoglobin produces a high signal intensity on T1-w and T2-w MRI sequences (Horger et al. 2009). This phase with its intrinsic contrast between tumor and native liver accurately demonstrates intratumoral hemorrhage induced by Sorafenib therapy. Tumor enhancement on the hepatic arterial phase of CE-MRI reflects the degree of neoangiogenesis. Internal enhancement of the tumor assessed before and after gadolinium administration can carefully show the response to therapy. Tumor necrosis is evident as a non-enhancing tumoral region that increases dimensionally compared to a previous examination, with an increase in the relationship between the necrotic tumor and still vital portion. However, in a small percentage of patients, tumoral necrosis can lead to a considerable increase (>20%) of the tumor volume, which

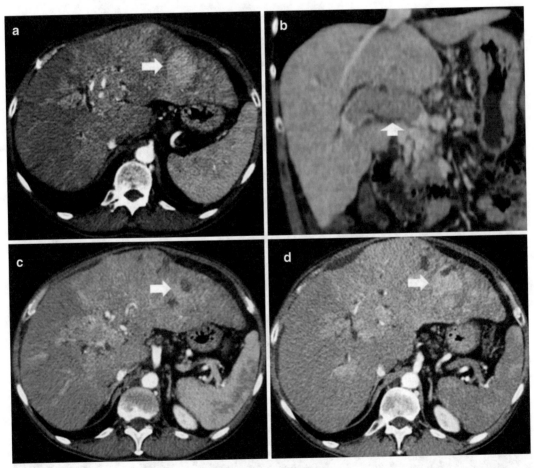

Fig. 11 (**a–d**) 61-years old man with multifocal HCC. Contrast-enhanced CT. Dominant nodule (long arrow) on the left liver lobe (**a**), and neoplastic thrombosis of the portal vein (short arrow) (**b**). Partial response after treatment. Contrast-enhanced CT, arterial phase, the same HCC nodule in the left hepatic lobe at 2 months (**c**) and 4 months (**d**) from the beginning of sorafenib therapy. A central hypodense region appears within the nodule after 2 months of treatment with mild reduction of tumoral vascularity due to anti angiogenetic effect of sorafenib (**c**)

should not be considered immediately as disease progression but as 'pseudoprogression' (Kwak et al. 2015).

On CE-MRI, tumoral perfusion can be estimated using kinetic models. Ktrans reflects capillary permeability. HCC treated with sorafenib showed a higher decrease in Ktrans and this finding reflects a decrease in tumor capillary permeability and correlates with longer progression-free survival and overall survival (Hsu et al. 2011; Yopp et al. 2011). Dynamic CE-MRI T2* - w sequences are affected by susceptibility effects of intravascular contrast medium and are much more sensitive to contrast than T1-w CE-MRI sequences. A reduction in the signal intensity ini-

tially occurs after contrast agent administration, with subsequent recovery of the signal intensity since the T1 effects overcomes the T2* effects.

Diffusion-weighted MR imaging (DWI) has been helpful in liver tumor detection, tumor characterization, and monitoring response to treatment (Figueiras et al. 2011) The apparent diffusion coefficient (ADC) value has been correlated with the tumor proliferation index and tumor grade before therapy, as well as with the presence of necrosis and tumor cell apoptosis after treatment (Padhani and Koh 2011; Anzidei et al. 2011). The ADC is a parameter used in DWI MRI sequences to quantify the water mobility due to Brownian motions through gradient

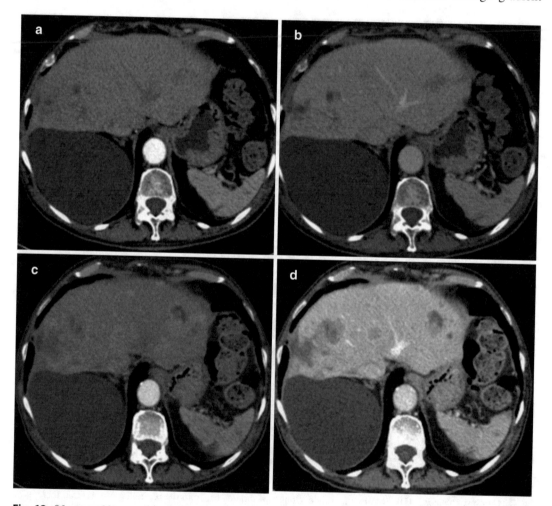

Fig. 12 86-years old man with multifocal HCC HCV related to treatment with second-line drugs (tivantinib). Disease progression. CE-CT on hepatic arterial phase and portal venous phase at 0 months (**a**, **b**), at 2 months (**c**, **d**) and 4 months (**e**, **f**) after begin of therapy shows disease progression with evidence of progressively increasing number of hypodense lesions

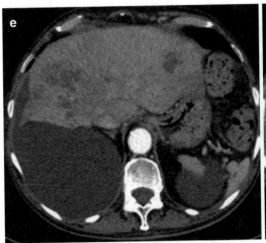
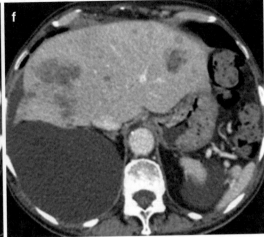

Fig. 12 (continued)

duration and amplitude (b-values). A lower ADC value is related to tumor viability (Heijmen et al. 2013). Successful therapy increases water diffusivity resulting in a higher ADC value, which reflects the derangement of tumor macromolecular architecture (e.g., due to necrosis) and increased water mobility. Studies have shown a potential to characterize malignant lesions and to differentiate viable tissue from necrosis on the basis of ADC cut-off values (Heijmen et al. 2013; Wagner et al. 2012). Early changes in ADC values in patients treated with Sorafenib generally show a contrary trend which is thought to be caused by shrinkage of extracellular space due to resorption of plasma and occurrence of hemoglobin degradation products (e.g., methemoglobin) after hemorrhage (Atlas et al. 2000). In fact, patients with HCC treated by Sorafenib have reported a transient decrease in tumor ADC value approximately 1 month after treatment, thus, suggesting hemorrhagic necrosis; however, a sustained decrease in ADC at 3-months follow-up may indicate a viable tumor or tumor progression (Schraml et al. 2009).

About other imaging, the value of CEUS for assessing the treatment response to Sorafenib in HCC has been validated by recent studies. Shiozawa et al. (2001) demonstrated that the intratumoral vascular architecture classified by microflow imaging and the contrast mean arrival time from the reference point to the tar-get lesion 2 weeks after treatment were correlated with overall survival (OS) (Shiozawa et al. 2001; Shiozawa et al. 2016). Moreover, CEUS is a more simple example to use noninvasive imaging technique that allows accurate evaluation of tumor vascularization and could be capable of selecting patients who will benefit from treatment with Sorafenib (Lamuraglia et al. 2006).

References

Abou-Alfa GK, Meyer T, Cheng AL et al (2018) Cabozantinib (C) vs. placebo (P) in patients (pts) with advanced hepatocellular carcinoma (HCC) who have received prior sorafenib: results from the randomized phase III CELESTIAL trial. J Clin Oncol 36:abstr 2017

Achenbach T, Seifert JK, Pitton MB et al (2002) Chemoembolization for primary liver cancer. Eur J Surg Oncol 28:37–41

Adam SZ, Miller FH (2015) Imaging of the liver following interventional therapy for hepatic neoplasms. Radiol Clin N Am 53:1061–1076

Ahmed M, Solbiati L, Brace CL et al (2014) Image-guided tumor ablation: standardization of terminology and reporting criteria—a 10-year update. Radiology 273(1):241–260

Ahn SS, Kim M-J, Lim JS et al (2010) Added value of gadoxetic acid-enhanced hepatobiliary phase MR imaging in the diagnosis of hepatocellular carcinoma. Radiology 255(2):459–466

Altenbernd J, Heusner TA, Ringelstein A et al (2011) Dual-energy-CT of hypervascular liver lesions in patients with HCC: investigation of image quality and sensitivity. Eur Radiol 21:738–743

American College of Radiology (ACR). Liver Imaging Reporting and Data System (LI-RADS); 2017. ACR website. https://www.acr.org/Clinical-Resources/Reporting-and-Data-Systems/LI-RADS

Anzidei M, Napoli A, Zaccagna F et al (2011) Liver metastases from colorectal cancer treated with conventional and antiangiogenetic chemotherapy: evaluation with liver computed tomography perfusion and magnetic resonance diffusion-weighted imaging. J Comput Assist Tomogr 35(6):690–696

Atassi B, Bangash AK, Bahrani A et al (2008) Multimodality imaging following ^{90}Y radioembolization: a comprehensive review and pictorial essay. Radiographics 28(1):81–99

Atlas SW, DuBois P, Singer MB et al (2000) Diffusion measurements in intracranial hematomas: implications for MR imaging of acute stroke. AJNR 21:1190–1194

Becker G, Allgaier HP, Olschewski M et al (2007) Long-acting octreotide versus placebo for treatment of advanced HCC; a randomized controlled double-blind study. Hepatology 45:9–15

Boas FE, Do B, Louie JD et al (2015) Optimal imaging surveillance schedules after liver-directed therapy for hepatocellular carcinoma. J Vasc Interv Radiol 26:69–73

Brandi G, de Rosa F, Agostini V et al (2013) Metronomic capecitabine in advanced hepatocellular carcinoma patients: a phase II study. Oncologist 18(12):1256–1257

Braschi-Amirfarzan M, Tirumani SH, Hodi FS et al (2017) Immune-checkpoint inhibitors in the era of precision medicine: what radiologists should know. Korean J Radiol 18(1):42–53

Brennan IM, Ahmed M (2013) Imaging features following transarterial chemoembolization and radiofrequency ablation of hepatocellular carcinoma. Semin Ultrasound CT MR 34:336–351

Brown KT, Do RK, Gonen M et al (2016) Randomized trial of hepatic artery embolization for hepatocellular carcinoma using doxorubicin-eluting microspheres compared with embolization with microspheres alone. J Clin Oncol 34:2046–2053

Bruix J, Qin S, Merle P et al (2017) Regorafenib for patients with hepatocellular carcinoma who progressed on sorafenib treatment (RESORCE): a randomised, double-blind, placebo-controlled, phase 3 trial. Lancet 389:56–66

Cabibbo G, Enea M, Attanasio M et al (2010) A meta-analysis of survival rates of untreated patients in randomized clinical trials of hepatocellular carcinoma. Hepatology 51:1274–1283

Cantisani V, Ricci P, Erturk M et al (2010) Detection of hepatic metastases from colorectal cancer: prospective evaluation of gray scale US versus SonoVue® low mechanical index real time-enhanced US as compared with multidetector-CT or Gd-BOPTA-MRI. Ultraschall Med 31:500–505

Cha CH, Lee FT Jr, Gurney JM et al (2000) CT versus sonography for monitoring radiofrequency ablation in a porcin liver. AJR Am J Roentgenol 175:705–711

Cheng AL, Kang YK, Chen Z et al (2009) Efficacy and safety of sorafenib in patients in the Asia-Pacific region with advanced hepatocellular carcinoma: a phase III randomised, double-blind, placebo-controlled trial. Lancet Oncol 10:25–34

Chiou VL, Burotto M (2015) Pseudoprogression and immune- related response in solid tumors. J Clin Oncol 33(31):3541–3543

Choi D, Lim HK, Kim MJ et al (2005) Liver abscess after percutaneous radiofrequency ablation for hepatocellular carcinomas: frequency and risk factors. J Hepatol 56:908–943

Choi MH, Park GE, Oh SN et al (2018) Reproducibility of mRECIST in measurement and response assessment for hepatocellular carcinoma treated by Transarterial chemoembolization. Acad Radiol 23:1363–1373

Chow PK, Tai BC, Tan CK et al (2002) High-dose tamoxifen in the treatment of inoperable hepatocellular carcinoma: a multicenter randomized controlled trial. Hepatology 36:1221–1226

Chung YE, Kim KW (2015) Contrast-enhanced ultrasonography: advance and current status in abdominal imaging. Ultrasonography 34:3–18

Dietrich CF, Kratzer W, Strobe D et al (2006) Assessment of metastaic liver disease in patients with primary extrahepatic tumors by contrast-enhanced sonography versus CT and MRI. World J Gastroenterol 12:1699–1705

Dromain C, de Baere T, Elias D et al (2002) Hepatic tumors treated with percutaneous radio-frequency ablation: CT and MR imaging follow-up. Radiology 223:255–262

Elsayes KM, Hooker JC, Agrons MM et al (2017) version of LI-RADS for CT and MR imaging: an update. Radiographics 37(7):1994–2017

Figueiras RG, Padhani AR, Goh VJ et al (2011) Novel oncologic drugs: what they do and how they affect images. Radiographics 31(7):2059–2091

Filice C, Calliada F, De Masi S et al (2011) Italian guidelines for noninvasive imaging assessment of focal liver lesions: development and conclusions. Eur J Gastroenterol Hepatol 23:343–353

Forner A, Ayuso C, Varela M et al (2009) Evaluation of tumor response after locoregional therapies in hepatocellular carcinoma: are response evaluation criteria in solid tumors reliable? Cancer 115:616–623

Galle PR, Forner A, Llovet JM et al (2018) EASL clinical practice guidelines: management of hepatocellular carcinoma. J Hepatol 69(1):182–236

Goldberg SN, Gazelle GS, Compton CC et al (2000) Treatment of intrahepatic malignancy with radiofrequency ablation: radiologic-pathologic correlation. Cancer 88:2452–2463

Golowa YS, Cynamon J, Reinus JF et al (2012) Value of noncontrast CT immediately after transarterial chemoembolization of hepatocellular carcinoma with drug-eluting beads. J Vasc Interv Radiol 23:1031–1035

Goodwin MD, Dobson JE, Sirlin CB et al (2011) Diagnostic challenges and pitfalls in MR imaging with hepatocyte- specific contrast agents. Radiographics 31(6):1547–1568

Heath VL, Bicknell R (2009) Anticancer strategies involving the vasculature. Nat Rev Clin Oncol 6: 395–404

Heijmen L, Ter Voert EE, Nagtegaal ID et al (2013) Diffusion-weighted MR imaging in liver metastases of colorectal cancer: reproducibility and biological validation. Eur Radiol 23(3):748–756

Horger M, Lauer UM, Schraml C et al (2009) Early MRI response monitoring of patients with advanced hepatocellular carcinoma under treatment with the multikinase inhibitor sorafenib. BMC Cancer 9:2087

Hsu CY, Shen YC, Yu CW et al (2011) Dynamic contrast-enhanced magnetic resonance imaging biomarkers predict survival and response in hepatocellular carcinoma patients treated with sorafenib and metronomic tegafur/uracil. J Hepatol 55(4):858–865

Jayson GC, Kerbel R, Ellis LM et al (2016) Antiangiogenic therapy in oncology: current status and future directions. Lancet 388:518–529

Karp DD, Falchook GS (2014) Handbook of targeted cancer therapy. Wolters Kluwer, Philadelphia, PA

Kim SH, Lim HK, Choi D et al (2004) Changes in bile ducts after radiofrequency ablation of hepatocellular carcinoma: frequency and clinical significance. AJR Am J Roentgenol 183(6):1611–1617

Kim MJ, Choi JI, Lee JS et al (2011) Computed tomography findings of sorafenib-treated hepatic tumors in patients with advanced hepatocellular carcinoma. J Gastroenterol Hepatol 26:1201–1206

Kubota K, Hisa N, Nishikawa T et al (2001) Evaluation of hepatocellular carcinoma after treatment with transcatheter arterial chemoembolization: comparison of Lipiodol-CT, power Doppler sonography, and dynamic MRI. Abdom Imaging 26:184–190

Kudo M, Kubo S, Takayasu K et al (2010) Response evaluation criteria in Cancer of the liver (RECICL) proposed by the liver Cancer study Group of Japan (2009 revised version). Hepatol Res 40(7):686–692

Kwak JJ, Tirumani SH, Van den Abbeele et al (2015) Cancer immunotherapy: imaging assessment of novel treatment response patterns and immune-related adverse events. Radiographics 35(2):424–437

Lamuraglia M, Escudier B, Chami L et al (2006) To predict progression-free survival and overall survival in metastatic renal cancer treated with sorafenib: pilot study using dynamic contrast-enhanced Doppler ultrasound. Eur J Cancer 42:2472–2479

Larsen LP, Rosenkilde M, Christensen H et al (2007) The value of contrast enhanced ultrasonography in detection of liver metastases from colorectal cancer: a prospective double-blinded study. Eur J Radiol 62:302–307

Lee DH, Lee JM, Baek JH et al (2015) Diagnostic performance of gadoxetic acid-enhanced liver MR imaging in the detection of HCCs and allocation of transplant recipients on the basis of the Milan criteria and UNOS guidelines: correlation with histopathologic findings. Radiology 274(1):149–160

Lee SR, Kilcoyne A, Kambadakone A et al (2016) Interventional oncology: pictorial review of post-ablation imaging of liver and renal tumors. Abdom Radiol Apr 41(4):677–705

Lencioni R (2010) Loco-regional treatment of hepatocellular carcinoma in the era of molecular targeted therapies. Oncology 78:107–112

Lencioni R, Llovet JM (2010) Modified RECIST (mRECIST) assessment for hepatocellular carcinoma. Semin Liver Dis 30(1):52–60

Li K, Lan Y, Wang J, Liu L (2017) Chimeric antigen receptor-engineered T cells for liver cancers, progress and obstacles. Tumor Biol 39(3):1010428317692229

Livraghi T, Goldberg SN, Monti F et al (1997) Saline-enhanced radio-frequency tissue ablation in the treatment of liver metastases. Radiology 202:205–210

Llovet JM, Bruix J (2008) Molecular targeted therapies in hepatocellular carcinoma. Hepatology 48:1312–1327

Llovet JM, Real MI, Montaña X et al (2002) Barcelona liver Cancer group. Arterial embolisation or chemoembolisation versus symptomatic treatment in patients with unresectable hepatocellular carcinoma: a randomised controlled trial. Lancet 359:1734–1739

Llovet JM, Ricci S, Mazzaferro V et al (2008) Sorafenib in advanced hepatocellular carcinoma. N Engl J Med 359:378–390

Lu DS, Raman SS, Limanond P et al (2003) Influence of large peritumoral vessels on outcome of radiofrequency ablation of liver tumors. J Vasc Interv Radiol 14:1267–1274

Maksimovic O, Schraml C, Hartmann JT et al (2010) Evaluation of response in malignant tumors treated with the multitargeted tyrosine kinase inhibitor sorafenib: a multitechnique imaging assessment. AJR Am J Roentgenol 194:5–14

Maleux G, van Malenstein H, Vandecaveye V et al (2009) Transcatheter chemoembolization of unresectable hepatocellular carcinoma: current knowledge and future directions. Dig Dis 27:157–163

Mauri G, Porazzi E, Cova L et al (2014) Intraprocedural contrast-enhanced ultrasound (CEUS) in liver percutaneous radiofrequency ablation: clinical impact and health technology assessment. Insights Imaging 5:209–216

Mellman I, Coukos G, Dranoff G (2011) Cancer immunotherapy comes of age. Nature 480(7378):480–489

Meloni MF, Goldberg SN, Livraghi T et al (2001) Hepatocellular carcinoma treated with radiofrequency ablation comparison of pulse inversion contrast-enhanced harmonic sonography, contrast-enhanced power Doppler sonography, and helical CT. AJR Am J Roentgenol 177:375–380

Meloni MF, Andreano A, Franza E et al (2012) Contrast enhanced ultrasound: should it play a role in immediate evaluation of liver tumors following thermal ablation. Eur J Radiol 81:897–902

Memon JK, Kulik L, Lewandowski RJ et al (2011) Radiographic response to locoregional therapy in hepatocellular carcinoma predicts patient survival times. Gastroenterology 141(2):526–535

Michot JM, Bigenwald C, Champiat S et al (2016) Immune-related adverse events with immune checkpoint blockade: a comprehensive review. Eur J Cancer 54:139–148

Mulier S, Mulier P, Ni Y et al (2002) Complications of radiofrequency coagulation of liver tumours. Br J Surg Oct 89(10):1206–1222

Padhani AR, Koh DM (2011) Diffusion MR imaging for monitoring of treatment response. Magn Reson Imaging Clin N Am 19(1):181–209

Park W, Chung YH, Kim JA et al (2013) Recurrences of hepatocellular carcinoma following complete remission by transarterial chemoembolization or radiofrequency therapy: focused on the recurrence patterns. Hepatol Res 43:1304–1312

Pesapane F, Nezami N, Patella F, Geschwind JF (2017) New concepts in embolotherapy of HCC. Med Oncol 34:58

Raman SS, Lu DS, Vodopich DJ et al (2000) Creation of radiofrequency lesions in a porcine model correlation with sonography, CT, and histopathology. AJR Am J Roentgenol 175:1253–1258

Riaz A, Memon K, Miller FH et al (2011) Role of the EASL, RECIST, and WHO response guidelines alone or in combination for hepatocellular carcinoma: radiologic-pathologic correlation. J Hepatol 54:695–704

Rostambeigi N, Taylor AJ, Golzarian J et al (2016) Effect of MRI versus MDCT on Milan criteria scores and liver transplantation eligibility. AJR Am J Roentgenol 206:726–733

Sahani DV, Holalkere NS, Mueller PR, Zhu AX (2007) Advanced hepatocellular carcinoma: CT perfusion of liver and tumor tissue—initial experience. Radiology 243:736–743

Sahin H, Harman M, Cinar C et al (2012) Evaluation of treatment response of chemoembolization in hepatocellular carcinoma with diffusion-weighted imaging on 3.0-T MR imaging. J Vasc Interv Radiol 23:241–247

Sainani NI, Gervais DA, Mueller PR et al (2013) Imaging after percutaneous radiofrequency ablation of hepatic tumors: part 2, abnormal findings. Am J Roentgenol 200(1):194–204

Salvaggio G, Campisi A, Lo Greco V et al (2010) Evaluation of posttreatment response of hepatocellular carcinoma; comparison of ultrasonography with second-generation ultrasound contrast agent and multidetector CT. Abdom Imaging 35:447–453

Schraml C, Schwenzer NF, Martirosian P et al (2009) Diffusion-weighted MRI of advanced hepatocellular carcinoma during sorafenib treatment: initial results. AJR Am J Roentgenol 193(4):W301–W307

Schuster M, Nechansky A, Kircheis R (2006) Cancer immunotherapy. Biotechnol J 1(2):138–147

Seymour L, Bogaerts J, Perrone A, RECIST working group et al (2017) iRECIST: guidelines for response criteria for use in trials testing immunotherapeutics. Lancet Oncol 18:143–152

Shankar S, vanSonnenberg E, Silverman SG et al (2003) Diagnosis and treatment of intrahepatic biloma complicating radiofrequency ablation of hepatic metastases. AJR Am J Roentgenol 181(2):475–477

Shiozawa K, Watanabe M, Ikehara T et al (2001) Evaluation of sorafenib for advanced hepatocellular carcinoma with low α-fetoprotein in arrival time parametric imaging using contrast-enhanced ultrasonography. J Med Ultrason 44:101–107

Shiozawa K, Watanabe M, Ikehara T et al (2016) Therapeutic evaluation of sorafenib for hepatocellular carcinoma using contrast-enhanced ultrasonography: preliminary result. Oncol Lett 12:579–584

Shropshire EL, Chaudhry M, Miller CM et al (2019) LI-RADS treatment response algorithm: performance and diagnostic accuracy. Radiology 292(1):226–234

Smith S, Gillams A (2008) Imaging appearances following thermal ablation. Clin Radiol 63:1–11

Solbiati L, Ierace T, Goldberg SN et al (1997) Percutaneous US-guided radiofrequency tissue ablation of liver metastases: treatment and follow-up in 16 patients. Radiology 202(1):195–203

Somarouthu B, Lee SI, Urban T et al (2018) Immune-related tumor response assessment criteria: a comprehensive review. Br J Radiol 91(1084):2017045

Vilana R, Bianchi L, Varela M et al (2006) B.C.L.C. group, is microbubble-enhanced ultrasonography sufficient for assessment of response to percutaneous treatment in patients with early hepatocellular carcinoma. Eur Radiol 16:2454–2462

Vogl TJ, Kummel S, Hammerstingl R et al (1996) Liver tumors: comparison of MR imaging with Gd-EOB-DTPA and Gd-DTPA. Radiology 200(1):59–67

Wagner M, Doblas S, Daire JL et al (2012) Diffusion-weighted MR imaging for the regional characterization of liver tumors. Radiology 264(2):464–472

Wang GX, Kurra V, Gainor JF et al (2017) Immune checkpoint inhibitor cancer therapy: spectrum of imaging findings. Radiographics 37(7):2132–2144

Westwood M, Joore M, Grutters J et al (2013) Contrast-enhanced ultrasound using SonoVue® (Sulphur hexafluoride microbubbles) compared with contrast-enhanced computed tomography and contrast-enhanced magnetic resonance imaging for the characterisation of focal liver lesions and detection of liver metastases: a systematic review and cost-effectiveness analysis. Health Technol Assess 17:1–243

Wilhelm SM, Carter C, Tang L et al (2004) BAY 43-9006 exhibits broad spectrum oral antitumor activity and targets the RAF/MEK/ERK pathway and receptor tyrosine kinases involved in tumor progression and angiogenesis. Cancer Res 64:7099–7109

Wilhelm SM, Dumas J, Adnane L et al (2011) Regorafenib (BAY 73-4506): a new oral multikinase inhibitor of angiogenic, stromal and oncogenic receptor tyrosine kinases with potent preclinical antitumor activity. Int J Cancer 129:245–255

Wilson SR, Burns PN (2010) Microbubble-enhanced US in body imaging: what role? Radiology 257(2010):24–39

Yaghmai V, Miller FH, Rezai P et al (2011) Response to treatment series: part 2, tumor response assessment-using new and conventional criteria. AJR Am J Roentgenol 197(1):18–27

Yim HJ, Suh SJ, Um SH (2015) Current management of hepatocellular carcinoma: an eastern perspective. World J Gastroenterol 21:3826–3842

Yopp AC, Schwartz LH, Kemeny N et al (2011) Antiangiogenic therapy for primary liver cancer: correlation of changes in dynamic contrast-enhanced magnetic resonance imaging with tissue hypoxia markers and clinical response. Ann Surg Oncol 18:2192–2199

Part IV
Special Topics

Hepatic Tumoral Pathology: The Pediatric Liver

Gabriele Masselli, Marianna Guida, Silvia Ceccanti, and Denis Cozzi

Contents

Abstract

Paediatric hepatic tumours are relatively rare with malignant lesions being twice as frequent as benign neoplasms and are mostly metastases.

G. Masselli (✉) · M. Guida
Radiology Department, Umberto I Hospital Sapienza University, Rome, Italy
e-mail: gabriele.masselli@uniroma1.it

S. Ceccanti · D. Cozzi
Pediatric Surgery Unit, Umberto I Hospital Sapienza University, Rome, Italy

Hepatic tumors in children include lesions that are unique to the pediatric age group and others that are more common in adults.

Important considerations when evaluating a child with a liver tumor are the age of the patient, laboratory findings, and specific imaging features.

Imaging has a significant role in the evaluation of most paediatric liver tumours. Differentiating benign from malignant tumours is important as it significantly affects treatment decisions.

The current emphasis is on imaging features, which are helpful not only for the initial

© Springer Nature Switzerland AG 2021
E. Quaia (ed.), *Imaging of the Liver and Intra-hepatic Biliary Tract,*
Medical Radiology Diagnostic Imaging, https://doi.org/10.1007/978-3-030-39021-1_16

diagnosis, but also for pre- and post-treatment evaluation and follow-up.

The role of advanced imaging test such as magnetic resonance imaging, which allow for non-invasive assessment of liver tumors, is of utmost importance in pediatric patients, especially when repeated imaging tests are needed and radiation exposure should be avoided.

Knowledge of the imaging features of these tumors can help radiologists offer an appropriate differential diagnosis and management plan.

Primary hepatic neoplasms account for 1–4% of all children solid tumors with approximately two-thirds of the primary hepatic neoplasms being malignant (Yikilmaz et al. 2017)

Metastatic disease is the most common neoplasm involving the liver in children (Chung et al. 2010)

Most of the focal hepatic masses cause abdominal pain or palpable abdominal mass or distention. Imaging evaluation is necessary for characterizing and managing pediatric patients with suspected focal hepatic masses. Although abdominal radiograph may provide helpful imaging findings that can suggest the presence of focal hepatic masses such as hepatomegaly, ultrasound is the first imaging modality because of its low cost and availability, without lack of ionizing radiation (Adeyiga et al. 2012)

Contrast-enhanced US (CEUS) is currently emerging as a promising modality in detecting and characterizing liver tumors (Anupindi et al. 2017)

CT was often performed for lesion characterization, staging, and surgical planning for liver masses and now remains the gold standard for detecting lung metastasis in malignant hepatic neoplasms. Parameters like kV, mAs, and pitch can be adjusted for decreasing children's exposure to radiation maintaining adequate diagnostic image quality. IV contrast agent is essential to characterizing tumor and vascular supply to both the tumor and the normal hepatic parenchyma.

Unlike adults, multiphase CT liver imaging should not be performed in pediatric patients to avoid excessive exposure to radiation. It is recommended a single portal-venous phase with a 50-second delay to initiate imaging after injection of IV contrast agent.

The diagnostic role of CT in characterization, staging, and surgical planning of hepatic tumors in the pediatric population has been reduced with recent advances in MR imaging.

MRI is becoming the modality of choice for the imaging of pediatric abdominal masses because of its very good multiplanar spacial resolution and excellent multiparametric tissue characterization without exposure to ionizing radiation. Newer and faster image sequences have also been developed for reducing motion artifact and for improving detailed visualization of vascular anatomy.

However, the disadvantages of MR imaging include longer imaging time and the frequent need for sedation or anesthesia in smaller children.

The imaging protocol employed should attempt to minimize scan time while maximizing image resolution (Rozell et al. 2014; Roebuck 2009).

An ideal MR imaging protocol should be performed with axial and coronal T2-weighted turbo spin-echo; axial in- and opposed-phase T1 gradient recalled echo, axial diffusion-weighted and axial/coronal post-contrast 3-dimensional fat-suppressed gradient recalled-echo sequences with arterial, portal venous, equilibrium and delayed post-contrast phases up to 20 min with the use of a hepatocyte-specific gadolinium-based contrast agent (such as gadoxetate disodium) (Shelmerdine et al. 2016; Chavhan et al. 2016; Mitchell and Vasanawala 2011; Meyers et al. 2011)

1 Benign Tumors

One-third of primary liver tumors are benign, which may be of mesenchymal or epithelial origin; the most common benign tumors are infantile hemangioma, mesenchymal hamartoma, focal nodular hyperplasia (FNH), nodular regenerative hyperplasia (NRH), and hepatocellular adenoma (Table 1) (Stocker 2001; Chung et al. 2010)

Table 1 Data from Lopez-Terrada 2014

Incidence of primary liver tumors in children	
Infantile hepatic hemangioma	15%
Mesenchymal hamartoma	7%
Focal nodular hyperplasia	5%
Hepatocellularadenoma	3%
Hepatoblastoma	37%
Hepatocellular carcinoma	21%
Undifferentiated embryonal sarcoma	8%
Other	4%

1.1 Infantile Hepatic Hemangioma

Infantile hepatic hemangiomas are the most common benign vascular tumor, which is composed of vascular endothelium, and are divided into three subtypes: focal, multifocal, and diffuse.

The congenital sub-type is well-formed at birth while infantile hemangiomas typically present 4–8 weeks after birth and continue to grow up to a year, followed by a slow phase of regression over 8–9 years and typically resolve by puberty. Clinicians and radiologists, to distinguish between infantile and congenital hemangiomas, have to know the timing of lesion presentation or GLUT-1 expression by tissue sampling (which is a sensitive and specific marker for infantile hemangiomas) (Masand 2018).

Solitary tumor size varies from 0.5 to 14 cm in maximum dimension while multifocal lesions are usually around 1 cm in diameter.

Multifocal lesions are small and uniform while large focal may present central hemorrhage, necrosis, fibrosis, and calcification. In diffuse disease, the liver is replaced by multiple large masses that cause mass effect on adjacent organs (Chung et al. 2010)

At postnatal US, infantile hemangioma appears as a well-demarcated mass, generally hypoechoic or of mixed echogenicity, relative to adjacent live, unlike adults hemangioma which is typically iperechoic (Keslar et al. 1993)

Large hemangiomas may be heterogeneous because of central hemorrhage, necrosis, or fibrosis.

On CT precontrast images infantile hemangioma presents as a well-defined hypoattenuating mass with calcifications in up to 50% of cases.

After contrast injection, it shows intense peripheral nodular enhancement on arterial phase enhancement with a progressive centripetal fill-in on portal venous and delayed phase images, similar to adult hemangioma. Small multifocal tumors enhance intensely and uniformly, whereas large focal tumors enhance centripetally and may never completely enhance in the center (Kassarjian et al. 2004)

On MRI congenital or infantile hemangiomas present as focal mass lesions with hypointense T1-weighted and avidly hyperintense T2-weighted signal. On post-contrast sequences, they usually demonstrate a peripheral, discontinuous, and nodular pattern of enhancement on the arterial phase images. On delayed post-contrast images, these lesions continue to fill in and exhibit hypointense signal relative to the liver parenchyma (hepatobiliary phase) using a hepatocyte-specific contrast (Masand 2018; Dickie et al. 2009; Christison-Lagay et al. 2007) (Fig. 1).

1.2 Mesenchymal Hamartoma

Mesenchymal hamartomas of the liver are the second most common benign tumors in childhood, that occur typically before 3 years of age and are composed of disorganized bile ducts, immature fluid-filled mesenchymal tissue, and hepatocytes (Moore et al. 2009)

The appearance of mesenchymal hamartoma depends on its components, which range from a predominantly cystic mass with thin or thick septa to a predominantly solid (stromal or mesenchymal) mass with a few small cysts.

On US, the cystic portions of the mass are anechoic or nearly anechoic with thin or thick echogenic septa while the solid portions appear echogenic (Chung et al. 2010)

On CT mesenchymal hamartoma appears like a multilocular low-attenuation cystic mass with enhancing thick or thin septae and solid component; calcification is rare (Yikilmaz et al. 2017)

On MRI the most common multiseptated cystic mass presents low signal intensity on T1-weighted and high signal intensity on T2-weighted images. The intervening septations are of intermediate signal intensity and display enhancement on the post-contrast sequences. Mesenchymal hamartomas can be solid or have a mixed solid/cystic appearance. Solid mesenchy- mal hamartoma cannot be differentiated from hepatoblastoma on imaging alone and demonstrates heterogeneously hyperintense T2-weighted signal, hypointense T1-weighted

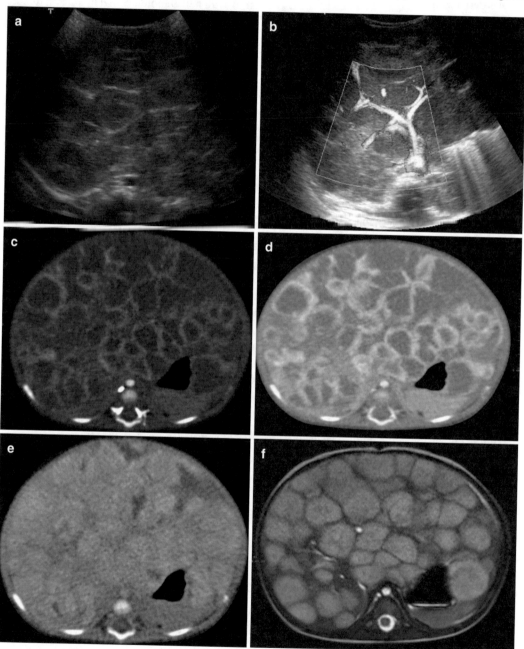

Fig. 1 4 months old female with hepatomegaly. US shows well-demarcated multiple hypoechoic nodular masses (**a**), without vascular signal on ECD (**b**). On CT (**c**, **d**, **e**) and on MRI (**f**, **g**, **h**) the liver is totally replaced by multiple hemangiomas with intense peripheral nodular enhancement on the arterial phase with a progressive cen- tripetal fill-in on portal venous and delayed phase images. Control after propranolol and corticosteroid therapy shows complete regression of hemangiomas 1 year later (**i**)

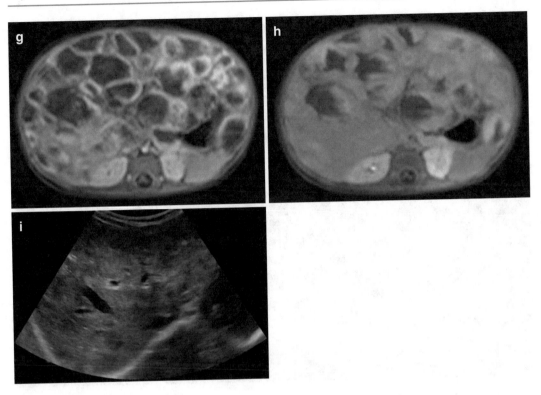

Fig. 1 (continued)

signal, and heterogeneous post-contrast enhancement within the mass (Masand 2018).

Hepatoblastoma is generally distinguished from mesenchymal hamartoma by marked elevation of the serum AFP level and the solid appearance and finding of calcification.

Undifferentiated embryonal sarcoma (UES) is similar to mesenchymal hamartoma for imaging and pathologic features but it occurs in an older age group (6–10 years of age) and often presents hemorrhage and necrosis with a frankly malignant stroma (Chung et al. 2010)

1.3 Focal Nodular Hyperplasia (FNH)

FNH represents 2% of all primary hepatic tumors in children from birth to age 20 years with a prevalence in the pediatric population between the ages of 2 and 5 years (Stocker 2001; Meyers 2007).

It has been supposed that focal nodular hyperplasia develops within a congenital vascular malformation or occurs secondary to iatrogenic hepatic vascular damage such as after chemotherapy (Masand 2018).

On US most FNH appears hypoechoic; however, they may be isoechoic and hyperechoic. The identification of isoechoic tumors may be difficult and recognizing indirect signs of compression adjacent to the mass may be helpful for the diagnosis. A hypoechoic halo is present in 32% of cases (Bartolotta et al. 2004; Wu et al. 2012).

On CT scan, FNH has more specific characteristics and typically demonstrates uniform enhancement with IV contrast during the arterial phase. In the later phases, FNH becomes isoattenuating to the liver (Ma et al. 2015).

A stellate scar, when present, is typically hypoattenuating on early contrast-enhanced images and demonstrates enhancement on delayed images.

MR imaging is the modality of choice for characterizing FNH, which appears isointense to slightly hypointense on T1-weighted and T2-weighted MR images, and enhances homogeneously. After contrast injection, the lesion

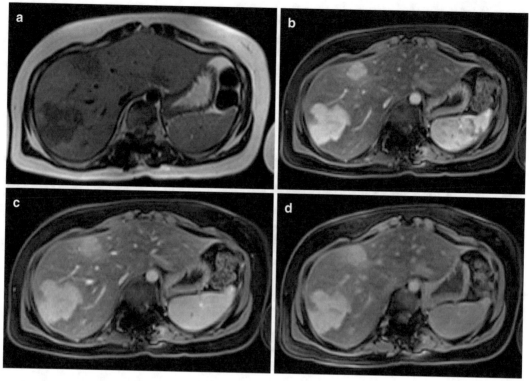

Fig. 2 10 years old female with a previous history of neuroblastoma. MRI shows multiple hypointense polilobulated lesions on T2-weighted images (**a**) which strongly enhance during the arterial phase and early portal venous phase (**b, c**). CE persisting during the hepatobiliary phase (**d**) allows differentiating FNH from metastatic disease

enhances strongly during the arterial phase and early portal venous phase, and becomes isointense to slightly hyperintense compared to the adjacent liver parenchyma during the late portal venous and delayed phase without a wash-out pattern. Enhancement during the hepatocyte phase using Gd-EOB-DTPA or Gd-BOPTA is a characteristic feature of FNH which allows differentiating FNH from other benign and malignant tumors of the liver (Yikilmaz et al. 2017)

In 80% of cases, there is a central scar that is typically hypointense on T1-weighted MR images and hyperintense on T2-weighted MR images. This scar enhances during the portal venous phase and delayed phases using extracellular contrast agents while it does not enhance during the hepatocyte phase using hepatocyte-specific contrast agents (Sutherland et al. 2014)

Fibrolamellar carcinoma may also demonstrate a collagenous central scar (unlike the vascular myxomatous scar of FNH) which is hypointense, rather than hyperintense, on T2-weighted images and does not enhance on delayed images (Fig. 2).

1.4 Nodular Regenerative Hyperplasia

Nodular regenerative hyperplasia is a rare disorder consisting of a diffuse micronodular transformation of hepatic parenchyma without intervening fibrous septa (Adeyiga et al. 2012).

There is typically no underlying cirrhotic liver disease or fibrosis. It occurs in many clinical conditions such as lymphoproliferative disease, autoimmune disorders, collagen vascular disease, portal hypertension, biliary atresia, and Budd-Chiari syndrome (Trenschel et al. 2000).

At US, the nodules may be invisible or may manifest only as heterogeneous echotexture or distortion of normal architecture. If visible, the nodules are generally well-circumscribed, homogeneous, and hypoechoic but may be hyperechoic compared with normal liver (Casillas et al. 1997; Dachman et al. 1987; Clouet et al. 1999).

On CT, small hepatic nodules may not be detected. They usually appear hypodense without significant enhancement after contrast injection. Sometimes there may be a diffuse or peripheral rim-like enhancement.

On MRI, the visible is often homogeneous and slightly hyperintense on T1-weighted images and variable on T2-weighted images. On fat-suppressed T1-weighted images a decreased signal intensity due to intracellular fat may be observed. After intravenous injection of gadolinium contrast material, the nodules may enhance preferentially in the portal venous phase like normal liver parenchyma (Chung et al. 2010)

1.5 Hepatocellular Adenoma

Hepatic adenoma is a rare benign tumor in childhood, accounting for 2–4% of all liver tumors. It is much more common in adults with a typical presentation in healthy young women with a history of oral contraceptives (Yikilmaz et al. 2017)

In recent years, four distinct subtypes of hepatocellular adenomas have been classified by Bordeaux classification: inflammatory adenoma (40–50%), hepatocyte nuclear factor-1 alpha-mutated adenoma (30–40%), beta-catenin-activated adenoma (10–15%), and unclassified adenoma (10–25%) (Masand 2018; Van Aalten et al. 2011)

US findings of hepatic adenoma are nonspecific and depend on the presence of fat, hemorrhage, and necrosis. Lesions with a high lipid content or hemorrhage may be hyperechoic to the normal liver. On doppler imaging, hepatic adenoma may show internal vascularity (Adeyiga et al. 2012)

On CT hepatic adenoma is usually hypodense because of the fat content; areas of hemorrhage appear hyperdense. After iodinated contrast injection hepatocellular adenomas demonstrate preferentially hepatic arterial enhancement and appear isoattenuating in the portal venous and delayed phases.

On MRI hepatic adenoma appears isointense to slightly hyperintense on T1-weighted sequences and hyperintense on T2-weighted sequences. There is usually early arterial enhancement after intravenous administration of gadolinium which becomes isointense to the liver on portal venous and delayed phase images (especially in inflammatory subtype). The enhancement may not continue during the portal venous phase and delayed phase in hepatocyte nuclear factor 1 alpha mutated type (Pugmire and Towbin 2016).

2 Malignant Tumors

Metastatic disease is the most common neoplasm affecting children's liver, especially from neuroblastoma, Wilms tumor, or lymphoma. Two-thirds of primary liver tumors in the pediatric population are malignant, and malignant primary hepatic tumors account for 1–2% of all childhood cancers (Chung et al. 2011).

The most common malignant tumors in decreasing order of frequency are hepatoblastoma, hepatocellular carcinoma (HCC), undifferentiated (embryonal) sarcoma (UES), angiosarcoma, and embryonal rhabdomyosarcoma. Epithelioid hemangioendothelioma (EHE) may also occur in adolescents (Table 1) (Ishak et al. 2001).

2.1 Hepatoblastoma

Hepatoblastoma is the most common malignant primary hepatic tumor in childhood. In many cases, it occurs in the first 2 years of life and causes a rapidly growing abdominal mass, hepatomegaly, pain, anorexia, and weight loss (Yikilmaz et al. 2017).

It usually occurs sporadically, but it may be associated with Beckwith-Wiedemann syndrome, hemihypertrophy, and familial adenomatous polyposis coli (McCarville and Roebuck 2012; Czauderna et al. 2014).

Serum alpha-fetoprotein levels are elevated in up to 90% of children with hepatoblastoma.

Metastatic disease most frequently involves the lungs, with pulmonary metastases seen in 10–20% of cases.

Histologically, hepatoblastoma is classified into the epithelial type and the mixed epithelial and mesenchymal type. Epithelial hepatoblastomas typically demonstrate a homogeneous appearance, while mixed epithelial and mesenchymal tumors appear more heterogeneous.

The appropriate initial diagnostic imaging in a patient with palpable abdominal mass is abdominal ultrasound (US). On US hepatoblastoma appears well-defined, lobulated, heterogeneous, and mildly echogenic masses. Calcifications, hemorrhage, and necrosis may be detected (Baheti et al. 2018)

On CT hepatoblastoma appears as a sharply circumscribed mass, slightly hypoattenuating on unenhanced and contrast-enhanced images. Epithelial hepatoblastomas are more homogeneous than a mixed tumor. About one half of hepatoblastomas appear lobulated or septated, especially on contrast-enhanced images. After contrast injection hepatoblastoma enhances slightly, less than the adjacent liver. In the arterial phase, it may present peripherical or septal enhancement (Chung et al. 2011)

On MRI hepatoblastoma can be unifocal or multifocal and typically appears hypointense on T1-weighted images, heterogeneously hyperintense on T2-weighted images, with variable characteristics based on the degree of bleeding and necrosis. After gadolinium injection, it enhances heterogeneously with possible areas of early washout from arteriovenous shunting. On the diffusion-weighted sequence (DWI), hepatoblastoma shows intense diffusion restriction (Masand 2018) (Figs. 3 and 4).

The International Childhood Liver Tumor Strategy Group (SIOPEL) designed the Pretreatment Assessment of Tumor Extension (PRETEXT) system for staging and risk stratification in liver tumors, particularly hepatoblastoma and HCC.

The PRETEXT system is made of two components: the PRETEXT group and the annotation factors. The PRETEXT group describes the extent of a tumor within the liver and is based on determining the number of contiguous tumor-free liver sections. The annotation factors help to describe associated features such as vascular involvement (either portal vein or hepatic vein/inferior vena cava), extrahepatic disease, multifocality, tumor rupture, and metastatic disease (to both the lungs and lymph nodes) (Towbin et al. 2018)

CT is the gold standard for evaluating pulmonary metastatic disease in children. MRI of the lungs is not yet considered sufficiently sensitive to identify small pulmonary nodules, the detection of which would impact the outcome. 18F-FDG PET/CT has no role in hepatoblastoma staging, although it.

might be useful in select cases of suspected relapse when AFP levels are elevated but no site of disease is revealed by conventional imaging (Voss 2018; Cistaro et al. 2013)

The main differential diagnosis includes infantile hemangioendothelioma, which occurs almost exclusively in children under 1 year of age and may also contain calcifications, but more fine and granular, with a high enhancement, more than adjacent liver, and mesenchymal hamartoma of the liver that manifests in the same age group as hepatoblastoma but presents normal serum AFP levels and is usually predominantly cystic (Chung et al. 2011) (Fig. 5).

2.2 Hepatocellular Carcinoma (HCC)

HCC is the most common primary hepatic malignancy in adolescence and the second most common primary pediatric malignancy of the liver. Pediatric HCC differs from adult-type because preexisting liver disease is seen in only 30–50% of pediatric patients (Shelmerdine et al. 2016)

Serum alpha-fetoprotein levels are elevated in 55–65% of the cases. Affected children usually present with an abdominal mass, constitutional symptoms, and abdominal pain (Murawski et al. 2016)

The most predisposing factors are biliary atresia, cholestatic syndromes, hemochromatosis, hereditary tyrosinemia, glycogen storage disorders, Wilson's disease, and hepatitis B infection.

On US, HCC is variable: smaller HCCs are predominantly hypoechoic to normal liver, although they may be isoechoic or hyperechoic while larger lesions may be more heterogeneous with hyperechoic areas representing fat or acute hemorrhage and anechoic areas due to necrosis or old hemorrhage. Infiltrative HCC may appear as a diffuse disruption of the normal liver echotexture (Helmberger et al. 1999)

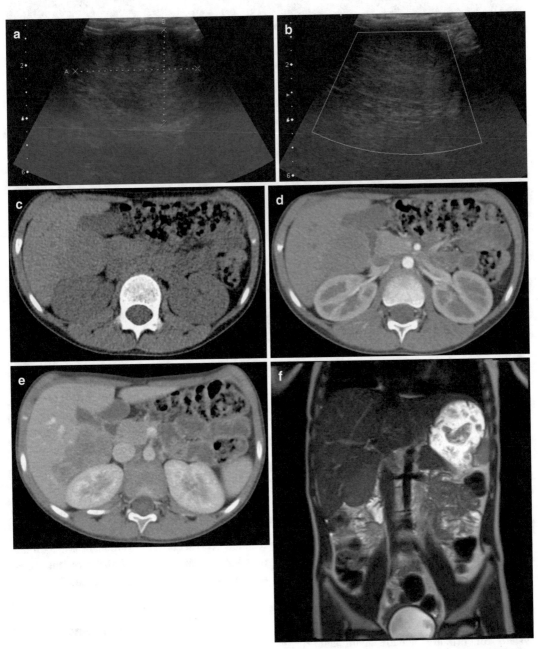

Fig. 3 Hepatoblastoma in a 5 years old male who presented with an abdominal mass, abdominal pain, and weight loss. US shows a well-defined solid mild echogenic mass (**a**) with a poor vascular spot on color-doppler (**b**). On CT the mass appears slightly hypoattenuating on unenhanced (**c**) and contrast-enhanced images (**d**, **e**), with areas of necrosis on venous phase (**e**). On MRI it appears iso-slightly iperintense on T2 coronal image (**f**) with a mild restriction on DWI (**g**) and shows poor contrast enhancement after gadolinium injection (**h**). Surgery specimen confirmed the diagnosis of hepatoblastoma (**i**)

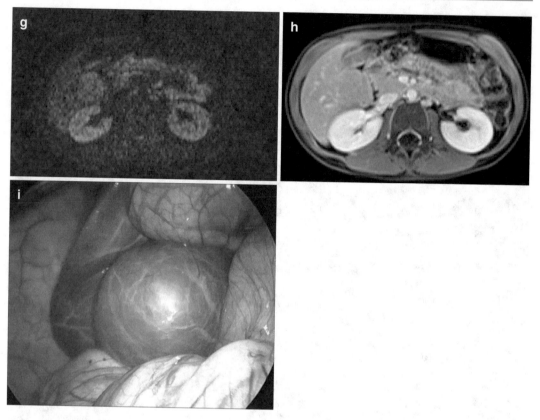

Fig. 3 (continued)

On CT, the mass is usually hypodense or isodense with well-defined or ill-defined margins and calcifications in 40% of HCC. After contrast injection, HCC presents early arterial enhancement with rapid wash-out. In delayed phases, it can present a peripherical capsule. CT is the gold standard for identifying vascular invasion and metastatic disease. Enlarged metastatic lymph nodes are seen at the porta hepatis in more than 50% of children's HCC. The most common metastatic disease spreads to the lungs, mediastinum, skeleton, and brain. Segmental liver involvement, vascular invasion, and distant metastatic spread are determinants of upfront resectability and are evaluated in PRETEXT, a radiologic staging system for primary hepatic malignancies of childhood (Yikilmaz et al. 2017; Jha et al. 2009)

On MRI, hepatocellular carcinoma is heterogeneously hyperintense on the T2-weighted sequences, hypointense on T1-weighted sequences and presents intense diffusion restriction on the diffusion-weighted sequence. On dynamic phases, HCC enhances heterogeneously on the arterial phase and shows washout on the portal venous phase because of arteriovenous shunting. Hemorrhagic areas present bright signals on the pre-contrast T1-weighted sequences while calcification or hemosiderin manifests as focal areas of susceptibility on the gradient recalled echo sequences. Tumor thrombus in the portal or hepatic veins enhances on the postcontrast T1-weighted images (Masand 2018).

2.3 Fibrolamellar Carcinoma

Fibrolamellar carcinoma is a rare variant of HCC, which primarily affects adolescents and young adults that occurs without predisposing factors such as cirrhosis or viral hepatitis.

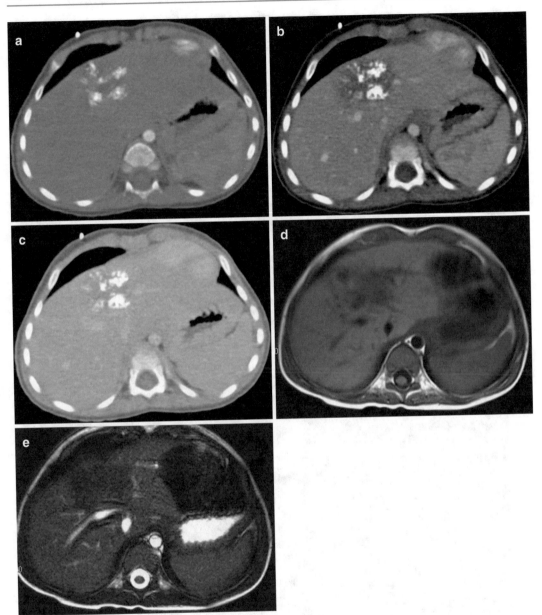

Fig. 4 One-year-old male patient with hepatoblastoma. CT shows a solid mass with coarse calcifications and poor contrast-enhancement after MDC (**a**, **b**, **c**). On MRI the mass appears slightly hypointense on T1 (**d**) and T2 (**e**) images

The tumor appears as a large, circumscribed, and nonencapsulated mass in 80–90% of cases (Levy 2002).

On US fibrolamellar carcinoma is heterogeneous, associated calcification may be seen as hyperechoic foci with posterior acoustic shadow-ing. A central scar appears as a hyperechoic focus (Yikilmaz et al. 2017)

On CT fibrolamellar carcinoma presents well-defined lobulated margins, it's hypoattenuating relative to the adjacent liver, frequently with a central scar with or without calcifications. After

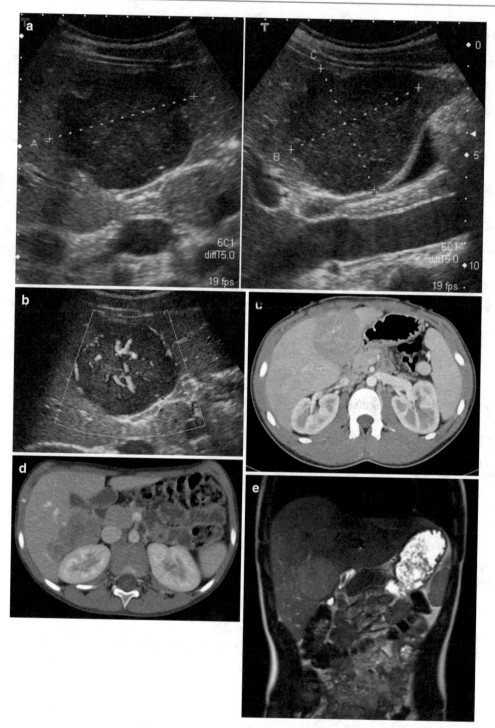

Fig. 5 5 years old male who presented with an abdominal palpable mass. US shows a polilobulated ipoechoic solid mass (**a**) with high peri- and intralesional vascular signal (**b**). On contrast-enhanced CT, it appears slightly ipodense with some intralesional vessels and small necrosis foci (**c**, **d**). MRI demonstrates a slightly hyperintense mass on T2-weighted images (**e**), with intense diffusion restriction on DWI images (**f**). On multiphase images, it appears slightly hypointense to the adjacent liver (**g**, **h**) and remarkably hypointense on epatobiliary phase (**i**). This lesion was first considered by radiologists as a hepatoblastoma but on surgical treatment, pathology revealed an inflammatory pseudotumor-like follicular dendritic cell sarcoma (FDC), a very rare low-grade sarcoma

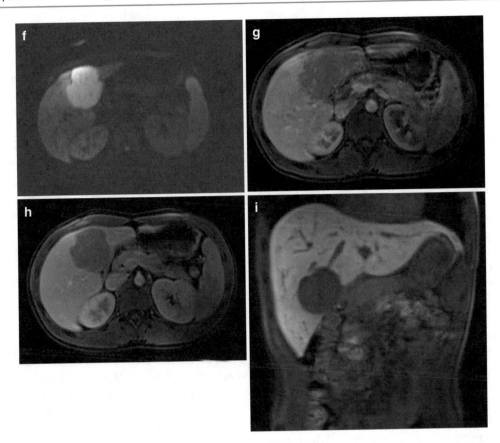

Fig. 5 (continued)

contrast administration, the tumor is hyperattenuating relative to the adjacent liver in the arterial phase with variable attenuation in the portal venous phase.

On MRI, the lesion is usually isointense or hypointense on T1-weighted MR images and hyperintense on T2-weighted MR images, and on dynamic phases, it shows avid contrast enhancement during the arterial phase with variable enhancement during the portal venous phase. The central scar is usually hypointense on both T1-weighted and T2-weighted MR without enhancement on dynamic phases not enhance unlike the scar of FNH (Smith et al. 2008)

2.4 Undifferentiated Embryonal Sarcoma (UES)

Undifferentiated embryonal sarcoma (UES) is the third most common hepatic malignancy of mesenchymal origin, accounting for 6% of all pediatric liver tumors and 10–15% of all malignant pediatric liver tumors and typically occurs in children 6–10 years of age. Serum AFP level is normal in UES.

On US, it appears as a large heterogeneous solid mass (>10 cm at diagnosis). While UES appears solid on US, paradoxically, it shows cystic aspect on CT and MR imaging because of its myxoid stroma which is a similar imaging feature of myxoid sarcoma and synovial sarcoma (Yikilmaz et al. 2017)

On CT, UES shows water attenuation (because of myxoid stroma) with soft tissue components, especially on the periphery of forming septa. A dense pseudocapsule with peripherical enhancement or hemorrhagic foci may be observed. After intravenous administration of iodinated contrast material, predominantly peripheral enhancement is noted on delayed images (Buetow et al. 1997)

On MRI, undifferentiated embryonal sarcoma appears as a large mixed solid and multicystic mass with central necrosis and areas of hemorrhage that present hyperintense T1-weighted signal. The cystic components have hypointense T1-weighted and hyperintense T2-weighted signal while the solid components show iso- to hypointense T1-weighted and heterogeneously hyperintense T2-weighted signal intensity. A T1- and T2-weighted hypointense pseudocapsule may be seen around the tumor. Post-contrast sequences demonstrate heterogeneous enhancement, usually peripherally and within the solid components of the mass (Masand 2018).

2.5 Epithelioid Hemangioendothelioma

Epithelioid hemangioendothelioma is an epithelial liver tumor classified under the category of malignant vascular tumors in the latest ISSVA classification (ISSVA 2014).

Epithelioid hemangioendothelioma occurs almost exclusively in young adults and appears, on imaging, as multiple discrete nodules ranging from 0.5 cm to 12 cm, or as confluent coalescent masses. Peripheral lesions may cause retraction of the liver capsule in up to 69% of the cases (Yikilmaz et al. 2017)

On US, epithelioid hemangioendothelioma may appear as individual nodules, confluent nodules, or diffusely heterogeneous echotexture of the liver. Nodules usually appear hypoechoic because of central myxoid stroma, but they may appear hyperechoic with or without a hypoechoic rim or isocheoic with a hypoechoic halo (Makhlouf et al. 1999; Miller et al. 1992; Buetow et al. 1994; Lyburn et al. 2003)

On CT, epithelioid hemangioendothelioma presents central hypodensity without contrast enhancement because of the presence of myxoid and hyalinized stroma or necrosis. It shows peripheral enhancement during the arterial phase with possible progressive centripetal enhancement during the portal venous and delayed phases; residual non-enhancing areas may persist (Yikilmaz et al. 2017)

ON MRI epithelioid hemangioendothelioma appears hypointense to the liver on T1-weighted images, with a possible more hypointense central portion, and heterogeneously hyperintense on T2-weighted images with a more hyperintense central portion. After contrast administration, there is a typical peripheral enhancement, although very large lesions may show more heterogeneous enhancement (Chung et al. 2011)

Fluorine 18 (18F) fluorodeoxyglucose positron emission tomography (PET) demonstrates moderate to intense uptake in the tumors and may demonstrate the involvement of adjacent lymph nodes and extrahepatic sites (Nguyen 2004).

2.6 Angiosarcoma

Angiosarcoma is a high-grade malignant tumor of the liver that is derived from endothelial cells, which occurs rarely in children. The mean presenting age is 3 years and the prognosis is poor.

Angiosarcoma may present multiple nodules or a large dominant mass or a mixture of a dominant mass and multiple nodules and, least commonly, diffuse micronodular infiltration of the liver (Koyama et al. 2002)

On US, angiosarcoma may appear as multiple nodules, a large mass, or both or diffuse heterogeneous echotexture of the entire liver. The echogenicity of the nodules depends on hemorrhagic or necrotic change.

On CT, lesions are usually hypoattenuating relative to the liver on arterial and venous phase images with foci of early heterogeneous, occasionally central enhancement or ring enhancement. On delayed images, persistent enhancement is observed without centripetal fill-in.

On MRI, angiosarcoma presents as a large mass hypointense on T1-weighted images and heterogeneously hyperintense on T2-weighted images and shows disorganized enhancement secondary to random vessel distribution on arterial phase imaging. On dynamic it presents markedly heterogeneous enhancement, which is progressive on the delayed phase, without central fill-in (Chung et al. 2011)

18F fluorodeoxyglucose PET/CT may demonstrate marked uptake in the liver tumors and can be helpful in localizing extrahepatic disease (Maeda et al. 2007)

2.7 Embryonal Rhabdomyosarcoma

Embryonal rhabdomyosarcoma is the only malignant tumor that arises in the biliary tree in children. It typically presents under the age of 5 years of age with jaundice, abdominal pain, nausea, vomiting, and fever.

The tumor usually involves major extrahepatic bile ducts but may originate in or grow into intrahepatic biliary ducts and invade the liver and causes biliary duct dilatation.

Biliary rhabdomyosarcoma typically shows an intraductal growth pattern and appears on US as a hypoechoic intraductal mass causing biliary duct dilatation (Kirli et al. 2012)

On CT, rhabdomyosarcoma appears as a heterogeneous mass filling the biliary tree with a grape-like or branching pattern, which shows variable enhancement after contrast administration (Yikilmaz et al. 2017)

On MRI, rhabdomyosarcoma presents T1 hypointense and T2 hyperintense signal or predominantly fluid-intensity signal and appears as a mass in the common duct or biliary radicals or a heterogeneous intrahepatic mass with large fluid-intensity areas. On CPRM it may appear as a partially cystic lesion in the common bile duct and as a mass adjacent to the duct that causes mural irregularity (Spunt et al. 2000; Kitagawa and Aida 2007; Lopez-Terrada and Finegold 2014; Nemade et al. 2007).

3 Conclusions

Imaging should aim to clarify the presence of a lesion, the likelihood of malignancy and potential for complete surgical resection.

US is the initial investigation modality of choice. Both CT and MRI may be used for evaluating the extent of the tumor for further evalua-

tion, to acquire additional information for differential diagnoses and to diagnose metastases to lung, lymph nodes or bone. CT requires less or no anesthesia due to faster scan times.

MRI has the advantage over CT of the absence of radiation exposure and the usage of mixed hepatocyte specific/extracellular contrast agents allows for better lesion characterisation and location, particularly with respect to the biliary system.

References

Adeyiga AO, Lee EY, Eisenberg RL (2012) Focal hepatic masses in pediatric patients. AJR Am J Roentgenol 199(4):W422–W440

Anupindi SA, Biko DM, Ntoulia A et al (2017) Contrast-enhanced US assessment of focal liver lesions in children. Radiographics 37(6):1632–1647

Baheti AD, Chapman T, Rudzinski E et al (2018) Diagnosis, histopathologic correlation and management of hepatoblastoma: what the radiologist needs to know. Clin Imaging 52:273–279

Bartolotta TV, Midiri M, Scialpi M et al (2004) Focal nodular hyperplasia in normal and fatty liver: a qualitative and quantitative evaluation with contrast-enhanced ultrasound. Eur Radiol 14:583–591

Buetow PC, Buck JL, Ros PR (1994) Malignant vascular tumors of the liver: radiologic pathologic correlation. Radiographics 14(1):153–166

Buetow PC, Buck JL, Pantongrag-Brown L et al (1997) Undifferentiated (embryonal) sarcoma of the liver: pathologic basis of imaging findings in 28 cases. Radiology 203(3):779–783

Casillas C, Martí-Bonmatí L, Galant J (1997) Pseudotumoral presentation of nodular regenerative hyperplasia of the liver: imaging in five patients including MR imaging. Eur Radiol 7(5):654–658

Chavhan GB, Shelmerdine S, Jhaveri K et al (2016) Liver MR imaging in children: current concepts and technique. Radiographics 36:1517–1532

Christison-Lagay ER, Burrows PE, Alomari A et al (2007) Hepatic hemangiomas: subtype classification and development of a clinical practice algorithm and registry. J Pediatr Surg 42:62–67

Chung EM, Cube R, Lewis RB et al (2010) From the archives of the AFIP: pediatric liver masses: radiologic-pathologic correlation part 1. Benign tumors. Radiographics 30(3):801–826

Chung EM, Lattin GE Jr, Cube R (2011) From the archives of the AFIP: pediatric liver masses: radiologic-pathologic correlation. Part 2. Malignant tumors. Radiographics 31(2):483–507

Cistaro A, Treglia G, Pagano M et al (2013) A comparison between (18F)F-FDG PET/CT imaging and biological and radiological findings in restaging of hepatoblastoma patients. Biomed Res Int 2013:709037

Clouet M, Boulay I, Boudiaf M et al (1999) Imaging features of nodular regenerative hyperplasia of the liver mimicking hepatic metastases. Abdom Imaging 24(3):258–261

Czauderna P, Lopez-Terrada D, Hiyama E et al (2014) Hepatoblastoma state of the art: pathology, genetics, risk stratification, and chemotherapy. Curr Opin Pediatr 26:19–28

Dachman AH, Ros PR, Goodman ZD et al (1987) Nodular regenerative hyperplasia of the liver: clinical and radiologic observations. AJR Am J Roentgenol 148(4):717–722

Dickie B, Dasgupta R, Nair R et al (2009) Spectrum of hepatic hemangiomas: management and outcome. J Pediatr Surg 44:125–133

Helmberger TK, Ros PR, Mergo PJ et al (1999) Pediatric liver neoplasms: a radiologic- pathologic correlation. Eur Radiol 9(7):1339–1347

Ishak KG, Goodman ZD, Stocker JT (2001) Tumors of the liver and intrahepatic bile ducts AFIP Atlas of Tumor Pathology, Third Series, Fascicle 31

ISSVA (International Society for the Study of Vascular Anomalies classification of vascular anomalies) (2014)

Jha P, Chawla SC, Tavri S et al (2009) Pediatric liver tumors–a pictorial review. Eur Radiol 19:209–219

Kassarjian A, Zurakowski D, Dubois J et al (2004) Infantile hepatic hemangiomas: clinical and imaging findings and their correlation with therapy. AJR Am J Roentgenol 182(3):785–795

Keslar PJ, Buck JL, Selby DM (1993) Infantile hemangioendothelioma of the liver revisited. Radiographics 13(3):657–670

Kirli EA, Parlak E, Oguz B et al (2012) Rhabdomyosarcoma of the common bile duct: an unusual cause of obstructive jaundice in a child. Turk J Pediatr 54:654–657

Kitagawa N, Aida N (2007) Biliary rhabdomyosarcoma. Pediatr Radiol 37(10):1059

Koyama T, Fletcher JG, Johnson CD et al (2002) Primary hepatic angiosarcoma: findings at CT and MR imaging. Radiology 222(3):667–673

Levy AD (2002) Malignant liver tumors. Clin Liver Dis 6(1):147–164

Lopez-Terrada D, Finegold MJ (2014) Tumors of the liver. In: Suchy FJ, Sokol RJ (eds) Liver disease in children, 4th edn. Cambridge University Press, Cambridge, pp 728–729

Lyburn ID, Torreggiani WC, Harris AC et al (2003) Hepatic epithelioid hemangioendothelioma: sonographic, CT, and MR imaging appearances. AJR Am J Roentgenol 180(5):1359–1364

Ma IT, Rojas Y, Masand PM et al (2015) Focal nodular hyperplasia in children: an institutional experience with review of the literature. J Pediatr Surg 50(3):382–387

Maeda T, Tateishi U, Hasegawa T et al (2007) Primary hepatic angiosarcoma on coregistered FDG PET and CT images. AJR Am J Roentgenol 188(6):1615–1617

Makhlouf HR, Ishak KG, Goodman ZD (1999) Epithelioid hemangioendothelioma of the liver: a clinicopathologic study of 137 cases. Cancer 85(3): 562–582

Masand PM (2018) Magnetic resonance imaging features of common focal liver lesions in children. Pediatr Radiol 48(9):1234–1244

McCarville MB, Roebuck DJ (2012) Diagnosis and staging of hepatoblastoma: imaging aspects. Pediatr Blood Cancer 59:793–799

Meyers RL (2007) Tumors of the liver in children. Surg Oncol 16(3):195–203

Meyers AB, Towbin AJ, Serai S et al (2011) Characterization of pediatric liver lesions with gadoxetate disodium. Pediatr Radiol 41:1183–1197

Miller WJ, Dodd GD 3rd, Federle MP et al (1992) Epithelioid hemangioendothelioma of the liver: imaging findings with pathologic correlation. AJR Am J Roentgenol 159(1):53–57

Mitchell CL, Vasanawala SS (2011) An approach to pediatric liver MRI. AJR Am J Roentgenol 196:W510 W526

Moore M, Anupindi SA, Mattei P et al (2009) Mesenchymal cystic hamartoma of the liver: MR imaging with pathologic correlation. J Radiol Case Rep 3:22–26

Murawski M, Weeda VB, Maibach R et al (2016) Hepatocellular carcinoma in children: does modified platinum and doxorubicin-based chemotherapy increase tumor resectability and change outcome: lessons learned from the SIOPEL 2 and 3 studies. J Clin Oncol 34:1050–1056

Nemade B, Talapatra K, Shet T et al (2007) Embryonal rhabdomyosarcoma of the biliary tree mimicking a choledochal cyst. J Cancer Res Ther 3(1): 40–42

Nguyen BD (2004) Epithelioid hemangioendothelioma of the liver with F-18 FDG PET imaging. Clin Nucl Med 29(12):828–830

Pugmire BS, Towbin AJ (2016) Magnetic resonance imaging of primary pediatric liver tumors. Pediatr Radiol 46:764–777

Roebuck DJ (2009) Assessment of malignant liver tumors in children. Cancer Imaging 9 (Special No A):S98–S103

Rozell JM, Catanzano P, Polansky SM et al (2014) Primary liver tumors in pediatric patients: proper imaging technique for diagnosis and staging. Semin Ultrasound CT MR 35(4):382–393

Shelmerdine SC, Roebuck DJ, Towbin AJ et al (2016) MRI of paediatric liver tumours: how we review and report. Cancer Imaging 16:21

Smith MT, Blatt ER, Jedlicka P et al (2008) Best cases from the AFIP: fibrolamellar hepatocellular carcinoma. Radiographics 28:609–613

Spunt SL, Lobe TE, Pappo AS et al (2000) Aggressive surgery is unwarranted for biliary tract rhabdomyosarcoma. J Pediatr Surg 35(2):309–316

Stocker JT (2001) Hepatic tumors in children. Clin Liver Dis 5(1):259–281

Sutherland T, Seale M, Yap K (2014) Part 1: MRI features of focal nodular hyperplasia with an emphasis on hepatobiliary contrast agents. J Med Imaging Radiat Oncol 58:50–55

Towbin AJ, Meyers RL, Woodley H (2018) 2017 PRETEXT: radiologic staging system for primary hepatic malignancies of childhood revised for the Paediatric hepatic international tumour trial (PHITT). Pediatr Radiol 48(4):536–554

Trenschel GM, Schubert A, Dries V et al (2000) Nodular regenerative hyperplasia of the liver: case report of a 13-year-old girl and review of the literature. Pediatr Radiol 30:64–68

Van Aalten SM, Thomeer MG, Terkivatan T et al (2011) Hepatocellular adenomas: correlation of MR imaging with pathologic subtype classification. Radiology 261:172–181

Voss SD (2018) Staging and following common pediatric malignancies: MRI versus CT versus functional imaging. Pediatr Radiol 48:1324–1336

Wu S, Tu R, Liu G et al (2012) The frequency and clinical significance of the halo sign in focal nodular hyperplasia of the liver. Med Ultrason 14:278–282

Yikilmaz A, George M, Lee EY (2017) Pediatric Hepatobiliary neoplasms: An Overview and Update. Radiol Clin North Am 55(4):741–766

Functional Imaging of the Liver

Simona Picchia, Martina Pezzullo,
Maria Antonietta Bali, Septian Hartono,
Choon Hua Thng, and Dow-Mu Koh

Contents

S. Picchia
Department of Radiology, University "La Sapienza",
Rome, Italy

M. Pezzullo
Department of Radiology, Erasme Hospital,
Université Libre de Bruxelles, Brussels, Belgium

M. A. Bali
Department of Radiology, Institut Jules Bordet,
Université Libre de Bruxelles, Brussels, Belgium

S. Hartono · C. H. Thng
Department of Diagnostic Imaging, National Cancer
Centre, Singapore, Singapore

D.-M. Koh (✉)
Department of Radiology, Royal Marsden Hospital,
London, UK
e-mail: dowmukoh@icr.ac.uk

© Springer Nature Switzerland AG 2021
E. Quaia (ed.), *Imaging of the Liver and Intra-hepatic Biliary Tract*,
Medical Radiology Diagnostic Imaging, https://doi.org/10.1007/978-3-030-39021-1_17

Abstract

Traditionally, imaging of focal and diffuse liver diseases has relied on morphological assessment on ultrasound, CT and MRI. However, morphological changes detectable on conventional imaging may be insensitive to early disease or therapeutic effects. For this reason, functional imaging techniques are increasingly used to evaluate liver diseases. The most widely investigated functional measurements include perfusion imaging (CT and MRI), diffusion-weighted MRI, MR elastography and quantitative T1-weighted gadoxetate-enhanced MRI of the liver. These techniques are used to improve disease detection, assess therapeutic effects and also evaluate liver function. The technical implementation, clinical utility and evidence for their deployment are discussed in this chapter.

1 Introduction

The liver is a large, richly vascularised, solid organ that is easily accessible to various imaging modalities such as ultrasonography (US), computed tomography (CT), magnetic resonance (MR) and positron emission tomography (PET) for detection, characterisation and monitoring of diffuse and focal hepatic diseases. Morphological imaging remains the cornerstone for radiological assessment of the liver, although functional imaging techniques are being increasingly deployed. Functional imaging techniques can reflect liver pathophysiology and allows quantitative measurements to be made, which are used to quantify changes associated with disease states. Studies have shown that functional imaging techniques can aid early disease detection, characterise disease behaviour, provide an early assessment of therapeutic effects or yield insights into disease prognosis.

In this chapter, we survey the functional imaging techniques that can be applied towards the assessment of both focal and diffuse liver diseases. A comprehensive survey of all functional liver imaging techniques is beyond the scope of this chapter. Hence, we focus our discussion on the use of functional imaging to study liver perfusion, tissue cellularity and microstructural organisation, liver stiffness and hepatocyte function. The clinical utility and limitations of these techniques is discussed, together with the evolving developments in the field.

2 Functional Imaging Techniques in the Liver

Functional CT, MRI and molecular imaging techniques can be applied to evaluate the liver. The most widely investigated functional CT technique is perfusion CT, which requires rapid and repeated scanning of the liver following intravenous contrast administration. This allows parameters that reflect blood flow in the liver to be derived. As CT perfusion studies can result in significant radiation burden, its adoption has been limited to clinical trials and specialised centsres. Some investigators regard the use of dual-energy CT image acquisition as a functional imaging technique, as data acquired using x-rays of different energies can be used to derive quantitative information, such as tissue iodine concentration following intravenous contrast injection, which is linked to tissue perfusion.

MRI is the most versatile functional liver technique for the liver, as different image acquisition techniques can be used to derive specific measurement parameters, each reflecting a different aspect of liver pathophysiology. Using dynamic contrast-enhanced MRI, perfusion MRI is performed, which is used to characterise blood flow in liver tumours and their response to treatment. Intrinsic susceptibility MRI (IS-MRI) can provide insights into tumour blood volume and tissue oxygenation, although the technique is not often applied in the liver. By contrast, diffusion-weighted imaging (DWI) is now widely used in the liver to study tissue cellularity and microstructural organisation. In clinical practice, DWI is most often used to highlight cellular disease from the rest of the normal liver parenchyma, without the need for exogenous contrast administration. The use of DWI has significantly enhanced the clinical diagnostic confidence for the detection of focal liver lesions and is a key sequence in emerging abbreviated liver imaging protocols, which aims to accelerate liver MR imaging without compromising diagnostic performance. MR elastography, which is used to measure liver stiffness, is a useful technique to assess for liver fibrosis and cirrhosis. The adoption of MR elastography requires hardware investment, which means that it is not often available beyond specialist liver centres, where there is a significant caseload to justify its deployment. More recently, there has been significant interest in the use of MRI to assess hepatic function. To achieve this, MR imaging is performed following the injection of a hepatocyte selective contrast medium, and temporal changes in the quantitative T1 relaxation time is used to estimate the hepatocyte function.

For molecular imaging, the most widely used radiotracer remains as 18F-deoxyglucose (18F-FDG), which is widely used in the cancer setting to detect hypermetabolic tumours; and to monitor their response to treatment. However, other molecular tracers, such as Ga68-DOTATAE and 18F-choline, have also their utility in a specific context, the former for the assessment of neuroendocrine liver metastases; and the latter for the assessment of liver tumours (e.g. hepatocellular carcinoma). Further discussion of molecular imaging techniques for liver assessment is beyond the scope of this chapter. The commonly used functional imaging techniques used to assess the liver are summarised in Table 1.

Table 1 Functional imaging techniques for liver imaging

Imaging Technique	Biological correlates	Examples of measurement parameters
CT		
Perfusion CT	Blood flow, vascular permeability, microvessel density	Non-quantitative: Shape of the enhancement curve Semiquantitative: Hepatic perfusion index, time to peak, slope of enhancement, area under the curve Quantitative: Blood flow, vascular permeability, relative hepatic artery and portal vein blood flow, extracellular volume
MRI		
Perfusion MRI	Blood flow, vascular permeability, microvessel density,	Non-quantitative: Shape of the enhancement curve Semiquantitative: Hepatic perfusion index, time to peak, slope of enhancement Quantitative: Blood flow, vascular permeability, relative arterial and portal vein blood flow, extracellular volume
Intrinsic susceptibility MRI	Blood volume, tissue oxygenation	Blood volume, T2* relaxivity
Diffusion-weighted MRI	Tissue cellularity, extracellular space tortuosity, microstructural organisation, fluid viscosity	Monoexponential model: Apparent diffusion coefficient (ADC) Non-monoexponential models: Intravoxel incoherent motion: Perfusion fraction, pseudodiffusion coefficient, diffusion coefficient Diffusion kurtosis: Kurtosis, diffusion coefficient
MR elastography	Tissue stiffness, tissue elasticity	Shear stiffness
Fat and water quantification	Intravoxel fat and iron	Percentage of fat and iron in the liver
Change in T1 relaxivity of the liver after hepatocyte selective contrast medium	Hepatocellular function	Change in T1 relaxation time, hepatocyte extraction ratio
Molecular imaging		
18F-FDG PET	Glucose metabolism	Standardised uptake values
18F-choline PET	Cellular membrane turnover	Standardised uptake values
68Ga-DOTATE PET	Expression of somatostatin receptor 2	Standardised uptake values

3 Assessing Liver Perfusion

3.1 Background Considerations

Imaging liver perfusion can be a challenging task because the liver has a unique dual vascular supply with approximately 25% of hepatic blood flow originating from the hepatic artery and 75% from the portal vein (Chiandussi et al. 1968). Both these afferent vascular systems communicate with each other through trans-sinusoidal and transvasal network and the peribiliary plexuses. The aim of perfusion imaging is to non-invasively obtain information on normal and pathologic hepatic microcirculation and to identify possible imaging biomarkers reflecting the underlying physiology/physiopathology that aids the detection and characterisation of pathological conditions and for predicting and monitoring response to treatment.

When primary tumours or metastatic deposits are present within the liver, they will lead to hemodynamic changes of the hepatic blood flow that can be detected by perfusion imaging. These changes are related to tumour neo-vascularisation which represents a key factor for tumour growth, progression and metastasis. Tumour neo-vascularisation is a complex process that is induced and mediated by tumour and host-related factors responsible for increased vessel density consisting of new non-endothelialised highly leaky capillaries and arteriovenous shunts (Dvorak et al. 1995; Lee et al. 2003). However, neo-vascularisation also means that tumours in the liver derive their blood supply predominantly from the hepatic artery rather than the portal vein. Tumours with high vascularity also show more aggressive behaviour and are associated with worse disease outcomes (Henderson et al. 2003).

Ideally, the following requirements should be considered when performing liver perfusion using imaging modalities: high temporal and spatial resolution images to correctly identify the kinetic properties of the tracer; accurate quantification of global or regional arterial and portal perfusion; calculation of tracer concentrations for an accurate quantitative study; robust modelling of liver perfusion physiology; and whole-liver coverage.

3.2 Computed Tomography Perfusion Imaging

The general principle of computed tomography perfusion imaging (CTPI) is based on monitoring changes of iodinated contrast agent concentration in the hepatic blood vessels and tissue as a function of time following intravenous injection. These contrast agent concentrations are linearly proportional to the CT attenuation changes within the vascular structures and the tissue expressed in Hounsfield units (Axel 1980). Therefore, temporal changes in attenuation can be analysed to provide several parameters that reflect the underlying vascular and tissue physiology/physiopathology.

The vascular and tissue attenuation curves versus time are obtained by placing a region of interest (ROI) respectively on the hepatic artery (or abdominal aorta), the portal vein and the tissue/lesion being analysed, on the dynamic CT images acquired with high temporal resolution (e.g. 1 image/sec for the first pass of contrast agent in the tissue) before, during and after the intravenous administration of an iodinated contrast agent using a power injector. In the presence of image misregistration, mainly due to respiratory motion, the use of motion correction tools is recommended (Miles et al. 2012). From these contrast concentration-time curves, CTPI parameters can be calculated using either a model-free or a model-based approach (Kim et al. 2014).

In the model-free approach, only the perfusion phase (first-pass of contrast material) is taken into account which allows calculation of the hepatic arterial and portal venous perfusion (PVP) and the hepatic perfusion index (HPI) (Miles et al. 1993). The model-based approach has moved towards a dual-input, dual compartment pharmacokinetic model, provided that there is good data support for such analysis. The dual-input model respects the dual vascular supply of the liver from the hepatic artery and the portal vein. However, when evaluating hepatic metastases or hepatocellular carcinoma (HCC), which are known to be predominantly supplied by the arterial network, a single-input model may be considered, given that the portal venous supply is typically very small.

A dual-compartment model assumes that the contrast agent is distributed between two compartments, the vascular space and the extravascular-extracellular space (EES), that is, interstitial space. In the normal liver, a single-compartment model could be considered, assuming that the interstitial space (space of Disse) communicates freely with the sinusoids through large fenestration. However, this assumption is not true for the diseased liver (Materne et al. 2000). For example, in liver fibrosis, the deposition of collagen causes an alteration in the sinusoidal architecture (loss of fenestration) and increases resistance to the sinusoidal flow, requiring a dual compartment model to describe the regional microcirculatory alterations (Pandharipande et al. 2005).

The model-based approach allows the calculation of quantitative parameters besides arterial and portal liver perfusion and hepatic perfusion index (HPI), such as regional blood flow (BF, blood flow per unit volume/mass of tissue),

regional blood volume (BV, a fraction of tissue that consists of flowing blood), mean transit time (MTT, averaged time for blood to traverse the tissue vasculature), permeability surface area product (PS, reflecting the diffusion of contrast agent across the capillary endothelium and the surface area of the endothelium) (Miles et al. 2012; Kim et al. 2014) (Fig. 1).

The use of such quantitative parameters as imaging biomarkers in longitudinal studies requires an important prerequisite which is the estimation of the measurement repeatability/reproducibility, which reflects the consistency of the acquisition technique, image post-processing and the data analysis (Bretas et al. 2017). The reported coefficient of variations from previous pre-clinical and clinical studies is less than 5% for perfusion measurements suggesting that this technique can provide robust quantitative parameters (Sahani et al. 2007; Kan et al. 2005; Stewart et al. 2008).

The disadvantages of liver CTPI include limited anatomical coverage and high radiation dose,

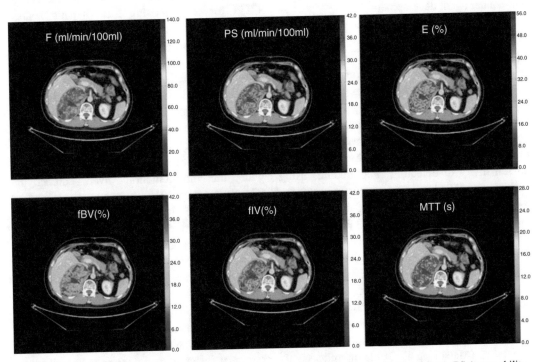

Fig. 1 A middle-age man with hepatocellular carcinoma in the right lobe of the liver underwent perfusion CT imaging. Parametric maps are generated using a dual-input, dual-compartment, distributed-parameter tracer kinetic model showing F (blood flow), PS (permeability–surface area product), E (extraction fraction), fractional intravascular volume (fBV), fractional interstitial volume (fIV) and mean transit time (MTT)

For this reason, dual-energy CT has been suggested as a potential surrogate for perfusion information. In comparative studies performed in patients with HCC, the quantitative parameter of iodine density determined at dual-energy CT showed good correlation with CTPI derived perfusion parameters (Gordic et al. 2016; Mule et al. 2018). Indeed, the advantage of dual-energy CT is the substantially lower radiation dose when compared to CTPI; however the disadvantage is that acquisition is usually obtained in a single phase, and the lack of information regarding lesion/tissue temporal and peak enhancement can lead to inaccurate results (Gordic et al. 2016).

3.2.1 Clinical Application

Since the first reports in the early 1990s on the usefulness of CTPI in the liver, there has been a wide interest, especially in oncology, for disease detection and characterisation, tumour staging, identification of prognostic biomarkers for patient outcome, assessment of treatment efficacy and in pharmacodynamic evaluation for anti-cancer agent development.

3.2.1.1 Focal Liver Lesions

In patients with chronic liver disease and at high risk for HCC, imaging is used to detect and characterise small hepatic nodules (< 2 cm). Increased arterialisation of early HCC can be detected by contrast-enhanced imaging, which contributes to the differentiating between benign/premalignant and malignant nodules. The overall sensitivity of detecting HCC nodules using multiphase CT has been reported between 54-87%, and this decreases to 45-57% for nodules less than 2 cm. By using CTPI to quantify lesion arterial and portal perfusion, a higher detection rate of 92-98% has been reported (Fischer et al. 2015).

During carcinogenesis, an increase in the hepatic arterial perfusion and HPI, together with a decrease hepatic venous perfusion are signs of malignant transformation of dysplastic nodules into HCC (Matsui et al. 2011; Ippolito et al. 2012). A sensitivity of 100% using a cut off of ≥99% HPI and a specificity of 100% using a cut off of ≥85% HPI for the diagnosis of HCC have

been reported (Fischer et al. 2015). The BF, BV and MTT also have prognostic value in patients with HCC: tumour with high BF and BV and low MTT, suggesting high vascularity and extensive arteriovenous shunts, are associated with poorer prognosis (Jiang et al. 2012; Petralia et al. 2011).

In livers with occult micro-metastases, increased hepatic arterial perfusion and HPI and decreased PVP have been observed due to the hemodynamic changes secondary to the formation of new, unpaired arterial vessels. These observations reported in both pre-clinical and clinical studies suggest that CTPI may be used to predict the presence of micro-metastases in patients at a high risk in whom conventional imaging modality may have limited diagnostic sensitivity because of the lack of associated morphologic changes (Tsushima et al. 2001; Cuenod et al. 2001). Indeed, early detection of liver metastasis can have important implications for treatment management and patient prognosis.

Several studies have investigated the use of CTPI for characterising focal hepatic lesions based on their perfusion properties. Hepatic metastases from colorectal cancer, for example, which receive their vascular supply principally through the arterial network, show an increased hepatic arterial perfusion and decreased portal venous perfusion at CTPI (Reiner et al. 2012). Hepatic metastases from neuroendocrine tumours demonstrate significantly higher HPI, BF, BV, PS, and significantly shorter MTT compared with the non-tumoural liver parenchyma (Guyennon et al. 2010). Moreover, there is anecdotal evidence that CTPI parameters such as increased HPI or decreased portal vein perfusion may confer a poor prognostic in patients with colorectal liver metastases although this requires further validation (Leggett et al. 1997; Miles et al. 1998).

Another application for CTPI is for the evaluation of treatment efficacy. Vascular targeting anti-cancer agents used in combination with conventional systemic treatment or as monotherapy, in several tumour types. These drugs arrest tumour progression by inhibiting vascular formation thus inducing a cytostatic more than a cytotoxic effect and as a consequence, there may be minimal morphologic or size measurement changes. Recent studies showed a significant reduction in the BF and BV and increased MTT in responders to therapy without significant size, in both the pre-clinical and clinical setting, suggesting that these parameters could be considered for monitoring treatment response and also as potential early predictive biomarkers of response (Ren et al. 2012; Ng et al. 2011; Yang et al. 2012; Ng et al. 2018). In both hepatic metastases and HCC nodules treated with radiofrequency ablation (RF), a decrease of HPI of more than 73% in the central necrotic zone and more than 76% in the transitional zone assessed 24 h after RF was associated with a complete response with an AUC of 0.911 (Marquez et al. 2017). Although highly promising, CTPI quantitative parameters cannot yet be used to direct patient management as further validation needs to be acquired from large and multicentric prospective studies (Kim et al. 2014).

3.2.1.2 Diffuse Liver Disease

Liver fibrosis is a diffuse cicatrisation process related to chronic liver damage, which can be induced by viral, genetic, metabolic and autoimmune aetiologies. The severity of liver damage is based on the histological analysis of the necroinflammatory activity present on liver biopsy specimens and is graded from A0 (absent) to A3 (severe), as well as fibrosis graded from F0 (absent) to F4 (cirrhosis) (Bedossa and Poynard 1996). Cirrhosis represents the end-stage of liver fibrosis progression and is a predisposing condition for liver failure and increases the risk for HCC (Schuppan and Afdhal 2008).

Important microcirculatory changes occur in liver fibrosis and cirrhosis. There is increased intrahepatic vascular resistance with a secondary decrease in portal venous inflow compensated by an increased arterial inflow (Lautt 1985; Tsushima et al. 1999). Hence, CTPI can be used to increased hepatic arterial perfusion and decreased portal venous perfusion, together with reduced total liver perfusion associated with cirrhosis (Miles et al. 1993; Materne et al. 2000; Van Beers et al. 2001). Moreover, for discrimi-

nating minimal (F1) from the intermediate stage of fibrosis (>F2), the MTT was found to be discriminatory in this setting (Ronot et al. 2010).

3.3 Dynamic Contrast-Enhanced MR Imaging (DCE-MRI)

Perfusion imaging can be undertaken using CT and MRI. For hepatic MR perfusion, several techniques may be deployed. Typically, intravenous contrast is administered for DCE-MRI and T1-weighted sequences are used to track the passage of gadolinium contrast media through tissues. However, there are also non-contrast techniques. Intra-voxel incoherent motion (IVIM) applies diffusion-sensitising magnetic field gradients to the MR imaging sequence, which does not require contrast agent administration. Likewise, the arterial spin labelling technique is based on observing magnetically labelled proximal endogenous water in arterial blood, as this water freely diffuses into the tissue.

Compared with CTPI, DCE-MRI has several advantages including the lack of radiation, higher contrast-to-noise ratios and multiparametric capabilities. DCE-MR imaging can provide information on the microcirculatory characteristics of the tissue by probing low molecular weight gadolinium (gd)-based contrast agents, as they leak from the vascular space into the extravascular extracellular space (EES) and is then eliminated by the kidneys. As the contrast agent transits through the tissue, changes in T1 signal are observed.

Semi-quantitative parameters can be extracted from the signal intensity-time curve and include area under the curve (AUC) which provides the amount of enhancement over a defined period, the peak enhancement ratio, time to peak, steepest slope and the mean transient time (MTT) (Evelhoch 1999). This approach although straightforward has a number of limitations: the calculated parameters do not accurately reflect contrast agent concentration in the tissue, they are highly dependent on the imaging acquisition protocols and the scanner properties and they provide no insight into the underlying physiology (Padhani 2002; Yankeelov and Gore 2009).

Conversion of signal intensity (SI) changes versus time into contrast agent concentration changes versus time curves allows the use of tracer kinetic modelling and the calculation of microcirculatory quantitative parameters. The general approach to model the changes of Gd-based contrast agent concentration is similar to that developed for the diffusible tracer. Since these contrast agents do not penetrate the cells, the exchange occurs between the vascular compartment and the interstitial space (EES). Hence, changes in the tissue of contrast agent concentration are given by combining the changes in the EES and the changes in the plasma concentration, namely the arterial (vascular) input function (AIF) (Tofts 1997).

There are some technical requirements that should be considered and respected when applying DCE-MR to investigate the liver/lesion perfusion that includes robust acquisition techniques using high temporal resolution, estimation of gd-based contrast agent concentration using multiples flip angles techniques and measuring both the arterial and the venous vascular inputs since, as said previously, the liver is supplied by the hepatic artery and the portal vein (Buckley 2002). To obtain high temporal resolution images (<3 s) of the liver, three-dimensional gradient-echo weighted sequences are most commonly used. However, more recently there is increased interest in motion-resistant sequences (i.e. Radial-VIBE or CAIPIRINHA-VIBE) which may provide high-quality images from free-breathing sequences. Low molecular weight (<1000 Da) chelates of gadolinium that exchange relatively fast with the interstitial space should be administered using a power injector to assure the reproducibility of the injection.

As for CTPI, from a modelling perspective, a dual-input function (dual-AIF) should be considered for the liver as the tracer input into the model will come from both the hepatic artery and the portal vein (Materne et al. 2002). By doing so, the use of a more complex modelling approach such as dual-input, dual-compartment and distributed parameter model can be applied

(46). The following quantitative parameters can be obtained using a dual vascular input and a bi-compartmental model (vascular and interstitial space): K_{trans} (transfer constant) which represents vascular permeability in a permeability-limited (high-flow) situation or blood flow in a flow-limited situation, the K_{ep} (reverse flux rate constant) which estimates the return process of the contrast agent from the EES to the intravascular space, and v_e, which reflects the volume fraction of EES (Thng et al. 2014; Sourbron 2010).

3.3.1 Clinical Applications: Diffuse and Focal Liver Diseases

DCE-MR has been widely used in clinical trials to provide imaging biomarkers for diffuse liver diseases such as liver fibrosis and cirrhosis and to monitor anti-angiogenic drug efficacy on hepatic metastases or hepatocellular carcinoma (Hagiwara et al. 2008; Liu and Matsui 2007). Most of these studies have used IAUC (model-free approach) (Fig. 2.) and/or a single-input, dual-compartment model (Tofts model) in which K_{trans} (transfer constant) and v_e were calculated.

DCE-MR imaging can provide non-invasive semi-quantitative and quantitative perfusion-related parameters that correlate with the stage of liver fibrosis: with increasing fibrosis, there is a decrease in the portal fraction and an increase in the arterial enhancement fraction to increase (Patel et al. 2010; Ou et al. 2013; Bonekamp et al. 2012; Kim et al. 2008). These microcirculatory changes become more marked in cirrhotic livers where they also correlate with the degree of liver dysfunction and portal hypertension (Annet et al. 2003). The diagnostic performance of DCE-MR increases with the severity of fibrosis (Petitclerc et al. 2017).

Similar to CTPI, DCE-MR has been used to assess the treatment efficacy of anti-cancer agents. Vascular targeting anti-cancer drugs such as anti-angiogenic and vascular-disruption agents act on the tumour vascularisation (Fig. 3). In advanced HCC treated with sorafenib combined with tegafur/uracil, a reduction of K_{trans} was associated with improved progression-free

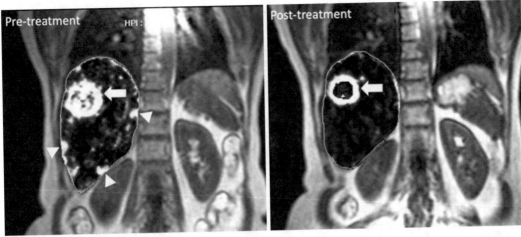

Fig. 2 Hepatic perfusion index. A woman with metastatic neuroendocrine tumour. Semi-quantitative hepatic perfusion index (HPI) maps obtained before and after 12 weeks of octreotide treatment. Pre-treatment HPI map shows a dominant metastasis (arrow) in the right lobe of the liver, with smaller metastases (arrowheads) in the peripheral of the liver showing high HPI values. Note the HPI reduction in the centre of the dominant metastasis after therapy, as well as in the smaller peripheral metastases

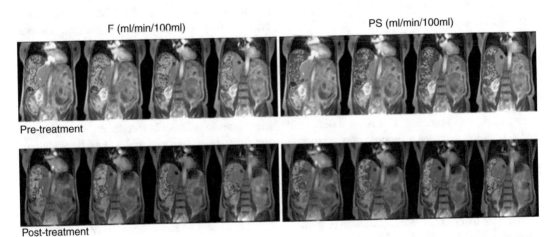

Fig. 3 Quantitative response of tumour to treatment. Parametric blood flow (F) and permeability-surface area product (PS) maps overlaid on T1-weighted images in a patient with hepatocellular carcinoma. Pre-treatment images show high F (58.11) and PS (33.16) values within the large tumour in the right lobe of the liver. Post-treatment images following targeted therapy shows a slight reduction in tumour size but significant reduction in the F (50.81) and PS (13.2) values, in keeping with treatment response

survival and overall survival (Hsu et al. 2011). Moreover, in HCC treated with sunitinib, perfusion parameters were more accurate to predict early response and progression-free survival than RECIST 1.1 and mRECIST (Sahani et al. 2013). In patients with colorectal liver metastases treated with Regorafenib monotherapy, DCE-MR derived parameters such as KEF (summarised median values of K_{trans} and EF (enhancing fraction)) demonstrated predictive value for response assessment and was significantly associated with progression-free and overall survival. Patients responding to the treatment demonstrated a significant drop of KEF on day 15 after treatment initiation and significantly better PFS and OS compared to non-responders where no changes in KEF were observed (Khan et al. 2018).

4 Assessing Cellularity and Microstructural Organisation

4.1 Background Considerations

Diffusion-weighted MRI (DWI) is now an established technique for imaging the liver (Taouli and Koh 2010). Using a single-shot echo-planar technique, DWI can be performed rapidly in the liver using a breath-hold, respiratory-triggered or free-breathing imaging technique, providing high contrast between areas of impeded diffusion against the normal liver parenchyma (Koh and Collins 2007). In clinical practice, DWI is widely used as an inherent contrast mechanism to help detect focal liver lesions, especially liver metastases and HCC, without the need for intravenous contrast administration. However, there is interest in developing quantitative DWI to improve disease assessment.

Depending on the number and the range of diffusion weightings (b-values) used for image acquisition, different quantitative parameters can be derived that can inform disease assessment. The most widely used quantitative parameter derived is the apparent diffusion coefficient (ADC), which assumes a monoexponential relationship between the image signal attenuation with increasing b-value. The ADC value is reduced in areas of increased cellularity (e.g. liver tumours) and/or increased microstructural complexity that impede water diffusion (e.g. liver fibrosis or cirrhosis) (Koh and Collins 2007).

However, by using multiple b-values (typically more than 5) including three or more at lower b-values ($\leq$150 s/mm²), a biexponential relationship between the image signal and b-values is observed in tissues. This occurs because of intravoxel incoherent motion (IVIM), which results in higher tissue signal attenuation at lower b-values due to the nulling of the protons associated with capillary perfusion (Koh et al. 2011). Hence, using IVIM technique enables the calculation of a diffusion coefficient (D) that reflects tissue diffusivity, a pseudo-diffusion coefficient (D*) that reflects the rate of tissue perfusion, as well as the perfusion fraction, which reflects the amount of tissue perfusion. More recently, there has also been an interest in diffusion kurtosis imaging (DKI), which requires diffusion-weighted imaging performed using multiple b-values but including at least one very high b-value (>1500 s/mm²) to study the non-Gaussian behaviour of water diffusion, which is likely to better reflect microstructural organisation, membrane integrity and intracellular water (Rosenkrantz et al. 2015). Using a DKI model, a diffusion coefficient (D) and the diffusion kurtosis (k) can be calculated (Fig. 4).

The ADC is a robust measurement that is highly repeatable in the liver. In well-conducted studies, the coefficient of repeatability of ADC in the normal liver is of the order of less than 10%, which increases to less than 15 to 20% in liver tumours, which may reflect the heterogeneous nature of liver tumours (Andreou et al. 2013; Winfield et al. 2017). The ADC value is also reproducible across vendor platforms. In one study, the coefficient of reproducibility of ADC across vendor systems was found to be approximately 14% for normal abdominal organs (Donati et al. 2014). By contrast, perfusion sensitive IVIM parameters generally show poor measurement repeatability and reproducibility, especially for focal liver lesions, which has limited their wider deployment in the clinical setting (Adreou et al. 2013). The perfusion fraction, f, has better measurement repeatability and reproducibility compared with the pseudo-diffusion coefficient D*. There may be some merits of using the perfusion fraction f to evaluate disease in specific disease settings, which will be discussed later. There has been limited experience in the measurement repeatability of k in the liver and more work is needed to determine its potential value for disease assessment.

4.2 Clinical Applications

4.2.1 Focal Liver Lesions

Diffusion-weighted MRI provides excellent contrast for the detection of focal liver lesions. The combination of DWI with gadoxetate-enhanced MRI has been shown to result in the

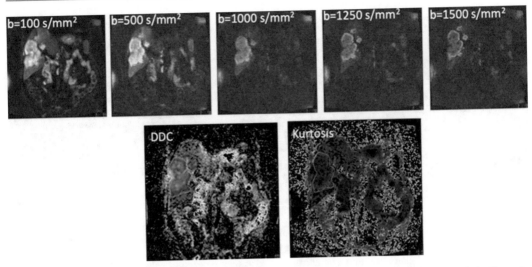

Fig. 4 Diffusion Kurtosis Imaging. Diffusion-weighted imaging using multiple b-values including high b-value ($\geq$1500 s/mm^2) allows the application of a diffusion kurtosis model to measure the direct diffusion coefficient (DDC) and the kurtosis (K) value. Note that in this patient with liver metastasis in the right lobe of the liver, the tumour returns slightly higher DDC and K values compared with the adjacent liver parenchyma. (Courtesy: Mihaela Rata, Royal Marsden Hospital, UK)

highest diagnostic accuracy for the detection of liver metastases (Vilgrain et al. 2016). DWI is also highly sensitive for visualising neuroendocrine liver metastases (Ronot et al. 2018) (Fig. 5). DWI facilitates the detection of HCC, including smaller (Park et al. 2012; Le Moigne et al. 2012) (<2 cm in size) and hypovascular (Di Pietropaolo et al. 2015) lesions, although lesion detection depends on the tumour grade and the severity of background cirrhosis (Jiang et al. 2017a).

The ADC value has been employed for the characterisation of focal liver lesions. Benign lesions have been shown to have higher ADC values than malignant lesions. Liver haemangiomas have been shown to have the highest ADC values amongst solid hepatic lesions. A threshold of approximately 1.7×10^{-3} mm^2/s has been found to have relatively high sensitivity and specificity (Taouli and Koh 2010). However, this threshold has to be applied with caution and in conjunction with all available imaging findings, as there is substantial overlap in the ADC values of solid liver lesions. For example, the ADC values of focal nodular hyperplasia and adenomas can overlap with the ADC values of HCC and cholangiocarcinomas.

The ADC value is potentially useful for assessing therapeutic effects (Fig. 6). Studies have shown that the ADC value increases in responders to chemotherapy, radiotherapy, embolisation therapy or minimally invasive treatments (Padhani and Koh 2011; Kokabi et al. 2015). Such an ADC increase has been shown to occur as early as 7 to 14 days following the commencement of treatment, providing an early biomarker to therapeutic effects. For this reason, the ADC value is being applied as a potential readout for assessing the effectiveness of novel therapeutics.

Using IVIM MRI, one study evaluated 74 patients with 75 lesions, of which 51 were malignant and 24 benign. The diffusion coefficient (D) and perfusion fraction (f) were found to be significantly lower in malignant than benign lesions. Nonetheless, D was found to be still more accurate than f for this purpose (Luo et al. 2017). IVIM MRI was also shown to help discriminate between different grades of HCC (Granata et al. 2016); as well as between HCC and intrahepatic cholangiomas (Shao et al. 2019). A recent meta-analysis (Wu et al. 2018) evaluated 484 patients with 582 liver lesions, including 381 malignant and 201 benign lesions. The authors found that ADC and

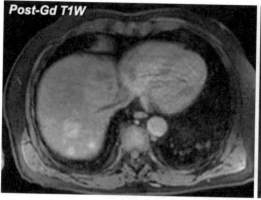

Fig. 5 Detection of neuroendocrine liver metastases. Diffusion-weighted imaging improves the detection of neuroendocrine liver metastases. Portovenous phase MRI following intravenous gadolinium contrast administration shows several enhancing metastases in the right lobe of the liver. However, diffusion-weighted imaging demonstrates many more lesions (arrows) within the liver, not visualised on contrast-enhanced MRI

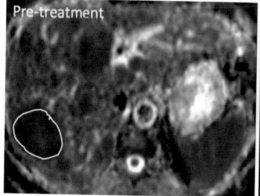
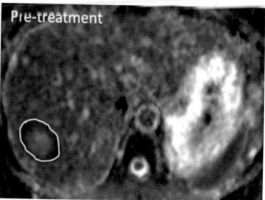

Fig. 6 Change in ADC in responders to treatment. ADC maps in a man with neuroendocrine liver metastasis before and after Y90-Dotatate treatment. The liver metastasis shows a mean ADC value of 0.89×10^{-3} s/mm^2 before treatment, increasing to 1.54×10^{-3} s/mm^2 after treatment, representing a 73% increase in the ADC value, in keeping with treatment response. Note that there is only a slight reduction in the tumour size after treatment

D values were significantly higher in benign lesions, while there was no significant difference in the $D*$ and f values between the benign and malignant lesions. The heterogeneity of the IVIM results may relate to the techniques applied which impacts the repeatability and reproducibility of the perfusion sensitive parameters. In this regard, meticulous technique to ensure good image signal-to-noise and careful choice of model fitting should be advocated in future studies. IVIM has also been used to evaluate the treatment response of liver metastases, which revealed a reduction in the perfusion fraction in responders to treatment (Granata et al. 2015; Kim et al. 2016).

4.2.2 Diffuse Liver Disease

Diffuse and focal steatosis can lead to a lowering of the ADC value of the liver parenchyma (Murphy et al. 2015; Dijkstra et al. 2014; Guiu et al. 2012). In patients with chronic liver disease, liver fibrosis and cirrhosis also lower the ADC value of hepatic parenchyma, which aids the detection of fibrosis/cirrhosis (Jiang et al. 2017b). It has been found that patients with higher grades of liver fibrosis (F3, F4) have lower ADC values than those with lower grades of liver fibrosis (F1, F2). However, the differences in the ADC values between these categories may be relatively small in relation to the measurement repeatability. This means that on a practicable basis, it is unclear to what extent the ADC value may have sufficient dynamic range to confidently discern between the different degrees of hepatic fibrosis.

IVIM DWI has been also applied to evaluate hepatic cirrhosis. The diffusion coefficient (D) and perfusion fraction (f) have been shown to decrease with fibrosis and cirrhosis (Franca et al. 2017; Ichikawa et al. 2015; Yoon et al. 2014). Using DKI, studies have also shown that the kurtosis value (k) is directly correlated with the degree of liver fibrosis (Yoon et al. 2019; Yang et al. 2018). However, the performance of IVIM DWI and DKI are poorer than MR elastography for the diagnosis and staging of liver fibrosis (Ichikawa et al. 2015).

More recently, it has been suggested that diffusion-weighted MRI may be used as a method to measure the elasticity of liver tissue (virtual elastogram), without the need for the use of an external drive. The calculation of the shifted ADC (sADC) has been shown to correlate with the shear modulus derived from MR elastography ($r2 = 0.9$). However, this approach requires further validation (Le Bihan et al. 2017).

5 Assessing Tissue Elasticity and Stiffness

5.1 Background Consideration

Magnetic resonance elastography (MRE) is a functional imaging technique that is used to quantify the elasticity of soft tissues by visualising the propagation of shear waves, usually generated using an external driver, using a modified phase-MRI sequence. The use of MRE is akin to "virtual palpation", which aims to differentiate tissues based on their tissue stiffness. MRE is an accurate method for the detection and staging of liver fibrosis, although its use is often limited to specialist centres as dedicated hardware and software are needed to implement the technique on MRI systems.

MRE can be performed at both 1.5 T and 3.0 T, although it appears to be more robust at 1.5 T across different vendor systems. MRE examination requires an actuator, which uses mechanical excitation positioned against the body to generate compression waves, which are translated into transverse shear waves in the body. The actuator used to generate the compression waves can be pneumatic, electromechanical or piezoelectric. The shear waves that are propagated in the body are imaged using a phase-contrast MRI technique that includes oscillating motion sensitising gradients, of which gradient-echo, spin-echo echo-planar sequences are frequently used. A meta-analysis revealed that both gradient-echo and spin-echo echo-planar techniques performed equally in the evaluation of liver fibrosis (Kim et al. 2018). The phase shift in the MRI signal in tissues is used to generate the wave image, and by using an inversion algorithm, the wave images are transformed into elastograms of tissue stiffness.

Studies have liver MRE has good measurement repeatability (intraclass coefficients) and inter-rater agreement (Shire et al. 2011; Lee et al. 2014). In one meta-analysis, a 22% or greater change in the mean liver stiffness evaluated over the same region using the same technique indicates that a real change has occurred with 95% confidence (Serai et al. 2017). MRE measurement of liver stiffness was not found to be influenced by age, gender, body-mass index (Singh et al. 2015) or the administration of gadolinium contrast medium (95). However, liver stiffness is affected by prandial state (Hines et al. 2011), and hence, liver MRE should be measured following a period of fasting. A good intra-class correlation coefficient (ICC) of 0.9 (95%CI: 0.78-0.96) and a within-subject coefficient of variation of 2.2%-11.4% have been reported for MRE liver stiffness measurements (Singh et al. 2015; Wang et al. 2018). The mean liver stiffness also showed good measurement reproducibility in a study across two vendor systems; showing a mean difference of 0.09 KPa, and a coefficient of repeatability of 0.25 KPa for the mean liver stiffness (Serai et al. 2015).

5.2 Clinical Applications

5.2.1 Focal Liver Lesions

MRE has been applied to characterise focal liver lesions. A preliminary study involving 44 liver tumours (which included metastases-14, hepatocellular carcinoma- 12, hemangioma-9, cholangiocarcinoma-5, focal nodular hyperplasia-3, and hepatic adenoma-1) found that MRE could distinguish tumours as malignant or benign with 100% accuracy, using a stiffness threshold of 5 kPa at 60 Hz (Venkatesh et al. 2008). More recently, in a study of 79 patients with 80 malignant and 44 benign focal liver lesions, MRE was found to be superior to diffusion-weighted imaging (DWI) for differentiating between malignant and benign pathologies (Hennedige et al. 2016). Malignant lesions showed a higher mean stiffness (7.9 kPa vs. 3.1 kPa) but lower mean ADC value (1.29 vs. 2.00 × 10^{-3} mm²/s) compared with benign lesions (100). However, ROC analysis showed higher diagnostic accuracy for MRE than DWI (0.986 vs. 0.82) (Hennedige et al. 2016).

5.2.2 Diffuse Liver Disease

The patients with suspected liver fibrosis, liver biopsy is confirmatory but is highly invasive and is associated with sampling errors and potential risk of complications. For this reason, non-invasive diagnosis of liver fibrosis is attractive, which can also be used to monitor the evolution of the disease. Biopsy can also be targeted towards where fibrosis is most severe on imaging (Perumpail et al. 2012).

Multiple studies have confirmed the value of MRE for the non-invasive evaluation of liver fibrosis (Fig. 7). In one recent meta-analysis of 26 studies with a total of 3200 patients, the authors found no significant difference in the pooled sensitivity and specificity of MRE using either a gradient-echo or a spin-echo EPI technique. The area under the receiver operator characteristic curve for the stage diagnosis of any ($F \geq 1$), significant ($F \geq 2$), advanced ($F \geq 3$), and cirrhosis ($F = 4$) on gradient-echo MRE and spin-echo echo-planar MRE were 0.93 versus 0.94, 0.95 versus 0.94, 0.94 versus 0.95, and 0.92

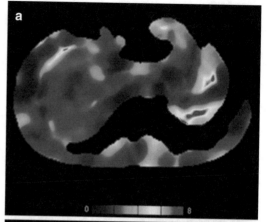

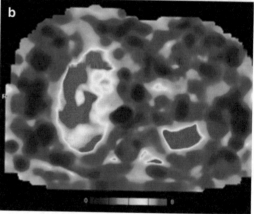

Fig. 7 Shear-wave elastography of (**a**) a normal liver and (**b**) man with Metavir grade F4 liver cirrhosis showing increased liver stiffness (in KPa) in the small cirrhotic liver (Courtesy: Dr. Albert Low, Singapore General Hospital)

versus 0.93, respectively (90). MRE was also more accurate for diagnosing liver fibrosis compared with transient elastography or point shear wave elastography (Perumpail et al. 2012). Using a threshold of 2.93 kPa at 60 Hz, Yin et al. (2007) found that MRE had 98% sensitivity, 99% specificity and 97% negative predictive value for liver fibrosis. Interestingly, the performance of MRE for staging liver fibrosis appears to be independent of the aetiology of the disease.

MRE has also been used to study the effects of treatment that modulates liver fibrosis. In one study (Jayakumar et al. 2019), 54 patients with MRE and liver biopsies at baseline and week 24 were treated with selonsertib, an inhibitor of apoptosis signal-regulating kinase 1 (ASK1), which has anti-inflammatory and anti-fibrotic properties. In that study, 18 (33%) had fibrosis improvement (≥1-stage reduction) after undergoing 24 weeks of treatment with the study drug. The area under the receiver operating characteristic curve of MRE-stiffness to identify improvement in the fibrosis score was 0.62 (95% CI 0.46-0.78) and the optimal threshold was a ≥0% relative reduction. Applying this threshold, MRE had 67% sensitivity, 64% specificity, 48% positive predictive value, 79% negative predictive value.

In addition, MRE has been applied to observe changes in liver stiffness in patients with non-alcoholic fatty liver disease (NAFLD). Several studies have demonstrated an increase in liver stiffness in patients with non-alcoholic steatohepatitis (NASH), in the absence of fibrosis. In one study, using a threshold of 2.74 kPa (Chen et al. 2011), MRE showed high diagnostic accuracy for identifying patients with NASH from patients with simple steatosis with an area under the ROC curve of 0.93. However, the practical application of MRE in this clinical context requires further validation.

6 Evaluation of Liver Function

6.1 Background

Chronic liver parenchymal disease leads to hepatocellular dysfunction, which eventually manifests as deranged serum liver function tests. However, the loss of normal liver function can be heterogeneous, segmental or sub-segmental, which may not be appreciated from serum findings. The ability to visualise the extent and distribution of liver dysfunction may be useful for treatment planning.

Following the administration of a hepatocyte selective contrast medium (e.g. gadoxetic acid), approximately 50% of gadoxetatic acid is taken up by hepatocytes during the transitional and hepatobiliary phase of contrast enhancement by transmembrane transporters such as the organic anion transporting polypeptides OATP1 B1/B3 present on the sinusoidal membrane of the hepa-

tocytes. The excretion of contrast into the biliary system occurs through the MRP2 transporters. Hence, the T1-enhancement of liver parenchyma following gadoxetic acid contrast administration can reflect hepatocyte function.

To measure hepatocyte function, quantification of the T1-relaxivity of hepatic parenchyma is performed before and at 10 to 20 min following gadoxetic acid contrast administration. There are several imaging sequences that have been applied, including a modified Look-Locker inversion recovery (MOLLI) technique or a variable flip angle (VFA) gradient-echo technique. These sequences may be executed with or without correction for the B1-field inhomogeneity. Studies have shown that the magnitude of change in the T1-relaxation time following contrast administration is highly reflective of the underlying liver excretory function, which can be used to produce parametric maps of hepatocellular function. Although the native T1 value of the liver is reduced in patients with liver cirrhosis (Cassinotto et al. 2015), this is not sufficiently discriminatory to identify patients with impaired liver function.

Measurement of the T1-relaxation time in the liver is highly repeatable (107). In one study, the within-subject coefficient of variance for T1 measurement of the liver was found to be 0.3% before gadoxetate contrast administration, and 1.1% after gadoxetate administration. However, significant variation is encountered in the T1-relaxation time of the liver when different T1-measurement techniques are applied. For example, there is significant variance in the T1 measurement between using MOLLI sequence versus the VFA technique (Yoon et al. 2016; Yoon et al. 2017).

6.2 Clinical Application

6.2.1 Evaluating Liver Function

Currently there is no consensus on which MR-derived parameters should be used to assess liver function by gadoxetate-enhanced MRI (Bae et al. 2012). Relative liver enhancement (RLE), contrast enhancement index and hepatic uptake index (HUI) are parameters based on single intensity (SI) measurements, which are relatively easy to derive (Watanabe et al. 2011). Measurement of the T1 relaxation time is more accurate than SI measurements, given the more direct relationship between T1 relaxation times and contrast agent concentration, although this relationship is more complex using gadoxetate, as the contrast is distributed in different compartments (i.e. intracellular and in the bile) (Besa et al. 2015). There is also considerable variation in the T1-relaxation time measurements depending on the imaging sequence/technique applied, the availability of these sequences varies across vendor systems. In addition, there is reportedly segmental variation of the liver T1 value across the liver, both before and after contrast administration (Haimerl et al. 2017). Furthermore, the T1-relaxation time varies with the magnetic field strength, being longer at higher field strength than at lower field strength. For these reasons, there is not yet a universally accepted method to measure or define liver tissue T1 relaxivity.

Nonetheless, it has been found that the change in the T1 relaxation time measured by the same imaging technique before and after gadoxetate contrast administration is highly correlated with liver function. Although the native T1 relaxation time of cirrhotic liver is longer compared with normal liver, this is not predictive of liver function. However, patients that show a small reduction in the T1 relaxation time (expressed as a percentage of the pre-contrast T1 relaxation time) after contrast administration are associated with impairment of liver function (Yoon et al. 2016; Besa et al. 2015; Katsube et al. 2011; Haimerl et al. 2013) (Fig. 8). Other quantitative parameters that have been used to identify patients with impaired liver function include the extracellular enhancement (by comparing with the enhancement of the spleen), functional liver-to-weight ratio and the hepatic uptake ratio (Yoon et al. 2019). One recent study at 3 T showed the hepatic uptake ratio was highly correlated with the ICG-r15 test, in patients with Child-Pugh class A or B liver cirrhosis (Yoon et al. 2019).

One potentially more sophisticated approach is dynamic hepatocyte-specific contrast-enhanced MRI which provides both semi-quantitative and quantitative parameters. Semi-quantitative parameters such as the maximum enhancement (Emax), time to peak (Tmax) and elimination half-life do not have any clear insight into the underlying physiology. The calculation of quantitative parameters implies the use of pharmacokinetic analysis of the parenchyma- and vascular-input concentration-time curves and include regional BF, regional BV, arterial and portal venous perfusion and hepatocyte extraction fraction (Sourbron et al. 2012). However, this approach requires sophisticated data acquisition and analysis, which can only be undertaken in specialist institutions.

Besides the microcirculatory changes, a decrease in the expression of the hepatocyte organic anion transporters has been observed in liver fibrosis, which can be inferred by using gadoxetate MRI. The reduction in OATP transporters will cause a decrease in the T1-shortening effect of the gadolinium contrast. Quantitative T1 mapping-based hepatocyte fraction demonstrated a strong correlation with fibrosis stages and also showed a good diagnostic performance in identifying patients with advanced liver fibrosis and cirrhosis (Pan et al. 2018).

7 Future Developments

There have been significant advances in MR hardware and software over the years, which have impacted our ability to derive functional imaging data from the liver. As compressed-sensing techniques become mainstream on all vendor MR systems, the ability to acquire high temporal and high spatial-resolution dynamic contrast-enhanced MR images significantly improve the way we perform perfusion MRI and possibly on how we assess liver function using MRI.

One of the major disruptors in imaging is artificial intelligence and deep learning, and there is no doubt that rapid developments in the field improve the speed of image reconstruction for functional imaging, disease segmentation and complex data analysis. One of the current limitations of applying functional imaging

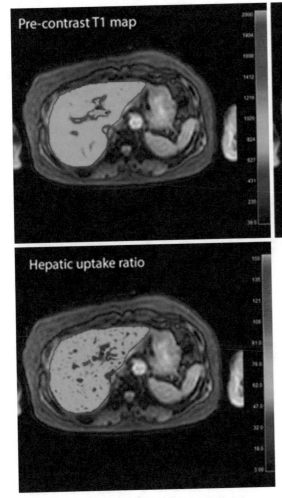

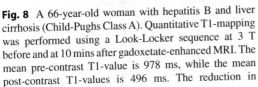

Fig. 8 A 66-year-old woman with hepatitis B and liver cirrhosis (Child-Pughs Class A). Quantitative T1-mapping was performed using a Look-Locker sequence at 3 T before and at 10 mins after gadoxetate-enhanced MRI. The mean pre-contrast T1-value is 978 ms, while the mean post-contrast T1-values is 496 ms. The reduction in T1-value after contrast indicates a good liver function test. These findings are corroborated with the hepatic uptake ratio map (normalised to splenic uptake), which shows a mean uptake ratio of 70 (Courtesy: Dr. Yoon Jeong Hee, Seoul National University Hospital)

techniques is that many of the image processing steps and data analysis are performed off-line by dedicated physicists and data scientists, which are not accessible to the majority of radiological departments. Using artificial intelligence and machine learning, it may be possible to generate new tools that can undertake in-line processing of complex functional imaging datasets automatically or semi-automatically, so that the quantitative results can be made available at the point of image reading for clinical decision making.

As radiomics analyses continue to generate promising biophysical properties from images that are linked to patients' treatment outcomes or prognosis, there is increasing interest in performing radiomics on MRI datasets. One of the limitations of using MR images for radiomics is that there may be substantial variations in the measured signal according to the patient position within the MRI scanner, which can lead to variations in the results. Currently, different approaches to signal normalisation are being applied to overcome some of these limitations, but there are advantages in performing radiomics analyses on quantitative maps derived from functional MR imaging measurements, as a way of overcoming the issue of MR signal variations across native acquired morphological images.

The speed of image acquisition can also be speeded up using artificial intelligence and machine learning. Hence, future liver MRI examination time is likely to decrease; which may allow more time to be spent acquiring functional imaging data. The routine use of a multiparametric functional imaging paradigm for liver imaging for patients within our daily clinical workflow may produce new insights into common diseases, and provide new knowledge for disease management.

References

Andreou A, Koh DM, Collins DJ, Blackledge M, Wallace T, Leach MO et al (2013) Measurement reproducibility of perfusion fraction and pseudodiffusion coefficient derived by intravoxel incoherent motion diffusion-weighted MR imaging in normal liver and metastases. Eur Radiol 23(2):428–434

Annet L, Materne R, Danse E, Jamart J, Horsmans Y, Van Beers BE (2003) Hepatic flow parameters measured with MR imaging and Doppler US: correlations with degree of cirrhosis and portal hypertension. Radiology 229(2):409–414

Axel L (1980) Cerebral blood flow determination by rapid-sequence computed tomography: theoretical analysis. Radiology 137(3):679–686

Bae KE, Kim SY, Lee SS, Kim KW, Won HJ, Shin YM et al (2012) Assessment of hepatic function with Gd-EOB-DTPA-enhanced hepatic MRI. Dig Dis 30(6):617–622

Bedossa P, Poynard T (1996) An algorithm for the grading of activity in chronic hepatitis C. the METAVIR cooperative study group. Hepatology 24(2):289–293

Besa C, Bane O, Jajamovich G, Marchione J, Taouli B (2015) 3D T1 relaxometry pre and post gadoxetic acid injection for the assessment of liver cirrhosis and liver function. Magn Reson Imaging 33(9):1075–1082

Bonekamp D, Bonekamp S, Geiger B, Kamel IR (2012) An elevated arterial enhancement fraction is associated with clinical and imaging indices of liver fibrosis and cirrhosis. J Comput Assist Tomogr 36(6):681–689

Bretas EAS, Torres US, Torres LR, Bekhor D, Saito Filho CF, Racy DJ et al (2017) Is liver perfusion CT reproducible? A study on intra- and interobserver agreement of normal hepatic haemodynamic parameters obtained with two different software packages. Br J Radiol 90(1078):20170214

Buckley DL (2002) Uncertainty in the analysis of tracer kinetics using dynamic contrast-enhanced T1-weighted MRI. Magn Reson Med 47(3):601–606

Cassinotto C, Feldis M, Vergniol J, Mouries A, Cochet H, Lapuyade B et al (2015) MR relaxometry in chronic liver diseases: comparison of T1 mapping, T2 mapping, and diffusion-weighted imaging for assessing cirrhosis diagnosis and severity. Eur J Radiol 84(8):1459–1465

Chen J, Talwalkar JA, Yin M, Glaser KJ, Sanderson SO, Ehman RL (2011) Early detection of nonalcoholic steatohepatitis in patients with nonalcoholic fatty liver disease by using MR elastography. Radiology 259(3):749–756

Chiandussi L, Greco F, Sardi G, Vaccarino A, Ferraris CM, Curti B (1968) Estimation of hepatic arterial and portal venous blood flow by direct catheterization of the vena porta through the umbilical cord in man. Preliminary results. Acta Hepatosplenol 15(3):166–171

Cuenod C, Leconte I, Siauve N, Resten A, Dromain C, Poulet B et al (2001) Early changes in liver perfusion caused by occult metastases in rats: detection with quantitative CT. Radiology 218(2):556–561

Di Pietropaolo M, Briani C, Federici GF, Marignani M, Begini P, Delle Fave G et al (2015) Comparison of diffusion-weighted imaging and gadoxetic acid-enhanced MR images in the evaluation of hepatocellular carcinoma and hypovascular hepatocellular nodules. Clin Imaging 39(3):468–475

Dijkstra H, Handayani A, Kappert P, Oudkerk M, Sijens PE (2014) Clinical implications of non-steatotic hepatic fat fractions on quantitative diffusion-weighted imaging of the liver. PLoS One 9(2):e87926

Donati OF, Chong D, Nanz D, Boss A, Froehlich JM, Andres E et al (2014) Diffusion-weighted MR imaging of upper abdominal organs: field strength and intervendor variability of apparent diffusion coefficients. Radiology 270(2):454–463

Dvorak HF, Brown LF, Detmar M, Dvorak AM (1995) Vascular permeability factor/vascular endothelial growth factor, microvascular hyperpermeability, and angiogenesis. Am J Pathol 146(5):1029–1039

Evelhoch JL (1999) Key factors in the acquisition of contrast kinetic data for oncology. J Magn Reson Imaging 10(3):254–259

Fischer MA, Kartalis N, Grigoriadis A, Loizou L, Stal P, Leidner B et al (2015) Perfusion computed tomography for detection of hepatocellular carcinoma in patients with liver cirrhosis. Eur Radiol 25(11):3123–3132

Franca M, Marti-Bonmati L, Alberich-Bayarri A, Oliveira P, Guimaraes S, Oliveira J et al (2017) Evaluation of fibrosis and inflammation in diffuse liver diseases using intravoxel incoherent motion diffusion-weighted MR imaging. Abdom Radiol (NY). 42(2):468–477

Gordic S, Puippe GD, Krauss B, Klotz E, Desbiolles L, Lesurtel M et al (2016) Correlation between dual-energy and perfusion CT in patients with hepatocellular carcinoma. Radiology 280(1):78–87

Granata V, Fusco R, Catalano O, Filice S, Amato DM, Nasti G et al (2015) Early assessment of colorectal

Cancer patients with liver metastases treated with Antiangiogenic drugs: the role of Intravoxel incoherent motion in diffusion-weighted imaging. PLoS One 10(11):e0142876

Granata V, Fusco R, Catalano O, Guarino B, Granata F, Tatangelo F et al (2016) Intravoxel incoherent motion (IVIM) in diffusion-weighted imaging (DWI) for hepatocellular carcinoma: correlation with histologic grade. Oncotarget 7(48):79357–79364

Guiu B, Petit JM, Capitan V, Aho S, Masson D, Lefevre PH et al (2012) Intravoxel incoherent motion diffusion-weighted imaging in nonalcoholic fatty liver disease: a 3.0-T MR study. Radiology 265(1):96–103

Guyennon A, Mihaila M, Palma J, Lombard-Bohas C, Chayvialle JA, Pilleul F (2010) Perfusion characterization of liver metastases from endocrine tumors: computed tomography perfusion. World J Radiol 2(11):449–454

Hagiwara M, Rusinek H, Lee VS, Losada M, Bannan MA, Krinsky GA et al (2008) Advanced liver fibrosis: diagnosis with 3D whole-liver perfusion MR imaging--initial experience. Radiology 246(3):926–934

Haimerl M, Verloh N, Zeman F, Fellner C, Muller-Wille R, Schreyer AG et al (2013) Assessment of clinical signs of liver cirrhosis using T1 mapping on Gd-EOB-DTPA-enhanced 3T MRI. PLoS One 8(12):e85658

Haimerl M, Verloh N, Zeman F, Fellner C, Nickel D, Lang SA et al (2017) Gd-EOB-DTPA-enhanced MRI for evaluation of liver function: comparison between signal-intensity-based indices and T1 relaxometry. Sci Rep 7:43347

Henderson E, Milosevic MF, Haider MA, Yeung IW (2003) Functional CT imaging of prostate cancer. Phys Med Biol 48(18):3085–3100

Hennedige TP, Hallinan JT, Leung FP, Teo LL, Iyer S, Wang G et al (2016) Comparison of magnetic resonance elastography and diffusion-weighted imaging for differentiating benign and malignant liver lesions. Eur Radiol 26(2):398–406

Hines CD, Lindstrom MJ, Varma AK, Reeder SB (2011) Effects of postprandial state and mesenteric blood flow on the repeatability of MR elastography in asymptomatic subjects. J Magn Reson Imaging 33(1):239–244

Hsu CY, Shen YC, Yu CW, Hsu C, Hu FC, Hsu CH et al (2011) Dynamic contrast-enhanced magnetic resonance imaging biomarkers predict survival and response in hepatocellular carcinoma patients treated with sorafenib and metronomic tegafur/uracil. J Hepatol 55(4):858–865

Ichikawa S, Motosugi U, Morisaka H, Sano K, Ichikawa T, Enomoto N et al (2015) MRI-based staging of hepatic fibrosis: comparison of intravoxel incoherent motion diffusion-weighted imaging with magnetic resonance elastography. J Magn Reson Imaging 42(1):204–210

Ippolito D, Capraro C, Casiraghi A, Cestari C, Sironi S (2012) Quantitative assessment of tumour associated neovascularisation in patients with liver cirrhosis and hepatocellular carcinoma: role of dynamic-CT perfusion imaging. Eur Radiol 22(4):803–811

Jayakumar S, Middleton MS, Lawitz EJ, Mantry PS, Caldwell SH, Arnold H et al (2019) Longitudinal correlations between MRE, MRI-PDFF, and liver histology in patients with non-alcoholic steatohepatitis: analysis of data from a phase II trial of selonsertib. J Hepatol 70(1):133–141

Jiang T, Kambadakone A, Kulkarni NM, Zhu AX, Sahani DV (2012) Monitoring response to antiangiogenic treatment and predicting outcomes in advanced hepatocellular carcinoma using image biomarkers, CT perfusion, tumor density, and tumor size (RECIST). Investig Radiol 47(1):11–17

Jiang H, Chen J, Gao R, Huang Z, Wu M, Song B (2017a) Liver fibrosis staging with diffusion-weighted imaging: a systematic review and meta-analysis. Abdom Radiol (NY). 42(2):490–501

Jiang T, Xu JH, Zou Y, Chen R, Peng LR, Zhou ZD et al (2017b) Diffusion-weighted imaging (DWI) of hepatocellular carcinomas: a retrospective analysis of the correlation between qualitative and quantitative DWI and tumour grade. Clin Radiol 72(6):465–472

Kan Z, Kobayashi S, Phongkitkarun S, Charnsangavej C (2005) Functional CT quantification of tumor perfusion after transhepatic arterial embolization in a rat model. Radiology 237(1):144–150

Katsube T, Okada M, Kumano S, Hori M, Imaoka I, Ishii K et al (2011) Estimation of liver function using T1 mapping on Gd-EOB-DTPA-enhanced magnetic resonance imaging. Investig Radiol 46(4):277–283

Khan K, Rata M, Cunningham D, Koh DM, Tunariu N, Hahne JC et al (2018) Functional imaging and circulating biomarkers of response to regorafenib in treatment-refractory metastatic colorectal cancer patients in a prospective phase II study. Gut 67(8):1484–1492

Kim H, Booth CJ, Pinus AB, Chen P, Lee A, Qiu M et al (2008) Induced hepatic fibrosis in rats: hepatic steatosis, macromolecule content, perfusion parameters, and their correlations--preliminary MR imaging in rats. Radiology 247(3):696–705

Kim SH, Kamaya A, Willmann JK (2014) CT perfusion of the liver: principles and applications in oncology. Radiology 272(2):322–344

Kim JH, Joo I, Kim TY, Han SW, Kim YJ, Lee JM et al (2016) Diffusion-related MRI parameters for assessing early treatment response of liver metastases to cytotoxic therapy in colorectal Cancer. AJR Am J Roentgenol 207(3):W26–W32

Kim YS, Jang YN, Song JS (2018) Comparison of gradient-recalled echo and spin-echo echo-planar imaging MR elastography in staging liver fibrosis: a meta-analysis. Eur Radiol 28(4):1709–1718

Koh DM, Collins DJ (2007) Diffusion-weighted MRI in the body: applications and challenges in oncology. AJR Am J Roentgenol 188(6):1622–1635

Koh DM, Collins DJ, Orton MR (2011) Intravoxel incoherent motion in body diffusion-weighted MRI: reality and challenges. AJR Am J Roentgenol 196(6):1351–1361

Kokabi N, Ludwig JM, Camacho JC, Xing M, Mittal PK, Kim HS (2015) Baseline and early MR apparent diffusion coefficient quantification as a predictor of response of Unresectable hepatocellular carcinoma to doxorubicin drug-eluting bead chemoembolization. JVIR 26(12):1777–1786

Lautt WW (1985) Mechanism and role of intrinsic regulation of hepatic arterial blood flow: hepatic arterial buffer response. Am J Phys 249(5 Pt 1):G549–G556

Le Bihan D, Ichikawa S, Motosugi U (2017) Diffusion and Intravoxel incoherent motion MR imaging-based virtual Elastography: a hypothesis-generating study in the liver. Radiology 285(2):609–619

Le Moigne F, Durieux M, Bancel B, Boublay N, Boussel L, Ducerf C et al (2012) Impact of diffusion-weighted MR imaging on the characterization of small hepatocellular carcinoma in the cirrhotic liver. Magn Reson Imaging 30(5):656–665

Lee TY, Purdie TG, Stewart E (2003) CT imaging of angiogenesis. Q J Nucl Med 47(3):171–187

Lee Y, Lee JM, Lee JE, Lee KB, Lee ES, Yoon JH et al (2014) MR elastography for noninvasive assessment of hepatic fibrosis: reproducibility of the examination and reproducibility and repeatability of the liver stiffness value measurement. J Magn Reson Imaging 39(2):326–331

Leggett DA, Kelley BB, Bunce IH, Miles KA (1997) Colorectal cancer: diagnostic potential of CT measurements of hepatic perfusion and implications for contrast enhancement protocols. Radiology 205(3):716–720

Liu Y, Matsui O (2007) Changes of intratumoral microvessels and blood perfusion during establishment of hepatic metastases in mice. Radiology 243(2):386–395

Luo M, Zhang L, Jiang XH, Zhang WD (2017) Intravoxel incoherent motion diffusion-weighted imaging: evaluation of the differentiation of solid hepatic lesions. Transl Oncol 10(5):831–838

Marquez HP, Puippe G, Mathew RP, Alkadhi H, Pfammatter T, Fischer MA (2017) CT perfusion for early response evaluation of radiofrequency ablation of focal liver lesions: first experience. Cardiovasc Intervent Radiol 40(1):90–98

Materne R, Van Beers BE, Smith AM, Leconte I, Jamart J, Dehoux JP et al (2000) Non-invasive quantification of liver perfusion with dynamic computed tomography and a dual-input one-compartmental model. Clin Sci (Lond) 99(6):517–525

Materne R, Smith AM, Peeters F, Dehoux JP, Keyeux A, Horsmans Y et al (2002) Assessment of hepatic perfusion parameters with dynamic MRI. Magn Reson Med 47(1):135–142

Matsui O, Kobayashi S, Sanada J, Kouda W, Ryu Y, Kozaka K et al (2011) Hepatocelluar nodules in liver cirrhosis: hemodynamic evaluation (angiography-assisted CT) with special reference to multi-step hepatocarcinogenesis. Abdom Imaging 36(3):264–272

Miles KA, Hayball MP, Dixon AK (1993) Functional images of hepatic perfusion obtained with dynamic CT. Radiology 188(2):405–411

Miles KA, Leggett DA, Kelley BB, Hayball MP, Sinnatamby R, Bunce I (1998) In vivo assessment of neovascularization of liver metastases using perfusion CT. Br J Radiol 71(843):276–281

Miles KA, Lee TY, Goh V, Klotz E, Cuenod C, Bisdas S et al (2012) Current status and guidelines for the assessment of tumour vascular support with dynamic contrast-enhanced computed tomography. Eur Radiol 22(7):1430–1441

Mule S, Pigneur F, Quelever R, Tenenhaus A, Baranes L, Richard P et al (2018) Can dual-energy CT replace perfusion CT for the functional evaluation of advanced hepatocellular carcinoma? Eur Radiol 28(5):1977–1985

Murphy P, Hooker J, Ang B, Wolfson T, Gamst A, Bydder M et al (2015) Associations between histologic features of nonalcoholic fatty liver disease (NAFLD) and quantitative diffusion-weighted MRI measurements in adults. J Magn Reson Imaging 41(6):1629–1638

Ng CS, Charnsangavej C, Wei W, Yao JC (2011) Perfusion CT findings in patients with metastatic carcinoid tumors undergoing bevacizumab and interferon therapy. AJR Am J Roentgenol 196(3):569–576

Ng CS, Wei W, Duran C, Ghosh P, Anderson EF, Chandler AG et al (2018) CT perfusion in normal liver and liver metastases from neuroendocrine tumors treated with targeted antivascular agents. Abdom Radiol (NY) 43(7):1661–1669

Ou HY, Bonekamp S, Bonekamp D, Corona-Villalobos CP, Torbenson MS, Geiger B et al (2013) MRI arterial enhancement fraction in hepatic fibrosis and cirrhosis. AJR Am J Roentgenol 201(4):W596–W602

Padhani AR (2002) Dynamic contrast-enhanced MRI in clinical oncology: current status and future directions. J Magn Reson Imaging 16(4):407–422

Padhani AR, Koh DM (2011) Diffusion MR imaging for monitoring of treatment response. Magn Reson Imaging Clin N Am 19(1):181–209

Pan S, Wang XQ, Guo QY (2018) Quantitative assessment of hepatic fibrosis in chronic hepatitis B and C: T1 mapping on Gd-EOB-DTPA-enhanced liver magnetic resonance imaging. World J Gastroenterol 24(18):2024–2035

Pandharipande PV, Krinsky GA, Rusinek H, Lee VS (2005) Perfusion imaging of the liver: current challenges and future goals. Radiology 234(3): 661–673

Park MJ, Kim YK, Lee MW, Lee WJ, Kim YS, Kim SH et al (2012) Small hepatocellular carcinomas: improved sensitivity by combining gadoxetic acid-enhanced and diffusion-weighted MR imaging patterns. Radiology 264(3):761–770

Patel J, Sigmund EE, Rusinek H, Oei M, Babb JS, Taouli B (2010) Diagnosis of cirrhosis with intravoxel incoherent motion diffusion MRI and dynamic contrast-enhanced MRI alone and in combination: preliminary experience. J Magn Reson Imaging 31(3): 589–600

Perumpail RB, Levitsky J, Wang Y, Lee VS, Karp J, Jin N et al (2012) MRI-guided biopsy to correlate tissue specimens with MR elastography stiffness readings in liver transplants. Acad Radiol 19(9):1121–1126

Petitclerc L, Sebastiani G, Gilbert G, Cloutier G, Tang A (2017) Liver fibrosis: review of current imaging and MRI quantification techniques. J Magn Reson Imaging 45(5):1276–1295

Petralia G, Fazio N, Bonello L, D'Andrea G, Radice D, Bellomi M (2011) Perfusion computed tomography in patients with hepatocellular carcinoma treated with thalidomide: initial experience. J Comput Assist Tomogr 35(2):195–201

Reiner CS, Goetti R, Burger IA, Fischer MA, Frauenfelder T, Knuth A et al (2012) Liver perfusion imaging in patients with primary and metastatic liver malignancy: prospective comparison between 99mTc-MAA spect and dynamic CT perfusion. Acad Radiol 19(5):613–621

Ren Y, Fleischmann D, Foygel K, Molvin L, Lutz AM, Koong AC et al (2012) Antiangiogenic and radiation therapy: early effects on in vivo computed tomography perfusion parameters in human colon cancer xenografts in mice. Investig Radiol 47(1):25–32

Ronot M, Asselah T, Paradis V, Michoux N, Dorvillius M, Baron G et al (2010) Liver fibrosis in chronic hepatitis C virus infection: differentiating minimal from intermediate fibrosis with perfusion CT. Radiology 256(1):135–142

Ronot M, Clift AK, Baum RP, Singh A, Kulkarni HR, Frilling A et al (2018) Morphological and functional imaging for detecting and assessing the Resectability of neuroendocrine liver metastases. Neuroendocrinology 106(1):74–88

Rosenkrantz AB, Padhani AR, Chenevert TL, Koh DM, De Keyzer F, Taouli B et al (2015) Body diffusion kurtosis imaging: basic principles, applications, and considerations for clinical practice. J Magn Reson Imaging 42(5):1190–1202

Sahani DV, Holalkere NS, Mueller PR, Zhu AX (2007) Advanced hepatocellular carcinoma: CT perfusion of liver and tumor tissue--initial experience. Radiology 243(3):736–743

Sahani DV, Jiang T, Hayano K, Duda DG, Catalano OA, Ancukiewicz M et al (2013) Magnetic resonance imaging biomarkers in hepatocellular carcinoma: association with response and circulating biomarkers after sunitinib therapy. J Hematol Oncol 6:51

Schuppan D, Afdhal NH (2008) Liver cirrhosis. Lancet 371(9615):838–851

Serai SD, Yin M, Wang H, Ehman RL, Podberesky DJ (2015) Cross-vendor validation of liver magnetic resonance elastography. Abdom Imaging 40(4):789–794

Serai SD, Obuchowski NA, Venkatesh SK, Sirlin CB, Miller FH, Ashton E et al (2017) Repeatability of MR Elastography of liver: a meta-analysis. Radiology 285(1):92–100

Shao S, Shan Q, Zheng N, Wang B, Wang J (2019) Role of Intravoxel incoherent motion in discriminating hepatitis B virus-related intrahepatic mass-forming Cholangiocarcinoma from hepatocellular carcinoma based on liver imaging reporting and data system v2018. Cancer Biother Radiopharm

Shire NJ, Yin M, Chen J, Railkar RA, Fox-Bosetti S, Johnson SM et al (2011) Test-retest repeatability of MR elastography for noninvasive liver fibrosis assessment in hepatitis C. J Magn Reson Imaging 34(4):947–955

Singh S, Venkatesh SK, Wang Z, Miller FH, Motosugi U, Low RN et al (2015) Diagnostic performance of magnetic resonance elastography in staging liver fibrosis: a systematic review and meta-analysis of individual participant data. Clin Gastroenterol Hepatol 13(3):440–51 e6

Sourbron S (2010) Technical aspects of MR perfusion. Eur J Radiol 76(3):304–313

Sourbron S, Sommer WH, Reiser MF, Zech CJ (2012) Combined quantification of liver perfusion and function with dynamic gadoxetic acid-enhanced MR imaging. Radiology 263(3):874–883

Stewart EE, Chen X, Hadway J, Lee TY (2008) Hepatic perfusion in a tumor model using DCE-CT: an accuracy and precision study. Phys Med Biol 53(16):4249–4267

Taouli B, Koh DM (2010) Diffusion-weighted MR imaging of the liver. Radiology 254(1):47–66

Thng CH, Koh TS, Collins D, Koh DM (2014) Perfusion imaging in liver MRI. Magn Reson Imaging Clin N Am 22(3):417–432

Tofts PS (1997) Modeling tracer kinetics in dynamic Gd-DTPA MR imaging. J Magn Reson Imaging 7(1):91–101

Tsushima Y, Blomley JK, Kusano S, Endo K (1999) The portal component of hepatic perfusion measured by dynamic CT: an indicator of hepatic parenchymal damage. Dig Dis Sci 44(8):1632–1638

Tsushima Y, Blomley MJ, Yokoyama H, Kusano S, Endo K (2001) Does the presence of distant and local malignancy alter parenchymal perfusion in apparently disease-free areas of the liver? Dig Dis Sci 46(10):2113–2119

Van Beers BE, Leconte I, Materne R, Smith AM, Jamart J, Horsmans Y (2001) Hepatic perfusion parameters in chronic liver disease: dynamic CT measurements correlated with disease severity. AJR Am J Roentgenol 176(3):667–673

Venkatesh SK, Yin M, Glockner JF, Takahashi N, Araoz PA, Talwalkar JA et al (2008) MR elastography of liver tumors: preliminary results. AJR Am J Roentgenol 190(6):1534–1540

Vilgrain V, Esvan M, Ronot M, Caumont-Prim A, Aube C, Chatellier G (2016) A meta-analysis of diffusion-weighted and gadoxetic acid-enhanced MR imaging for the detection of liver metastases. Eur Radiol 26(12):4595–4615

Wang XM, Zhang XJ, Ma L (2018) Diagnostic performance of magnetic resonance technology in detecting steatosis or fibrosis in patients with nonalcoholic fatty liver disease: a meta-analysis. Medicine (Baltimore) 97(21):e10605

Watanabe H, Kanematsu M, Goshima S, Kondo H, Onozuka M, Moriyama N et al (2011) Staging hepatic fibrosis: comparison of gadoxetate disodium-enhanced and diffusion-weighted MR imaging--preliminary observations. Radiology 259(1):142–150

Winfield JM, Tunariu N, Rata M, Miyazaki K, Jerome NP, Germuska M et al (2017) Extracranial soft-tissue tumors: repeatability of apparent diffusion coefficient estimates from diffusion-weighted MR imaging. Radiology 284(1):88–99

Wu H, Liang Y, Jiang X, Wei X, Liu Y, Liu W et al (2018) Meta-analysis of intravoxel incoherent motion magnetic resonance imaging in differentiating focal lesions of the liver. Medicine (Baltimore) 97(34):e12071

Yang L, Zhang XM, Tan BX, Liu M, Dong GL, Zhai ZH (2012) Computed tomographic perfusion imaging for the therapeutic response of chemoembolization for hepatocellular carcinoma. J Comput Assist Tomogr 36(2):226–230

Yang L, Rao S, Wang W, Chen C, Ding Y, Yang C et al (2018) Staging liver fibrosis with DWI: is there an added value for diffusion kurtosis imaging? Eur Radiol 28(7):3041–3049

Yankeelov TE, Gore JC (2009) Dynamic contrast enhanced magnetic resonance imaging in oncology: theory, data acquisition, analysis, and examples. Curr Med Imaging Rev 3(2):91–107

Yin M, Talwalkar JA, Glaser KJ, Manduca A, Grimm RC, Rossman PJ et al (2007) Assessment of hepatic fibrosis with magnetic resonance elastography. Clin Gastroenterol Hepatol 5(10):1207–13 e2

Yoon JH, Lee JM, Baek JH, Shin CI, Kiefer B, Han JK et al (2014) Evaluation of hepatic fibrosis using intravoxel incoherent motion in diffusion-weighted liver MRI. J Comput Assist Tomogr 38(1):110–116

Yoon JH, Lee JM, Paek M, Han JK, Choi BI (2016) Quantitative assessment of hepatic function: modified look-locker inversion recovery (MOLLI) sequence for T1 mapping on Gd-EOB-DTPA-enhanced liver MR imaging. Eur Radiol 26(6):1775–1782

Yoon JH, Lee JM, Kim E, Okuaki T, Han JK (2017) Quantitative liver function analysis: volumetric T1 mapping with fast multisection B1 inhomogeneity correction in hepatocyte-specific contrast-enhanced liver MR imaging. Radiology 282(2):408–417

Yoon JH, Lee JM, Kang IIJ, Ahn SJ, Yang H, Kim E et al (2019) Quantitative assessment of liver function by using Gadoxetic acid-enhanced MRI: hepatocyte uptake ratio. Radiology 290(1):125–133

Printed in the United States
by Baker & Taylor Publisher Services